Treatment of Skin Diseases: A Practical Guide

Treatment of Skin Diseases: A Practical Guide

Editor: Derek Kennedy

AMERICAN
MEDICAL PUBLISHERS
www.americanmedicalpublishers.com

AMERICAN
MEDICAL PUBLISHERS
www.americanmedicalpublishers.com

Cataloging-in-Publication Data

Treatment of skin diseases : a practical guide / edited by Derek Kennedy.
p. cm.
Includes bibliographical references and index.
ISBN 979-8-88740-535-3
1. Skin--Diseases--Treatment. 2. Skin--Diseases. 3. Skin--Diseases--Diagnosis.
4. Dermatology. I. Kennedy, Derek.
RL110 .T74 2023
616.5--dc23

American Medical Publishers,
41 Flatbush Avenue,
1st Floor, New York,
NY 11217, USA

ISBN 979-8-88740-535-3 (Hardback)

Contents

Preface

I am honored to present to you this unique book which encompasses the most up-to-date data in the field. I was extremely pleased to get this opportunity of editing the work of experts from across the globe. I have also written papers in this field and researched the various aspects revolving around the progress of the discipline. I have tried to unify my knowledge along with that of stalwarts from every corner of the world, to produce a text which not only benefits the readers but also facilitates the growth of the field.

Skin diseases are a group of conditions that affect the skin. There are several types of skin diseases, which include vitiligo, acne, rosacea, skin cancer, Raynaud's phenomenon, psoriasis, alopecia areata, etc. Skin diseases can be caused by bacteria trapped in pores or hair follicles, conditions that affect thyroid, kidneys or immune system, and fungus or parasites living on the skin. They can also be caused by medications, such as the ones used to treat inflammatory bowel disease (IBD), genetics, and contact with environmental triggers such as allergens or another person's skin. The signs and symptoms of skin diseases vary according to the type of condition. A person with skin diseases generally experiences symptoms like abnormal pigmentation, dry skin, rashes, itchiness or pain, and red, white or pus-filled bumps. On the basis of the condition of the skin, treatments like antibiotics, laser skin resurfacing, steroid pills, creams or injections, and surgical procedures can be used. This book is a practical guide for the treatment of skin diseases. It consists of contributions made by international experts. This book will prove to be immensely beneficial to students and researchers engaged in the diagnosis and treatment of skin diseases.

Finally, I would like to thank all the contributing authors for their valuable time and contributions. This book would not have been possible without their efforts. I would also like to thank my friends and family for their constant support.

Editor

1

A Traditional Chinese Medicine Formula Danshen Baibixiao Ameliorates Imiquimod-Induced Psoriasis-Like Inflammation in Mice

*Xiaoqi Jin[1†], Hongfeng Xu[2†], Chuanqi Huang[2], Haoran Ma[2], Xin Xiong[2], Lu Cheng[2], Fuqian Wang[2], Yan Feng[3] and Geng Zhang[1,2]**

[1]School of Pharmacy, Hubei University of Chinese Medicine, Wuhan, China, [2]Department of Pharmacy, Wuhan Hospital of Traditional Chinese and Western Medicine, Wuhan, China, [3]Department of Pathology, Wuhan Hospital of Traditional Chinese and Western Medicine, Wuhan, China

***Correspondence:**
Geng Zhang
zhanggen888@126.com

†These authors have contributed equally to this work and share first authorship

Background: Danshen Baibixiao (DB) is a traditional Chinese medicine formula, which has been used to treat psoriasis for decades. Although DB shows good efficacy in clinical practice, the pharmacological effects and underlying mechanisms of DB remain elusive. This study aimed to evaluate the anti-psoriatic effects of DB and explore its underlying mechanisms in an imiquimod (IMQ)-induced psoriasis-like mouse model.

Materials and methods: DB was orally administered on IMQ-induced psoriatic mice. Psoriasis area severity index (PASI) was used to evaluate the severity of the inflammation in skin, and histological changes were evaluated by hematoxylin and eosin (H and E) staining. Levels of inflammatory cytokines, such as tumor necrosis factor α (TNF-α), interleukin (IL)-17A, IL-23, IL-6, IL-1β and IL-22 in serum were assessed by enzyme-linked immunosorbent assay (ELISA). mRNA expressions of IL-17A, IL-23, IL-6 and IL-22 were determined by real-time polymerase chain reaction (PCR). Expression levels of proteins related to NF-κB, STAT3 and MAPKs signaling pathways were measured by western blotting (WB).

Results: DB significantly ameliorated the psoriatic symptoms in IMQ-induced mice. The serum levels of inflammatory cytokines (TNF-α, IL-17A, IL-23, IL-6, IL-1β and IL-22) were decreased, and mRNA expressions of IL-17A, IL-23, IL-6 and IL-22 in skin tissues were down-regulated. Moreover, WB analysis indicated that DB inhibited the activation of NF-κB, STAT3 and MAPKs signaling pathways.

Abbreviations: ANOVA, analysis of variance; cDNA, complementary deoxyribonucleic acid; DB, Danshen Baibixiao; DCs, dendritic cells; ELISA, enzyme-linked immunosorbent assay; ERK, extracellular regulating kinase; GAPDH, glyceraldehyde-3-phosphate dehydrogenase; H&E, hematoxylin and eosin; IL, interleukin; IMQ, imiquimod; JAK, Janus-activated kinase; JNK, c-Jun N-terminal kinases; MAPK, mitogen-activated protein kinase; MTX, methotrexate; NC, normal control; NF-κB, nuclear factor-kappa B; PASI, psoriasis area severity index; PCR, polymerase chain reaction; SD, standard deviation; STAT3, signal transducer and activator of transcription 3; TCM, traditional Chinese medicine; TH, T helper; TLR, toll-like receptor; TNF, tumor necrosis factor; UVA, ultraviolet a; UVB, ultraviolet b.

Conclusion: This study confirms the anti-psoriatic activity of DB in IMQ-induced psoriasis-like mice. The possible mechanism may relate to the activities of regulating the IL-23/TH-17 axis and suppressing the activation of NF-κB, STAT3 and MAPKs signaling pathways.

Keywords: traditional Chinese medicine, IL-23/TH-17 axis, NF-κB, STAT3, MAPK

INTRODUCTION

Psoriasis is a chronic auto-immune inflammatory disease, usually manifesting silvery scales, thickened *epidermis* and erythema on different parts of body. Pathologically, it is characterized by abnormal proliferation and differentiation of keratinocytes, infiltration of inflammatory cells and release of inflammatory cytokines (Greb et al., 2016; Chiang et al., 2020). It is reported that psoriasis affects approximately 2,3% of the global population (Armstrong and Read, 2020). What's worse, patients with psoriasis often suffer from comorbidities, such as cardiovascular disease, metabolic syndrome, cancer and depression, which synergistically increase the physical and psychological burden on patients (Boehncke and Schön, 2015; Kuai et al., 2020).

Although the pathogenesis of psoriasis is not totally understood, interleukin-23 (IL-23)/T helper 17 (TH-17) axis is believed to be critically involved in the development and maintenance of psoriasis (Gaffen et al., 2014; Schinocca et al., 2021). Upon aberrant activation, dendritic cells (DCs) secrete pro-inflammatory mediators, such as IL-23, IL-6 and TNF-α. TH-17 cells induced by IL-23 and IL-1β, can produce inflammatory cytokines, such as IL-17A, IL-22, TNF-α, IL-6 (Greb et al., 2016; Hou et al., 2018; Rai et al., 2020). These inflammatory factors jointly promote keratinocyte proliferation and other hallmarks of psoriasis. Numerous studies have demonstrated that inflammation related pathways, such as nuclear factor-kappa B (NF-κB) pathways, signal transducer and activator of transcription 3 (STAT3) pathways and mitogen-activated protein kinase (MAPKs) pathways were involved in psoriasis (Haase et al., 2001; Sun et al., 2017; Nguyen et al., 2018; Wang et al., 2019; Xu et al., 2019). NF-κB can mediate gene encoding of many pro-inflammatory and inflammatory cytokines (García-Pérez et al., 2014; Xu et al., 2018). STAT3 is a key transcription factors, participating in T cells' activation and proliferation, differentiation of keratinocytes and synthesis of inflammatory cytokines (Palanivel et al., 2014). MAPKs, including p38, JNK and ERK1/2, are activated to produce many important inflammatory cytokines, such as TNF-α, IL-23 and IL-6 (Mavropoulos et al., 2013; Hammouda et al., 2020).

Currently, treatment of psoriasis involves topical medicines (corticosteroids, vitamin D analogs and acitretin), systemic drugs (methotrexate, dexamethasone and cyclosporine), phototherapy (UVA and UVB), and biological medicines (TNF-α antagonists, Janus kinase inhibitors, anti-IL-23 agents and anti-IL-17 agents) (Greb et al., 2016). However, none of them can cure psoriasis, and a number of side effects associated with these medications remain a concern (Rapalli et al., 2018; Li et al., 2019b). Therefore, new anti-psoriatic medicine with improved efficacy and safety should be developed. Traditional Chinese medicine (TCM) with a long history of treating psoriasis can be a possible source of new anti-psoriatic medicine.

Danshen Baibixiao (DB), a traditional Chinese medicinal formula comprised of 15 kinds of traditional Chinese medicine ingredients (**Table 1**), has been used to treat psoriasis for over 30 years in Wuhan Hospital of Traditional Chinese and Western Medicine. The efficacy of DB was widely recognized by doctors and patients. (Xuan and Zhang, 2003; Lin et al., 2005). DB, previously named as Xiaobiwan, was developed by Professor Changfa Hu, a famous TCM doctor specialized in skin diseases. He defined the ingredients and amounts of ingredients used in the formula based on TCM theory and anti-psoriatic medicines recorded in ancient Chinese medicine literatures (Lin et al., 2005). This formula has been developed into a hospital preparation, renamed as Danshen Baibixiao, and has been used to treat psoriasis in the dermatology department of our hospital since 1990s. Among the ingredients, Salvia miltiorrhizae served as the monarch drug of the formula, which was thought to play a major role in the therapeutic action of the formula (Lin et al., 2005). According to TCM theory, Salvia miltiorrhizae has the efficacy to clear blood heat, promote blood circulation and remove blood stasis. Thus, Salvia miltiorrhizae is frequently used in the prescriptions to treat psoriasis (Zhang et al., 2014; Jia et al., 2020). A wide spectrum of secondary metabolites has been identified from Salvia miltiorrhizae. Diterpenoid quinones and hydrophilic phenolic acids are the major bioactive constituents (Su et al., 2015). Several chemical constituents of Salvia miltiorrhizae, such as tanshinone II, danshensu, salvianolic acid B and cryptotanshinone were reported to show anti-psoriatic effects (Li et al., 2012; Tang et al., 2018; Jia et al., 2020; Wang et al., 2020). In clinical observations of DB treatment, total effective rate of therapy with DB was 73.7% (Lin et al., 2005), and total effective rate of combination therapy of DB and phototherapy (UVA) on psoriasis vulgaris was 95.2% (Xuan and Zhang, 2003). Although DB shows good efficacy in clinical practice, the pharmacological effects and underlying mechanisms of DB remain elusive. In this investigation, we evaluated the anti-psoriatic effect in IMQ-induced psoriasis-like mice model and explored the mechanism of DB through its regulation on IL-23/TH-17 axis, and NF-κB, STAT3, MAPK signaling pathways.

MATERIALS AND METHODS

Chemicals and Reagents

Imiquimod cream (containing 5% imiquimod) was obtained from Meheco Keyi Pharma Co. Ltd (Hubei, China, batch number: 190301). Depilatory cream was purchased from

TABLE 1 | Composition of danshen baibixiao.

Ingredients	Source	Medicinal parts	Pocessing method	Mass ratio
Salvia miltiorrhizae radix et rhizome (丹參)	*Salvia miltiorrhiza* Bge	Root and Rhizome	Thick sliced and dried	4
Scorpio (全蝎)	*Buthus martensii* Karsch	Whole body	Dried	2
Zaocys (烏梢蛇)	*Zaocys dhumnades* (Cantor)	Whole body	Segmented and dried	2
Rhei radix et rhizome (大黃)	*Rheum officinale* Baill	Root and Rhizome	Thick sliced and dried	2
Cicadae periostracum (蟬蛻)	*Cryptotympana pustulata* Fabricius	cot	Dried	2
Eupolyphaga steleophaga (土鱉蟲)	*Eupolyphaga sinensis* Walker	Whole body	Dried	2
Cynanchi paniculati radix et rhizome (徐長卿)	*Cynanchum paniculatum* (Bge.)Kitag	Root and Rhizome	Segmented and dried	2
Crataegi fructus (山楂)	*Crataegus pinnatifida* Bge. Var. major N. E. Br	Mature fruit	Thick sliced and dried	6
Isatidis radix (板藍根)	*Isatis indigotica* Fort	Root	Thick sliced and dried	6
Carthami flos (紅花)	*Carthamus tinctorius* L	Flower	Dried	2
Saposhnikoviae radix (防風)	*Saposhnikovia divaricate* (Turcz.)Schischk	Root	Thick sliced and dried	4
Sophorae flavescentis radix (苦參)	*Sophora flavescens* Ait	Root	Thick sliced and dried	2
Phellodendri amurensis cortex (關黃柏)	*Phellodendron amurense* Rupr	Bark	Shredded and dried	4
Scolopendra (蜈蚣)	*Scolopendra subspinipes mutilans* L.Koch	Whole body	Dried	1
Glycyrrhizae radix et rhizome (甘草)	*Glycyrrhiza uralensis* Fisch	Root and Rhizome	Thick sliced and dried	1

Reckitt Benckiser (London, United kingdom). Methotrexate and chemical references (salvianolic acid B, tanshinone IIA, berberine hydrochloride, prim-O-glucosylcimifugin, sophocarpidine, and ammonium glycyrrhetate) were purchased from National Institutes for Food and Drug Control of China (Beijing, China). ELISA kits for IL-17A, IL-23, IL-22, IL-6, TNF-α, IL-1β were purchased from Invitrogen (Carlsbad, CA, United States). Primary antibodies used in western blotting analysis were obtained from Cell Signaling Technology (Danvers, MA, United States).

Plant Materials and Preparation of DB Extract

All DB ingredients were commercially available TCM decoction pieces, bought from Tianji pharmaceutical company (Hubei, China). The ingredients were authenticated by Professor Hezhen Wu from Hubei University of Chinese Medicine through morphological identification according to Chinese Pharmacopoeia. The specimens of the 15 ingredients were deposited in the herbarium of Wuhan Hospital of Traditional Chinese and Western Medicine for future reference (voucher number from 20190301 to 20190315 for all ingredients). Detailed information on medicinal parts and processing methods of the materials was listed in **Table 1**. According to traditional use of TCM prescriptions, the ingredients were mixed together and soaked with 10x weight of distilled water, followed by boiled for 1 h. The decoction was filtrated with gauze, and the medicines were boiled with another 10x weight of distilled water for 1 h. The decoctions from the two cycles were mixed and then concentrated to a solution containing 0.228 g/ml of crude drugs with a rotary evaporator (IKA, Staufen, Germany). Concentrated solution containing 0.228 g/ml of crude drugs was used to treat mice of the high-dosage DB group. The solutions of low-dosage (0.114 g/ml) and middle-dosage (0.057 g/ml) DB were diluted from the high-dose solution with distilled water. The solutions were stored at −20°C before use.

The dosages of DB used in our experiment were calculated from human dosage based on body surface area as described by Xu et al. (2002). Body surface area ratio of mouse (20 g) to human (70 kg) is 0.0026. Recommend dose of DB for an adult was 22 g per day. For a 20 g mouse, the equivalent dose of DB was 22 g × 0.0026 ÷ 0.02 kg = 2.86 g/kg, which was set to be the middle dosage in our experiment. The volume of drug administrated to mice was 0.5 ml, thus the concentration of solution for middle dosage was 2.86 g/kg × 0.02 kg ÷ 0.5 ml = 0.114 g/ml of crude drugs. The low dosage and high dosage were set at half or 2 times of middle dosage. Thus, the concentration of the solution for low, middle and high dosage was 0.057, 0.114, 0.228 g/ml of crude drugs, respectively.

HPLC-MS/MS Analysis

HPLC-MS/MS method was used to analyze the chemical constituents of DB. According to Chinese Pharmacopoeia, salvianolic acid B and tanshinone IIA are used as reference compounds for quality control of Salvia miltiorrhizae radix et rhizome. Berberine hydrochloride, prim-O-glucosylcimifugin, sophocarpidine and ammonium glycyrrhetate are used as reference compounds for Phellodendri amurensis cortex, Saposhnikoviae radix, Sophorae flavescentis radix, Glycyrrhizae radix et rhizoma, respectively (Chinese-Pharmacopoeia-Commission, 2020). And these compounds were reported to be active compounds of these ingredients, respectively (Su et al., 2015; Kreiner et al., 2017; Pastorino and Cornara, 2018; Sun and Lenon, 2019; Zhu and Hou, 2021). Therefore, salvianolic acid B, tanshinone IIA, berberine hydrochloride, prim-O-glucosylcimifugin, sophocarpidine, and ammonium glycyrrhetate were used as standard references. An appropriate amount of each standard compounds were dissolved in a known volume of methanol individually to make the standard stock solutions. The standard working solutions were prepared by diluting the stock solutions with methanol. Then, an appropriate amount of each standard working solution were mixed and diluted with a known volume of methanol to make the mixed standard working solution.

The DB extract was prepared as described above and was filtered through a 0.45 μm filter for the HPLC-MS/MS analysis. The analysis was performed on a Shimadzu LC-20AD liquid chromatography system coupled with an API 4000 mass spectrometer (AB SCIEX, Foster City, United States). A Sunfire C18 column (2.1*150 mm,

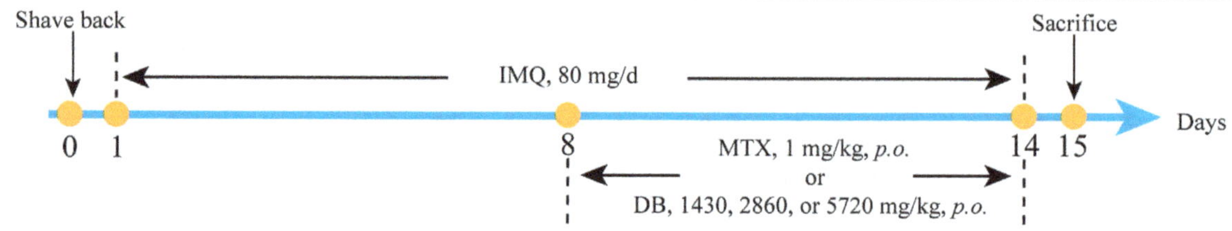

FIGURE 1 | Scheme of the animal experimental procedure.

3.5 μm particle size, Waters, Milford, United States) was used for the separation of the components. Water and acetonitrile [both containing 0.1% (v/v) formic acid] were used as mobile phase A and B. HPLC analysis was carried out at a flow rate of 0.2 ml/min with a gradient elution (10–30% B from 0 to 20 min; 30–100% B from 20 to 35 min; 100% B from 35 to 40 min).

The quantifications of the chemical constituents of DB were performed with the multiple reaction monitoring (MRM) mode. The turbo spray ion source was operated in the positive ion mode. The source parameters (ion-spray voltage, temperature, gas1, gas2, curtain gas, collision gas) used in the analysis were 5000 V, 500°C, 55, 55, 35, 6 psi. Ion pairs used for multiple reaction monitoring were 741.3/561.3 (salvianolic acid B), 295.3/277.2 (tanshinone IIA), 336.3/321.2 (berberine hydrochloride), 469.1/307.4 (prim-O-glucosylcimifugin), 249.6/148.3 (sophocarpidine) and 840.6/823.6 (ammonium glycyrrhetate). Compounds in the DB were quantified using the standard calibration curves.

Animals

Male C57BL/6 mice of 20–25 g weight and 8-weeks age were obtained from Laboratory Animal Center of Huazhong University of Science and Technology (Hubei, China). A total number of 60 mice were used in this experiment. The mice were housed in plastic cages under specific pathogen-free conditions of 24–26°C temperature, 55% relative humidity on 12 h light/dark cycles with abundant food and water. All of them were acclimatized for 1 week and kept in good health condition before use. Animal handling and institutional approval were supported and approved by the Institutional Animal Care and Use Committee at Tongji Medical College of Huazhong University of Science and Technology (approval number: 2,520). All experiments were conducted in accordance with the National Institutes of Health Guide for the Care and Use of Laboratory Animals (the seventh edition, United States).

Animals Treatment and Sample Collection

Backs of the mice were shaved and depilated with depilatory cream to expose the back skin. Sixty mice were randomly divided into six groups (n = 10): the normal control (NC) group, the model group (IMQ group), the methotrexate (MTX) treated group, and three groups treated with low, middle and high dosage of DB. Five groups except for NC group received application of 80 mg IMQ cream daily on their back skins for 14 consecutive days. For the last 7 days, the low-dosage DB group (DB-L), middle-dosage DB group (DB-M) and high-dosage DB group (DB-H) received orally 1.43, 2.86, 5.72 g/kg DB (calculated from the human dosage) after IMQ application daily, while the MTX group received 1 mg/kg MTX daily, IMQ and NC groups received distilled water. On day 15, the mice were sacrificed by cervical dislocation after narcotized by inhalation of diethyl ether, the blood samples and back skin tissues were collected. The animal experimental procedure was shown in **Figure 1**.

Behavior Observation and Psoriasis Area and Severity Index Assessment

During the experiment, body weight of the mice was recorded every day. Behaviors, such as activity, mental state, daily intake of water and food, defecation and urination of the mice were also observed. PASI was used to evaluate the severity of the inflammation in skin. Degrees of erythema, scaling and thickening were scored independently on a scale of 0–4: 0 for none; one for slight; two for moderate; three for severe; four for very severe. The severity of the inflammation was measured by the cumulative score (erythema plus scaling plus thickening) on a scale of 0–12 (van der Fits et al., 2009).

Histological Analysis

On day 15, the back skin samples were collected and fixed in 10% buffered formalin and embedded in paraffin. Then the samples were cut into 3 μm sections and stained with hematoxylin and eosin (H and E). The samples were examined with an optical microscope (Olympus BX53, Tokyo, Japan). Epidermal thickness was measured in three randomly selected spots.

Enzyme-Linked Immunosorbent Assay

The serum samples were separated by centrifugation from the blood samples at 12000 g, 4°C for 15 min. Levels of the cytokines IL-17A, IL-23, IL-22, IL-6, TNF-α, IL-1β in serum samples were measured using ELISA kits (Invitrogen, Carlsbad, CA, United States) according to manufacturer's instructions.

Quantitative Real-Time PCR Assay

The skin samples were extracted with Trizol reagent (Invitrogen, Carlsbad, CA, United States) to obtain the total RNA. Then the RNAs were reverse transcribed into cDNA with M-MLV reverse transcriptase (Promega, Madison, United States). Quantitative PCR was performed with SYBR Green qPCR Supermix (Invitrogen, Carlsbad, CA, United States) on an ABI 7500 real-time quantitative PCR system (Applied Biosystems, Foster City,

TABLE 2 | Primers used for qPCR assays.

Gene	Forward primer	Reverse primer
IL-23	5′-CTC ACC GTG ACG TTT AGG GA-3′	5′-ACT AGA ACT CAG GCT GGG CAT C-3′
IL-17A	5′-TCA TGT GGT GGT CCA GCT TTC-3′	5′-GAA GGC CCT CAG ACT ACC TCA A-3′
IL-22	5′-TTT CCT GAC CAA ACT CAG CA-3′	5′-CTG GAT GTT CTG GTC GTC AC-3′
IL-6	5′-AGA GTA GTG AG GAA CAA GCC-3′	5′-TAC ATT TGC CGA AGA GCC CT-3′
GAPDH	5′-GGT TGT CTC CTG CGA CTT CA-3′	5′-TGG TCC AGG GTT TCT TAC TCC-3′

United States). The PCR cycle parameters were as follows: denature at 95°C for 5 min, followed by 40 cycles of 95°C for 15 s (denature) and 60°C for 32 s (annealing). Data were analyzed with the $2^{-\Delta\Delta CT}$ method. Primers used were listed in **Table 2**.

Western Blotting

Total protein was extracted from skin samples with RIPA buffer (Beyotime Biotechnology, Shanghai, China). After determination of the protein concentration by BCA kit (Jiancheng Bioengineering Institute, Nanjing, Jiangsu, China), the protein was separated by 10% sodium dodecyl sulfate-polyacrylamide gel electrophoresis (SDS-PAGE) and transferred onto polyvinylidene fluoride membranes (0.45 mm, Millipore, Boston, MA, United States). After blocking with 5% fat-free milk, the membranes were incubated with primary antibodies against NF-κB p65, IκB, p38 MAPK, JNK, ERK, p-p38 MAPK, p-JNK, p-ERK and STAT3 (dilution ratio of 1:1,000, Cell Signaling Technology, Danvers, United States) at 4°C overnight. After washing, the membranes were incubated with horseradish peroxidase (HRP) conjugated secondary antibodies with dilution ratio of 1:4,000 at 37°C for 1 h. Then the membranes were washed for 3 times with Tris buffer saline containing 0.1% (v/v) Tweens 20, and incubated with enhanced chemiluminescence reagent (Millipore, Boston, MA, United States). The signals were captured with X-ray films and quantified with the ImageJ software (NIH, Bethesda, MD, United States). GADPH was used as internal reference protein.

Statistical Analysis

All data were expressed as mean ± standard deviation (SD). Data were analyzed with SPSS 20.0. Statistical significance was assessed using the one-way analysis of variance (ANOVA). Differences were considered statistically significant at $p < 0.05$.

RESULTS

Analysis of the Chemical Constituents of DB Extract

In TCM theory, ingredients in the formula could be divided into four categories, as monarch, minister, assistant and guide drugs. Salvia miltiorrhizae radix et rhizome was the monarch drug of the formula. Phellodendri amurensis cortex and Sophorae flavescentis radix were the minister drug, Saposhnikoviae radix was the assistant drug, and Glycyrrhizae radix et rhizome was the guide drug. These ingredients are the representatives of the four categories in the DB formula, so reference compounds of these ingredients were chosen in the analysis of DB. MRM chromatograms of both DB and referential substances were shown in **Figure 2**. The retention times of salvianolic acid B, tanshinone IIA, berberine hydrochloride, prim-O-glucosylcimifugin, sophocarpidine, and ammonium glycyrrhetate were 23.2, 32.7, 16.6, 11.6, 1.8 and 27.2 min, respectively. The concentrations of these six components in DB were 12.3, 0.13, 6.71, 3.04, 49.5, 5.96 μg/mg.

DB Ameliorated IMQ-Induced Psoriasis-like Skin Lesions in Mice

During the experiment, no significant differences in body weight, activity, mental state, daily intake of water and food, defecation and urination were observed between the mice in different groups. Typical signs of erythema, scaling and epidermal thickening appeared after 7 days of IMQ application compared with NC group. From day 8 to day 14, DB treatment significantly attenuated the symptoms of psoriasis compared with IMQ-group (**Figure 3A**).

PASI score was determined for assessing the severity of skin inflammation for all mice. In **Figures 3B–E**, the PASI scores continually increased after IMQ application from day 1 to day 7. However, the PASI scores decreased gradually after MTX or DB treatment from day 8 to day 14. The PASI scores of DB and MTX-treated groups were significantly lower compared to IMQ group ($p < 0.01$).

Histopathological Analysis

Histological changes in the skin tissues after DB treatment were evaluated with H and E staining. In **Figure 4**, the IMQ-treated group displayed remarkable elevation in epidermal hyperplasia, hyperkeratosis, acanthosis and inflammatory cells' infiltration. After application of DB, the psoriatic symptoms were alleviated significantly, especially in the high-dosage DB treated group. The epidermal thickness of the mice was measured in three randomly selected spots. In **Figure 3F**, the IMQ-treated group showed significant thickening of *epidermis* compared to the NC group ($p < 0.01$), while epidermal thickness was significantly reduced in DB and MTX-treated groups ($p < 0.01$).

DB Decreased the Levels of Inflammatory Cytokines in the Peripheral Blood of IMQ-Induced Psoriatic Mice

ELISA assays were used to evaluate the effects of DB on the levels of the cytokines in serum. According to **Figures 5A–F**, TNF-α, IL-17A, IL-23, IL-22, IL-1β, IL-6 levels were significantly increased in the IMQ group compared to NC group ($p < 0.01$). DB treatment significantly decreased levels of these cytokines compared to IMQ group ($p < 0.01$). Levels of TNF-α, IL-23 and IL-6 were decreased with a dose-dependent manner.

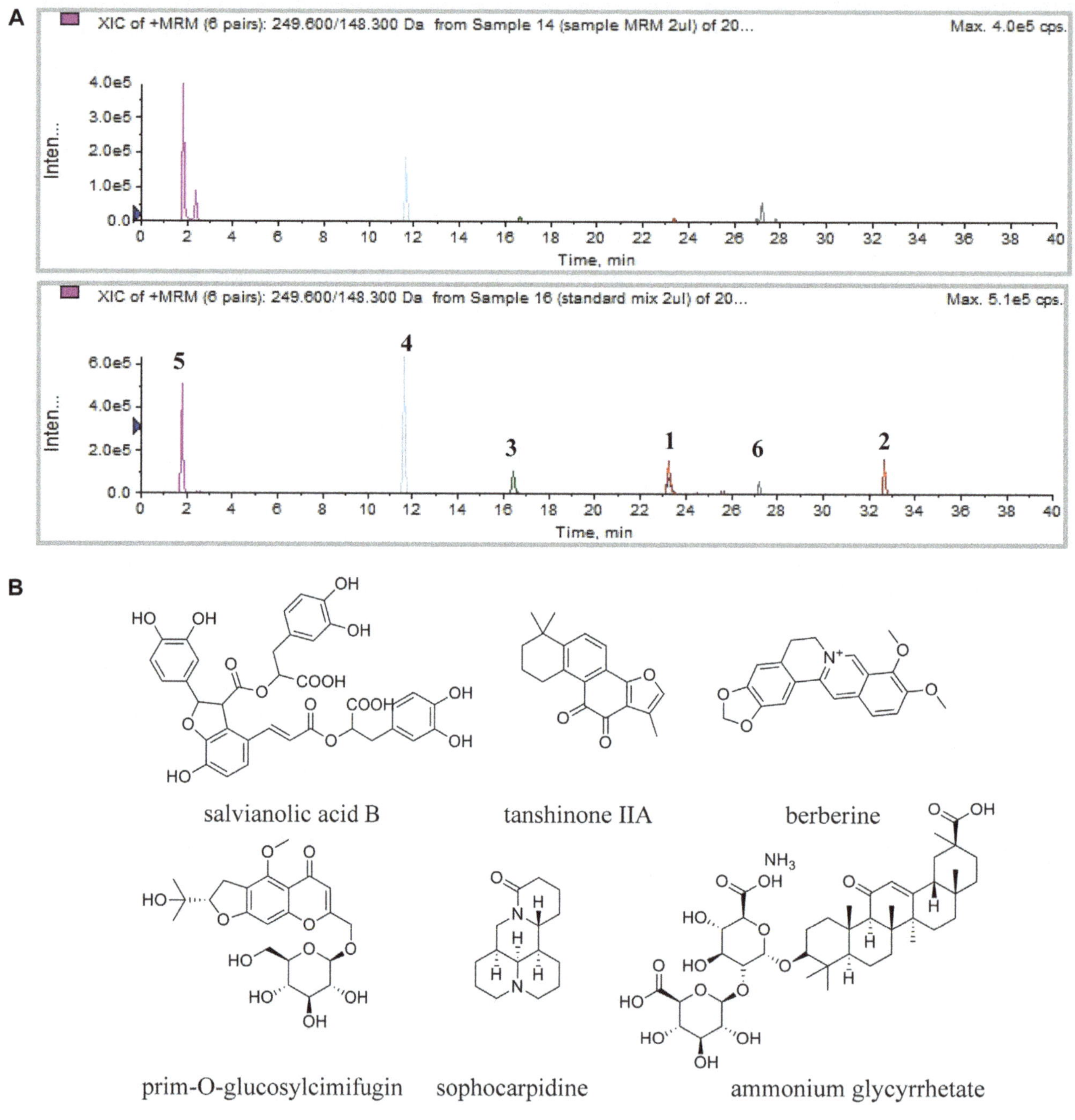

FIGURE 2 | HPLC-MS/MS analysis of the chemical constituents in the DB. **(A)** MRM chromatogram of DB **(upper)** and MRM chromatogram of the referential substances **(lower)**. Salvianolic acid B (1), tanshinone IIA (2), berberine hydrochloride (3), prim-O-glucosylcimifugin (4), sophocarpidine (5) and ammonium glycyrrhetate (6). **(B)** Chemical structures of salvianolic acid B, tanshinone IIA, berberine hydrochloride, prim-O-glucosylcimifugin, sophocarpidine and ammonium glycyrrhetate.

DB Down-Regulated the mRNA Expressions of Inflammatory Cytokines in IMQ-Induced Psoriatic Mice

The mRNA expressions of inflammatory cytokines in skin tissues after DB treatment were evaluated by real-time PCR. In **Figures 6A–D**, IMQ treatment significantly increased the mRNA expressions of IL-17, IL-23, IL-22 and IL-6 compared with NC group ($p < 0.01$). However, the mRNA levels of these cytokines dose-dependently declined in the DB-treated groups ($p < 0.01$).

DB Inhibited the Activations of NF-κB, MAPKs and STAT3 Signaling Pathways

Western blotting analysis were performed to evaluate the expression levels of the proteins related to NF-κB, MAPKs

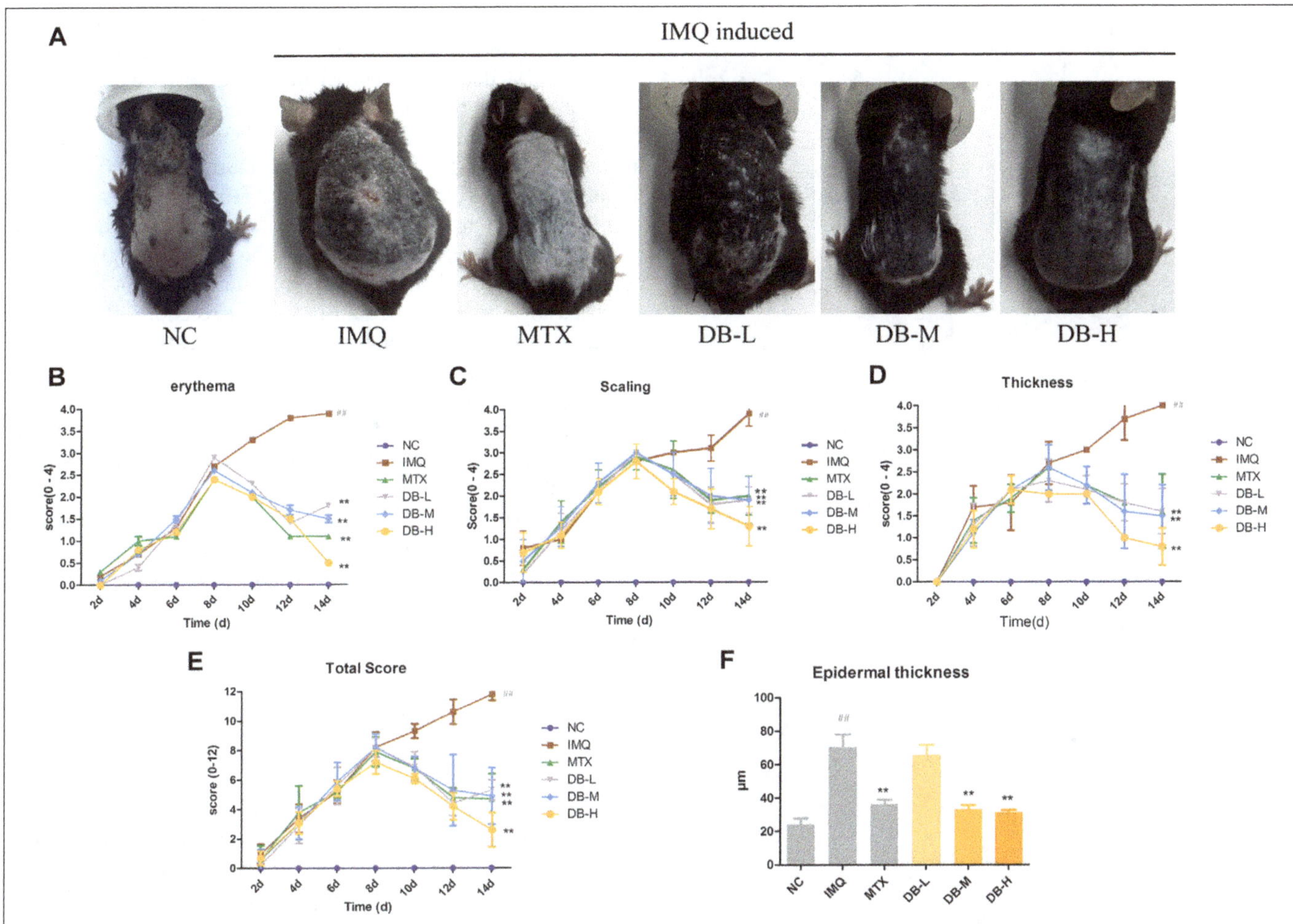

FIGURE 3 | Effects of DB treatment against the psoriasis-like symptoms. **(A)** Images of psoriatic skin lesions in six different groups. **(B–D)** PASI intensity scores (erythema, scaling, epidermal thickness) of skin lesions in six different groups. **(E)** cumulated PASI scores in six different groups. **(F)** Epidermal thickness of back skin was measured in three randomly selected spots. Values are expressed as mean ± SD (n = 10). Where $^{\#}p < 0.05$ and $^{\#\#}p < 0.01$ versus NC group, $^{*}p < 0.05$ and $^{**}p < 0.01$ versus IMQ group.

and STAT3 signaling pathways in the skin tissues after DB treatment. As shown in **Figures 7A,B**, the expressions of NF-κB p65 were up-regulated and the degradation of IκB was increased after IMQ application compared to the NC group ($p < 0.01$). DB significantly suppressed the expressions of NF-κB p65 and the degradation of IκB in a dose-dependent manner ($p < 0.01$).

In **Figures 7C–E**, IMQ treatment increased the expressions of p38, JNK and ERK significantly ($p < 0.01$), and these IMQ-induced enhancements in the expressions were markedly prevented by DB ($p < 0.01$). Meanwhile, DB suppressed the phosphorylation of p38 and ERK ($p < 0.01$), though the phosphorylation of JNK were not suppressed by DB (**Figures 7F–H**).

In **Figure 7I**, IMQ up-regulated the expression level of STAT3 ($p < 0.01$) while the expression of STAT3 was suppressed significantly after DB treatment in a dose-dependent manner ($p < 0.01$).

DISCUSSION

Psoriasis is one of the most common inflammatory skin disorders, affecting an estimated 125 million people worldwide (Armstrong and Read, 2020). As a systemic autoimmune disease, psoriasis may also affect nails, joints and other organs, resulting in poor quality of life (Greb et al., 2016). Moreover, people with psoriasis are at higher risk for comorbidities such as obesity, cardiovascular disease, metabolic syndrome and depression. The pathogenesis of psoriasis is complex and not fully understood. Both genetic factors and environmental factors are thought to be involved in the development of psoriasis (Kamiya et al., 2019). Current medications for psoriasis include topical medicines, oral systemic drugs and biologics (Armstrong and Read, 2020). However, treatment of psoriasis remains a challenge due to the low efficacy, side effects or high costs of the medications. New treatment of efficacy and less side effects should be developed.

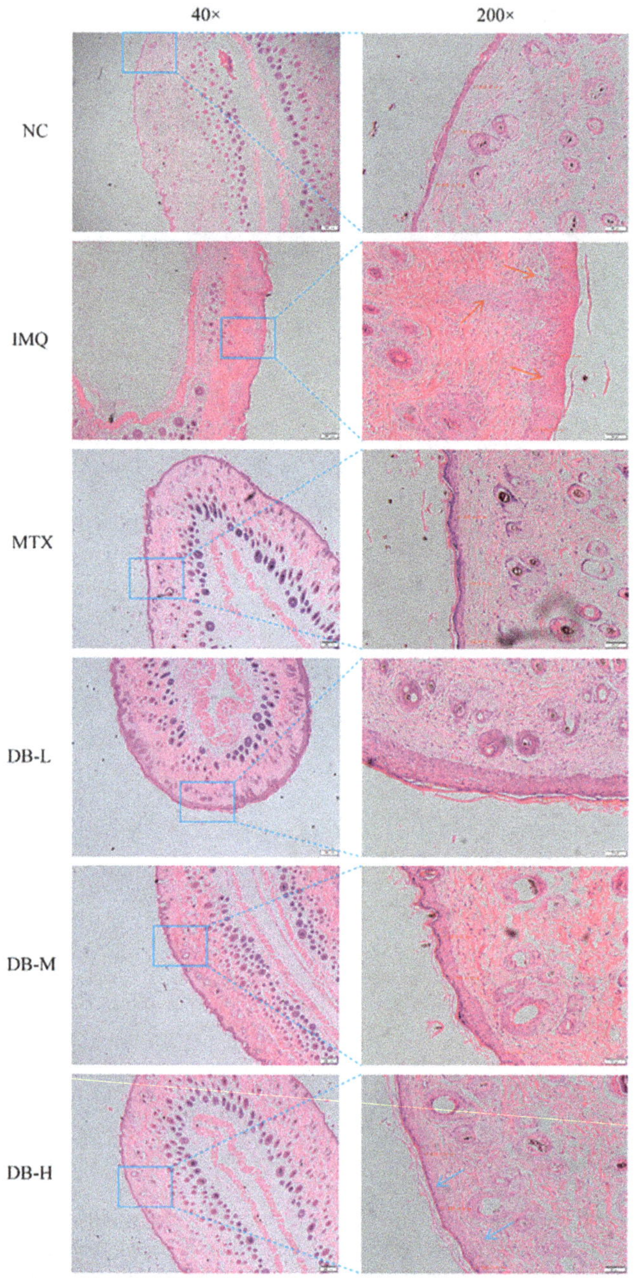

FIGURE 4 | Histopathological images of back skins of the mice (images magnified × 40 and × 200).

Traditional Chinese medicine has a long history for the treatment of psoriasis. The earliest record of psoriasis may date back to Sui Dynasty (581–618 AD) in an ancient medical book named Various Pathogenic Designate Theory (諸病源候論) (Cao et al., 2015). In TCM theory, treatment should be based on syndrome differentiation. For psoriasis, syndrome differentiation should base on blood-related symptoms, and treatment should focus on blood. Traditional Chinese doctors differentiate psoriasis into three basic syndromes including blood-heat, blood-dryness and blood-stasis (Deng et al., 2006; Li et al., 2021). Different formulae were formed based on the syndrome differentiation and clinical medication experiences. DB was developed by a famous TCM doctor specialized in skin diseases, and has been efficiently used to treat psoriasis for 30 years in Wuhan Hospital of Traditional Chinese and Western Medicine. DB contains ingredients which have the efficacy to clear blood heat, moisten dryness, promote blood circulation and remove blood stasis, thus DB is used to treat three basic syndrome differentiations of psoriasis (Lin et al., 2005). However, the pharmacological effects and underlying mechanisms of DB remain unclear. In this study, we tried to investigate the anti-psoriatic effects of DB on IMQ-induced psoriasis-like mice model and elucidate the possible underlying mechanisms of DB.

IMQ, an agonist of toll-like receptor (TLR) 7/8, can induce psoriasis on mice skin. IMQ-induced psoriasis-like mice model closely resembles human psoriasis, which critically depends upon the IL-23/TH-17 cytokine axis (van der Fits et al., 2009; Bocheńska et al., 2017). After 7 days of IMQ application, all the mice developed prominent characteristics of psoriasis. After DB treatment, the psoriasis-like symptoms including erythema, white scales, wrinkles and thicken skins, were ameliorated visibly (**Figure 3A**). The PASI scores of the mice treated with DB decreased significantly compared to the IMQ-group (**Figure 3E**). Furthermore, histological analysis revealed smoother, fewer inflammatory cells' infiltration and thinner *epidermis* in DB-treated groups (**Figure 4**). These results suggested that DB showed obvious anti-psoriatic effects in IMQ-induced psoriatic mice.

The pathogenesis of psoriasis involves the interaction of a variety of cell types, including dendritic cells, macrophages, keratinocytes and T cells (Georgescu et al., 2019; Rendon and Schäkel, 2019). Typically, upon aberrant activation, dendritic cells secrete pro-inflammatory mediators, such as IL-23, IL-6 and TNF-α. These pro-inflammatory mediators induce the proliferation and activation of T cells, such as TH1, TH22 and TH17 cells, which leads further production of cytokines, such as TNF-α, IL-17 and IL-22. These cytokines lead to the recruitment of additional inflammatory cells into the lesion, proliferation and activation of keratinocytes, and other hallmark features of psoriasis. Among these pathways, IL-23/TH17 axis is thought to play a predominant role (Hawkes et al., 2018). Upon stimulation of IL-23, TH17 cells are differentiated from naive T cells and produce IL-17, IL-22, and TNF-α. IL-17 and IL-22 induce proliferation of keratinocytes and release of cytokines from keratinocytes, such as TNF-α, IL-6 and IL-17, which can act back on the DCs and T cells to form a positive feedback loop (Lowes et al., 2014; Deng et al., 2016). TNF-α is a pro-inflammatory cytokine, produced by different cell types including T cells, DCs, macrophages and keratinocytes. TNF-α can induce the production of cytokines to amplify inflammation in psoriasis (Boehncke and Schön, 2015). IL-1β and IL-6 also contribute on the differentiation and activation of Th17 (Parmar et al., 2017). In our present study, application of DB significantly reduced the serum levels of TNF-α, IL-17A, IL-23, IL-22, IL-1β and IL-6 in the DB treated groups compared with the IMQ group (**Figure 5**). mRNA levels of IL-17A, IL-23, IL-22 and IL-6 were also suppressed by DB compared with the IMQ group (**Figure 6**),

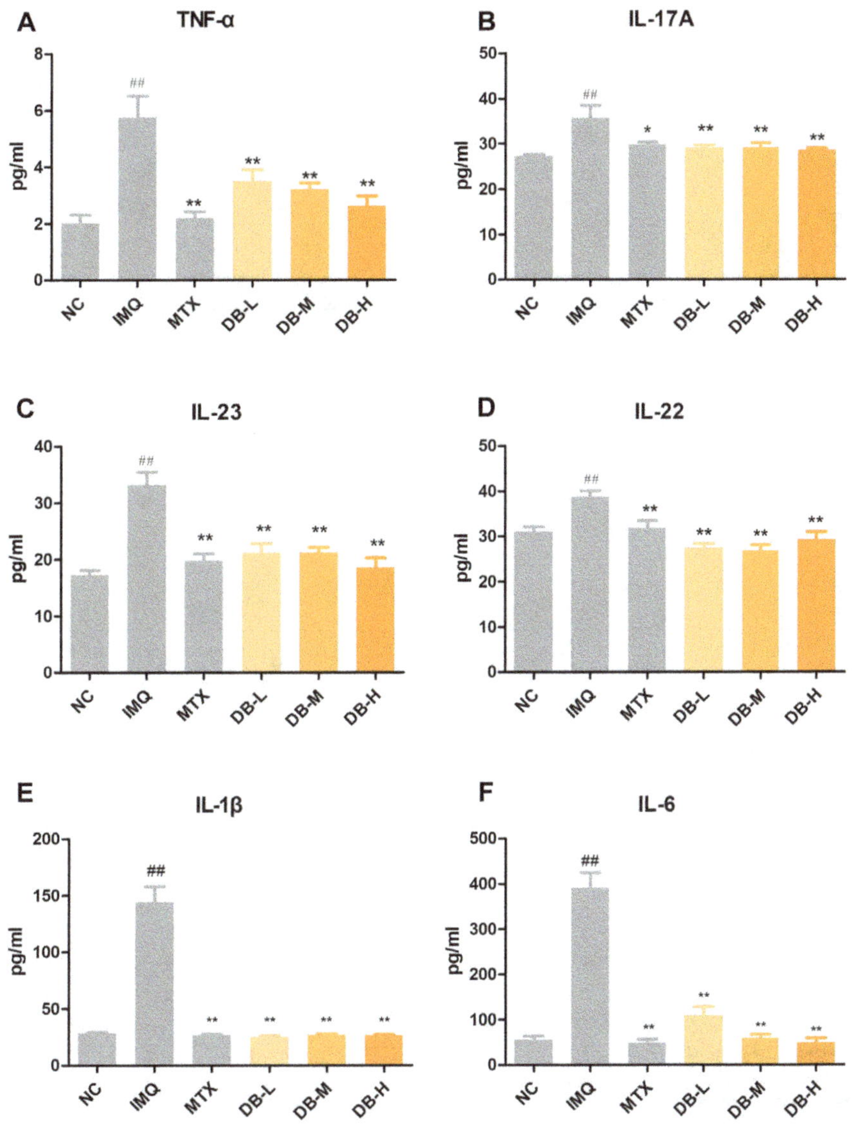

FIGURE 5 | Effects of DB on serum levels of the inflammatory cytokines in IMQ-induced psoriatic mice. The concentrations of TNF-α **(A)**, IL-17A **(B)**, IL-23 **(C)**, IL-22 **(D)**, IL-6 **(E)**, IL-1β **(F)** were measured with ELISA. Values are expressed as mean ± SD (n = 10). Where $^{\#}p < 0.05$ and $^{\#\#}p < 0.01$ versus NC group,$^{*}p < 0.05$ and $^{**}p <$ 0.01 versus IMQ group.

which are in consistent with the ELISA experiments. These results showed that DB could inhibit psoriatic inflammation by regulating the IL-23/TH-17 axis.

Recently, roles of several signaling pathways in pathogenesis of psoriasis have attracted increased attention. NF-κB is a transcription factor, mediating in a variety of inflammatory pathways, cellular proliferation and differentiation, and apoptosis. Under normal conditions, the NF-κB dimer p50/p65 is located in the cytosol and bound to IκB proteins. When NF-κB is activated, IκB is phosphorylated and degraded, p50/p65 is accumulated in the nucleus and activates transcription of target genes. In psoriasis, numerous cell types, including DCs, T cells and keratinocytes, are dependent on NF-κB signaling pathway. NF-κB activates the expressions of TNF-α, IL-6 and IL-1β, and induces inflammatory cells' infiltration (Pasparakis, 2012; Goldminz et al., 2013; Rai et al., 2020). In our study, DB significantly down-regulated the expressions of NF-κB p65 and up-regulated the expressions of IκB in a dose-dependent manner compared with IMQ group (**Figure 7**), which suggested that DB could suppress the expressions of NF-κB and degradation of IκB, thus to suppress the activation of NF-κB signaling pathway.

STAT3 is another key transcription factor involved in psoriasis. STAT3 mediates the signal of most cytokines in pathogenesis of psoriasis, including IL-23, IL-17A, IL-22. These cytokines rely on STAT3 pathways to induce the proliferation and activation of TH-17 and keratinocytes. In fact, STAT3 hyperactivation has been found in numerous cell types involved in psoriasis (Calautti et al., 2018; Li et al., 2019a). In our investigation, DB significantly

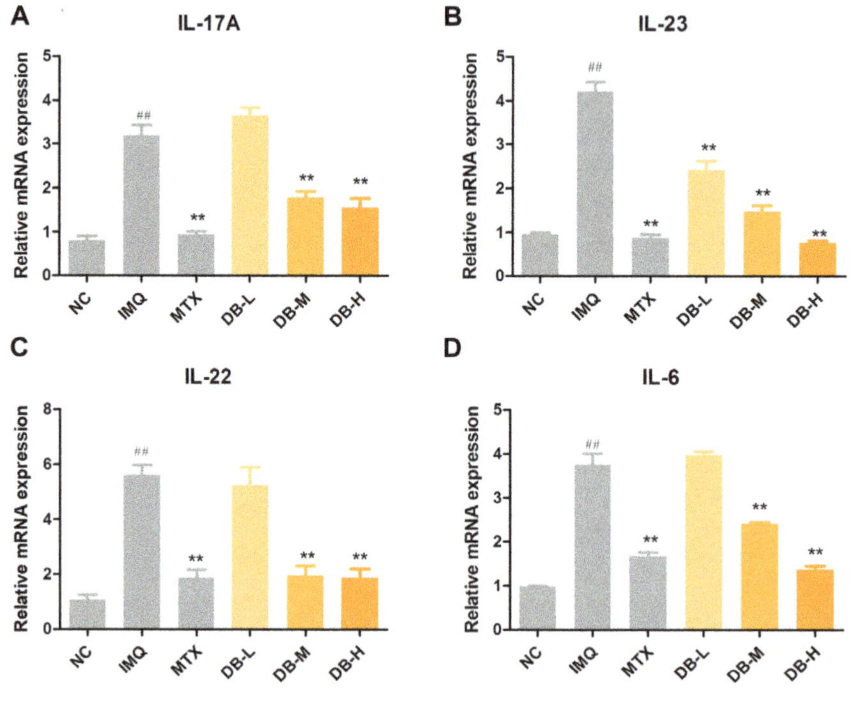

FIGURE 6 | DB reduces the mRNA expressions of IL-17A **(A)**, IL-23 **(B)**, IL-22 **(C)** and IL-6 **(D)** in IMQ-induced psoriatic mice. The mRNA levels in the back skins were detected by real-time PCR. Values are expressed as mean ± SD (n = 3). Where $^{\#}p < 0.05$ and $^{\#\#}p < 0.01$ versus NC group, $^{*}p < 0.05$ and $^{**}p < 0.01$ versus IMQ group.

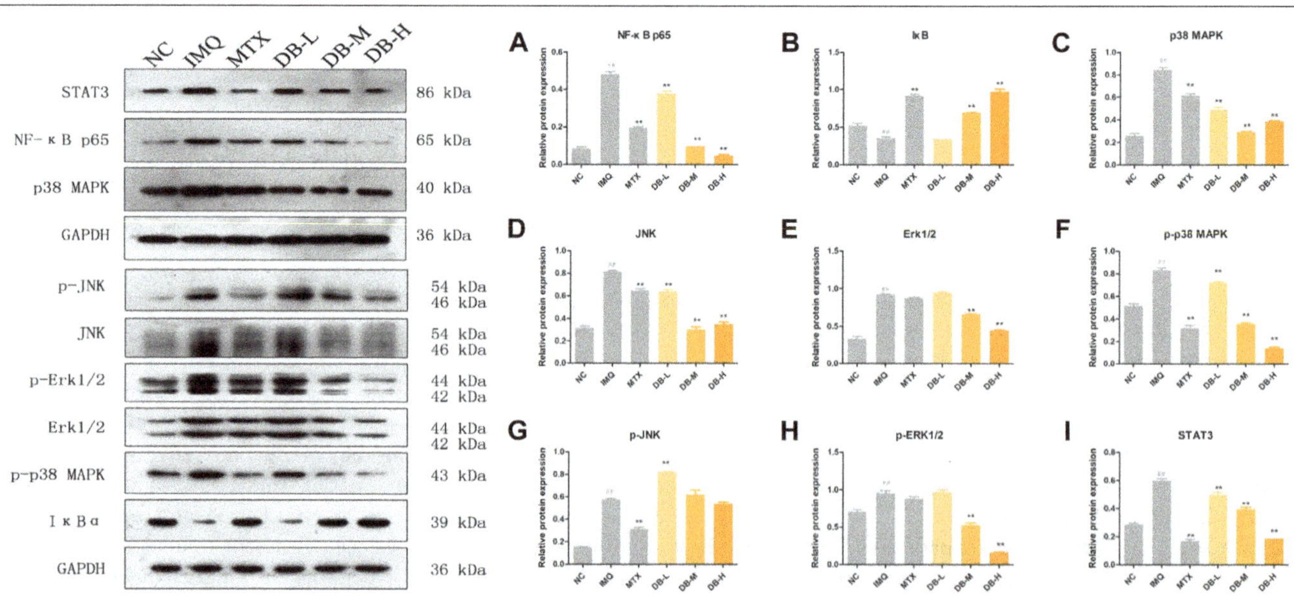

FIGURE 7 | Effects of DB on the NF-κB (NF-κB p65, IκBα), MAPKs (p38, JNK, ERK1/2) and STAT3 signaling pathways. The expression levels of p65 **(A)**, IκBα **(B)**, p38 **(C)**, JNK **(D)**, ERK1/2 **(E)**, p-p38 **(F)**, p-JNK **(G)**, p-ERK1/2 **(H)**, STAT3 **(I)** in the back skin tissues were detected using western blotting. Values are expressed as mean ± SD (n = 3). Where $^{\#}p < 0.05$ and $^{\#\#}p < 0.01$ versus NC group, $^{*}p < 0.05$ and $^{**}p < 0.01$ versus IMQ group.

decreased the expressions of STAT3 compared with IMQ group (**Figure 7**). This result showed DB had ability to suppress STAT3 pathways, especially at high dosage.

Emerging data suggests MAPK signaling pathways play a role in the development of psoriasis. MAPKs, including p38, JNK and ERK signaling pathways, regulate a variety of cellular activities,

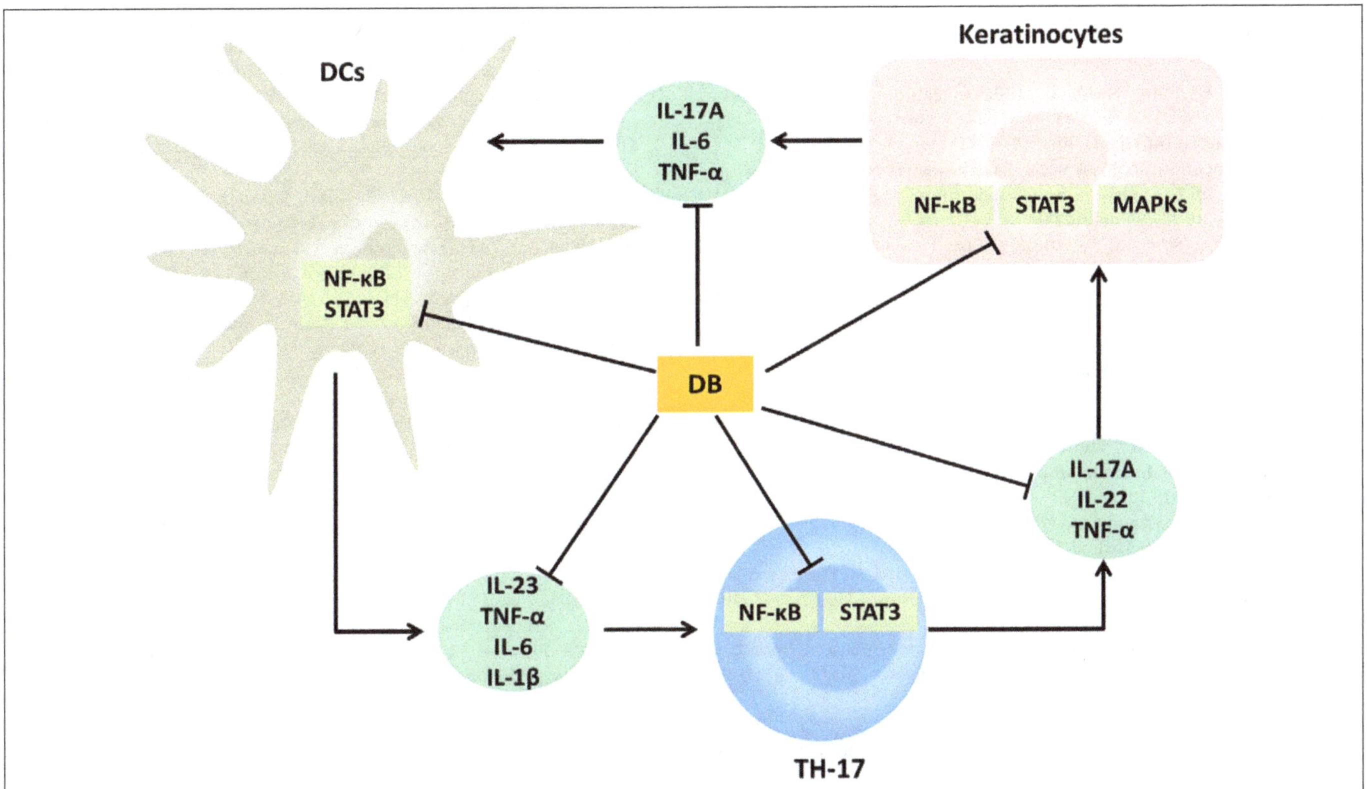

FIGURE 8 | Schematic diagram of proposed mechanisms of the anti-psoriatic effects of DB.

including cell proliferation, gene expression, apoptosis and inflammation. MAPKs are activated by phosphorylation, and phosphorylate downstream target proteins. MAPKs are reported to be related to the differentiation of Th1 and Th2, secretion of TNF-α, IL-6 and IL-1β, and excessive proliferation of keratinocytes (Mavropoulos et al., 2013; Hammouda et al., 2020). In our present study, except for p-JNK, the expressions of p38, JNK, ERK, p-p38 and p-ERK were significantly decreased by DB (**Figure 7**). These results indicated that DB could regulate the expressions of p38, JNK, ERK and suppress the phosphorylation of p38 and ERK to inhibit the activations of MAPK signaling pathways.

TCM are thought to have the character of multi-targets and multiple-pathways due to complex constituents. Some ingredients or chemical constituents of DB were reported to have anti-inflammatory activities. For example, salvianolic acid B, major active compounds in Salvia miltiorrhizae radix et rhizome, can suppress NF-κB triggered by TNF-α and the phosphorylation of JNK and ERK1/2 (Dong et al., 2016). Berberine, main active compounds in Phellodendri amurensis cortex, inhibits the inflammatory factors (IL-1, IL-6, COX-2, iNOS) and NF-κB, MAPK signaling pathway to suppress the inflammation (Lin and Lin, 2011; Zou et al., 2017). Cimicifugin of Saposhnikoviae radix is used to treat inflammatory diseases for its activities of inhibition of Th17 and suppression of JAK-STAT and NF-κB signaling pathways (Rahal et al., 2013). Though the whole is not the sum of its parts, the anti-inflammatory activities of ingredients partially explain the anti-psoriatic activity of DB. The therapeutic action of TCM prescription was the whole function of the ingredients. Therefore, we evaluated the anti-psoriatic effects of the whole formula in this study. As the monarch drug of the formula, anti-psoriatic effect of Salvia miltiorrhizae or active compounds of Salvia miltiorrhizae has been reported in several literatures. However, the anti-psoriatic effects of other ingredients and what are the main active compounds of DB still need our further investigation.

CONCLUSION

Our results revealed that DB had obvious anti-psoriatic effects in the IMQ-induced psoriatic mice. Its anti-psoriatic effects were related to the regulation of IL-23/TH-17 axis and inhibition on the activation of NF-κB, MAPKs and STAT3 signaling pathways (**Figure 8**). These findings clarify the therapeutic effects and mechanism of DB, thus provide crucial evidences to support the clinical use of DB.

AUTHOR CONTRIBUTIONS

XJ, HX, and GZ conceived the study. XJ and HX participated in most of experiments. XJ wrote the manuscript. HM and FW performed the LC-MS/MS analysis. CH and XX participated in the animal experiments and qPCR analysis. LC performed the ELISA analysis. YF performed the histological examination. All authors have read and approved the manuscript.

REFERENCES

Armstrong, A. W., and Read, C. (2020). Pathophysiology, Clinical Presentation, and Treatment of Psoriasis: A Review. *JAMA* 323 (19), 1945–1960. doi:10.1001/jama.2020.4006

Bocheńska, K., Smolińska, E., Moskot, M., Jakóbkiewicz-Banecka, J., and Gabig-Cimińska, M. (2017). Models in the Research Process of Psoriasis. *Int. J. Mol. Sci.* 18 (12). doi:10.3390/ijms18122514

Boehncke, W. H., and Schön, M. P. (2015). Psoriasis. *Lancet* 386 (9997), 983–994. doi:10.1016/s0140-6736(14)61909-7

Calautti, E., Avalle, L., and Poli, V. (2018). Psoriasis: A STAT3-Centric View. *Int. J. Mol. Sci.* 19 (1). doi:10.3390/ijms19010171

Cao, X. X., Xu, R., Li, F. L., Li, F., Chen, J., and Li, B. (2015). The Chinese Traditional Treatment of Psoriasis. *Med. Recapitulate* 21, 117–118.

Chiang, C. C., Cheng, W. J., Lin, C. Y., Lai, K. H., Ju, S. C., Lee, C., et al. (2020). Kan-Lu-Hsiao-Tu-Tan, a Traditional Chinese Medicine Formula, Inhibits Human Neutrophil Activation and Ameliorates Imiquimod-Induced Psoriasis-like Skin Inflammation. *J. Ethnopharmacol* 246, 112246. doi:10.1016/j.jep.2019.112246

Chinese-Pharmacopoeia-Commission (2020). *Pharmacopoeia of People's Republic of China.* Beijing: China Medical Science Press.

Deng, B. X., Jiang, C. Y., Wang, P., and Liu, W. L. (2006). Rule of Distribution and Development of TCM Syndromes of Psoriasis. *J. Traditional Chin. Med.* 47 (10), 770–772.

Deng, Y., Chang, C., and Lu, Q. (2016). The Inflammatory Response in Psoriasis: a Comprehensive Review. *Clin. Rev. Allergy Immunol.* 50 (3), 377–389. doi:10.1007/s12016-016-8535-x

Dong, Z., Ma, D., Gong, Y., Yu, T., and Yao, G. (2016). Salvianolic Acid B Ameliorates CNS Autoimmunity by Suppressing Th1 Responses. *Neurosci. Lett.* 619, 92–99. doi:10.1016/j.neulet.2016.01.008

Gaffen, S. L., Jain, R., Garg, A. V., and Cua, D. J. (2014). The IL-23-IL-17 Immune axis: from Mechanisms to Therapeutic Testing. *Nat. Rev. Immunol.* 14 (9), 585–600. doi:10.1038/nri3707

García-Pérez, M. E., Allaeys, I., Rusu, D., Pouliot, R., Janezic, T. S., and Poubelle, P. E. (2014). Picea Mariana Polyphenolic Extract Inhibits Phlogogenic Mediators Produced by TNF-α-Activated Psoriatic Keratinocytes: Impact on NF-Kb Pathway. *J. Ethnopharmacol* 151 (1), 265–278. doi:10.1016/j.jep.2013.10.034

Georgescu, S. R., Tampa, M., Caruntu, C., Sarbu, M. I., Mitran, C. I., Mitran, M. I., et al. (2019). Advances in Understanding the Immunological Pathways in Psoriasis. *Int. J. Mol. Sci.* 20 (3). doi:10.3390/ijms20030739

Goldminz, A. M., Au, S. C., Kim, N., Gottlieb, A. B., and Lizzul, P. F. (2013). NF-κB: an Essential Transcription Factor in Psoriasis. *J. Dermatol. Sci.* 69 (2), 89–94. doi:10.1016/j.jdermsci.2012.11.002

Greb, J. E., Goldminz, A. M., Elder, J. T., Lebwohl, M. G., Gladman, D. D., Wu, J. J., et al. (2016). Psoriasis. *Nat. Rev. Dis. Primers* 2, 16082. doi:10.1038/nrdp.2016.82

Haase, I., Hobbs, R. M., Romero, M. R., Broad, S., and Watt, F. M. (2001). A Role for Mitogen-Activated Protein Kinase Activation by Integrins in the Pathogenesis of Psoriasis. *J. Clin. Invest.* 108 (4), 527–536. doi:10.1172/jci12153

Hammouda, M. B., Ford, A. E., Liu, Y., and Zhang, J. Y. (2020). The JNK Signaling Pathway in Inflammatory Skin Disorders and Cancer. *Cells* 9 (4). doi:10.3390/cells9040857

Hawkes, J. E., Yan, B. Y., Chan, T. C., and Krueger, J. G. (2018). Discovery of the IL-23/IL-17 Signaling Pathway and the Treatment of Psoriasis. *J. Immunol.* 201 (6), 1605–1613. doi:10.4049/jimmunol.1800013

Hou, Y., Zhu, L., Tian, H., Sun, H. X., Wang, R., Zhang, L., et al. (2018). IL-23-induced Macrophage Polarization and its Pathological Roles in Mice with Imiquimod-Induced Psoriasis. *Protein Cell* 9 (12), 1027–1038. doi:10.1007/s13238-018-0505-z

Jia, J., Mo, X., Liu, J., Yan, F., Wang, N., Lin, Y., et al. (2020). Mechanism of Danshensu-Induced Inhibition of Abnormal Epidermal Proliferation in Psoriasis. *Eur. J. Pharmacol.* 868, 172881. doi:10.1016/j.ejphar.2019.172881

Kamiya, K., Kishimoto, M., Sugai, J., Komine, M., and Ohtsuki, M. (2019). Risk Factors for the Development of Psoriasis. *Int. J. Mol. Sci.* 20 (18). doi:10.3390/ijms20184347

Kreiner, J., Pang, E., Lenon, G. B., and Yang, A. W. H. (2017). Saposhnikoviae Divaricata: a Phytochemical, Pharmacological, and Pharmacokinetic Review. *Chin. J. Nat. Med.* 15 (4), 255–264. doi:10.1016/s1875-5364(17)30042-0

Kuai, L., Song, J. K., Zhang, R. X., Xing, M., Luo, Y., Ru, Y., et al. (2020). Uncovering the Mechanism of Jueyin Granules in the Treatment of Psoriasis Using Network Pharmacology. *J. Ethnopharmacol* 262, 113214. doi:10.1016/j.jep.2020.113214

Li, B., He, S., Liu, R., Huang, L., Liu, G., Wang, R., et al. (2019a). Total Glucosides of Paeony Attenuates Animal Psoriasis Induced Inflammatory Response through Inhibiting STAT1 and STAT3 Phosphorylation. *J. Ethnopharmacol* 243, 112121. doi:10.1016/j.jep.2019.112121

Li, F. L., Xu, R., Zeng, Q. C., Li, X., Chen, J., Wang, Y. F., et al. (20122012). Tanshinone IIA Inhibits Growth of Keratinocytes through Cell Cycle Arrest and Apoptosis: Underlying Treatment Mechanism of Psoriasis. *Evid. Based Complement. Alternat Med.* 2012, 927658. doi:10.1155/2012/927658

Li, X. Q., Chen, Y., Zhou, H. M., Shi, H. L., Yan, X. N., Lin, L. P., et al. (2019b). Anti-psoriasis Effect of Water-Processed Rosin in Mice. *J. Ethnopharmacol* 242, 112073. doi:10.1016/j.jep.2019.112073

Li, Y. J., Zhou, T., Zhang, J., Zhang, L., Ke, H., Zhang, C., et al. (2021). Clinical Trait-Connected Network Analysis Reveals Transcriptional Markers of Active Psoriasis Treatment with Liangxue-Jiedu Decoction. *J. Ethnopharmacol* 268, 113551. doi:10.1016/j.jep.2020.113551

Lin, S. H., Zhou, L. P., and Yu, N. C. (2005). Preparation of Concentrated Xiaobiwan and its Clinical Application. *Chin. J. Hosp. Pharm.* 25 (02), 86.

Lin, W. C., and Lin, J. Y. (2011). Berberine Down-Regulates the Th1/Th2 Cytokine Gene Expression Ratio in Mouse Primary Splenocytes in the Absence or Presence of Lipopolysaccharide in a Preventive Manner. *Int. Immunopharmacol* 11 (12), 1984–1990. doi:10.1016/j.intimp.2011.08.008

Lowes, M. A., Suárez-Fariñas, M., and Krueger, J. G. (2014). Immunology of Psoriasis. *Annu. Rev. Immunol.* 32, 227–255. doi:10.1146/annurev-immunol-032713-120225

Mavropoulos, A., Rigopoulou, E. I., Liaskos, C., Bogdanos, D. P., and Sakkas, L. I. (2013). The Role of P38 MAPK in the Aetiopathogenesis of Psoriasis and Psoriatic Arthritis. *Clin. Dev. Immunol.* 2013, 569751. doi:10.1155/2013/569751

Nguyen, L. T. H., Ahn, S. H., Nguyen, U. T., and Yang, I. J. (2018). Dang-Gui-Liu-Huang Tang a Traditional Herbal Formula, Ameliorates Imiquimod-Induced Psoriasis-like Skin Inflammation in Mice by Inhibiting IL-22 Production. *Phytomedicine* 47, 48–57. doi:10.1016/j.phymed.2018.04.051

Palanivel, J. A., Macbeth, A. E., Chetty, N. C., and Levell, N. J. (2014). An Insight into JAK-STAT Signalling in Dermatology. *Clin. Exp. Dermatol.* 39 (4), 513–518. doi:10.1111/ced.12273

Parmar, K. M., Itankar, P. R., Joshi, A., and Prasad, S. K. (2017). Anti-psoriatic Potential of Solanum Xanthocarpum Stem in Imiquimod-Induced Psoriatic Mice Model. *J. Ethnopharmacol* 198, 158–166. doi:10.1016/j.jep.2016.12.046

Pasparakis, M. (2012). Role of NF-Kb in Epithelial Biology. *Immunol. Rev.* 246 (1), 346–358. doi:10.1111/j.1600-065X.2012.01109.x

Pastorino, G., Cornara, L., Soares, S., Rodrigues, F., and Oliveira, M. B. P. P. (2018). Liquorice (Glycyrrhiza Glabra): A Phytochemical and Pharmacological Review. *Phytother Res.* 32 (12), 2323–2339. doi:10.1002/ptr.6178

Rahal, A., Kumar, A., Chakraborty, S., Tiwari, R., Sk, L., and Dhama, K. (2013). Cimicifuga: A Revisiting Indigenous Herb with Multi-Utility Benefits for Safeguarding Human Health – A Review. *Int. J. Agron. Plant Prod.* 4, 1590–1601.

Rai, V. K., Sinha, P., Yadav, K. S., Shukla, A., Saxena, A., Bawankule, D. U., et al. (2020). Anti-psoriatic Effect of Lavandula Angustifolia Essential Oil and its Major Components Linalool and Linalyl Acetate. *J. Ethnopharmacol* 261, 113127. doi:10.1016/j.jep.2020.113127

Rapalli, V. K., Singhvi, G., Dubey, S. K., Gupta, G., Chellappan, D. K., and Dua, K. (2018). Emerging Landscape in Psoriasis Management: From Topical Application to Targeting Biomolecules. *Biomed. Pharmacother.* 106, 707–713. doi:10.1016/j.biopha.2018.06.136

Rendon, A., and Schäkel, K. (2019). Psoriasis Pathogenesis and Treatment. *Int. J. Mol. Sci.* 20 (6). doi:10.3390/ijms20061475

Schinocca, C., Rizzo, C., Fasano, S., Grasso, G., La Barbera, L., Ciccia, F., et al. (2021). Role of the IL-23/IL-17 Pathway in Rheumatic Diseases: An Overview. *Front. Immunol.* 12, 637829. doi:10.3389/fimmu.2021.637829

Su, C. Y., Ming, Q. L., Rahman, K., Han, T., and Qin, L. P. (2015). Salvia Miltiorrhiza: Traditional Medicinal Uses, Chemistry, and Pharmacology. *Chin. J. Nat. Med.* 13 (3), 163–182. doi:10.1016/s1875-5364(15)30002-9

Sun, Y., Zhang, J., Zhai, T., Li, H., Li, H., Huo, R., et al. (2017). CCN1 Promotes IL-1β Production in Keratinocytes by Activating P38 MAPK Signaling in Psoriasis. *Sci. Rep.* 7, 43310. doi:10.1038/srep43310

Sun, Y., Lenon, G. B., and Yang, A. W. H. (2019). Phellodendri Cortex: A Phytochemical, Pharmacological, and Pharmacokinetic Review. *Evidence-Based Complement. Altern. Med.* 2019, 1–45. doi:10.1155/2019/7621929

Tang, L., He, S., Wang, X., Liu, H., Zhu, Y., Feng, B., et al. (2018). Cryptotanshinone Reduces Psoriatic Epidermal Hyperplasia via Inhibiting the Activation of STAT3. *Exp. Dermatol.* 27 (3), 268–275. doi:10.1111/exd.13511

van der Fits, L., Mourits, S., Voerman, J. S., Kant, M., Boon, L., Laman, J. D., et al. (2009). Imiquimod-induced Psoriasis-like Skin Inflammation in Mice Is Mediated via the IL-23/IL-17 axis. *J. Immunol.* 182 (9), 5836–5845. doi:10.4049/jimmunol.0802999

Wang, A., Wei, J., Lu, C., Chen, H., Zhong, X., Lu, Y., et al. (2019). Genistein Suppresses Psoriasis-Related Inflammation through a STAT3-NF-κb-dependent Mechanism in Keratinocytes. *Int. Immunopharmacol* 69, 270–278. doi:10.1016/j.intimp.2019.01.054

Wang, S., Zhu, L., Xu, Y., Qin, Z., and Xu, A. (2020). Salvianolic Acid B Ameliorates Psoriatic Changes in Imiquimod-Induced Psoriasis on BALB/c Mice by Inhibiting Inflammatory and Keratin Markers via Altering Phosphatidylinositol-3-Kinase/protein Kinase B Signaling Pathway. *Korean J. Physiol. Pharmacol.* 24 (3), 213–221. doi:10.4196/kjpp.2020.24.3.213

Xu, F., Xu, J., Xiong, X., and Deng, Y. (2019). Salidroside Inhibits MAPK, NF-Kb, and STAT3 Pathways in Psoriasis-Associated Oxidative Stress via SIRT1 Activation. *Redox Rep.* 24 (1), 70–74. doi:10.1080/13510002.2019.1658377

Xu, J., Duan, X., Hu, F., Poorun, D., Liu, X., Wang, X., et al. (2018). Resolvin D1 Attenuates Imiquimod-Induced Mice Psoriasiform Dermatitis through MAPKs and NF-Kb Pathways. *J. Dermatol. Sci.* 89 (2), 127–135. doi:10.1016/j.jdermsci.2017.10.016

Xu, S. Y., Bian, R. L., and Chen, X. (2002). *Experimental Methodology of Pharmacology.* Beijing: People's Medical Publishing House.

Xuan, P. H., and Zhang, J. Z. (2003). Preliminary Clinical Observation on the Combination Therapy Effects of Psoriasis with Chinese Medicine Formula Xiaobiwan. *J. Clin. Dermatol. (Chinese)* 32 (06), 360–361.

Zhang, C. S., Yu, J. J., Parker, S., Zhang, A. L., May, B., Lu, C., et al. (2014). Oral Chinese Herbal Medicine Combined with Pharmacotherapy for Psoriasis Vulgaris: a Systematic Review. *Int. J. Dermatol.* 53 (11), 1305–1318. doi:10.1111/ijd.12607

Zhu, N., and Hou, J. (2021). Molecular Mechanism of the Anti-inflammatory Effects of Sophorae Flavescentis Aiton Identified by Network Pharmacology. *Sci. Rep.* 11 (1), 1005. doi:10.1038/s41598-020-80297-y

Zou, K., Li, Z., Zhang, Y., Zhang, H. Y., Li, B., Zhu, W. L., et al. (2017). Advances in the Study of Berberine and its Derivatives: a Focus on Anti-inflammatory and Anti-tumor Effects in the Digestive System. *Acta Pharmacol. Sin* 38 (2), 157–167. doi:10.1038/aps.2016.125

2

Efficacy and Safety of Socheongryong-Tang Among Atopic Dermatitis Patients with Respiratory Disorders

*Ju Hyun Lee[1], Eun Heui Jo[2], Jee Youn Jung[3], Young-Eun Kim[4], Mi-Ju Son[3], Su Jin Kang[5], Geum Jin Yang[6], Yu Hwa Shim[6] and Min Cheol Park[7]**

[1]Department of Korean Medicine Ophthalmology and Otolaryngology and Dermatology, Wonkwang University Korean Medicine Hospital, Iksan, South Korea, [2]Department of Acupuncture and Moxibustion, Wonkwang University Korean Medicine Hospital and Research Center of Traditional Korean Medicine, Wonkwang University, Deokjingu, South Korea, [3]Clinical Medicine Division, Korea Institute of Oriental Medicine, Daejeon, South Korea, [4]Future Medicine Division, Korea Institute of Oriental Medicine, Daejeon, South Korea, [5]Department of Korean Medicine Obstetrics and Gynecology, Wonkwang University Korean Medicine Hospital, Iksan, South Korea, [6]Korean Medicine Dermatology Clinical Research Center of Wonkwang University, Iksan, South Korea, [7]Department of Korean Medicine Ophthalmology and Otolaryngology and Dermatology, Wonkwang University Korean Medicine Hospital and Research Center of Traditional Korean Medicine, Wonkwang University, Iksan, South Korea

***Correspondence:**
Min Cheol Park
spinx11@wonkwang.ac.kr

Atopic dermatitis is a chronic inflammatory skin disease that affects the growth and development of children. The prevalence of atopic dermatitis has been continually increasing, and this has also been accompanied by rising socioeconomic costs. Interest has been growing in alternative medicine as a means of alleviating the burden of atopic dermatitis. This was a single-center, double-blinded, randomized, placebo-controlled investigator-led clinical trial including 60 atopic dermatitis patients. The participants were classified into an experimental group (30 persons) and a control group (30 persons), who were administered, respectively, socheongryong-tang or a placebo for 4 weeks. After 4 weeks of treatment, the participants visited the trial center again and assess their efficacy and safety. The researchers performed statistical comparisons of the changes in the SCORAD Index, amount and frequency of ointment use, and height and weight to assess the efficacy. To assess the safety, diagnostic tests and vital sign checks were performed at each visit, and the presence or absence of adverse events was observed. As a result, the frequency and the amount of steroid ointment application in both groups increased, but the experimental group showed less tendency ($p = 0.081$). Results of analyzing the children in the experimental group in relation to growth showed a significantly greater height growth than the control group ($p < 0.05$). In addition, all study participants did not show any remarkable abnormal signs in the safety evaluation. In conclusion, compared to the control group, the experimental group, who took socheongryong-tang showed a tendency to be less dependent on steroid ointment and statistically significant increase in height.

Keywords: allergy, atopic dermatitis, clinical trials, height growth, socheongryong-tang

INTRODUCTION

Atopic dermatitis (AD, also called atopic eczema) is a chronic relapsing inflammatory skin disorder that is accompanied by itching, is caused by genetic and environmental factors (Nutten, 2015; Otsuka et al., 2017), and is common in infants (Eichenfield et al., 2013). Due to the "allergic march", patients who suffered from AD in infancy are more likely to develop respiratory disorders such as allergic asthma or rhinitis in childhood (Bantz et al., 2014). Several studies on allergic disease have reported that atopic disease affects the growth and development of children. Although the mechanisms by which allergic diseases impair height growth have not yet been elucidated (Kristmundsdottir and David, 1987), children with a history of respiratory allergy or AD are more likely to be shorter than their peers (Ferguson et al., 1982; Kristmundsdottir and David, 1987; Sant'Anna et al., 1996).

The prevalence of AD has been persistently increasing to date (Deckers et al., 2012; Nutten, 2015), and this has been accompanied by rising socioeconomic costs. There has been growing interest in alternative medicine as a means of reducing the socioeconomic burden of AD. However, excluding a study analyzing the growth-promoting ingredients in boyangsungjang-tang (Hong et al., 2012) or studies demonstrating the efficacy of gamisasangja-tang (Park et al., 2015) and taeumjowi-tang (Park et al., 2019) for alleviating AD, there have been hardly any clinical studies demonstrating the efficacy of alternative medicine for AD and growth.

Socheongryong-tang (SCRT, also known as Sho-Seiru-To and Xiao-Qing-Long-Tang) is a type of herbal medicine that has been used for centuries to treat respiratory and allergic diseases in countries across East Asia (Ko et al., 2004; Das et al., 2009). However, in spite of these effects of SCRT, there have been almost no studies demonstrating its effects on AD and childhood growth. This research aims to evaluate the efficacy and safety of SCRT, vs. placebo, for the treatment of AD with respiratory disorders and as a growth promoter for short children.

MATERIALS AND METHODS

Sample Size Calculation

To evaluate SCRT efficacy in AD patients, we used SCORAD scores. In SCRT and placebo groups, It was hypothesized that the mean SCORAD scores change after intervention will be 7.9 (μc) and 13.8 (μt), respectively, with a standard deviation of 8.2. Based on the estimated dropout rate (20%), 60 participants in total were needed to achieve significance level of 0.05 in a 2-tailed test and a statistical power of 80%.

Study Design and Participants

This study was designed as a single-center, double-blinded, randomized, placebo-controlled, investigator-led clinical trial. The participants were divided into an experimental group (30 persons) and a control group (30 persons), who were administered SCRT or placebo, respectively, for 4 weeks. After 4 weeks of medication, the participants visited the trial center again, and the efficacy and safety of the treatments were assessed. The trial design of this study has already been published in the form of a protocol paper (Kang et al., 2020). This clinical trial was conducted from June 13, 2019 (first registration date) to December 13, 2019 (last visit date).

Patient Enrollment

A total of 65 persons were enrolled in the study, of which five persons were excluded during screening. The reasons for exclusion were contravening the exclusion criteria (two persons), contravening the inclusion criteria (two persons), and withdrawal of consent (one person). Investigator-led clinical trials were for trend search rather than statistical and clinical significance, and n number was selected as 30 cases per group considering 20% dropout rate.

Inclusion and Exclusion Criteria

Among patients who had heard and fully understood a thorough explanation of the study, voluntarily decided to participate, and gave written consent to adhere to the study precautions, those who satisfied all the following inclusion criteria and did not fit any of the exclusion criteria were defined as participants.

Inclusion Criteria

(1) Male or female individuals aged 7–65 years, having mild-moderate atopic dermatitis (SCORAD score ≥15 and <50), and with ≥3 major clinical symptoms and ≥3 minor clinical symptoms according to the Hanifin & Rajka diagnostic criteria (Hanifin and Rajka, 1980)
(2) Individuals who checked ≥1 respiratory disease or related symptom corresponding to the allergy march in the questionnaire for symptom classification

Exclusion Criteria

(1) Patients receiving intensive drug treatment for severe AD
(2) Patients who have used oral antihistamines, steroids, antibiotics, systemic photochemotherapy, or other immune-suppressants less than 4 weeks before the start of the trial
(3) Patients with a systemic infection or receiving systemic antibiotic therapy, or taking interferon therapy
(4) Patients with severe skin disease or pigment deposition other than AD, or with extensive scarring in the region of AD
(5) Patients with liver disease, kidney disease, severe acute cardiovascular disease, gastrointestinal disorders, excessive sweating, voiding dysfunction, or chronic disease
(6) Patients with a platelet count ≤100,000/mm^3 due to liver dysfunction caused by chronic hepatitis
(7) Patients who have taken potassium-containing agents, licorice-containing agents, glycyrrhizic acid, salt-containing agents, loop diuretics (furosemide, ethacrynic acid), thiazide diuretics (trichlormethiazide), ephedra/ephedrine-containing agents, MAO inhibitors, thyroid-related drugs, catecholamines, or xanthines less than 4 weeks before the start of the trial

TABLE 1 | Ingredients of the SCRT granules and placebo.

	Ingredient name	Amount (g)	Extract (g)		Ingredient name	Amount (g)
Main Ingredient	*Pinellia ternata* (Thunb.) Makino	2.00	1.05	Excipient	Lactose hydrate	1.490
	Ephedra sinica Stapf	1.00			Corn starch	1.490
	Paeonia lactiflora Pall.	1.00		Colorant	Caramel pigment	0.010
	Glycyrrhiza uralensis Fisch.	1.00		Fragrance	Ginseng flavor powder	0.010
	Cinnamomum cassia (L.) J. Presl	1.00		–	–	–
	Asiasarum heterotropoides var. *mandshuricum* (Maxim.) F. Maek.	1.00		–	–	–
	Zingiber officinale Roscoe	1.00		–	–	–
	Schisandra chinensis (Turcz.) Baill.	1.00		–	–	–
–				–	–	–
Excipient	Lactose hydrate	–	0.82	–	–	–
	Cornstarch	–	1.13	–	–	–
Total	–	–	3.00	Total	–	3.00

(8) Patients who have taken antipsychotic drugs less than 2 months before screening
(9) Patients who have participated in another clinical trial within the last 4 months
(10) Patients with a history of drug/alcohol abuse, hypersensitivity to any drugs used in this clinical trial or ingredients in those drugs
(11) Women who are pregnant, breastfeeding or capable of childbearing (i.e., women who have not undergone surgical sterilization) and do not accept the use of appropriate contraceptive methods
(12) Patients with thyroid dysfunction, indicated by thyroid-stimulating hormone (TSH) ≤0.1 or ≥10.0 μU/ml in screening

Investigated Drug and Placebo

The experimental group took SCRT granules (Batch number: 18423; Hanpoong Pharm and Foods, Jeonju, Jeollabuk-do, South Korea) and the control group took a placebo (Batch number: 18001; Hanpoong Pharm and Foods), which are all water extracted brown granules (**Table 1**). The participants took SCRT or the placebo three times per day for 4 weeks, taking one sachet before each meal. The one-time dose of SCRT or placebo was determined with reference to the regulations on reporting product licenses for herbal medicines published by the Korean Food and Drug Administration, differentiating according to age. The participants aged 7–14 years took a dose of 6.0 g per day, and the participants aged 15–65 years took a dose of 9.0 g per day.

To provide the minimal treatment for AD, all participants were supplied with Lacticare (Hydrocortisone acetate 1%) ointment, which is a Class 7 steroid, corresponding to the classification of "the least potent agent" (Ference and Last, 2009). Lacticare is a white lotion manufactured by Korea Pharma Co., Ltd. (Hwaseong, Gyeonggi-do, South Korea). All the participants were instructed to rub a thin layer of the ointment broadly into the affected area, in accordance with their physician's guidance. Each drug was stored at room temperature (20–30°C) in a sealed container, and storage, management, and distribution of the drugs was conducted under the guidance of the principal investigator and a traditional Korean medicine physician acting as a trial administrator.

Randomization and Blinding

Randomization

The participants who gave written consent to participate in the trial were allocated a screening number by researchers according to the order in which they gave consent. Of these, participants who satisfied the inclusion/exclusion criteria were assigned a randomization number in the order in which they visited. Treatment prescribed to the participants was based on these numbers assigned to the participants.

The randomization table contains information about the administration group assigned to the participants according to the randomization number. A block randomization method was used to randomize based on a 1:1 allocation ratio within a block of a certain size (e.g., 4, 6, 8). After generating the randomization table, for each participant, the corresponding drug was packaged, a label with the randomization number was attached, and the drug was sent to the pharmacist or traditional Korean medicine physician administrator at the trial center before the start of the trial.

Blinding

To ensure scientific results for the trial, double-blinding was performed, so that the investigators and participants were both unaware of the group allocation of each participant. In the event of unblinding due to adverse events, this was to be reported to the IRB and the petitioner was to be informed in accordance with the unblinding protocol.

Efficacy Assessment

SCORAD Index

The SCORAD Index is a scale for assessing AD that was developed in 1996 and has been used to date (European Task Force on Atopic Dermatitis, 1993). The investigators used the SCORAD Index to ascertain objective symptoms, such as the extent and severity of lesions, used the VAS to quantify and calculate subjective symptoms, such as pruritus and sleep disorders. Based on this data, the changes in the SCORAD Index were compared statistically between the two groups.

Ointment Application

Drugs that were prescribed for treatment purposes and could affect the results, such as antihistamines, steroids, and NSAIDs, were thoroughly banned. However, in order to provide the minimal treatment for AD, all participants were provided with the steroid ointment Lacticare. The study participants were instructed to apply an appropriate amount of steroid ointment to the skin lesion with a cotton swab whenever atopic dermatitis symptoms occurred. To prevent adverse reactions, the maximum number of applications per day of steroid ointment was limited to 1 to 3 times. The participants recorded their own frequency of ointment use every day in a notebook, and based on this record, they visited the research institute again on Week 4 to calculate the total number of times they used the ointment. The total amount of ointment used was measured using scales when the patients visited the trial center again 4 weeks after the start of the trial. Based on these measurements, the change in ointment use was compared statistically between the two groups.

Body Measurement

The investigators measured and recorded the participants' height and body weight when they visited the trial center at baseline and in Week 4. Based on these measurements, changes in height and weight were compared between the two groups.

Safety Assessment

Adverse Reaction

In this study, all harmful, unintended signs, symptoms, and diseases that the participants developed after receiving a drug in the trial were defined as adverse reactions. In the event of an adverse reaction, the investigators compiled a case record form including the name of the adverse reaction, the date of onset and recovery, by severity, relatedness to the drug taken, related procedures and treatments, and treatment outcomes. Abnormal laboratory results or vital signs that were considered to be clinically significant were also recorded as adverse reactions.

Diagnostic Test

For safety assessment, all participants were subjected to laboratory tests for a total of 20 items, including complete blood cell (CBC), renal function test (RFT), liver function test (LFT), blood lipid, and urine PH. The tests were performed twice, at baseline and in Week 4.

Vital Sign Monitoring

The investigators measured all participants' body temperature, pulse rate, and blood pressure when they visited the trial center at baseline and in Week 4. Changes in vital signs were monitored before and after taking the prescribed drug, and judged to be normal or abnormal based on the results.

Statistical Analyses

SAS for Windows was used for statistical analysis; the statistical significance level was set at 5% and the power at 80%, and 95% confidence intervals were provided for the differences between the groups. For test results, means, standard deviations, and frequencies were shown. Paired *t*-tests were used to compare the efficacy outcome variables between baseline and Week 4, and independent *t*-tests were used to analyze differences between the two groups. However, when normality was not satisfied through the normality test, nonparametric analysis was performed using Wilcoxon signed-rank test and Mann-Whitney test. The participants' gender and ratio of participants who developed adverse reactions was calculated and compared between the two groups using a chi-square test. The chi-square test, Fisher's exact test, and independent *t*-test were used for comparative analysis of factors that influence height growth. Means and standard deviations were shown for laboratory test results and vital signs, and independent t-tests and paired t-tests were used to compare the results, respectively, within groups between baseline and Week 4, and between groups. Missing values (e.g., due to dropout) were imputed using last observation carried forward (LOCF).

RESULTS

Demographic Information

There were no statistically significant differences in sex or age between the two groups. Statistical analysis in this study included a total of 49 participants, excluding the four participants who dropped out and seven participants who, in a MAST test for around 60 allergens to test for respiratory allergies, diverged from the normal distribution for an item on the statistically significant boundary between the two groups. The seven participants showing differences in the MAST test were all in the experimental group, and showed allergic reactions to garlic (one person), Cladosporium (three persons), *Alternaria alternata* (one person), and dog (two persons).

In order to precisely ascertain the extent of growth, participants who were aged <18 years were classified as children. A total of 30 children were recruited (15 in the experimental group and 15 in the control group). Among the children, there were no statistically significant differences in sex or age between the two groups (**Table 2**). One person in the experimental group and three persons in the control group dropped out during the trial. The reason for dropout in the experimental group was concomitant medication with a banned drug, and TSH outside the normal range in the placebo group. Among the children, one participant of the experimental group dropped out due to violation of exclusion criteria. Excluding the patients who dropped out, 56 patients completed the whole clinical trial in accordance with the prepared protocol (**Figure 1**).

TABLE 2 | Demographic information.

		Experimental group (n = 30)	Control Group (n = 30)	Total (n = 60)	*p*-value[a]
Total participants	Sex (M/F)	16/14	9/21	25/35	0.067[b]
	Age (years)	22.53 ± 14.67	25.47 ± 16.89	24.00 ± 15.75	0.476
		Experimental group (n = 15)	**Control group (n = 15)**	**Total (n = 30)**	***p*-value[a]**
Children participants	Sex (M/F)	9/6	6/9	15/15	0.273[b]
	Age (years)	10.00 ± 1.96	10.13 ± 2.10	10.07 ± 2.00	0.859

[a]*Values are presented as mean ± SD: analyzed by independent t-test.*
[b]*Values are presented as mean ± SD: analyzed by chi-square test.*

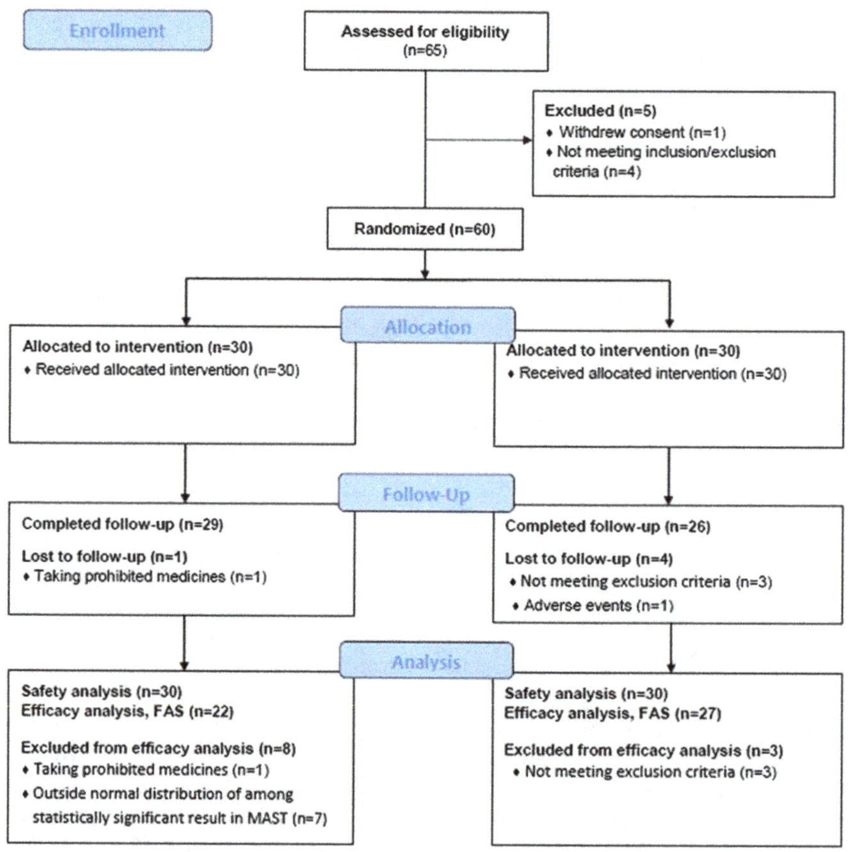

FIGURE 1 | Study flow chart describing the randomized controlled trial.

Compliance

The experimental group took a mean of 76.97 ± 12.01 doses of the prescribed drug, showing 94.55 ± 5.18% compliance. The control group took a mean of 76.33 ± 18.16 doses of the prescribed drug, showing 93.67 ± 6.21% compliance. Compliance was over 90% in both groups, and there was no statistically significant different between the two groups.

Efficacy Evaluation

SCORAD Index

In the efficacy evaluation in Week 4, the objective, subjective, and total SCORAD scores all showed statistically significant decreases compared to baseline in both the experimental group and the control group ($p < 0.05$). However, there were no significant differences when SCORAD scores were compared between the two groups (**Table 3**).

Ointment Application

The mean amount of ointment used in the experimental group increased by 2.50 ± 7.63 g at Week 4 compared to baseline, and the frequency of use increased by 3.00 ± 12.17. Meanwhile, the amount of ointment used in the control group increased by 11.85 ± 21.93 g, and the frequency of use increased by 7.33 ± 11.63. There were no statistically significant differences

TABLE 3 | Changes in the SCORAD index.

	Experimental group (n = 22)				Control group (n = 27)				*p*-value[b]
	Baseline	Week 4	Change value	*p*-value[a]	Baseline	Week 4	Change value	*p*-value[a]	
Extent of lesion	33.14 ± 12.13	23.77 ± 11.41	−9.36 ± 10.30	0.0003***	32.41 ± 15.86	23.37 ± 12.75	−9.04 ± 8.39	<0.0001***	0.903
Severity of lesion	4.27 ± 1.39	3.18 ± 1.40	−1.09 ± 0.92	<0.0001***	4.19 ± 1.44	3.11 ± 1.45	−1.07 ± 0.83	<0.0001***	0.947
Subjective symptoms	9.36 ± 3.37	6.59 ± 3.32	−2.77 ± 2.49	<0.0001***	8.52 ± 3.62	6.26 ± 3.72	−2.26 ± 2.46	<0.0001***	0.473
Total score	30.95 ± 7.72	22.48 ± 9.07	−8.46 ± 5.93	<0.0001***	29.65 ± 9.44	21.82 ± 9.06	−7.83 ± 5.53	<0.0001***	0.699

[a]*Values are presented as mean ± SD: analyzed by paired t-test.*
[b]*Values are presented as mean ± SD: analyzed by independent t-test.*
****p < 0.001.*

TABLE 4 | Changes in the amount and frequency of ointment use.

	Experimental group (n = 22)				Control group (n = 27)				*p*-value[b]
	Baseline	Week 4	Change value	*p*-value[a]	Baseline	Week 4	Change value	*p*-value[a]	
Frequency of use (times)	3.68 ± 3.98	6.18 ± 8.70	2.50 ± 7.63	0.139	5.93 ± 8.81	13.26 ± 14.55	7.33 ± 11.63	0.003**	0.100
Amount of use (g)	7.59 ± 10.83	10.59 ± 13.00	3.00 ± 12.17	0.260	6.59 ± 14.35	18.44 ± 21.68	11.85 ± 21.93	0.009**	0.081

[a]*Values are presented as mean ± SD: analyzed by paired t-test.*
[b]*Values are presented as mean ± SD: analyzed by independent t-test.*
***p < 0.01.*

TABLE 5 | Changes in children's height and weight.

	Experimental group (n = 14)				Control group (n = 15)				*p*-value[b]
	Baseline	Week 4	Change value	*p*-value[a]	Baseline	Week 4	Change value	*p*-value[a]	
Height (cm)	146.43 ± 16.20	147.00 ± 16.10	0.57 ± 0.65	0.006**	146.80 ± 11.93	146.87 ± 11.78	0.07 ± 0.26	0.334	0.015*
Weight (kg)	40.21 ± 10.52	40.53 ± 10.73	0.31 ± 0.95	0.239	45.91 ± 14.30	46.47 ± 14.38	0.56 ± 1.66	0.212	0.632
BMI (kg/m^2)	18.56 ± 2.82	18.55 ± 2.89	−0.01 ± 0.39	0.946	20.84 ± 4.86	21.09 ± 4.83	0.25 ± 0.74	0.205	0.243

[a]*Values are presented as mean ± SD: analyzed by paired t-test.*
[b]*Values are presented as mean ± SD: analyzed by independent t-test.*
**p < 0.05.*
***p < 0.01.*

between the two groups in the amount or frequency of ointment use. However, there was a trend for a less amount of ointment use in the experimental group compared to the control group (p = 0.08; **Table 4**).

Body Measurement

The mean height of the children in the experimental group was 146.43 ± 16.20 cm at baseline, and the mean growth after medication was 0.57 ± 0.65 cm. The mean height of the children in the control group was 146.80 ± 11.93 cm at baseline, and the mean growth after medication was 0.07 ± 0.26 cm. In statistical analysis, the height of the experimental group and the control group at baseline did not show a statistically significant difference. However, at Week 4, the experimental group showed a significant level of height growth, while the control group did not show any significant change. As a result, the experimental group showed significantly more growth than the control group ($p < 0.05$). On the other hand, there were no significant differences between the two groups in changes in body weight or BMI (**Table 5**).

In the analysis of the children and their parents, such as the parents' age, parents' education level, parents' occupation, family income, weight and height at birth, breastfeeding experience, which can affect height growth, no statistically significant difference was observed between the experimental group and the control group (**Table 6**). In addition, residential life (type of resident, residential environment, construction period, new/repaired house or new furniture, etc.), eating habits and other matters (cooking method, whether to take dietary supplements, number and type of eating out, type of snack, the number of exercise, participants' ethnicity etc.) did not show any significant difference between both groups (**Table 6**).

Safety Evaluation

Adverse Reaction

The adverse reactions reported by the participants were mild abdominal pain (two persons), acute palmoplantar vesicular eczema (one person), and fever and coughing (one person). Of these, the eczema and fever and coughing were considered to be unrelated to the prescribed drug, and disappeared promptly after monitoring. The two cases of abdominal pain were both in the

TABLE 6 | Analysis of influencing factors related to children's height growth.

			Experimental group (n = 15)	Control group (n = 15)	*p*-value
General characteristics of parents	Parent's age	Under 30	1 (6.67%)	0 (0.00%)	1.000[a]
		30–34	1 (6.67%)	1 (6.67%)	
		35–39	4 (26.67%)	4 (26.67%)	
		Over 40	9 (60.00%)	10 (66.67%)	
	Education level	High school graduate	5 (33.33%)	7 (46.67%)	0.456[b]
		College graduate	10 (66.67%)	8 (53.33%)	
	Occupation	Employed	11 (73.33%)	12 (80.00%)	1.000[a]
		Unemployed	4 (26.67%)	3 (20.00%)	–
	Family income (US dollor)	Under 200	2 (13.33%)	1 (6.67%)	0.582[a]
		200–300	1 (6.67%)	2 (13.33%)	
		300–400	6 (40.00%)	3 (20.00%)	
		Over 400	6 (40.00%)	9 (60.00%)	
General characteristics of children	Weight at birth (kg)	–	3.34 ± 0.38	3.26 ± 0.49	0.592[c]
	Height at birth (cm)	–	50.37 ± 1.60	49.93 ± 1.98	0.519[c]
	Breastfeeding experience	No lactation	3 (20.00%)	2 (13.33%)	0.775[a]
		Colostrum lactation	2 (13.33%)	2 (13.33%)	
		Under 6 months	6 (40.00%)	4 (26.67%)	
		Over 1 year	4 (26.67%)	7 (46.67%)	

[a]*Values are presented as mean ± SD or number (%): analyzed by Fisher's exact test.*
[b]*Values are presented as mean ± SD or number (%): analyzed by chi-square test.*
[c]*Values are presented as mean ± SD or number (%): analyzed by independent* t-*test.*

TABLE 7 | Changes in children's TSH and Vital sign.

	Experimental group (n = 14)				Control group (n = 15)				*p*-value[b]
	Baseline	Week 4	Change value	*p*-value[a]	Baseline	Week 4	Change value	*p*-value[a]	
TSH (uIU/ml)	1.46 ± 0.48	1.21 ± 0.36	−0.25 ± 0.32	0.012*	1.40 ± 0.68	1.89 ± 1.23	0.49 ± 1.08	0.103	0.022*
SBP (mmHg)	100.86 ± 10.73	100.79 ± 10.36	−0.07 ± 10.20	0.980	103.93 ± 14.56	106.27 ± 15.10	2.33 ± 11.33	0.438	0.554
DBP (mmHg)	59.93 ± 7.15	59.57 ± 9.47	−0.36 ± 12.07	0.911	63.00 ± 11.96	63.27 ± 12.04	0.27 ± 8.42	0.904	0.872
Body temperature (°C)	36.79 ± 0.21	36.78 ± 0.32	−0.01 ± 0.38	0.890	36.67 ± 0.22	36.77 ± 0.22	0.09 ± 0.28	0.224	0.396
Pulse (times/min)	85.57 ± 5.46	82.36 ± 5.88	−3.21 ± 8.34	0.146	81.33 ± 6.79	83.67 ± 5.05	2.33 ± 5.14	0.100	0.039*

[a]*Values are presented as mean ± SD: analyzed by paired* t-*test.*
[b]*Values are presented as mean ± SD: analyzed by independent* t-*test.*
$^*p < 0.05$.

placebo group, and one of these patients showed recovery without separate treatment. The other patient withdrew their consent and dropped out of the clinical trial due to the abdominal pain.

Diagnostic Test and Vital Sign Monitoring

In blood tests and vital sign monitoring after 4 weeks of medication, pulse and TSH levels of the children in the experimental group showed a significantly greater decrease from baseline compared to the control group ($p < 0.05$). The body temperature, SBP, DBP of the children in the experimental group also showed a decrease compared to the baseline. However, this change in TSH and vital sign was within the normal range, and all study participants did not show any abnormal signs in laboratory tests or vital sign monitoring throughout the study (**Table 7**).

DISCUSSION

AD is a relapsing, pruritic, inflammatory skin disease, reported to be caused by interactions between the immune system, microbial exposure, genetic and environmental factors, and skin barrier dysfunction (Flohr and Mann, 2014; Otsuka et al., 2017). For treatment of AD, depending on the etiology and the severity of symptoms, methods such as avoidance strategies, topical anti-inflammatory therapy, and phototherapy are used (Wollenberg et al., 2018a; Wollenberg et al., 2018b). Of these, application of steroidal ointment is the most commonly recommended treatment method to alleviate symptoms (Arellano et al., 2007). However, long-term steroid use can cause adverse reactions such as acne, steroid rosacea, telangiectasia, perioral dermatitis, and atrophy. For patients who do not respond to steroid treatment, AD can recur (Fukaya, 2000; Atherton, 2003).

The incidence of AD has been gradually increasing over several centuries, and currently affects around 20% of the world population (Bantz et al., 2014). The need to develop new therapeutic agents has become prominent due to the increasing socioeconomic costs of AD (Carroll et al., 2005; Suh et al., 2007), and this has been accompanied by growing interest in the potential of alternative medicine.

SCRT is a herbal medicine that has been used in East Asia to treat diseases related to the allergic march, such as allergic rhinitis and asthma, for hundreds of years (Shin et al., 2018). SCRT is reported to have an "anti-allergic effect" (Ikeda et al., 2002) and an "anti-inflammatory effect" (Shin et al., 2018). However, to date, there have been almost no clinical studies investigating the effects of SCRT for AD.

With the aim of verifying the efficacy of SCRT for AD, this study evaluated efficacy and safety in patients taking SCRT or a placebo. In the efficacy assessment, there were no statistically significances between the two groups in objective, subjective, and total SCORAD scores. This is thought to be due to the effects of the steroidal ointment supplied to all participants to provide the minimal treatment.

There were also no statistically significant differences between the two groups in the change in amount and frequency of ointment use. However, the experimental group showed a trend for less ointment use than the control group ($p = 0.081$). The reason for this phenomenon seems to be that the previously reported anti-allergic effect such as inhibiting IL-4 and $CD4^+$ of SCRT and its ingredients (Ikeda et al., 2002) affected the progression and remission of atopic dermatitis. This indicates that medication with SCRT could reduce AD patients' dependency on steroidal ointment.

In anthropometric analysis only including children (participants aged <18 years), the experimental group showed a significantly greater increase in height from baseline to Week 4 than the control group ($p < 0.05$). Most of the children in this study belonged to the school-age (7–12 years old), and in the statistical analysis conducted on these participants (13 from the experimental group and 12 from the control group), the experimental group showed a statistically significant height growth compared to the control group ($p = 0.016$). The remaining five participants (two from the experimental group and three from the control group) belonged to adolescence (over 13 years old), and in the height growth, no statistically significant difference was shown between the experimental group and control group. However, because the number of adolescence participants was too small, it was judged to have no statistical significance. In addition, as a result of investigating and comparing factors that can affect height growth such as parents' socioeconomic environment, physical information of the children, residential life, eating habits, participants' ethnicity and exercise, the experimental group and the control group didn't show any statistically significant differences in these items. This suggests that SCRT has a significant effect as a growth promoter for children with AD.

In blood tests and vital sign monitoring after 4 weeks of medication, TSH levels of the children in the experimental group showed a significantly greater decrease from baseline compared to the control group ($p < 0.05$). Thyroid hormones are known to have a major effect on children's growth and development (Tarım, 2011). The fact that the experimental group of this study showed height growth and TSH reduction after 4 weeks of SCRT administration suggests that there may be some association between SCRT, TSH, and children's height growth. However, considering the fact that the relationship between SCRT and TSH has not been clearly identified, further studies are needed to clarify this association.

In adverse reaction monitoring, vital sign monitoring, and laboratory tests to evaluate the safety of SCRT, there were no abnormal findings. Considering that previous studies have reported allergic diseases, such as allergic asthma and AD, leading to short stature in children (Ferguson et al., 1982; Kristumundsdottir and David, 1987; Snat'Anna et al., 1996), the growth-promoting effects of SCRT are thought to be mediated not only by hormones, but also by amelioration of allergic disease. The results of this study provide evidence to support claims that SCRT is a safe treatment method without adverse effects that can be used in children with AD as an alternative to growth hormone, which is controversial.

The mechanisms behind the growth-promoting effects of SCRT are unclear, and other factors affecting growth such as parental height could not be actively controlled. In addition, it is difficult to generalize the results as the number of research participants analyzed for height growth is relatively small. However, if independent studies of SCRT or a long-term, large-scale study of the effects on AD relief and growth factors such as T3, T4, and IGF-1 were performed, the mechanisms could be revealed more precisely.

CONCLUSION

The experimental group that took SCRT showed a trend for reduced dependence on steroidal ointment compared to the control group. In addition, SCRT treatment resulted in a significant promotion of height growth in children with AD. Also in safety evaluation, all study participants did not show any abnormal signs including laboratory tests or vital sign monitoring throughout the study.

AUTHOR CONTRIBUTIONS

JL: Conceptualization, Visualization, Writing of the original draft. EJ: Methodology, Revision and editing of the draft. JJ: Methodology, Revision and editing of the draft. Y-EK: Methodology. M-JS: Methodology. SK: Resources. GY: Resources. YS: Data curation, Resources. MP: Conceptualization, Project administration, Supervision, Revision and editing of the draft.

ACKNOWLEDGMENTS

We would like to express our gratitude to Ho-Seop Lee and Yoon-Jung Lee for their support of the research project. We would also like to thank Editage (www.editage.co.kr) for English language editing.

REFERENCES

Arellano, F. M., Wentworth, C. E., Arana, A., Fernández, C., and Paul, C. F. (2007). Risk of lymphoma following exposure to calcineurin inhibitors and topical steroids in patients with atopic dermatitis. *J. Invest. Dermatol.* 127, 808–816. doi:10.1038/sj.jid.5700622.

Atherton, D. J. (2003). Topical corticosteroids in atopic dermatitis. *BMJ* 327, 942–943. doi:10.1136/bmj.327.7421.942.

Bantz, S. K., Zhu, Z., and Zheng, T. (2014). The atopic march: progression from atopic dermatitis to allergic rhinitis and asthma. *J. Clin. Cell. Immunol.* 5 (2), 202. doi:10.4172/2155-9899.1000202.

Carroll, C. L., Balkrishnan, R., Feldman, S. R., Fleischer, A. B., Jr, and Manuel, J. C. (2005). The burden of atopic dermatitis: impact on the patient, family, and society. *Pediatr. Dermatol.* 22, 192–199. doi:10.1111/j.1525-1470.2005.22303.x.

Das, A. K., Mizuguchi, H., Kodama, M., Dev, S., Umehara, H., Kitamura, Y., et al. (2009). Sho-seiryu-to suppresses histamine signaling at the transcriptional level in TDI-sensitized nasal allergy model rats. *Allergol. Int.* 58, 81–88. doi:10.2332/allergolint.o-07-526.

Deckers, I. A. G., McLean, S., Linssen, S., Mommers, M., van Schayck, C. P., and Sheikh, A. (2012). Investigating international time trends in the incidence and prevalence of atopic Eczema 1990-2010: a systematic review of epidemiological studies. *PLoS One* 7, e39803. doi:10.1371/journal.pone.0039803.

Eichenfield, L. F., Tom, W. L., Chamlin, S. L., Feldman, S. R., Hanifin, J. M., Simpson, E. L., et al. (2014). Guidelines of care for the management of atopic dermatitis: section 1. Diagnosis and assessment of atopic dermatitis. *J. Am. Acad. Dermatol.* 70, 338–351. doi:10.1016/j.jaad.2013.10.010.

European Task Force on Atopic Dermatitis (1993). Severity scoring of atopic dermatitis: the SCORAD index. *Dermatology* 186, 23–31.

Ference, J. D., and Last, A. R. (2009). Choosing topical corticosteroids. *Am. Fam. Physician.* 79, 135–140.

Ferguson, A., Murray, A., and Tze, W. (1982). Short stature and delayed skeletal maturation in children with allergic disease. *J. Allergy Clin. Immunol.* 69, 461–466. doi:10.1016/0091-6749(82)90122-1.

Flohr, C., and Mann, J. (2014). New insights into the epidemiology of childhood atopic dermatitis. *Allergy* 69, 3–16. doi:10.1111/all.12270.

Fukaya, M. (2000). Why do patients with atopic dermatitis refuse to apply topical corticosteroids? *Dermatology* 201, 242–245. doi:10.1159/000018495.

Hanifin, J. M., and Rajka, G. (1980). Diagnostic features of atopic dermatitis. *Acta Derm. Venereol. Suppl.* 59, 44–47. doi:10.2340/00015555924447

Hong, H.-S., Lee, J.-Y., and Kim, D.-G. (2012). Analysis of factors enhancing growth effect of Boyangsungjang-Tang. *J. Korean Oriental Pediatr.* 26, 62–71. doi:10.7778/jpkm.2012.26.2.062.

Ikeda, Y., Kaneko, A., Yamamoto, M., Ishige, A., and Sasaki, H. (2002). Possible involvement of suppression of Th2 differentiation in the anti-allergic effect of Sho-seiryu-to in mice. *Jpn. J. Pharmacol.* 90, 328–336. doi:10.1254/jjp.90.328.

Kang, S.-J., Cho, H.-B., Jo, E.-H., Yang, G.-J., Hong, J.-E., Lee, J.-H., et al. (2020). Efficacy and safety of So-Cheong-Ryong-Tang in patients with atopic dermatitis and respiratory disorders. *Medicine*, 99. e18565. doi:10.1097/MD.0000000000018565.

Ko, E., Rho, S., Cho, C., Choi, H., Ko, S., Lee, Y., et al. (2004). So-cheong-ryong-tang, tradititional Korean medicine, suppresses Th2 lineage development. *Biol. Pharm. Bull.* 27, 739–743. doi:10.1248/bpb.27.739.

Kristmundsdottir, F., and David, T. J. (1987). Growth impairment in children with atopic eczema. *J. R. Soc. Med.* 80, 9–12. doi:10.1177/014107688708000106.

Nutten, S. (2015). Atopic dermatitis: global epidemiology and risk factors. *Ann. Nutr. Metab.* 66, 8–16. doi:10.1159/000370220.

Otsuka, A., Nomura, T., Rerknimitr, P., Seidel, J. A., Honda, T., and Kabashima, K. (2017). The interplay between genetic and environmental factors in the pathogenesis of atopic dermatitis. *Immunol. Rev.* 278, 246–262. doi:10.1111/imr.12545.

Park, B.-K., Park, Y.-C., Jung, I. C., Kim, S.-H., Choi, J. J., Do, M., et al. (2015). Gamisasangja-tang suppresses pruritus and atopic skin inflammation in the NC/Nga murine model of atopic dermatitis. *J. Ethnopharmacol.* 165, 54–60. doi:10.1016/j.jep.2015.02.040.

Park, J., Youn, D.-H., Kang, J., Ahn, K. S., Kwak, H. J., and Um, J.-Y. (2019). Taeumjowi-tang, a traditional Korean Sasang remedy, improves obesity-atopic dermatitis comorbidity by regulating hypoxia-inducible factor 1 alpha. *Front. Pharmacol.* 10, 1458. doi:10.3389/fphar.2019.01458.

Sant'Anna, C. A., Solé, D., and Naspitz, C. K. (1996). Short stature in children with respiratory allergy. *Pediatr. Allergy Immunol.* 7, 187–192. doi:10.1111/j.1399-3038.1996.tb00131.x.

Shin, N.-R., Kim, C., Seo, C.-S., Ko, J.-W., Cho, Y.-K., Kim, J.-C., et al. (2018). So-Cheong-Ryoung-Tang attenuates pulmonary inflammation induced by cigarette smoke in bronchial epithelial cells and experimental mice. *Front. Pharmacol.* 9, 1064. doi:10.3389/fphar.2018.01064.

Suh, D.-C., Sung, J., Gause, D., Raut, M., Huang, J., and Choi, I.-S. (2007). Economic burden of atopic manifestations in patients with atopic dermatitis–analysis of administrative claims. *J. Manag. Care Pharm.* 13, 778–789. doi:10.1 8553/jmcp.2007.13.9.778.

Tarım, Ö. (2011). Thyroid hormones and growth in health and disease. *J. Clin. Res. Pediatr. Endocrinol.* 3 (2), 51–55. doi:10.4274/jcrpe.v3i2.11.

Wollenberg, A., Barbarot, S., Bieber, T., Christen-Zaech, S., Deleuran, M., Fink-Wagner, A., et al. (2018a). Consensus-based European guidelines for treatment of atopic eczema (atopic dermatitis) in adults and children: part I. *J. Eur. Acad. Dermatol. Venereol.* 32, 657–682. doi:10.1111/jdv.14891.

Wollenberg, A., Barbarot, S., Bieber, T., Christen-Zaech, S., Deleuran, M., Fink-Wagner, A., et al. (2018b). Consensus-based European guidelines for treatment of atopic eczema (atopic dermatitis) in adults and children: part II. *J. Eur. Acad. Dermatol. Venereol.* 32, 850–878. doi:10.1111/jdv.14888.

3

Dihydroartemisinin Alleviates Imiquimod-Induced Psoriasis-Like Skin Lesion in Mice Involving Modulation of IL-23/Th17 Axis

Jiang-Min Liu[1†], *Quan-Xin Jin*[1†], *Manabu Fujimoto*[2], *Fang-Fang Li*[1], *Lin-Bo Jin*[1], *Ran Yu*[1], *Guang-Hai Yan*[3], *Lian-Hua Zhu*[4], *Fan-Ping Meng*[1], *Qing-Gao Zhang*[5] *and Gui-Hua Jin*[1*]

[1]Department of Immunology and Pathogenic Biology, Yanbian University Medical College, Yanji, China, [2]Department of Dermatology, Graduate School of Medicine, Osaka University; Laboratory of Cutaneous Immunology, Osaka University Immunology Frontier Research Center, Osaka, Japan, [3]Jilin Key Laboratory for Immune and Targeting Research on Common Allergic Diseases, Yanbian University Medical College, Yanji, China, [4]Department of Dermatology, Yanbian University Hospital, Yanji, China, [5]Chronic Disease Research Center, Dalian University, Dalian, China

Correspondence:
Gui-Hua Jin
ghjin@ybu.edu.cn

†These authors contributed equally to this work and share first authorship

Background: Psoriasis is a T help 17 (Th17) cell-mediated chronic inflammatory skin disease. Recent studies have shown that dihydroartemisinin (DHA) can significantly reduce experimental autoimmune encephalomyelitis and rheumatoid arthritis by regulating Th17 cells.

Objective: To verify whether DHA can improve the symptoms of psoriasis and to further explore the possible mechanism.

Methods: The efficiency of DHA was preliminary detected on human keratinocytes (HaCaT) cells in psoriatic condition. Then, imiquimod-induced psoriasis-like model in BALB/c mice was established to evaluate the effects of DHA *in vivo*.

Results: Under the stimulation of tumor necrosis factor-α (TNF-α) and interferon-γ (IFN-γ), DHA inhibited the proliferation of HaCaT cells and significantly affected the mRNA expression levels of IFN-γ, interleukin (IL), IL-17A and IL-23. DHA treatment reduced the severity of psoriasis-like skin and resulted in less infiltration of immune cells in skin lesions. DHA restored the expression of IFN-γ, IL-17A, and IL-23 in skins, as well as a decrease of cytokines and chemokines in skin supernatant. DHA also altered the cellular composition in the spleen, which is the makeup of the T cells, dendritic cells (DCs), and macrophages. DHA recovered Th17-related profile with decreased frequency of IL-$17^{+}CD4^{+}$T cells from splenocyte of mice. Furthermore, DHA also inhibited the concentration of IL-17 from Th17 cells and the expression of Th17 cell-related transcription factors retinoid-related orphan receptor-gamma t (ROR-γt) *in vitro*. In addition, phosphorylation of signal transducer and activator of transcription-3 (STAT3)

Abbreviations: CCR6, CCR6 C-C chemokine receptor 6; CXCL-1, chemokine (C-X-C motif) Ligand 1 Protein; DCs, dendritic cells; HaCaT, human keratinocytes; HSF, Human skin fibroblasts; IFN-γ, interferon-γ; IL-, interleukin-; IL-23R, IL-23 receptor; mTOR, mammalian target of rapamycin; ROR-γt, retinoid-related orphan receptor-gamma t; STAT3, signal transducer and activator of transcription 3; Th17, T help 17 cells; TNF, tumor necrosis factor; Treg, regulatory T cells.

was significantly reduced in DHA treatment mice, suggesting that the IL-23/Th17 axis plays a pivotal role.

Conclusion: DHA inhibits the progression of psoriasis by regulating IL-23/Th17 axis and is expected to be an effective drug for the treatment of psoriasis.

Keywords: dihydroartemisinin, psoriasis, Il-23/th17 axis, cytokines, T cells

INTRODUCTION

Psoriasis is an immune-related chronic inflammatory disease characterized by excessive growth and aberrant differentiation of keratinocytes (Lowes et al., 2007). Interleukin-23/T help 17 cells (IL-23/Th17) axis was found to have a potential function in the pathogenesis of psoriasis. Dendritic cells (DCs) secrete IL-23 to bind IL-23 receptor (IL-23R) presented on Th1, Th17, and Th22 cells, which in turn act on keratinocytes (Di Cesare et al., 2009; Raychaudhuri et al., 2015), ultimately leading to excessive proliferation of the cutaneous keratinocyte to form psoriasis (Chan et al., 2006). Intradermal injection of IL-23 in mouse skin induces several features of psoriatic skin (Gauld et al., 2018). Th17 cells can initiate the proliferation, maturation, and differentiation of neutrophils to result in the inflammatory reaction, stimulate keratinocyte proliferation, and have a synergistic stimulation effect on T cell activation (Teunissen et al., 1998; Fujishima et al., 2010). Th17 cells predominantly produce IL-17, but also emerge IL-21, IL-22, interferon-γ (IFN-γ), and tumor necrosis factor (TNF) and can express C-C chemokine receptor 6 (CCR6), a chemokine (CC motif) ligand 20 (CCL20) receptor that directs IL-17 and guide cells to epithelial barrier sites (Bedoya et al., 2013).

Recent studies have indicated that the IL-23/Th17 axis plays a significant role in psoriasis. Therefore, IL-23/Th17 axis has become a potential drug treatment target. At present, the anti-IL-17 antibody antagonists are approved by the Food and Drug Administration (FDA) in the United States for clinical use, including secukinumab and ixekizumab, which are superior to TNF-α antagonists in the treatment of moderate to severe plaque psoriasis, and have good safety and tolerance (Wong et al., 2016; Dubash et al., 2019). Several IL-23 antagonists, Risankizumab (Gordon et al., 2018), guselkumab (Reich et al., 2017), and tildrakizumab (Reich et al., 2020), have completed phase III clinical trials. Although antibodies are highly desirable, the application is difficult to popularize premium prices, serious side effects, and limited corresponding sites of action (Blauvelt et al., 2015; Teraki et al., 2018; Wendling et al., 2019). Direct inhibition of IL-17 by monoclonal antibodies in patients with psoriasis or psoriatic arthritis has been shown to increase the risk of Candida infection. Similarly, latent tuberculosis infection reactivation was observed in patients treated with TNF inhibitors (Souto et al., 2014; Saunte et al., 2017).

Dihydroartemisinin (DHA) is the main active metabolite of artemisinin compounds. Some studies have found that DHA has a potent effect on the treatment of autoimmune diseases and tumors without obvious toxic and side effects. DHA inhibits the activation of Toll-like receptor 4 signal transduction pathway and the production of type I interferon and anti-ds-DNA in splenocytes from MRL/lpr lupus mice to improve the pathological damage of lupus nephritis (Huang et al., 2014). Zhao YG et al. has demonstrated the immune regulatory function of DHA in reciprocally regulating Th and regulatory T cells (Treg) generation through the modulating mammalian target of rapamycin (mTOR) pathway so as to prevent the onset of experimental autoimmune encephalomyelitis (EAE) by modestly inhibiting the proliferation of activated T cells and particularly virtually abolishing Th17 differentiation (Zhao et al., 2012). Moreover, DHA derivative DC32 inhibits the immune system imbalance and lymphocytic infiltration in synovitis of rheumatoid arthritis (RA) by restoring Treg/Th17 balance through inhibition of IL-6 (Fan et al., 2018). Nevertheless, whether DHA has an effect on psoriasis has not been reported.

Based on the above research, we hypothesized the inhibitory effect of DHA on psoriasis and preliminarily explored the possible mechanism of DHA regulating psoriasis based on the IL-23/Th17 axis for providing a potential therapeutic agent for psoriasis.

MATERIALS AND METHODS

Cell Lines and Culture

Human keratinocytes (HaCaT cells) were purchased from FuDan IBS Cell Center (FDCC-HPN096, FDCC, Shanghai, China). Human skin fibroblasts (HSF) were established from FuHeng Cell Center (FH0186, Shanghai, China). They were maintained in DMEM medium (Gibco, United States) supplemented with 10% fetal bovine serum and 1% penicillin and streptomycin (BI, Israel). The cells were cultured at 37°C in 5% CO_2 atmosphere.

The proliferation of keratinocytes in psoriatic conditions was induced by 10 ng/ml recombinant human TNF-α and 10 ng/ml IFN-γ to further study the effects of DHA on the expression of cytokines on HaCaT cells.

Mice

BALB/c female mice (8–10 w) were healthy and fertile and did not display evidence of infection or disease. All mice were housed in a specific pathogen-free barrier facility and screened regularly for pathogens. All studies and procedures were approved by the Experimental Animal Ethical Committee of Yanbian University (SYXK (ji) 2020–0009).

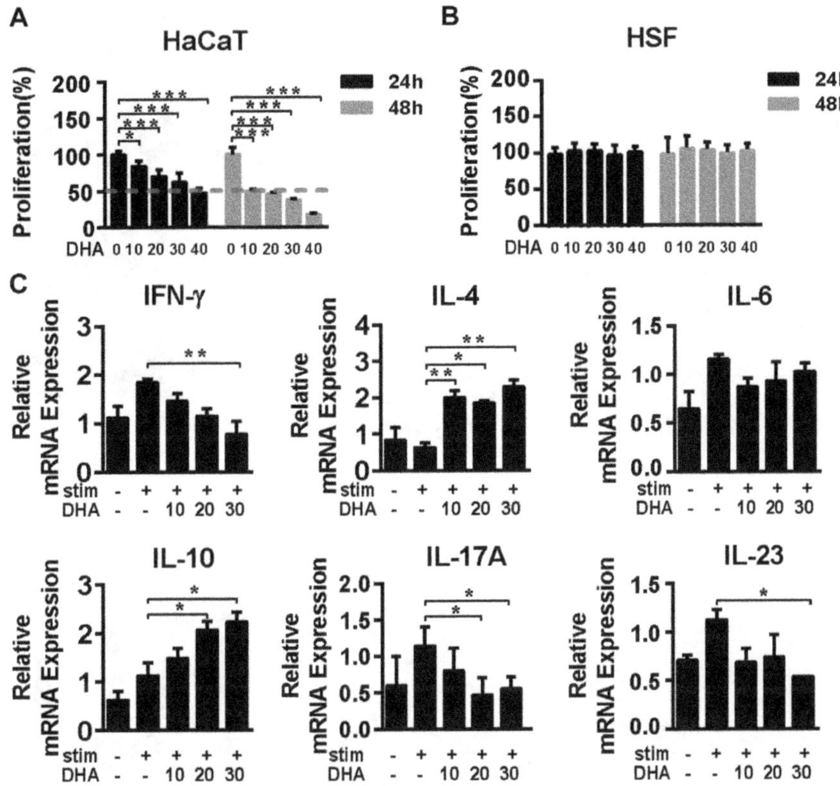

FIGURE 1 | The effect of DHA on the proliferation of HaCaT cells and the expression of cytokines. **(A,B)** The cell viability of HaCaT cells and HSF cells was detected by MTT assay being treated with different concentrations of DHA for 24 and 48 h (*$p = 0.0318$, ***$p < 0.001$). **(C)** After treatment on HaCaT cells with 0, 10, 20, 30 μg/ml DHA for 24 h with the stimulation of IFN-γ (10 ng/ml) and TNF-α (10 ng/ml), the mRNA expression of inflammation-related cytokines IFN-γ, IL-4, IL-6, IL-10, IL-17A, and IL-23 was detected by RT-PCR (IFN-γ, **$p = 0.0094$; IL-4, *$p = 0.0292$, **$p < 0.05$; IL-6, *NS*. Not significant; IL-10, *$p < 0.05$; IL-17A, *$p < 0.05$; IL-23, *$p = 0.0335$). The significant difference was compared relatively to the DHA untreated group. Statistical analysis was carried out using One-way ANOVA analysis of variance followed by Dunnett's test (n = 5–7).

Psoriasis-like Model and Dihydroartemisinin Treatment

62.5 mg 5% imiquimod (IMQ, Aldara, 3M Pharmaceuticals) cream was smeared to the shaved back of mice for 5 days to induce psoriasis-like skin lesions (IMQ group). Dihydroartemisinin (DHA, National Institutes for Food and Drug Control, Beijing, China) was applied i.g. at a dose of 25 mg/kg/d (DHA-L group) and 50 mg/kg/d (DHA-H group) 3 days in advance for 8 days. As for the control group (Con. Group), they were treated similarly with control vehicle cream and phosphate-buffered saline.

The inflammation skins were graded according to the clinical Psoriasis Area and Severity Index (PASI). Erythema, scaling, and thickening were scored independently on a scale from 0 to 4: 0, none; 1, slight; 2, moderate; 3, marked; 4, very marked. The cumulative PASI score served as a measure of the severity of inflammation (scale 0–12).

Cell Viability

HaCaT cells were placed into 96-well plates at a density of 2×10^4 cells per well, then incubated overnight at 37°C in 5% CO_2 atmosphere, and treated with different concentrations of DHA for 24 and 48 h. Cell viability was determined using MTT assays (Solarbio, China). The absorbance was measured at a wavelength of 490 nm using a microplate reader (Tecan Infinite M200 Pro, Switzerland).

Flow Cytometry

Fluorescein isothiocyanate-, R-phycoerythrin (PE)-, peridinin chlorophyll protein (PerCP)-, PE-Cy5-, PE-Cy7-, allophycocyanin (APC)-conjugated mAbs in this study include those to CD3 (17A2), CD4 (RM4-5), CD8 (53-6.7), F4/80 (BM8), CD11c (N418) from Biolegend, IFN-γ (XMG1.2), and IL-17 (eBio17B7) from eBioscience. For intracellular staining, cells were fixed and permeabilized using Cytofix/Cytoperm kit (BD Biosciences). Dead cells were detected by LIVE/DEAD Fixable Green Dead Cell Kit (Invitrogen-Molecular Probes). Multiparameter flow cytometric analysis was performed on the FACS Verse (BD Biosciences, San Jose, Calif) and CytoFLEX (Beckman Coulter, China). Data were analyzed using FlowJo software (Ver. 8.8.7).

Cell Isolation and Activation

Splenic T cells were purified using a $CD4^+$T cell isolation kit (Miltenyi Biotec, Germany; Stemcell, Canada), $CD4^+$T cells (5×10^4)

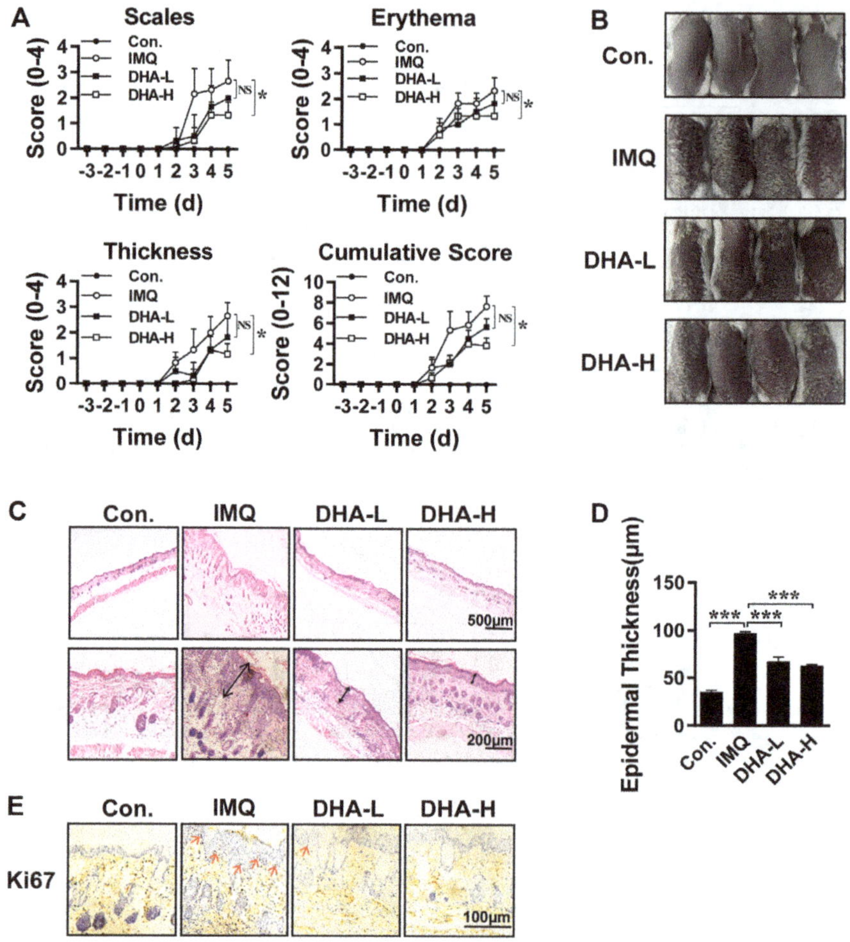

FIGURE 2 | DHA treatment attenuated psoriasis severity. **(A)** These selected mice were classified into four groups as described above, clinical indicators scales, erythema, and skin thickness for PASI clinical evaluation to assess the severity of psoriasis and the efficacy of DHA ($^*p < 0.05$, *NS*. Not significant). **(B)** Representative macroscopic skin lesion symptoms in each group. **(C)** H&E staining was performed to observe the pathological changes in mice's skin. Original magnifications, top ×40; bottom × 200. **(D)** Epidermal thickness was measured after DHA treatment in the psoriasis model ($^{***}p < 0.001$). **(E)** Keratinocyte proliferation was analyzed by detecting the expression of Ki67. Original magnifications, ×400. Statistical analysis was carried out using One-way ANOVA analysis of variance followed by Dunnett's test (n = 5–7).

were activated by 10 μg/ml anti-CD3 (17A2, Biolegend) and 2 μg/ml anti-CD28 (37.51, Biolegend) for 48 or 96 h with or without 0.5 μg/ml DHA. PMA (50 ng/ml; Sigma-Aldrich) and ionomycin (500 ng/ml; Sigma-Aldrich) were included in the culture medium for the last 5 h of incubation.

Histochemical Staining

Tissues were harvested using a disposable, sterile 6 mm punch biopsy blade (Maruho, Osaka, Japan) and assessed for tissue damage and the number of infiltrating T cells, DCs, and macrophages. Four-micrometer sections were stained using haematoxylin and eosin (H&E) to identify histologic changes of dermal tissues. To identify keratinocyte proliferation, rabbit anti-mouse Ki67 mAb (D3B5) were, respectively, used on paraffin-embedded sections by immunohistochemical (IHC) staining.

All cells were counted from the infection site in five serial skin sections. The numbers of infiltration cells were averaged in more than five power microscopic fields (HPFs, 0.07 mm^2). Each section was examined independently by three investigators in a blinded fashion, and the meaning was used for analysis.

Reverse Transcription Polymerase Chain Reaction

The total RNA was extracted from skin lesions and HaCaT cells using RNeasy Mini Kit (Qiagen, Hilden, Germany). Isolated RNA was reverse-transcribed to cDNA by using the M-MLV Reverse transcriptase system (Promega). cDNA was amplified with the ExTaq enzyme system. The sequences of primers were as follows: IFN-γ F: 5′-CGGCACAGTCATTGAAAGCCTA-3′, R: 5′-GTTGCTGATGGCCTGGATTGTC-3′; IL-4 F: 5′-ACGGAGATGGATGTGCCAAAC-3′, R: 5′-AGCACCTTGGAAGCCCTACAGA-3′; IL-6 F: 5′-CCACTTCACAAGTCGGAGGCTTA-3′, R: 5′-TGCAAGTGCATCATCGTTGTTC-3′; IL-10 F: 5′-GCCAGAGCCACATGCTCCTA-3′, R: 5′-GATAAGGCTTGGCAA

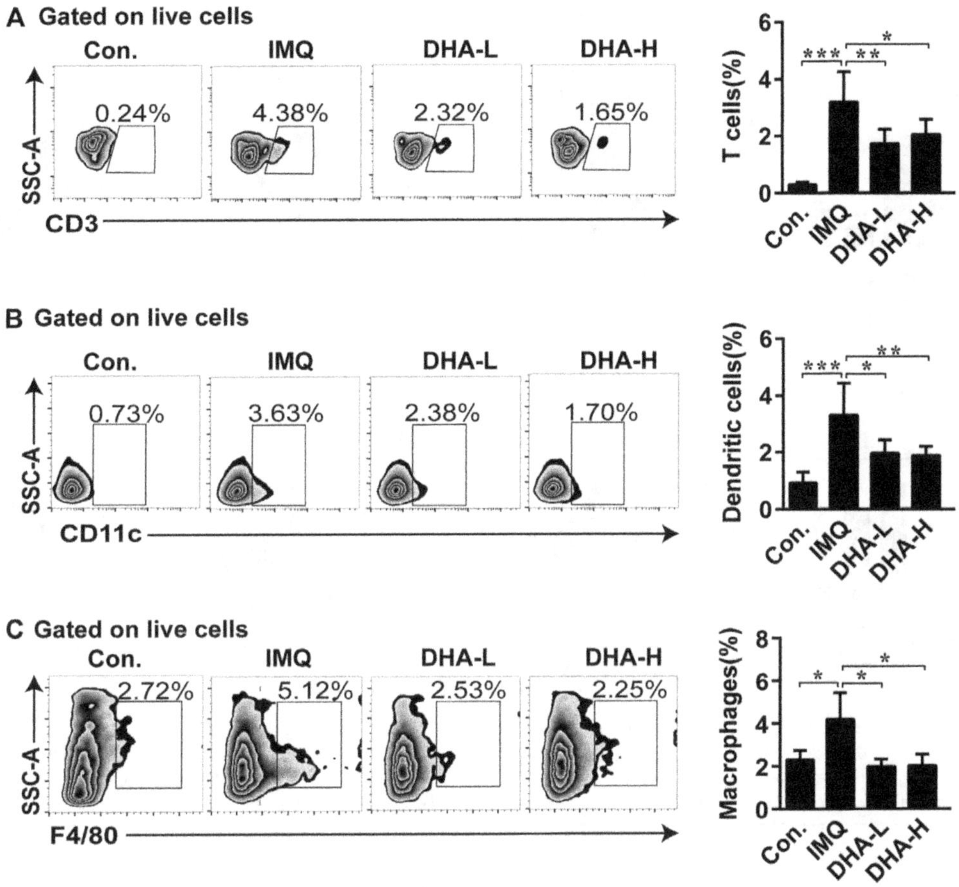

FIGURE 3 | DHA treatment decreased immune cells infiltration into skins. **(A–C)** Percentages of T cells, macrophages, and DCs among total live cells were determined by flow cytometry (T cells, $^{*}p = 0.0328$, $^{**}p = 0.0074$, $^{***}p < 0.001$; macrophages cells, $^{*}p < 0.05$; DCs, $^{*}p = 0.0141$, $^{**}p = 0.0097$, $^{***}p < 0.001$). Statistical analysis was carried out using One-way ANOVA analysis of variance followed by Dunnett's test (n = 4–6).

CCCAAGTAA-3′; IL-17A F: 5′-GAAGGCCCTCAGACTACC TCAA-3′, R: 5′-TCATGTGGTGGTCCAGCTTTC-3′; IL22 F: 5′-CCTTCCCCAGTCACCAGTTG-3′, R: 5′-CTCCACTCT CTCCAAGCTTTT-3′; IL23R F: 5′-GCTCTGAAGTGGAAT TATGTGC-3′, R: 5′-CTTCTTCTGTCTCTAAACTCTTCAC-3′; IL-23 F: 5′-GACTCAGCCAACTCCTCCAGCCAG-3′, R: 5′-TTGGCACTAAGGGCTCAGTCAGA-3′; Retinoid-related orphan receptor-gammat (ROR-γt) F: 5′-A-GCTAGGTGC AGAGCTTCAG-3′, R: 5′-ATTTGTGTTCTCATGACTGAG CC-3′; β-actin F: 5′-AGGTCATCACTATTGGCAACGA-3′, R: 5′-CACTTCATGATGGAATTGAATGTAGTT-3′. The relative expression levels of genes were compared with β-actin.

Western Blotting Assays

30 mg spleen tissue was minced and homogenated, and the proteins were treated and then incubated with primary antibodies against mouse STAT3 and phosphorylation of STAT3 Ab (Cell Signaling Technology) at 4°C overnight, followed by incubation with fluorescent secondary antibodies. Finally, the membranes were scanned using a Bio-Rad Gel imaging system (Bio-Rad, United States) after visualization treatment using the ECL reagent. Protein expressions were analyzed with ImageJ software.

Enzyme-Linked Immunosorbent Assay (ELISA)

50 mg depilated back skin was homogenated in PBS and 5% FBS medium, and the supernatant was obtained by centrifugation at 5000 rpm for 15 min. IL-1β, IL-6, IL-18, and Chemokine (C-X-C motif) Ligand 1 Protein (CXCL-1) in the supernatant were determined by an ELISA kit (Mbbiology biological, China).

IL-17 secretion from purified $CD4^{+}$T cells in the culture supernatant fluid was determined by ELISA kits (Mbbiology biological, China).

Statistical Analysis

All data were analyzed with GraphPad Prism 9.0 (GraphPad Software, La Jolla, United States) and exhibited as the means ± SD

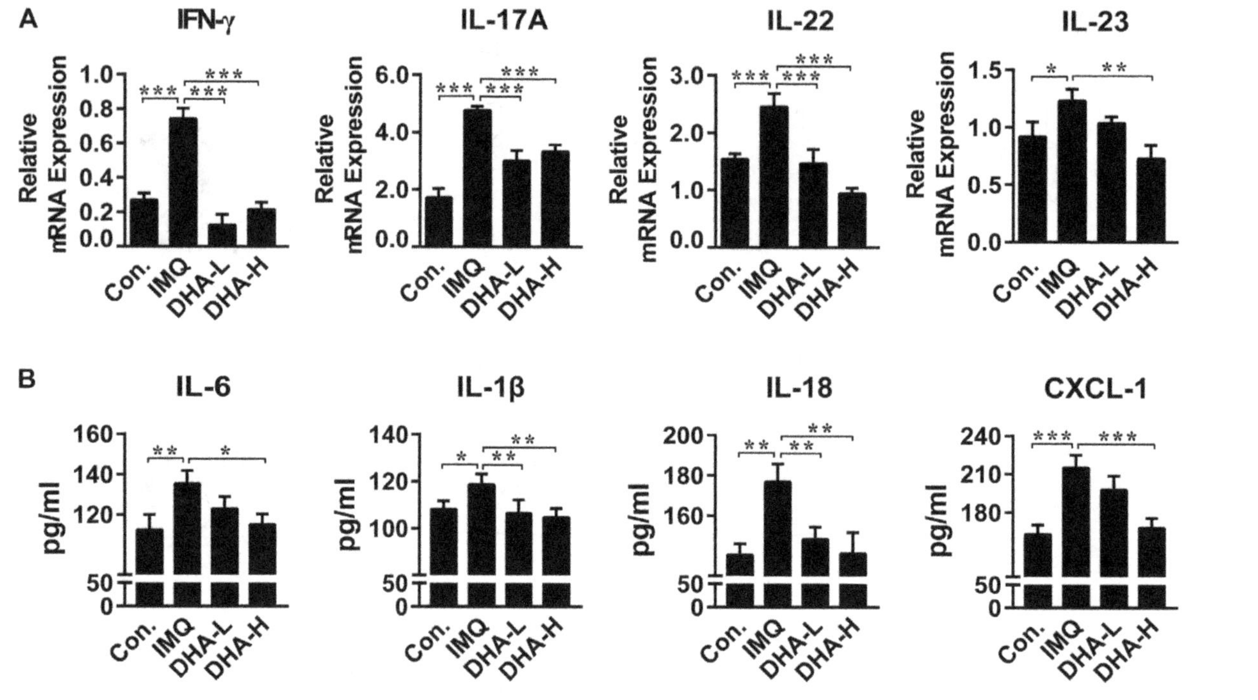

FIGURE 4 | DHA affected cytokines expression in psoriasis mice skin lesions. **(A)** IFN-γ, IL-17A, IL-22 and IL-23 mRNA levels in skin sections (30 mg) were analyzed by RT-PCR (IFN-γ, ***$p < 0.001$; IL-17A, ***$p < 0.001$; IL-22, ***$p < 0.001$; IL-23, *$p = 0.017$, **$p = 0.0010$). **(B)** IL-6, IL-18, IL-1β and CXCL-1 secretion in the supernatant from skins (50 mg) were measured by ELISA (IL-6, *$p = 0.011$, **$p = 0.0056$; IL-18, **$p < 0.01$; IL-1β, *$p = 0.0295$, **$p < 0.01$; CXCL-1, ***$p < 0.001$). Statistical analysis was carried out using One-way ANOVA analysis of variance followed by Dunnett's test (n = 4–6).

($n \geq 4$ mice/group). The significance of differences was determined using the Student's t test and one-way ANOVA analysis of variance followed by Dunnett's test.

RESULTS

Dihydroartemisinin Inhibited the Proliferation and Affected the Expression of Cytokines in Human Keratinocyte Cells

First, we clarified the inhibitory effect of DHA on keratinocytes and cytokines associated with inflammation. The effects of DHA on the proliferation of HaCaT cells and HSF cells were initially detected. MTT results showed that DHA inhibited the proliferation of HaCaT cells ($p < 0.05$); the IC50 values of 24 and 48 h were, respectively, 32.51 μg/ml and 8.23 μg/ml. Moreover, DHA did not affect the proliferation of human skin fibroblasts HSF cells (**Figures 1A,B**). The psoriatic condition of HaCaT cells is mainly induced by the TNF-α/IFN-γ-stimuli. The results showed that mRNA expression of IFN-γ, IL-17A, and IL-23 was significantly decreased, while IL-4 and IL-10 were accelerated in the DHA-treated group. In contrast, DHA treatment did not change IL-6 mRNA expression levels (**Figure 1C**). Thus, DHA adjusted inflammation-related cytokines expression in HaCaT cells.

Dihydroartemisinin Ameliorated Psoriasis-like Skin Lesions

To investigate the therapeutic effect of DHA *in vivo*, IMQ-induced psoriasis-like models were established. The symptoms of erythema, scales, and skin thickness were evidently mitigated in DHA-treated mice (**Figures 2A,B**). Histopathological analysis revealed that keratinization, the protrusion of the epidermis, the dilatation and congestion of capillaries, and cellular infiltration were markedly enhanced in psoriasis mice compared with wild-type mice. When compared with IMQ mice, mice receiving treatment with DHA showed marked recovery pathological changes (**Figures 2C,D**). Moreover, the proliferation of keratinocytes was monitored by IHC staining. As shown in **Figure 2E**, DHA treatment significantly reduced Ki67 positive cells compared with that in IMQ mice epidermis. Overall, these data suggested that DHA suppresses augmented psoriasis-like skin reactions.

Dihydroartemisinin Treatment Resulted in Decreased Accumulation of Immune Cells in Skin Lesions

Consistent with the report (Van der Fits et al., 2009), in the H&E sections of IMQ-treated back skin, abundant infiltrates of mononuclear cells were observed. In order to further confirm that DHA treatment can inhibit the infiltration of inflammatory cells, flow cytometry was applied. DHA-treated mice exhibited a significant decrease in T cells, macrophages, and DCs infiltration in skins compared to IMQ mice (**Figure 3**). The histopathological analysis also revealed that the degree of edema and cellular infiltration was markedly improved in DHA-treated mice compared with IMQ administration mice (**Supplementary Figure 1**). These results showed that DHA administration results in effects on the composition of the inflammatory cell.

Dihydroartemisinin Treatment Normalized Levels of Interleukin-23/T Help 17 Cells Axis-Related Cytokines and Inflammation-Related Cytokines and Chemokines in Skins

The critical role of the IL-23/Th17 axis in the development of psoriasis has been demonstrated. To further explore the effect of DHA on the IL-23/Th17 axis, we first determined mRNA expression levels of cytokines in each group. mRNA expression of IFN-γ was significantly decreased in the DHA administration group compared with the IMQ group. Likewise, IL-23/Th17 axis-related cytokines IL-17A, IL-22, and IL-23 were dramatically dropped in the DHA-treated groups (**Figure 4A**). Furthermore, we assessed expressions of inflammation-related cytokines and chemokines such as IL-1β, IL-6, IL-18, and CXCL-1 in skin tissues 6 days after DHA treatment, and the results showed that DHA significantly decreased expression of them (**Figure 4B**). Thus, DHA inhibited the expression of cytokines and chemokines in psoriasis-like skin damage.

Dihydroartemisinin Treatment Affected the Immune Cellular Composition in Spleens

The observed trends in spleens were also verified by flow cytometry. When compared with the control group, the frequency of DCs and macrophages was higher in the IMQ group. DHA treatment distinctly decreased the frequency of DCs and macrophages with a dose-dependent effect (**Figure 5A**). As shown in **Figure 5B**, the CD4^{+}/CD8^{+}T cells ratio was significantly reversed in the IMQ mice, which was recovered after DHA treatment. Furthermore, the percentage of IFN-γ^{+}CD8^{+}T cells significantly decreased in high-dose DHA-treated mice than that of IMQ mice (**Figure 5C**). Therefore, DHA treatment decreased inflammatory infiltration in the spleen of psoriasis mice.

Dihydroartemisinin Relieved Psoriasis-like Inflammation Dependent on Interleukin-23/T Help 17 cells Axis

It has been confirmed that DHA regulated Th17 cells generation to prevent the onset of EAE (Zhang et al., 2016). To evaluate whether DHA treatment influences the Th17 cells in psoriasis, the percentage of Th17 cells and expression of differentiation-related transcription factors were detected. Indeed, DHA

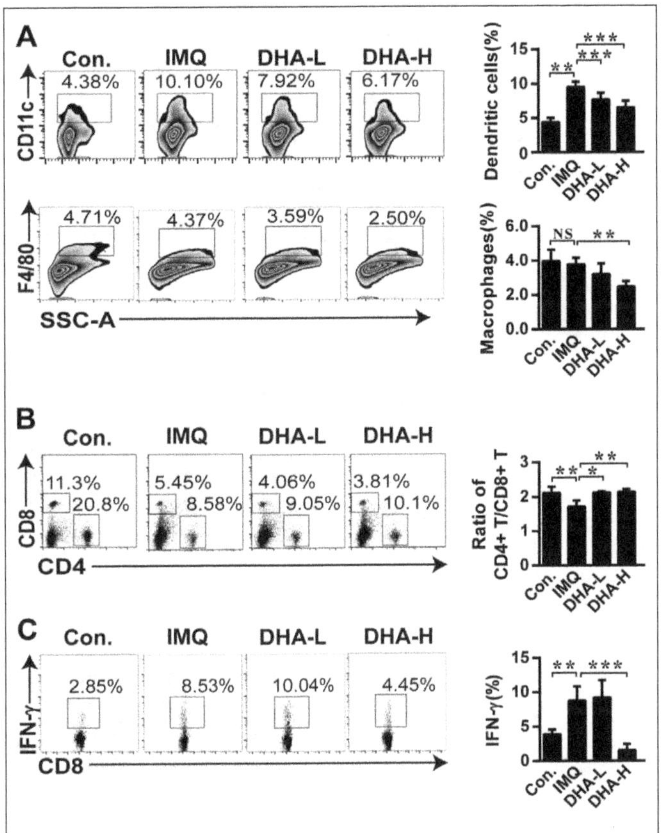

FIGURE 5 | DHA treatment altered immune cellular composition in spleens. **(A)** The frequencies of DCs, and the frequencies of macrophages. **(B)** Ratio of CD4^{+}/CD8^{+} T cells was analyzed by flow cytometry. **(C)** Splenocytes were stimulated by PMA and ionomycin for 4 h in the presence of brefeldin A, then frequency of IFN-γ^{+}CD8^{+}T cells was determined by flow cytometry (DCs, $^{**}p = 0.0027$, $^{***}p < 0.001$; macrophages, $^{**}p = 0.0011$; Ratio of CD4^{+}/CD8^{+} T cells, $^{*}p = 0.0117$, $^{**}p < 0.01$; IFN-γ^{+}CD8^{+}T cells, $^{**}p = 0.0056$, $^{***}p < 0.001$). Statistical analysis was carried out using One-way ANOVA analysis of variance followed by Dunnett's test (n = 4–6).

treatment significantly reduced the frequency of IL-17^{+}CD4^{+}T cells (**Figure 6A**). To evaluate Th17 cytokine production in spleens, CD4^{+}T cells were stimulated with anti-CD3 and anti-CD28 for 48 or 96 h *in vitro*, and the expression of IL-17 was performed. IL-17 production from Th17 cells was significantly inhibited by DHA treatment after 96 h. Additionally, ROR-γt, the Th17 cell-specific nuclear transcription factor, was also reduced after DHA treatment (**Figures 6B,C**). Furthermore, DHA also inhibited the mRNA expression of the IL-23 receptor compared with the IMQ group. (**Figure 6D**). STAT3 has emerged as an important transcription factor of keratinocytes to regulate cytokine expression and Th17 cell differentiation. Phosphorylation of STAT3 was significantly decreased after DHA administration (**Figure 6E**). These results showed that DHA affects the IL-23/Th17 axis composed of IL-23, IL-17, STAT3, and Th17 cells. Moreover, as shown in **Figure 6F**, the number of IFN-γ^{+}CD4^{+}T cells dropped after DHA treatment, indicating that Th1 cells were also affected by DHA, suggesting that the process of DHA alleviating psoriasis likely counted on Th1/Th17 polarization, which could turn into the subsequent target.

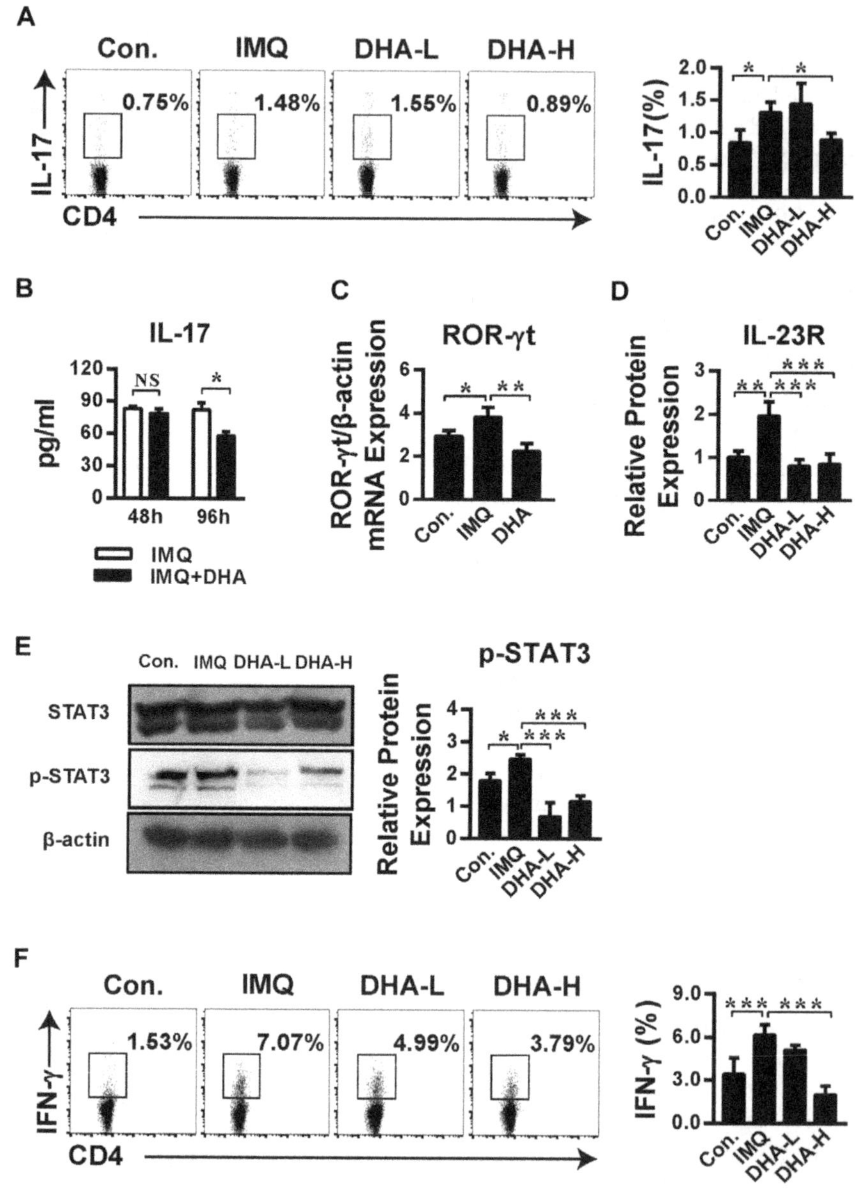

FIGURE 6 | DHA restrained psoriasis dependent on IL-23/Th17 axis. **(A)** The frequency of IL-17$^+$CD4$^+$T cells was analyzed by flow cytometry ($^*p < 0.05$). **(B,C)** Splenic single cell suspensions were stimulated as described in the Materials and Methods. **(B)** The concentration of IL-17 from purified CD4$^+$ T cells in the culture supernatant was measured by ELISA. Statistical analysis was carried out using unpaired *t*-test ($^*p = 0.0304$, NS. Not significant, $n = 5$–6). **(C)** ROR-γt mRNA level from Th17 cells was detected by RT-PCR ($^*p = 0.0448$, $^{**}p = 0.0038$). **(D)** IL-23R mRNA levels in skin sections (30 mg) were analyzed by RT-PCR ($^{**}p = 0.0026$, $^{***}p < 0.001$). **(E)** STAT3 phosphorylation in splenocytes from control, IMQ-, and DHA-treated mice was assessed by western blotting ($^*p = 0.0396$, $^{***}p < 0.001$). **(F)** IFN-γ production by CD4$^+$T cells from spleens was measured by flow cytometric analysis ($^{***}p < 0.001$). Statistical analysis was carried out using One-way ANOVA analysis of variance followed by Dunnett's test (A, C–F; $n = 4$–6).

DISCUSSION

In this study, we demonstrated that DHA treatment significantly inhibited the proliferation and cytokines expression of HaCaT cells. Moreover, DHA treatment significantly reduced psoriasis severity as determined by both skin score and histopathology. DHA restored IL-23/Th17 axis-related cytokine and chemokine expression and recovered polarization of Th17 cells. Therefore, the study demonstrated that DHA suppresses psoriasis-like skin lesions by regulating IL-23/Th17 axis.

The IL-23/Th17 axis is considered to play a major role in psoriasis (Gauld et al., 2019). Activated DCs and macrophages are the main source of IL-23 in psoriasis (Singh et al., 2016; Huang et al., 2018). Injection of IL-23 into the skin can induce dermal acanthosis, neutrophil aggregation, and infiltration of IL-

17^{+}T cells. Moreover, IL-23 inhibitors can significantly reduce the expression of IL-17 and IL-22 in psoriatic lesions (Krueger et al., 2016; Puig, 2017). In this article, we show that DC_S and macrophages were largely relieved after DHA treatment in skin lesions (**Figure 3**). In the meantime, treatment with DHA also markedly decreased DCs and macrophages infiltration in the spleen (**Figure 5**). Thus, DHA affects DCs and macrophages activation in psoriasis, and DCs were the main source of myeloid cell-derived IL-23.

IL-23 can induce the expression of IL-17 and assist the proliferation and survival of differentiated Th17 cells. In the absence of the IL-23 signaling pathway, Th17 cells stagnated in the early activation stage and could not regulate the encephalitis-inducing effect of EAE (Zheng et al., 2007). About 1/3 of patients with psoriasis develop psoriatic arthritis, while the number of Th17 cells in synovial fluid and synovial tissue is significantly increased, and the expression of IL-17 is also significantly increased, which demonstrates that there is a significant correlation between the level of IL-17 and joint injury. Multiple studies have demonstrated an increased expression of IL-17A and IL-17F in psoriatic skin in contrast to the nonlesion psoriatic skin, and the upregulation of IL-17A illustrated a positive association with disease severity (Lowes et al., 2008; Johansen et al., 2009). IL-17A gene could induce the proliferation of IL-$17RA^{+}CD11b^{+}Gr1^{low}$ osteoclast precursors, and the biomarkers of bone resorption also increased by transferring the IL-17A gene into the CIA model, which indicated that IL-17A could induce pathological bone resorption (a crux feature of psoriatic arthritis) through direct activation of osteoclast precursors (Marinoni et al., 2014; Adamopoulos et al., 2015; Sakkas and Bogdanos, 2017). Vitamin D has been applied in the treatment of moderately severe psoriasis because DCs treated with vitamin D have lower expression of MHC-II and costimulatory molecules CD80, CD86, and CD40L, which can reduce the production of IL-12 while secreting IL-10 and ultimately inhibit the proliferation of T cells and the secretion of IFN-γ and IL-17 (Hau et al., 2018).

DHA is the main active metabolite of artemisinin, which can significantly inhibit the release of proinflammatory cytokines (IL-6, IL-1β, IL-10, TNF-α, and so on) and affect T cell differentiation, which has a favorable application prospect in anti-inflammation (Yan et al., 2019), anticancer (Dong et al., 2019), and so on (Jagannathan et al., 2016). The natural plant antimicrobial solution could significantly reduce the gene expression and inflammatory cytokines production of macrophage-derived chemokine (MDC), IL-8, and IL-6 in TNF-α/IFN-γ-induced HaCaT cells (Dou et al., 2017). Artemisinin can improve the symptoms of experimental autoimmune myasthenia gravis by regulating the balance of Thl/Th17 and influencing the function of Treg (Chen et al., 2018). DHA can similarly inhibit the secretion of TNF-α in BXSB mice and improve the pathological damage of lupus nephritis (Li et al., 2006). DHA treatment was shown to induce a decrease in IL-23, IFN-γ, and IL-17 production *in vitro* and *in vivo* (**Figures 1, 4**). Moreover, increased $CD3^{+}$T cells and IFN-$\gamma^{+}CD8^{+}$T cells population in control groups were inhibited by DHA treatment (**Figures 3, 5**).

During the differentiation of Th17 cells, the signal of cytokines is transduced through STAT3, thus initiating the specific transcription program of Th17 cells. STAT3 can directly bind to IL-17A and IL-21 loci and regulate the expression of ROR-γt and IL-23R. Studies have confirmed that heterozygous STAT3 gene mutation can reduce the utilization rate of functional STAT3 dimer by 25% and consequently reduce the expression of ROR-γt by four times. The latter is a specific nuclear transcription factor necessary for Th17 cell differentiation. ROR-$\gamma t^{-/-}$ mice do not have Th17 cells, so leading to the immune diseases abatement (Ivanov et al., 2006; Yang et al., 2015). In the current study, the expression of phosphorylation of STAT3 was significantly inhibited by DHA administration, paralleled by a significant decrease in the expression of ROR-γt and IL-17 production from Th17 cells (**Figure 6**). Moreover, the IL-$17^{+}CD4^{+}$T cells population in psoriasis groups was significantly inhibited by DHA administration (**Figure 6**). Thus, our data showed that DHA effectively attenuates psoriasis-like skin lesions. DHA may partially regulate the IL-23/Th17 axis and polarization of Th17 cells in the psoriasis-like model. Consequently, DHA is expected to become a drug for the treatment of psoriasis in humans.

AUTHOR CONTRIBUTIONS

G-HJ designed the study; J-ML, Q-XJ, and L-BJ performed the experiments; J-ML, F-FL, and RY analyzed and plotted the data; Q-XJ validated the data; J-ML and F-FL drafted the manuscript; G-HY, F-PM, and L-HZ reviewed and edited the manuscript; MF and G-HJ supervised the project; G-HJ and Q-GZ funded the experiments for the study. All authors edited and approved the final version of the manuscript.

REFERENCES

Adamopoulos, I. E., Suzuki, E., Chao, C.-C., Gorman, D., Adda, S., Maverakis, E., et al. (2015). IL-17A Gene Transfer Induces Bone Loss and Epidermal Hyperplasia Associated with Psoriatic Arthritis. *Ann. Rheum. Dis.* 74 (6), 1284–1292. doi:10.1136/annrheumdis-2013-204782

Bedoya, S. K., Lam, B., Lau, K., and Larkin, J. (2013). Th17 Cells in Immunity and Autoimmunity. *Clin. Develop. Immunol.* 2013, 1–16. doi:10.1155/2013/986789

Blauvelt, A., Prinz, J. C., Gottlieb, A. B., Kingo, K., Sofen, H., Ruer-Mulard, M., et al. (2015). Secukinumab Administration by Pre-filled Syringe: Efficacy, Safety and Usability Results from a Randomized Controlled Trial in Psoriasis (FEATURE). *Br. J. Dermatol.* 172, 484–493. doi:10.1111/bjd.13348

Chan, J. R., Blumenschein, W., Murphy, E., Diveu, C., Wiekowski, M., Abbondanzo, S., et al. (2006). IL-23 Stimulates Epidermal Hyperplasia via TNF and IL-20R2-dependent Mechanisms with Implications for Psoriasis Pathogenesis. *J. Exp. Med.* 203 (12), 2577–2587. doi:10.1084/jem.20060244

Chen, W., Li, F. F., Li, C., Sui, J. K., Meng, Q. F., Li, X. L., et al. (2018). Artemisinin Ameliorates the Symptoms of Experimental Autoimmune Myasthenia Gravis by Regulating the Balance of TH1 Cells, TH17 Cells and Treg Cells. *J. Biol. Regul. Homeost Agents* 32 (5), 1217–1223.

Di Cesare, A., Di Meglio, P., and Nestle, F. O. (2009). The IL-23/Th17 axis in the Immunopathogenesis of Psoriasis. *J. Invest. Dermatol.* 129, 1339–1350. doi:10.1038/jid.2009.59

Dong, L., Wang, C., Zhen, W., Jia, X., An, S., Xu, Z., et al. (2019). Biodegradable Iron-Coordinated Hollow Polydopamine Nanospheres for Dihydroartemisinin

Delivery and Selectively Enhanced Therapy in Tumor Cells. *J. Mater. Chem. B* 7 (40), 6172–6180. doi:10.1039/c9tb01397k

Dou, R., Liu, Z., Yuan, X., Xiangfei, D., Bai, R., Bi, Z., et al. (2017). PAMs Ameliorates the Imiquimod-Induced Psoriasis-like Skin Disease in Mice by Inhibition of Translocation of NF-κB and Production of Inflammatory Cytokines. *PLoS One* 12 (5), e0176823. doi:10.1371/journal.pone.0176823

Dubash, S., Bridgewood, C., McGonagle, D., and Marzo-Ortega, H. (2019). The Advent of IL-17A Blockade in Ankylosing Spondylitis: Secukinumab, Ixekizumab and beyond. *Expert Rev. Clin. Immunol.* 15 (2), 123–134. doi:10.1080/1744666X.2019.1561281

Fan, M., Li, Y., Yao, C., Liu, X., Liu, X., and Liu, J. (2018). Dihydroartemisinin Derivative DC32 Attenuates Collagen-Induced Arthritis in Mice by Restoring the Treg/Th17 Balance and Inhibiting Synovitis through Down-Regulation of IL-6. *Int. Immunopharmacol.* 65, 233–243. doi:10.1016/j.intimp.2018.10.015

Fujishima, S., Watanabe, H., Kawaguchi, M., Suzuki, T., Matsukura, S., Homma, T., et al. (2010). Involvement of IL-17F via the Induction of IL-6 in Psoriasis. *Arch. Dermatol. Res.* 302 (7), 499–505. doi:10.1007/s00403-010-1033-8

Gauld, S. B., Gauvin, D., Olson, L., Leys, L., Paulsboe, S., Liu, Z., et al. (2018). Mechanistic and Pharmacological Assessment of Murine IL-23 Mediated Psoriasiform Dermatitis; Implications for Drug Discovery. *J. Dermatol. Sci.* 92 (1), 45–53. doi:10.1016/j.jdermsci.2018.08.001

Gauld, S. B., Jacquet, S., Gauvin, D., Wallace, C., Wang, Y., McCarthy, R., et al. (2019). Inhibition of Interleukin-23-Mediated Inflammation with a Novel Small Molecule Inverse Agonist of RORγt. *J. Pharmacol. Exp. Ther.* 371 (1), 208–218. doi:10.1124/jpet.119.258046

Gordon, K. B., Strober, B., Lebwohl, M., Augustin, M., Blauvelt, A., Poulin, Y., et al. (2018). Efficacy and Safety of Risankizumab in Moderate-To-Severe Plaque Psoriasis (UltIMMa-1 and UltIMMa-2): Results from Two Double-Blind, Randomised, Placebo-Controlled and Ustekinumab-Controlled Phase 3 Trials. *Lancet* 392 (10148), 650–661. doi:10.1016/S0140-6736(18)31713-6

Hau, C. S., Shimizu, T., Tada, Y., Kamata, M., Takeoka, S., Shibata, S., et al. (2018). The Vitamin D3 Analog, Maxacalcitol, Reduces Psoriasiform Skin Inflammation by Inducing Regulatory T Cells and Downregulating IL-23 and IL-17 Production. *J. Dermatol. Sci.* 92 (2), 117–126. doi:10.1016/j.jdermsci.2018.08.007

Huang, T., Gao, Z., Zhang, Y., Fan, K., Wang, F., Li, Y., et al. (2018). CRL4DCAF2 Negatively Regulates IL-23 Production in Dendritic Cells and Limits the Development of Psoriasis. *J. Exp. Med.* 215 (8), 1999–2017. doi:10.1084/jem.20180210

Huang, X., Xie, Z., Liu, F., Han, C., Zhang, D., Wang, D., et al. (2014). Dihydroartemisinin Inhibits Activation of the Toll-like Receptor 4 Signaling Pathway and Production of Type I Interferon in Spleen Cells from Lupus-Prone MRL/lpr Mice. *Int. Immunopharmacol.* 22 (1), 266–272. doi:10.1016/j.intimp.2014.07.001

Ivanov, I. I., McKenzie, B. S., Zhou, L., Tadokoro, C. E., Lepelley, A., Lafaille, J. J., et al. (2006). The Orphan Nuclear Receptor RORγt Directs the Differentiation Program of Proinflammatory IL-17+ T Helper Cells. *Cell* 126 (6), 1121–1133. doi:10.1016/j.cell.2006.07.035

Jagannathan, P., Bowen, K., Nankya, F., McIntyre, T. I., Auma, A., Wamala, S., et al. (2016). Effective Antimalarial Chemoprevention in Childhood Enhances the Quality of CD4+T Cells and Limits Their Production of Immunoregulatory Interleukin 10. *J. Infect. Dis.* 214 (2), 329–338. doi:10.1093/infdis/jiw147

Johansen, C., Usher, P. A., Kjellerup, R. B., Lundsgaard, D., Iversen, L., and Kragballe, K. (2009). Characterization of the Interleukin-17 Isoforms and Receptors in Lesional Psoriatic Skin. *Br. J. Dermatol.* 160 (2), 319–324. doi:10.1111/j.1365-2133.2008.08902.x

Krueger, J., Clark, J. D., Suárez-Fariñas, M., Fuentes-Duculan, J., Cueto, I., Wang, C. Q., et al. (2016). Tofacitinib Attenuates Pathologic Immune Pathways in Patients with Psoriasis: A Randomized Phase 2 Study. *J. Allergy Clin. Immunol.* 137 (4), 1079–1090. doi:10.1016/j.jaci.2015.12.1318

Li, W.-d., Dong, Y.-j., Tu, Y.-y., and Lin, Z.-b. (2006). Dihydroarteannuin Ameliorates Lupus Symptom of BXSB Mice by Inhibiting Production of TNF-Alpha and Blocking the Signaling Pathway NF-Kappa B Translocation. *Int. Immunopharmacol.* 6 (8), 1243–1250. doi:10.1016/j.intimp.2006.03.004

Lowes, M. A., Bowcock, A. M., and Krueger, J. G. (2007). Pathogenesis and Therapy of Psoriasis. *Nature* 445 (7130), 866–873. doi:10.1038/nature05663

Lowes, M. A., Kikuchi, T., Fuentes-Duculan, J., Cardinale, I., Zaba, L. C., Haider, A. S., et al. (2008). Psoriasis Vulgaris Lesions Contain Discrete Populations of Th1 and Th17 T Cells. *J. Invest. Dermatol.* 128 (5), 1207–1211. doi:10.1038/sj.jid.5701213

Marinoni, B., Ceribelli, A., Massarotti, M. S., and Selmi, C. (2014). The Th17 axis in Psoriatic Disease: Pathogenetic and Therapeutic Implications. *Autoimmun. Highlights* 5 (1), 9–19. doi:10.1007/s13317-013-0057-4

Puig, L. (2017). The Role of IL 23 in the Treatment of Psoriasis. *Expert Rev. Clin. Immunol.* 13 (6), 525–534. doi:10.1080/1744666X.2017.1292137

Raychaudhuri, S. K., Saxena, A., and Raychaudhuri, S. P. (2015). Role of IL-17 in the Pathogenesis of Psoriatic Arthritis and Axial Spondyloarthritis. *Clin. Rheumatol.* 34, 1019–1023. doi:10.1007/s10067-015-2961-7

Reich, K., Armstrong, A. W., Foley, P., Song, M., Wasfi, Y., Randazzo, B., et al. (2017). Efficacy and Safety of Guselkumab, an Anti-interleukin-23 Monoclonal Antibody, Compared with Adalimumab for the Treatment of Patients with Moderate to Severe Psoriasis with Randomized Withdrawal and Retreatment: Results from the Phase III, Double-Blind, Placebo- and Active Comparator-Controlled VOYAGE 2 Trial. *J. Am. Acad. Dermatol.* 76 (3), 418–431. doi:10.1016/j.jaad.2016.11.042

Reich, K., Warren, R. B., Iversen, L., Puig, L., Pau-Charles, I., Igarashi, A., et al. (2020). Long-term Efficacy and Safety of Tildrakizumab for Moderate-to-severe Psoriasis: Pooled Analyses of Two Randomized Phase III Clinical Trials (Re SURFACE 1 and Re SURFACE 2) through 148 Weeks. *Br. J. Dermatol.* 182 (3), 605–617. doi:10.1111/bjd.18232

Sakkas, L. I., and Bogdanos, D. P. (2017). Are Psoriasis and Psoriatic Arthritis the Same Disease? The IL-23/IL-17 axis Data. *Autoimmun. Rev.* 16 (1), 10–15. doi:10.1016/j.autrev.2016.09.015

Saunte, D. M., Mrowietz, U., Puig, L., and Zachariae, C. (2017). Candida Infections in Patients with Psoriasis and Psoriatic Arthritis Treated with Interleukin-17 Inhibitors and Their Practical Management. *Br. J. Dermatol.* 177 (1), 47–62. doi:10.1111/bjd.15015

Singh, T. P., Zhang, H. H., Borek, I., Wolf, P., Hedrick, M. N., Singh, S. P., et al. (2016). Monocyte-derived Inflammatory Langerhans Cells and Dermal Dendritic Cells Mediate Psoriasis-like Inflammation. *Nat. Commun.* 7, 13581. doi:10.1038/ncomms13581

Souto, A., Maneiro, J. R., Salgado, E., Carmona, L., and Gomez-Reino, J. J. (2014). Risk of Tuberculosis in Patients with Chronic Immune-Mediated Inflammatory Diseases Treated with Biologics and Tofacitinib: A Systematic Review and Meta-Analysis of Randomized Controlled Trials and Long-Term Extension Studies. *Rheumatology (Oxford)* 53, 1872–1885. doi:10.1093/rheumatology/keu172

Teraki, Y., Takahashi, A., Inoue, Y., and Takamura, S. (2018). Eyelid Dermatitis as a Side Effect of Interleukin-17A Inhibitors in Psoriasis. *Acta Derm. Venerol.* 98 (4), 456–457. doi:10.2340/00015555-2871

Teunissen, M. B. M., Bos, J. D., Koomen, C. W., de Waal Malefyt, R., and Wierenga, E. A. (1998). Interleukin-17 and Interferon-γ Synergize in the Enhancement of Proinflammatory Cytokine Production by Human Keratinocytes. *J. Invest. Dermatol.* 111 (4), 645–649. doi:10.1046/j.1523-1747.1998.00347.x

Van der Fits, L., Mourits, S., Voerman, J. S. A., Kant, M., Boon, L., Laman, J. D., et al. (2009). Imiquimod-induced Psoriasis-like Skin Inflammation in Mice Is Mediated via the IL-23/IL-17 axis. *J. Immunol.* 182 (9), 5836–5845. doi:10.4049/jimmunol.0802999

Wendling, D., Prati, C., Chouk, M., and Verhoeven, F. (2020). Effects of anti-IL-23 and anti-IL-17: The Hidden Side of Spondyloarthritis Polymorphism? *Jt. Bone Spine* 87 (19), 5–7. doi:10.1016/j.jbspin.2019.06.012

Wong, I. T., Shojania, K., Dutz, J., and Tsao, N. W. (2016). Clinical and Economic Review of Secukinumab for Moderate-To-Severe Plaque Psoriasis. *Expert Rev. Pharmacoeconomics Outcomes Res.* 16 (2), 153–166. doi:10.1586/14737167.2016.1133301

Yan, S. C., Wang, Y. J., Li, Y. J., Cai, W. Y., Weng, X. G., Li, Q., et al. (2019). Dihydroartemisinin Regulates the Th/Treg Balance by Inducing Activated CD4+ T Cell Apoptosis via Heme Oxygenase-1 Induction in Mouse Models of Inflammatory Bowel Disease. *Molecules* 24 (13), 2475. doi:10.3390/molecules24132475

Yang, Y., Winger, R. C., Lee, P. W., Nuro-Gyina, P. K., Minc, A., Larson, M., et al. (2015). Impact of Suppressing Retinoic Acid-Related Orphan Receptor gammat(ROR)γt in Ameliorating central Nervous System Autoimmunity. *Clin. Exp. Immunol.* 179 (1), 108–118. doi:10.1111/cei.12441

Zhang, L., Li, Y., Yang, X., Wei, J., Zhou, S., Zhao, Z., et al. (2016). Characterization of Th17 and FoxP3+Treg Cells in Paediatric Psoriasis Patients. *Scand. J. Immunol.* 83 (3), 174–180. doi:10.1111/sji.12404

Zhao, Y. G., Wang, Y., Guo, Z., Gu, A.-d., Dan, H. C., Baldwin, A. S., et al. (2012). Dihydroartemisinin Ameliorates Inflammatory Disease by its Reciprocal Effects on Th and Regulatory T Cell Function via Modulating the Mammalian Target of Rapamycin Pathway. *J. Immunol.* 189 (9), 4417–4425. doi:10.4049/jimmunol.1200919

Zheng, Y., Danilenko, D. M., Valdez, P., Kasman, I., Eastham-Anderson, J., Wu, J., et al. (2007). Interleukin-22, a TH17 Cytokine, Mediates IL-23-induced Dermal Inflammation and Acanthosis. *Nature* 445 (7128), 648–651. doi:10.1038/nature05505

4

Systems Pharmacology Approach and Experiment Evaluation Reveal Multidimensional Treatment Strategy of LiangXueJieDu Formula for Psoriasis

Jingxia Zhao[1,2†], *Yan Wang*[1,2†], *Weiwen Chen*[1], *Jing Fu*[1,2], *Yu Liu*[1,2,3], *Tingting Di*[1,2], *Cong Qi*[1,2], *Zhaoxia Chen*[1,2] *and Ping Li*[1,2*]

[1]Beijing Hospital of Traditional Chinese Medicine, Capital Medical University, Beijing, China, [2]Beijing Key Laboratory of Clinic and Basic Research with Traditional Chinese Medicine on Psoriasis, Beijing Institute of Traditional Chinese Medicine, Beijing, China, [3]Beijing University of Chinese Medicine, Beijing, China

***Correspondence:**
Ping Li
liping@bjzhongyi.com

[†]These authors have contributed equally to this work

Clinical studies have demonstrated the anti-psoriatic effect of the LiangXueJieDu (LXJD) herbal formula. However, the systemic mechanism and the targets of the LXJD formula have not yet been elucidated. In the present study, a systems pharmacology approach, metabolomics, and experimental evaluation were employed. First, by systematic absorption-distribution-metabolism-excretion (ADME) analysis, 144 active compounds with satisfactory pharmacokinetic properties were identified from 12 herbs of LXJD formula using the TCMSP database. These active compounds could be linked to 125 target proteins involved in the pathological processes underlying psoriasis. Then, the networks constituting the active compounds, targets, and diseases were constructed to decipher the pharmacological actions of this formula, indicating its curative effects in psoriasis treatment and related complications. The psoriasis-related pathway comprising several regulatory modules demonstrated the synergistic mechanisms of LXJD formula. Furthermore, the therapeutic effect of LXJD formula was validated in a psoriasis-like mouse model. Consistent with the systems pharmacology analysis, LXJD formula ameliorated IMQ-induced psoriasis-like lesions in mice, inhibited keratinocyte proliferation, improved keratinocyte differentiation, and suppressed the infiltration of CD3+ T cells. Compared to the model group, LXJD formula treatment remarkably reduced the expression of inflammatory cytokines and factors, such as IL-1β, IL-6, TNF-α, Cox2, and inhibited the phosphorylation of p-P65, p-IκB, p-ERK, p-P38, p-PI3K, p-AKT, indicating that LXJD formula exerts its therapeutic effect by inhibiting the MAPK, PI3K/AKT, and NF-κB signaling pathways. The metabolic changes in the serum of psoriasis patients were evaluated by liquid chromatography coupled with orbitrap mass spectrometry (LC-MS). The LXJD formula improved two perturbed metabolic pathways of glycerophospholipid metabolism and steroid hormone biosynthesis. Overall, this study revealed the complicated anti-psoriatic mechanism of LXJD formula and also offered a reliable strategy to elucidate the complex therapeutic mechanism of this Chinese herbal formula in psoriasis from a holistic perspective.

Keywords: traditional Chinese medicine, systems pharmacology, psoriasis, liangxuejiedu formula, inflammation cytokines

INTRODUCTION

Psoriasis is an immune-mediated, chronic skin condition that follows a relapsing and remitting course. It poses a significant public health challenge with a high prevalence rate of 0.09–11.43% worldwide and multiple co-morbidities, including arthritis, cardiovascular disease, obesity, diabetes mellitus, reduced quality of life, and depression/anxiety (World health organization, 2016). Psoriasis vulgaris is the most common form of psoriasis, encompassing about 80% of psoriasis patients. Clinical manifestations comprise well-demarcation, scaling, and erythematous plaques that appear anywhere on the body. Histologically, psoriasis is characterized by parakeratosis, acanthosis with downward elongation of rete ridges, thin/no granular cell layer, Munro's microabscesses (neutrophils in parakeratotic scale), increased mitotic figures above basal layer, and mixed dermal infiltrate of lymphocytes and neutrophils.

Current treatments for psoriasis are categorized as follows: topical therapies (topical corticosteroids, tar-based preparations, dithranol, vitamin D analogs, salicylic acid, and topical retinoids), oral medication (methotrexate, acitretin, and cyclosporine), biological agents (infliximab, adalimumab, etanercept, and ustekinumab), and Ultraviolet phototherapy (UV-B and psoralen-UV-A) (Heng et al., 2000; Gamret et al., 2018). However, 52.3% of patients with psoriasis reported dissatisfaction with their medical treatment because of the inefficacy of the methods and adverse effects (Kurd et al., 2008). Thus, the utilization of complementary and alternative medicine among psoriasis patients is common, with prevalence varying between 42 and 69% (Ben-Arye et al., 2003; Damevska et al., 2014; Talbott and Duffy, 2015). These methods constitute herbal therapies and traditional Chinese medicine (TCM) that have gained popularity in recent years. The application of TCM in the treatment of psoriasis has a long history. According to the theory of TCM, psoriasis vulgaris is classified as three main blood-related syndromes: blood heat, blood stasis, and blood dryness. The blood-heat syndrome is frequently observed at the active stage, accounting for 53.8% of the condition in psoriasis vulgaris (Zhang et al., 2009). LiangXueJieDu (LXJD) formula is commonly used to treat psoriasis vulgaris with blood-heat syndrome and has proven to be a safe remedy with better efficacy compared to conventional therapy in a multicenter randomized controlled study (Sun et al., 2020). However, the mechanisms underlying LXJD formula-alleviated psoriasis remain unclear.

TCM is based on its own theory of medicine with multiple ingredients' interactions. Relative to Western medicine, TCM treats the function and dysfunction of the body using a holistic approach. However, the complexity of the ingredients and their *in vivo* activity could interfere with identifying the targets and understanding the mechanisms of TCM. Systems pharmacology is an emerging systematic methodology that combines oral bioavailability screening, multiple drug targets prediction and validation, and network pharmacology, providing a holistic approach to explore the targets and mechanisms of TCM. In recent years, systems pharmacology has been widely used to reveal the potential mechanism of TCM formulas (Liu et al., 2016; Yuan et al., 2020).

Based on the proved clinical efficacy, we applied the systems pharmacology method to explore the pharmacological targets and mechanisms of LXJD formula in the treatment of psoriasis in this study. Next, we verified the mechanism of LXJD formula on the main targets and those integrated by systemic pharmacology in the samples from psoriasis patients and psoriasis-like mice.

MATERIALS AND METHODS

Reagents

High performance liquid chromatography (HPLC)-grade acetonitrile and methanol were purchased from Merck (Darmstadt, Germany). Purified water (18.2 MΩ) was obtained from a Milli-Q water purification system (Millipore, United States). Formic acid was obtained from Sigma-Aldrich (St. Louis, United States). Chlorogenic acid, caffeic acid, paeoniflorin, taxifolin, astilbin, albiflorin, resveratrol, rosmarinic acid, 5-O-methylvisammioside, quercetin, naringenin, luteolin, kaempferol, and isorhamnetin (all 98%, pure) were purchased from the National Institutes for Food and Drug Control (Beijing, China) (**Table 1**). All other chemicals were of analytical grade. CD3, Ki67, and loricrin antibodies were purchased from Abcam (Cambridge, MA, United States).

Database Construction

A total of 864 chemical ingredients of 12 herbs in LXJD formula were collected manually from PubMed, the China National Knowledge Infrastructure (CNKI), and the Traditional Chinese Medicines Systems Pharmacology (TCMSP) databases (http://lsp.nwsuaf.edu.cn/) (Ru et al., 2014).

Screening of Active Compounds

We employed an *in silico* integrative model-ADME (absorption, distribution, metabolism, and excretion of drugs) to screen out the compounds with favorable pharmacokinetics properties. Oral bioavailability (OB) is one of the most desirable attributes of new drugs representing the ratio of the orally administered dose that reaches the circulation system with unaltered activity.

In the present study, the OBioavail1.1 model was utilized to estimate the OB values. The compounds from LXJD formula which satisfy the criteria of OB ≥ 30% were selected as candidate active molecules for further screening (Ru et al., 2014; Yuan et al., 2020). Drug-likeness (DL) is a major factor in the absorption, distribution, metabolism, and elimination of the molecules in the human body. It is estimated from the molecular structure before the substance is synthesized and tested. Herein, a compound with

TABLE 1 | Identification of the chemical constituents of LXJD formula by UHPLC-ESI-MS analysis.

No	Retention time (min)	Selected ion	Measured mass (m/z)	Error (ppm)	Identification	Formula	Chemical structure
1	20.41	(M–H)	353.0878	–0.02	Chlorogenic acid	$C_{16}H_{18}O_9$	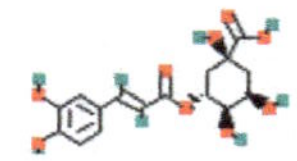
2	20.68	(M–H)	179.0351	0.63	Caffeic acid	$C_9H_8O_4$	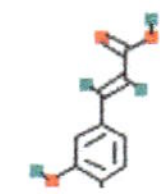
3	21.24	(M + H)	481.1712	–0.63	Paeoniflorin	$C_{23}H_{28}O_{11}$	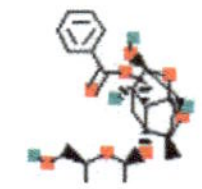
4	23.90	(M–H)	303.0510	–0.001	Taxifolin	$C_{15}H_{12}O_7$	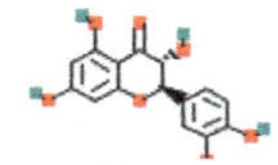
5	25.23	(M–H)	449.1090	0.03	Astilbin	$C_{21}H_{22}O_{11}$	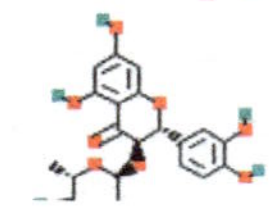
6	25.95	(M + H)	481.1713	–0.56	Albiflorin	$C_{23}H_{28}O_{11}$	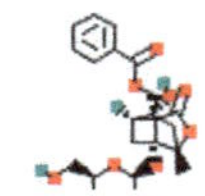
7	26.43	(M–H)	227.0714	–0.08	Resveratrol	$C_{14}H_{12}O_3$	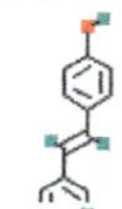
8	26.72	(M-H)	359.077	0.76	Rosmarinic acid	$C_{18}H_{16}O_8$	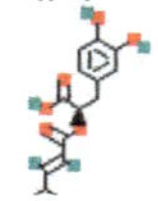
9	27.74	(M + H)	453.1760	1.04	5-O-methylvisammioside	$C_{22}H_{28}O_{10}$	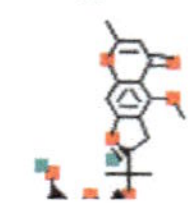
10	29.45	(M–H)	301.0352	–0.63	Quercetin	$C_{15}H_{10}O_7$	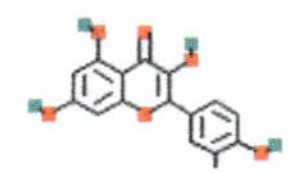
11	29.58	(M–H)	271.0612	–0.03	Naringenin	$C_{15}H_{12}O_5$	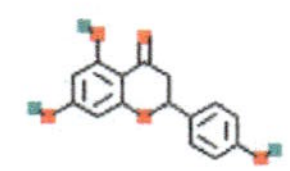

(Continued on following page)

TABLE 1 | (*Continued*) Identification of the chemical constituents of LXJD formula by UHPLC-ESI-MS analysis.

No	Retention time (min)	Selected ion	Measured mass (m/z)	Error (ppm)	Identification	Formula	Chemical structure
12	30.23	(M–H)	285.0403	−0.73	Luteolin	$C_{15}H_{10}O_6$	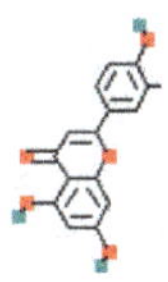
13	31.24	(M–H)	285.0404	−0.20	Kaempferol	$C_{15}H_{10}O_6$	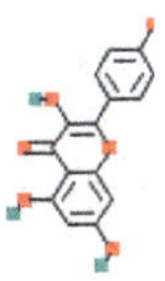
14	31.66	(M–H)	315.0510	−0.10	Isorhamnetin	$C_{16}H_{12}O_7$	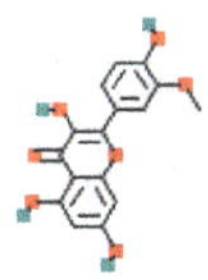

DL ≥ 0.18 was selected as the active compound of herbs for subsequent studies (Ru et al., 2014; Yuan et al., 2020). The oral absorption of drugs was realized *via* intestinal epithelial cells (IECs). In this study, a computer Caco-2 permeability prediction model was applied to predict the intestinal permeability of the components in TCMSP (Lv et al., 2019). The chemical ingredients with Caco-2 cell permeability ≥−0.4 were filtered out as candidate active compounds. The oil-water partition coefficient AlogP is the logarithm of the ratio of the partition coefficient of the substance in n-octanol and water. Lipophilicity is a leading physical and chemical parameter reflecting the permeability in biofilms. ALOGPS2.1 software was used to calculate AlogP, and the threshold was set to <5 according to Lipinski's rule of five (Lipinski et al., 2001; Tetko and Bruneau, 2004).

Target Fishing

A weighted ensemble similarity (WES) model was implemented to predict the potential target molecules of the candidate active compounds in LXJD formula. Then, a similarity search based on chemical fingerprinting was applied to obtain potential targets (http://sea.bkslab.org/search/). Finally, the targets from different sources were analyzed against the Pharmacogenomics knowledgebase (PharmGKB, https://www.pharmgkb.org/), Therapeutic Targets Database (TTD, http://database.idrb.cqu.edu.cn/TTD/), and Comparative Toxicogenomics Database (CTD, http://ctdbase.org/) to eliminate redundant and erroneous molecules, thereby guaranteeing the accuracy of the database.

Gene Ontology Enrichment and Clustering Analysis for Targets

To identify the targets associated with the physiological features of psoriasis, a Gene Ontology (GO) enrichment analysis was performed using DAVID (http://david.abcc.ncifcrf.gov) for classification. In this section, the GOBP (biological process) analysis result was highlighted. Then, functional annotation clustering analysis was carried out based on the GOBP enrichment data. *p*-value <0.05 indicated statistical significance.

Network Construction

TCM is a complex system consisting of multiple effective compounds, multiple targets of action, and related diseases. To illustrate the pharmacological mechanisms of LXJD formula in psoriasis treatment and clarify the complicated associations among the active compounds, targets, and diseases at a systems level, the network visualization analysis Cytoscape software was used to establish the compound-target network, target-disease network, and target-pathway network, respectively. In order to further interpret the molecular mechanism of LXJD formula against psoriasis, an integrated map of "psoriasis-related pathways" was constructed by integrating the key pathway obtained from the Kyoto Encyclopedia of Genes and Genomes (KEGG) database (http://www.kegg.jp/) using target-pathway network analysis.

Preparation of LiangXueJieDu Formula

LXJD formula, consisting of Tu Fu Ling (*Smilax glabra* Roxb.) (ratio 1:5), Huai Hua (Styphnolobium japonicum (L.) Schott syn. Sophora japonica L.) (ratio 1:10), Di Huang (Rehmannia glutinosa (Gaertn.) DC.) (ratio 1:10), Zi Cao (Arnebia euchroma (Royle ex Benth.) I.M.Johnst.) (ratio 1:15), Quan Shen (Bistorta officinalis Delarbre syn. Polygonum (Isatis tinctoria L.) (ratio 1: 15), Bai Mao Gen (Imperata cylindrica (L.) P.Beauv.) (ratio 1:15), Bai Xian Pi (Dictamnus dasycarpus Turcz.) (ratio 1:15), Bai Hua She She Cao (Scleromitrion diffusum (Willd.) R.J.Wang syn. Hedyotis diffusa Willd.) (ratio 1:15), Fang Feng (Saposhnikovia varzcata (Turcz.) Schischk.) (ratio 1:15), and Mu Dan Pi (Paeonia x suffruticosa Andr), were decocted and provided by the TCM Pharmacy of Beijing Hospital of Traditional Chinese Medicine. Briefly, 150 g of the crude drugs of LXJD formula were soaked and decocted in 400 ml of pure water for 30 min. Then, the water decoction was concentrated to 200 ml, and the final dosage of crude drugs was 0.75 g/ml.

All raw herbs were purchased from Beijing Xinglin Pharmaceutical (Beijing, China, Voucher number 20150301). The voucher specimen, identified by Professor Wei He, was deposited in our laboratory at Beijing Traditional Chinese Medical Hospital.

Preparation of Standard Solutions and Liquid Chromatography

A standard working solution of the 14 reference substances (**Table 1**, purities>98%) were prepared in concentrations ranging from 0.032 to 0.058 mg/ml in methanol and stored at 4°C. The 14 reference substances were used as standard control to identify the major components of LXJD formula by the UPLC-MS method.

The UPLC separation was performed on an ACQUITY UPLC™ BEH C18 column (100 × 2.1, 1.7 mm). Both negative and positive modes were examined. A gradient elution was used with 0.1% formic acid in methanol as solvent A and 0.1% formic acid in water as solvent B, at a flow rate of 0.2 ml min^{-1}. The following gradient elution scheme was used: 0–2 min, 100–100% B; 2–10 min, 100–93% B; 10–40 min, 93–0% B; 40–45 min, 0–0% B; 45–45.1 min, 0–100% B; and 45.1–60 min, 100–100% B. The injection volume was 10 µl.

Mass Spectrometric Conditions

A Thermo Q Exactive™ Plus Orbitrap™ mass spectrometer was used for the qualitative analysis of the constituents in LXJD formula. Mass spectrometric parameters were: sheath gas flow rate of 35; aux gas flow rate of 10; sweep gas flow rate of 0; S-lens RF level of 50. The spray voltage was 3.5 kV for the positive and −4.5 kV for the negative ion mode. The capillary temperature and aux gas heater temperature were set to 320 and 350 °C, respectively. The m/z ranged from 100–1200 and 150–2000 for the positive and negative ion modes, respectively.

Study Design

A total of 40 psoriasis patients were recruited from the Beijing Traditional Chinese Medical Hospital according to the specified inclusion and exclusion criteria.

The inclusion criteria were as follows: 1) Psoriasis vulgaris was diagnosed according to the "Clinical Guidelines of Psoriasis 2008" reported by the Chinese Medical Association; 2) age 18–65 years; 3) willing to sign a written informed consent; 4) psoriasis patients were diagnosed with blood-heat syndrome based on the theory of TCM; 4) PASI score >5.

Exclusion criteria (patients who met one of the following conditions were excluded): 1) Those who were allergic to LXJD formula or the composition; 2) women who were pregnant or in the lactation stage; 3) those who had been treated with steroids orally in the past 2 weeks or with retinoid orally or steroid topically in the past week; 4) arthropathic, pustular, or erythrodermic psoriasis; 5) those with severe heart, cerebrovascular, liver, kidney, hematopoietic system, cancer, or psychosis diseases.

The treatment group received the Chinese herbal medicine LXJD formula for 8 weeks. Each dose of LXJD formula (150 g of crude drugs) was decocted in 400 ml of water. Then, the water decoction was concentrated to 200 ml, and the final dosage of crude drugs was 0.75 g/ml. In total, 100 ml of the decoction was taken orally 30 min before breakfast and the other 100 ml 30 min before dinner. Serum samples were collected from each patient before and 8 weeks after LXJD formula treatment.

The study duration was 8 weeks. Patients were evaluated before the start of treatment and were followed up every 2 weeks during the trial period. Clinical symptoms, examination of psoriatic skin lesions, and psoriasis area and severity index (PASI) scores were documented. The PASI is a composite index of the severity of the three main characteristics of psoriatic plaques (erythema, scaling, and thickness) weighted by the amount of coverage of these plaques in the four main body areas (i.e., head, trunk, upper extremities, and lower extremities). PASI scores can range from 0 to 72, wherein higher scores indicate greater severity.

Out of a total of 40 potentially eligible patients, 15 patients were subsequently excluded from this study, of which 7 patients were excluded from the Chinese medicine treatment group for failing to adhere to the clinical trial protocol and eight patients were excluded because of the progression and evolution of patients' symptoms.

Of the remaining 25 patients, 52% of patients (13 in 25) after LXJD treatment achieved PASI60 and were considered as responders to LXJD treatment. Serum metabolomics were analyzed in these 13 responders' samples only.

Ethics Statement

Informed consent was given by the patients and this study was approved by the Ethics Committee of Beijing Traditional Chinese Medical Hospital (NO. 2017BL-073-01).

Sample Preparation

Serum (100 µl) was added into methanol (400 µl), vortex-mixed for 30 s, and the proteins were precipitated by centrifugation at 12,000 rpm for 15 min. Subsequently, the dried residue was reconstituted in 100 µl of acetonitrile-water (10:90, v/v) and then injected for LC-MS analysis.

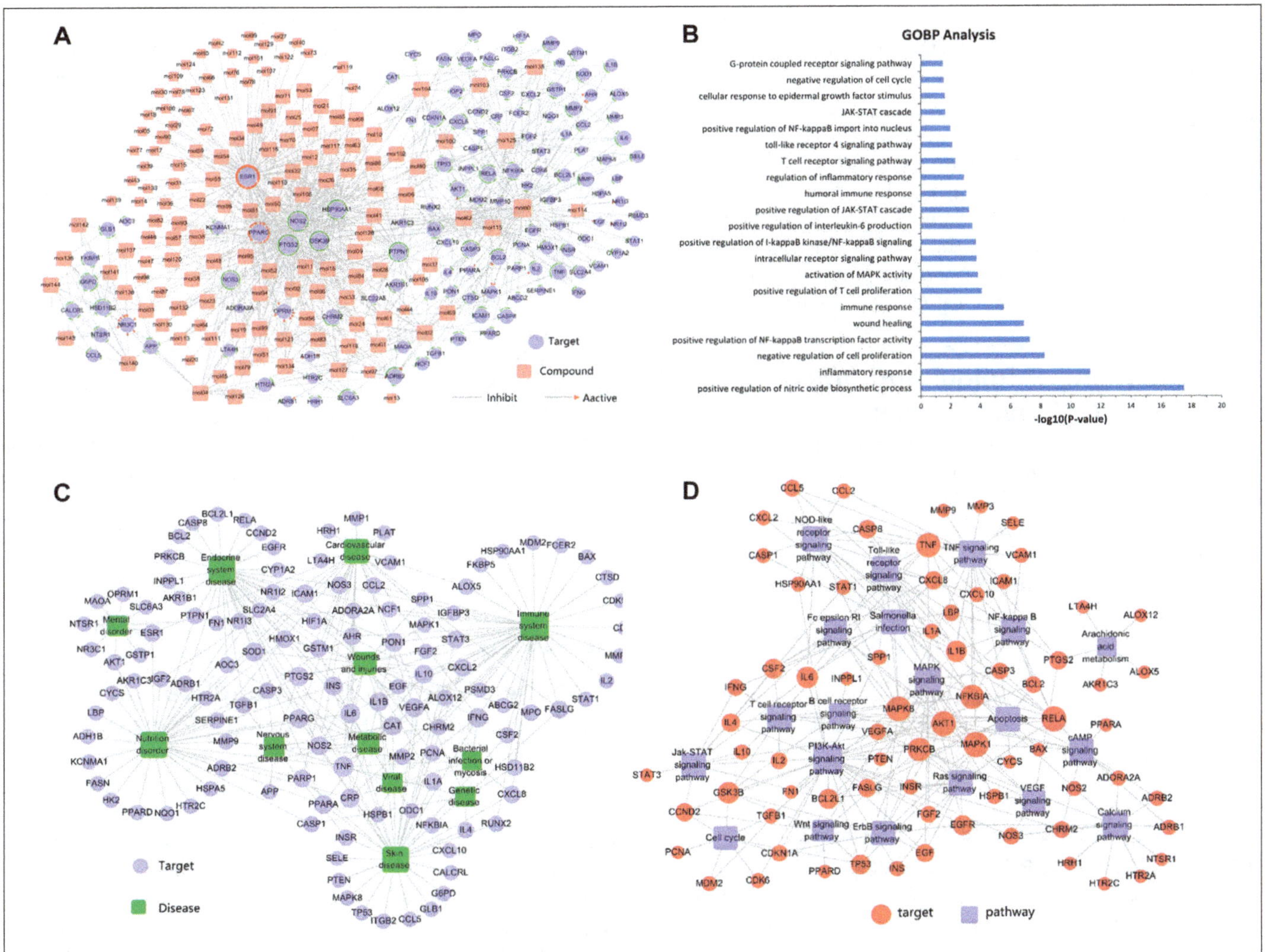

FIGURE 1 | (A) Compound-target network analysis. A compound and a target are linked if the target protein is hit by the corresponding compound. Node size is proportional to its degree. The pink square represents the compounds and the purple circle represents the targets. **(B)** GO enrichment analysis of the predicted protein targets. The top 21 enriched biological processes related to the targets are shown ($p < 0.05$). **(C)** Target-disease network. Target proteins are linked to their corresponding diseases and those diseases are linked to the corresponding disease categories they belong to. The purple circle represents the target and the green square represents the disease. **(D)** The target-pathway network was constructed by linking active compounds to their related pathways. Node size is related to the degree. The red circle represents the target and the purple square represents the pathway.

Metabolic Profiling

The chromatographic analysis of the serum sample was performed in a Thermo LC system (Thermo, Ultimate 3000 LC, Orbitrap Elite) equipped with a Hypergod C18 column (4.6 mm × 100 mm, 3.0 μm). The column was maintained at 40°C, and the flow rate was set at 0.30 ml/min. The mobile phase was composed of water (A) and acetonitrile (B), each containing 0.1% formic acid. The linear gradient program was optimized as follows: 0–2.0 min, 5% B; 2.0–12 min, 5–95% B; 12–15 min, washing with 95% B for 15–17 min, and equilibration with 5% B. A volume of 4 μl was injected in all the cases and analyzed on a Thermo mass spectrometer equipped with an electrospray ionization source (ESI) operating in positive and negative ion modes. The optimized parameters of TOF were set as follows: the spray voltage was 3.0 kV (ES+) and 3.2 kV (ES−) with the capillary temperature at 350°C, and sheath gas flow and auxiliary gas flow were set at 45 and 15, respectively. The mass range was set at 100–1000 m/z with 70,000 mass resolution at 400 m/z. The accepted scientific names must be updated using Medicinal Plant Name Service - KEW (https://mpns.science.kew.org/mpns-portal/).

The MS raw data of serum samples were processed using SIEVE software (Thermo Corp., Manchester, United Kingdom). This process included deconvolution, normalization, and alignment, and a dataset including retention time and mass pairs with the corresponding intensities of each metabolite was obtained. Then, the processed dataset was introduced into the SIMCA-P software package (v13.0, Umetric, Umeå, Sweden) to perform principal component analysis (PCA) and orthogonal to partial least squares-discriminate analysis (OPLS-DA). In the

OPLS-DA model, the variable importance of project (VIP) value and *S*-plot were employed as standards to select potential biomarkers.

Animals

Eight-week-old male C57BL/6 mice were purchased from Beijing Huafukang Biological Technology Co., Ltd. (Beijing, China) and maintained under specific pathogen-free conditions. All experiments adhered to the principles of the Declaration of Helsinki and were conducted using the protocols approved by the Beijing Institute of Traditional Chinese Medicine.

Establishment of Imiquimod (IMQ)-Induced Psoriasis-like Mouse Models

Mice were divided into four groups (10 mice/group): Control group, model group, MTX group, and LXJD group. All mice except those in the control group received a daily topical application of 42 mg of IMQ cream (5%) (MedShine, Chengdu, China) on their shaved back for seven consecutive days to establish a model of psoriasiform lesions. LXJD and MTX treatment started with the application of IMQ. From days 1–7, mice in the LXJD and MTX (positive control) groups were treated with LXJD (29.4 g herb/kg/day) and MTX (1 mg/kg/day) by gavage, respectively. Mice in the control group (control) and model group (model) were given saline by intragastric administration. On day seven, the animals were sacrificed, and skin samples were collected from their backs.

Histology, Immunohistochemistry, and Immunofluorescence Staining

The mouse back skin was fixed in formalin and embedded in paraffin. Partial sections were stained with hematoxylin-eosin (H&E) for pathological observation by microscopy. Partial sections were stained with anti-Rabbit CD3 (1:100, Abcam, United States) and anti-Loricrin (1:200, Abcam, United States), and Diaminobezidin (DAB) (Zhongshan Golden Bridge Biotechnology, China) was used for color development. For immunofluorescence, Ki-67 (proliferation) level was evaluated in skin sections using anti-Ki67 antibody (1:200, Abcam), following the manufacturer's instructions. For $CD3^+$, Ki-67+, and Loricrin+ cells, three areas in three sections of each sample were selected randomly, and the number of positive cells was calculated.

Quantitative RT-PCR Analysis (qRT-PCR)

Total RNA was extracted from the skin lesion and cultured cells using an ultrapure RNA extraction kit (Kang Biotechnology, China). Reverse transcription was carried out using the HiFi-MMLV cDNA first-strand synthesis kit (Kang Biotechnology). Quantitative real-time PCR amplification was performed on ABI 7500 Real-Time PCR Systems (Applied Biosystems, United States). A housekeeping gene was utilized as an internal reference standard. The relative gene expression was calculated using the $2^{-\Delta\Delta Ct}$ method.

Western Blot

The tissue extracts were prepared using RIPA buffer (50 mM of Tris-HCl pH 7.4, 150 mM of NaCl, 1 mM of EDTA, 1% Triton X-100, 0.1% SDS, 0.5% deoxycholate) supplemented with a complete protease inhibitor cocktail (Roche) and a PhosSTOP phosphatase inhibit or cocktail (Roche). Samples were subjected to SDS-PAGE and the resolved proteins were then transferred onto a polyvinylidene difluoride (PVDF) membrane (Millipore). The immunoblots were probed with indicated antibodies and visualized using a SuperSignal West Pico chemiluminescence ECL kit (Pierce). GAPDH was used as an internal control.

Statistical Analysis

All quantitative data are presented as means ± SD and analyzed for statistical significance using GraphPad Prism 5.0 (GraphPad Software Inc., San Diego, CA, United States). One-way analysis of variance (ANOVA) followed by Tukey's post hoc test and unpaired Student's t-test was used to analyze the statistical significance among multiple groups and between two groups, respectively. A two-tailed Student's *t*-test was performed in a clinical study using the Statistical Package for Social Science program (SPSS 20.0, Chicago, IL, United States). $p < 0.05$ indicated statistically significant difference.

RESULTS

Bioactive Compounds Identification for Each Herb in LiangXueJieDu Formula

In the current study, 864 chemical ingredients and their pharmaceutical properties in the LXJD formula were obtained from the TCMSP database. A combination of OB (≥30%), Caco-2 permeability (Caco-2) (>−0.4), prediction of permeability (AlogP <5), and drug-likeness (DL) ≥0.18 properties was applied to identify the active compounds of LXJD formula. Based on a previous report, some compounds that did not agree with the threshold of compounds screening were also likely to produce therapeutic effects, and hence, retained as active compounds in this study, such as palmitic acid (Dogra et al., 2018), sitosterol (REISS and JAIMOVICH, 1958), stigmasterol (Srivastava, 2014), trametenolic acid (Ma et al., 2013), lignoceric acid (Tsoukalas et al., 2019), tirucallane (Mireku et al., 2015), etc. These compounds have bioactivity and are reported as anti-psoriatic or anti-inflammatory molecules. Finally, 144 active compounds (**Supplementary Table S1**), including 37 in Isatis tinctoria, 8 in Scleromitrion diffusum, 10 in Dictamnus dasycarpus, 9 in Paeonia lactiflora, 11 in Rehmannia glutinosa, 14 in Arnebia euchroma, 3 in Paeonia x suffruticosa, 18 in Saposhnikovia varzcata, 5 in Smilax glabra, 8 in Imperata cylindrica, 7 in Bistorta officinalis, and 14 in Paeonia lactiflora, were obtained.

Target Identification and Analysis

TCM formulas exert their pharmacological activities through synergistic interactions between multiple compounds and targets. To identify the relevant targets of the potential compounds in LXJD formula, the TCMSP database and WES algorithms were used. A final list of 125 potential targets for 144 bioactive compounds was obtained. These targets were further subject to PharmGkb, CTD, and TTD for sanity checks. As shown

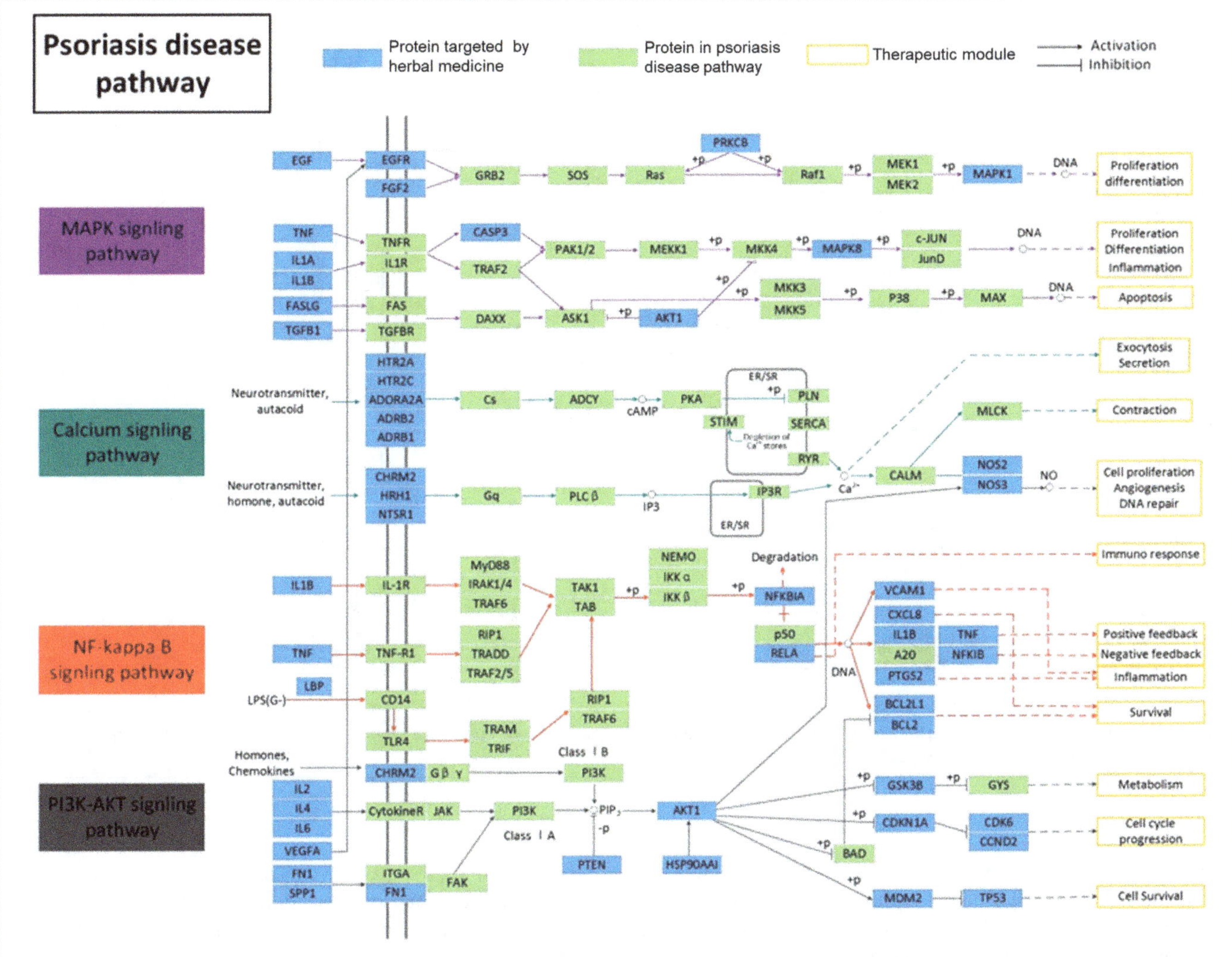

FIGURE 2 | Distribution of target proteins of LXJD formula in integrated psoriasis-related pathways, which includes the MAPK, calcium, NF-κB, and PI3K/AKT signaling pathways.s

in **Supplementary Table S2**, most active compounds could act on multiple targets simultaneously, and one target could also be linked to multiple active compounds. PTGS2, also known as cyclooxygenase-2 (COX-2), is one of the potential targets that play a critical role in inflammation (Yalçin et al., 2007). It was predicted that PTGS2 is linked to 86 active compounds in the LXJD formula to exert therapeutic effect synergistically. The active compound quercetin (MOL60) was found to be connected to 79 targets, reflecting the multiple targets of herbal medicine.

Gene Ontology Enrichment Analysis for Potential Targets

To validate whether the 125 potential targets in the network are associated with psoriasis, we performed GO term (BP) enrichment analysis. The top 21 significant GO terms responsible for psoriasis were enriched. As shown in **Figure 1B**, inflammatory response, positive regulation of NF-κB transcription factor activity, positive regulation of T cell proliferation, regulation of inflammatory response, and IL-6 production was intricately linked to the pathogenesis of psoriasis. These results suggested that the potential targets were significantly involved in the pathogenesis of psoriasis.

Compound-Target Network Analysis

Figure 1A shows that the compound-target network consisted of 144 active compounds, 125 targets, and 901 compound-target interactions (269 nodes and 901 edges). The results displayed an average of 7.2° per compound and 6.3° per target protein, respectively. In the correlations between compounds and targets (**Supplementary Table S3**), MOL60 exhibited the highest number of target interactions (79°), followed by MOL125 (35°), MOL115 (34°), and MOL62 (33°), which was consistent with the multi-component and multi-target traits of herbal medicines. Regarding the candidate targets, estrogen

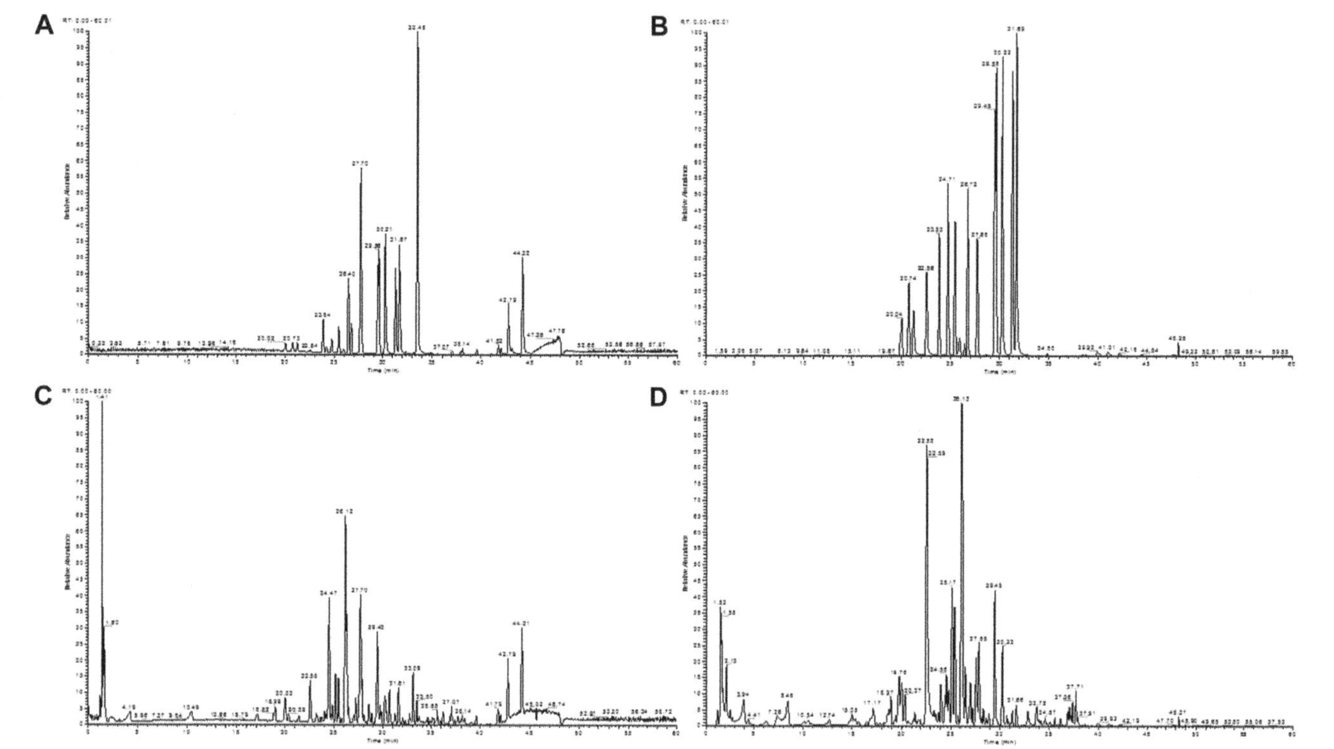

FIGURE 3 | Total ion chromatograms of a mixture of 14 standards obtained from the negative **(A)** and positive **(B)** ion scan modes. LXJD formula extract obtained from the negative **(C)** and positive **(D)** ion scan modes.

receptor (ESR1) showed the highest degree (113°), followed by PTGS2 (86°), NOS2 (81°), PPARG (60°), and GSK3B (56°), which demonstrated the potential therapeutic effect of each drug in LXJD formula for ameliorating psoriasis.

Target-Disease Network

In order to elucidate the correlation between LXJD formula and diseases, a target-disease network, including 122 target proteins and 12 corresponding diseases, was constructed based on the DrugBank, TTD, and PharmGKB databases. As shown in **Figure 1C**, LXJD formula was related to 12 types of diseases, including immune system disease (41°), endocrine system disease (37°), skin disease (35°), nutrition disorder (35°), cardiovascular disease (27°) wounds and injuries (29°), metabolic disease (14°), nervous system disease (10°), mental disorder (9°), genetic disease (7°), viral disease (7°), and bacterial infection or mycosis (4°). The target-disease network might explain the theory of "homotherapy for heteropathy" in TCM.

Target-Pathway Network Analysis

To further elucidate the therapeutic mechanisms underlying the LXJD formula in the treatment of psoriasis, all the predicted target proteins were mapped to enrich the relevant pathways. The target-pathway network containing 73 targets and 20 corresponding pathways is shown in **Figure 1D**. The majority of the target proteins were involved in multiple pathways, indicating that the target proteins of the LXJD formula interplayed with each other in different pathways and exerted synergistic effects in the treatment of psoriasis. As shown in **Supplementary Table S4**, the crucial target protein-associated pathways included the PI3K/AKT signaling pathway (27°), TNF signaling pathway (21°), MAPK signaling pathway (16°), toll-like receptor signaling pathway (15°), NOD-like receptor signaling pathway (13°), *salmonella* infection pathway (13°), Ras signaling pathway (13°), apoptosis pathway (12°), calcium signaling pathway (12°), NF-κB signaling pathway (11°), T cell receptor signaling pathway (11°), and JAK-STAT signaling pathway (11°). These results suggested that multiple targets affect various pathways regulating the pathological processes underlying psoriasis, thereby promoting a potent therapeutic approach for these diseases.

Psoriasis-Related Pathway Analysis

Based on the complex mechanism of the LXJD formula in the treatment of psoriasis, an integrated map of "psoriasis-related pathways" was constructed by integrating the key pathways obtained from the KEGG database using target-pathway network analysis. As shown in **Figure 2**, psoriasis-related pathways consist of four important pathways: the MAPK signaling pathway, calcium signaling pathway, PI3K/AKT signaling pathway, and NF-κB signaling pathway. These pathways were associated with several biological functions,

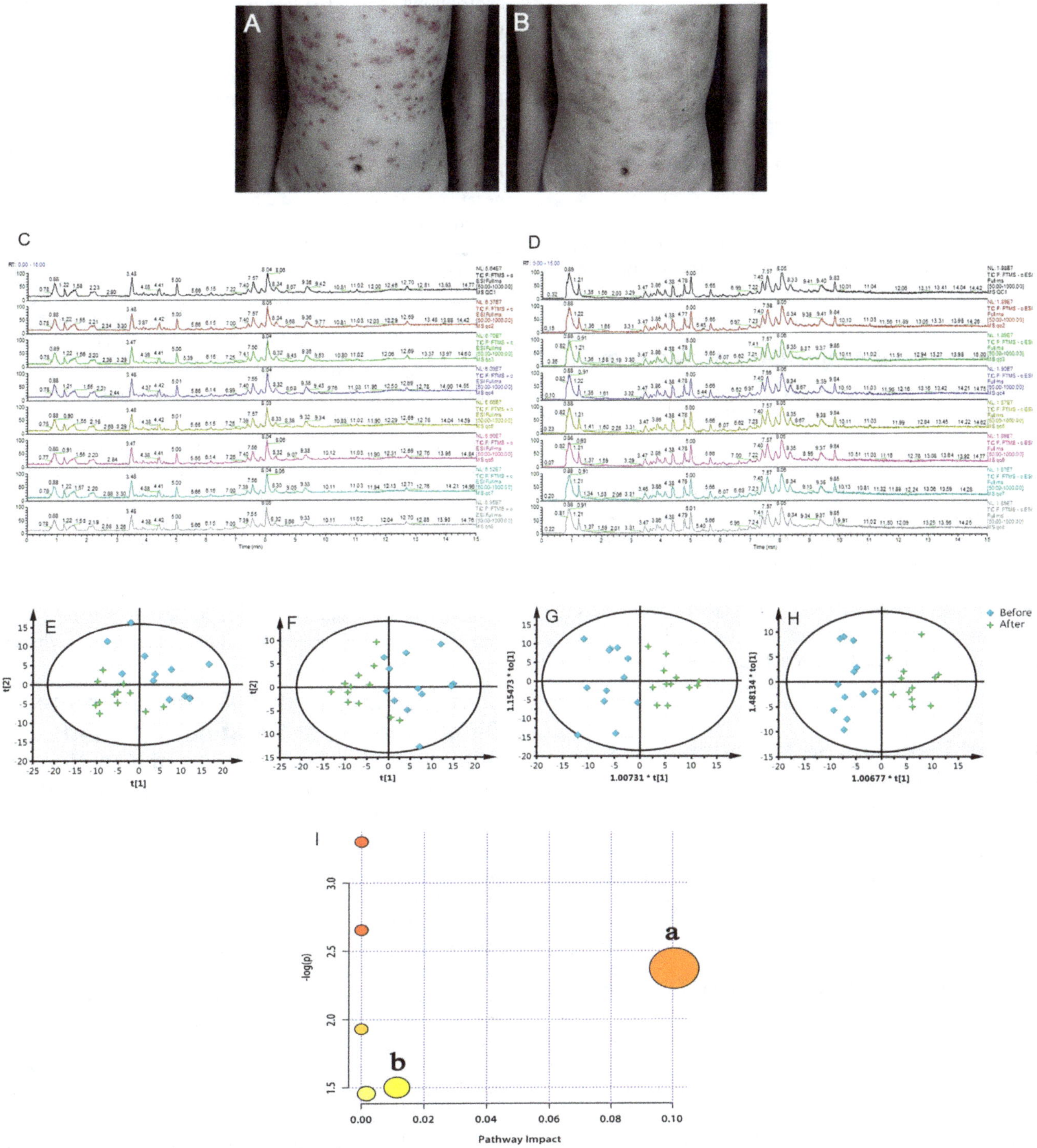

FIGURE 4 | (A, B) Representative photographs of the patient with psoriasis taken at baseline (week 0, A) and after 8 weeks **(B)** of treatment with LiangxueJiedu formula. Total ions chromatogram of QC samples from the positive **(C)** and negative **(D)** ion scan modes. **(E, F)** PCA score plots of serum samples collected from psoriasis patients before and after 8 weeks of LiangxueJiedu formula treatment measured in **(E,** $R^2X = 0.724$, $Q^2 = 0.495$**)** positive and **(F,** $R^2X = 0.574$, $Q^2 = 0.371$**)** negative mode. **(G, H)** OPLS-DA score plots of serum samples collected from psoriasis patients before and after 8 weeks of LiangxueJiedu formula treatment based on UPLC-Q-TOF/MS technology in (G, $R^2X = 0.557$, $R^2Y = 0.782$, $Q^2 = 0.671$) positive and (H, $R^2X = 0.410$, $R^2Y = 0.852$, $Q^2 = 0.453$) negative mode. **(I)** Summary of pathway analysis with MetPA, a: glycerophospholipid metabolism; b: steroid hormone biosynthesis.

TABLE 2 | Characteristics of the study cohorts.

	Before treatment	After treatment
Gender	7/6	7/6
PASI	13.6 ± 5.97	3.8 ± 2.1**

*Values are reported as the mean ± SD. Units for cholesterol and triglycerides are mmol/L, PASI, psoriasis area, and severity index. Gender balance: male/female. p < 0.05 indicated statistical significance for PASI scores before and after treatment (**p < 0.01).*

such as inflammation, proliferation, metabolism, cell survival, cell cycle, and immune response, indicating the therapeutic effect of the LXJD formula in psoriasis.

Identification of Major Components of LiangXueJieDu Formula

The total ion chromatograms of the LXJD formula extracted in both the positive and negative ion modes are shown in **Figure 3**. The MS data exhibited high precision with the mass accuracy within 5 ppm. Based on the MS spectra and fragmentation pattern using public databases (Chemspider and MassBank) or literature, 14 compounds were identified (**Table 1**). Chlorogenic acid, caffeic acid, paeoniflorin, taxifolin, astilbin, albiflorin, resveratrol, rosmarinic acid, 5-O-methylvisammioside, quercetin, naringenin, luteolin, kaempferol, and isorhamnetin were the main components of the LXJD formula extract, which was consistent with the systems pharmacology prediction. These results also demonstrated that the UPLC-MS method was suitable for identifying these compounds.

Effect of LiangXueJieDu Formula in Psoriasis Patients

After 8 weeks of treatment with LXJD formula, the skin symptoms of all patients improved. In addition, psoriasis area and severity index (PASI) scoring, a critical index to evaluate psoriasis in the clinic, decreased significantly ($p < 0.05$) following LXJD formula treatment (**Figures 4A,B** and **Table 2**).

Serum Metabolomics Study of Psoriasis Patients

Serum metabolic profiling of psoriasis patients was acquired to explore the protective effect of the LXJD formula. UPLC/Q-TOF-MS was applied for analysis. The quality-control (QC) sample was used to monitor the precision, repeatability, and reliability of the LC-MS measurements and peak intensity data (**Figures 4C,D**). These results indicated that methods were suitable for subsequent sample analysis. Principal component analysis (PCA) was employed to obtain unsupervized multivariate statistical analysis of serum metabolomics. In **Figures 4E,F**, serum metabolites in positive and negative ion modes were displayed by score plots, the cluster of psoriasis patients before LXJD formula treatment was clearly separated from those after 8 weeks of LXJD formula treatment in both modes. The OPLS-DA models were established to identify the discriminating ions contributing to the classification before and after LXJD formula treatment patients (**Figures 4G,H** and **Table 3**). The score plots based on the serum metabolomics of these two groups in positive and negative ion modes are shown in **Figures 4G,H**, the values of R^2X, R^2Y, and Q^2 were 0.557, 0.782, and 0.671 in the positive ion mode, 0.410, 0.852, and 0.453 in the negative ion mode, indicating the classification was well suited for the models. A total of 11 metabolites in the positive mode and seven metabolites in the negative mode were altered after LXJD formula treatment. These included cortisone (S1), L-urobilinogen (S2), PA[15:1(9Z)/22:4(7Z,10Z,13Z,16Z)] (S3), PC[18:0/18:4(6Z,9Z,12Z,15Z)] (S4), PC[18:1(9Z)/4:0] (S5), PC[20:0/14:1(9Z)] (S6), PC[20:4(8Z,11Z,14Z,17Z)/18:3(6Z,9Z,12Z)] (S7), PG[12:0/20:5(5Z,8Z,11Z,14Z,17Z)] (S8), PG[P-18:0/20:4(5Z,8Z,11Z,14Z)] (S9), phenyllactic acid (S10), traumatic acid (S11), 16-hydroxy hexadecanoic acid (S12), 4-hydroxybutanoic acid (S13), L-gamma-glutamyl-L-isoleucine (S14), MG[0:0/16:1(9Z)/0:0] (S15), PA[20:4(5Z,8Z,11Z,14Z)/18:4(6Z,9Z,12Z,15Z)] (S16), PG[20:3(8Z,11Z,14Z)/20:0] (S17), and PS[21:0/18:3(6Z,9Z,12Z)] (S18). To probe the associations between the key metabolic pathways and the regulatory effects of LXJD formula, metabolic pathway analysis (MetPA) (software of MetaboAnalyst 3.0; http://www.metaboanalyst.ca/) was performed by the integration of all serum potential metabolites. As a result, two disturbed metabolic pathways, glycerophospholipid metabolism and steroid hormone biosynthesis were considered as the most relevant pathways involved in psoriasis (**Figure 4I**). LXJD formula treatment improved both perturbed metabolic pathways.

LiangXueJieDu Formula Improved the Differentiation of Keratinocytes and Alleviated the Proliferation of Keratinocytes in an Establishment of Imiquimod-Induced Psoriasis-Like Mouse Model

To assess whether LXJD formula exerts therapeutic effects in a psoriasis mouse model, we applied IMQ on the shaved back skin of the animals for seven consecutive days. Subsequently, the skin developed typical erythema, scaling, and thickening. Consistent with the systems pharmacology analysis, mice treated with LXJD formula had smoother skin, less erythema, and sparser scales (**Figure 5A**). H&E staining of the skin lesion in the model group showed increased epidermal thickening, parakeratosis, and residual condensation of nuclei in the stratum corneum, representing typical characteristics of psoriasis-like skin lesions. These pathological features were ameliorated by LXJD formula (**Figures 5B,F**).

Loricrin is a keratinocyte differentiation marker that is mainly expressed in the cytoplasm and distributed throughout the stratum corneum of normal mouse skin. In the model group, low levels of loricrin indicated abnormal keratinocyte differentiation, which was reversed in animals treated with LXJD ($p < 0.01$) (**Figures 5D,H**). The expression of Ki-67, a marker strongly associated with cell proliferation and immune dysregulation (Alhosaini et al., 2021), was dramatically decreased in the LXJD-treated groups ($p < 0.01$) (**Figures 5E,I**), indicating that the IMQ-induced uncontrolled proliferation of basal keratinocytes was ameliorated.

TABLE 3 | Potential metabolites characterized in the serum profile and the altered trends in different groups.

NO.	Metabolites	VIP	m/z	Rt	*p*-value	Fold-change (B/A)
S1	Cortisone	1.025	360.1936	4.487	0.018	0.268
S2	L-Urobilinogen	1.111	596.3528	7.711	0.009	−0.854
S3	PA[15:1(9Z)/22:4(7Z,10Z,13Z,16Z)]	1.187	708.4561	3.832	0.005	−0.229
S4	PC[18:0/18:4(6Z,9Z,12Z,15Z)]	1.122	781.5589	10.116	0.008	0.899
S5	PC[18:1(9Z)/4:0]	1.075	591.3974	7.707	0.012	−0.672
S6	PC[20:0/14:1(9Z)]	1.070	759.5765	11.030	0.013	0.486
S7	PC(20:4[8Z,11Z,14Z,17Z)/18:3(6Z,9Z,12Z)]	1.103	803.5414	10.122	0.010	1.014
S8	PG[12:0/20:5(5Z,8Z,11Z,14Z,17Z)]	1.031	712.4401	8.479	0.017	−0.701
S9	PG[P-18:0/20:4(5Z,8Z,11Z,14Z)]	1.159	782.5629	10.828	0.006	0.650
S10	Phenyllactic acid	1.037	166.0626	4.306	0.016	0.633
S11	Traumatic acid	1.145	228.1364	6.101	0.007	−0.489
S12	16-hydroxy hexadecanoic acid	1.015	272.2349	7.480	0.019	−0.424
S13	4-hydroxybutanoic acid	1.106	104.0476	1.624	0.010	−0.694
S14	L-gamma-glutamyl-L-isoleucine	1.004	258.1369	5.235	0.021	−0.758
S15	MG[0:0/16:1(9Z)/0:0]	1.133	328.2605	11.324	0.008	−0.576
S16	PA[20:4(5Z,8Z,11Z,14Z)/18:4(6Z,9Z,12Z,15Z)]	1.043	716.4334	8.207	0.016	−0.756
S17	PG[20:3(8Z,11Z,14Z)/20:0]	1.030	828.5686	11.208	0.017	0.481
S18	PS[21:0/18:3(6Z,9Z,12Z)]	1.048	827.5646	11.112	0.015	0.508

Potential metabolites are characterized in the serum profile and their altered trends in different groups. Fold-change (B/A) represents the changing trend before and after LXJD formula treatment based on log 2 (B/A).

LiangXueJieDu Formula Inhibited T Cell Infiltration in an Establishment of Imiquimod-Induced Psoriasis-Like Mouse Model

We further examined the effect of LXJD formula on CD3+ T cell infiltration in the dermis. The control mice showed fewer CD3+ T cells in the dermis. The T cell infiltration in the dermis and epidermis was markedly higher in the model group than in the control group. On the other hand, LXJD and MTX groups showed reduced CD3+ T cell infiltration in the skin ($p < 0.01$) (**Figures 5C,G**).

LiangXueJieDu Formula Regulated the Expression of Inflammatory Cytokines and Factors in an Establishment of Imiquimod-Induced Psoriasis-Like Mouse Model

We determined the mRNA expression of several inflammatory cytokines and factors in the skin lesions and found that the levels of *Il1b*, *Il6*, *Tnfa*, *Cox2*, *Nos2*, and *Gsk3b* were significantly increased, while those of *Esr1* and *Pparg* mRNAs were suppressed in the lesions of the model group. Moreover, compared to the model group, the expression of *Il1b*, *Il6*, *Tnfa*, *Cox2*, *Nos2*, and *Gsk3b* mRNA declined in the LXJD group ($p < 0.01$ or $p < 0.05$), and that of *Esr1* and *Pparg* mRNAs reversed after LXJD formula administration ($p < 0.01$ or $p < 0.05$) (**Figure 6**).

LiangXueJieDu Formula Improved the Establishment of Imiquimod-Induced Psoriasis-Like Dysfunction Pathway

To further validate the prediction of systematic pharmacological analysis, we examined the effect of LXJD formula on key proteins in integrated psoriasis-related pathways, including MAPK, calcium, PI3K/AKT, and NF-κB signaling pathways using Western blot. IMQ application significantly increased the level of p-P65, p-IκB, p-ERK, p-P38, p-JNK, p-PI3K, p-AKT, and p-CAMKII in skin lesions. Compared to the model group, LXJD formula treatment remarkably inhibited the phosphorylation of p-P65, p-IκB, p-ERK, p-P38, p-PI3K, and p-AKT ($p < 0.01$ or $p < 0.05$), but showed a negligible inhibitory effect on p-JNK and p-CAMKII phosphorylation, indicating that LXJD formula exerts its therapeutic effect by inhibiting the MAPK, PI3K/AKT, and NF-κB signaling pathways to a large extent (**Figure 7**).

DISCUSSION

TCM has been used in clinical treatment in China for more than 2000 years and has accumulated a wealth of experience in the treatment of psoriasis. Our previous study has shown that the administration of LXJD formula in psoriasis vulgaris patients with blood-heat syndrome was associated with significantly better outcomes and a lower recurrence rate compared to standard Western medicine (cetirizine hydrochloride, vitamin C, and vitamin B complex) (Sun et al., 2020). However, bioactive ingredients with potential anti-psoriatic activities and specific targets have not yet been identified. TCM is a complex material system encompassing multiple active compounds, multiple targets of action, and related diseases; while it does not correspond to the theory of "single gene, single target, and single disease" (Lv et al., 2019). Therefore, exploring the targets and mechanism of LXJD formula in the treatment of psoriasis through a systems pharmacology method combined with a screening of active compounds, drug targets, and network analysis is essential.

In this study, we identified 144 compounds in the active fractions of LXJD formula using an *in silico* integrative model-ADME system with the following thresholds: OB ≥ 30%, DL ≥

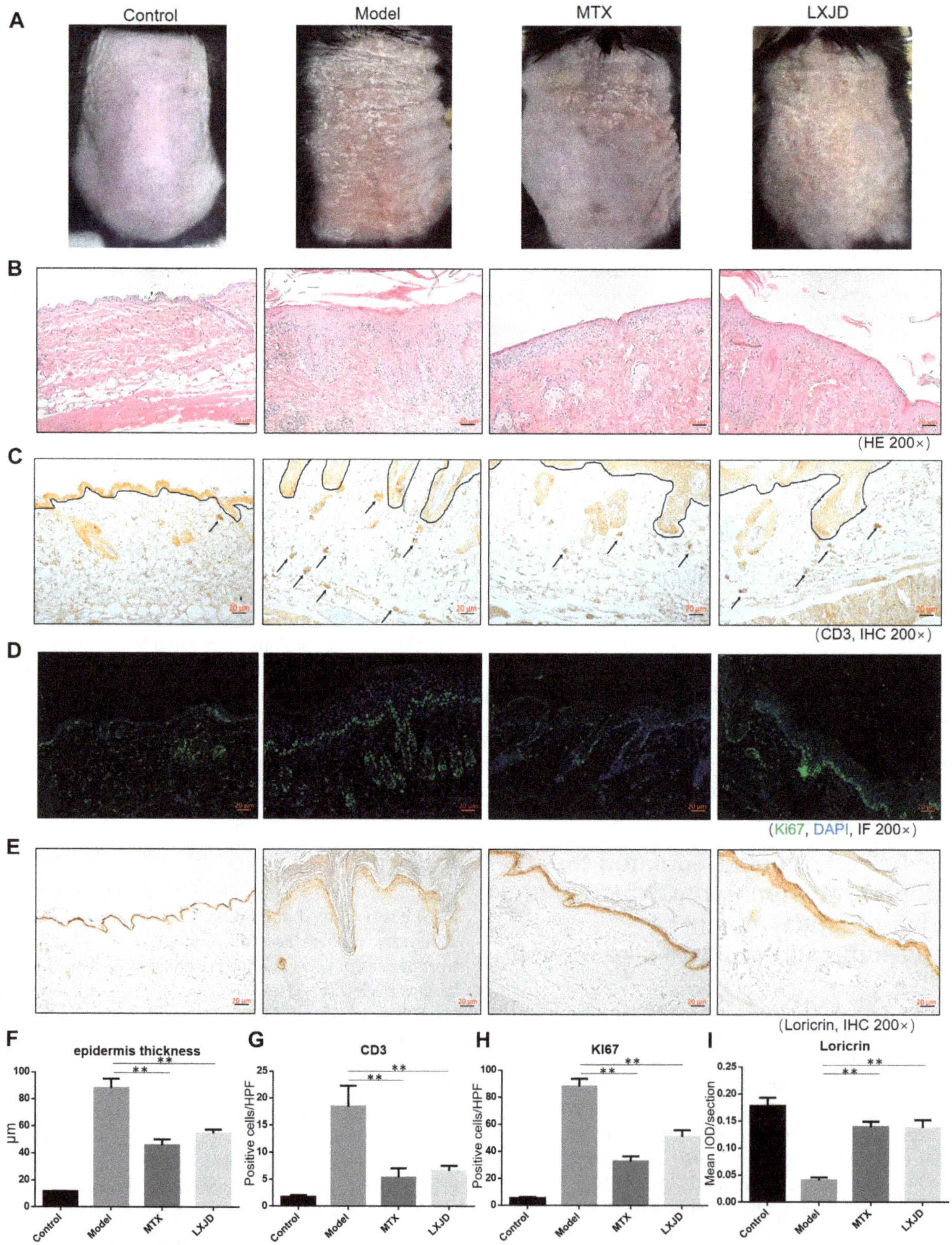

FIGURE 5 | C57 BL/6 mice were treated daily with IMQ cream on the shaved back skin to induced psoriasis-like dermatitis, while the control group (CTRL) was treated with matrix. The IMQ-treated mice were administered saline (model) [methotrexate (MTX) serves as a positive control] or LXJD formula for a total of 7 days. **(A)** Phenotypic presentation of the back skin on day 7 after IMQ treatment. **(B)** Histological analyses of mouse back skin by H&E staining. **(C)** Immunohistochemical staining of CD3+ cells in skin lesions. Mouse back skin was stained for Ki67 **(D)** and loricrin **(E)**. **(F–I)** Quantification analysis for epidermis thickness, CD3+ and Ki-67+, and loricrin was performed. Data are shown as mean ± SD. n = 5 mice. $^{*}p < 0.05$ and $^{**}p < 0.01$ vs. model group.

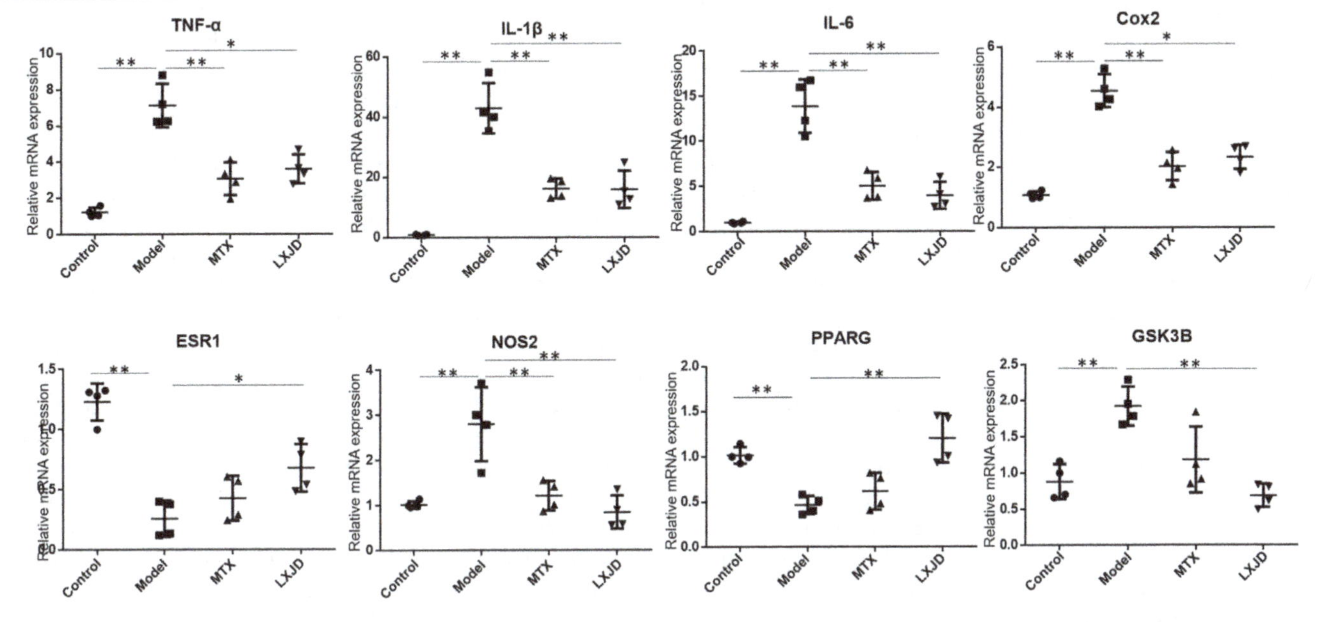

FIGURE 6 | The mRNA expression of key inflammatory cytokines and predicted genes in the skin lesion of the psoriasis-like mouse model. Values were normalized to β-actin and expressed relative to the control group. Data are shown as mean ± SD. n = 4 mice. *$p < 0.05$ and **$p < 0.01$ vs. model group.

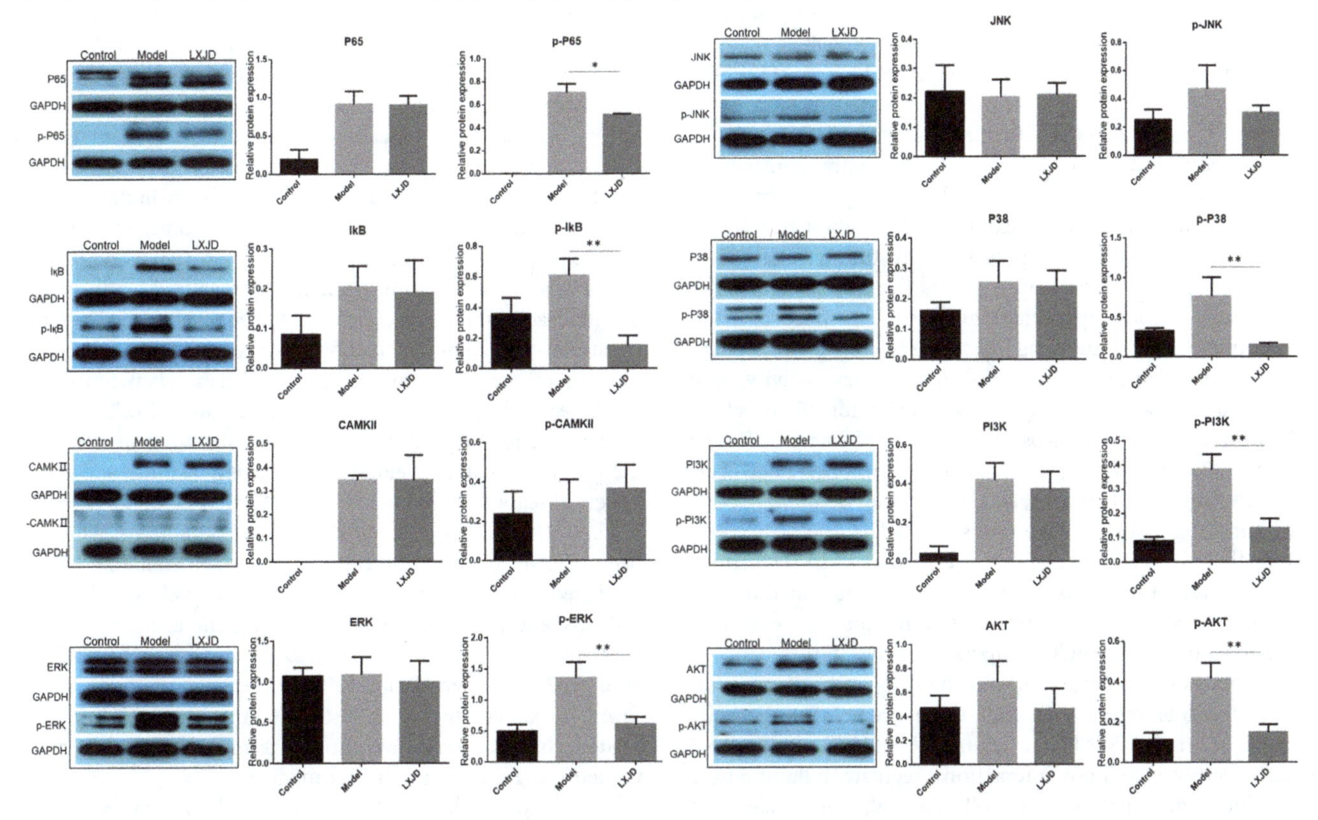

FIGURE 7 | Effects of LXJD formula on IMQ-induced psoriasis-like dysfunction pathway. Levels of P65, p-P65, IκB, p-IκB, CAMKII, p-CAMKII, ERK, p-ERK, P38, p-P38, JNK, p-JNK, PI3K, p-PI3K, AKT, and p-AKT proteins in skin lesions are detected by Western blot. Semiquantitative analysis was performed. *$p < 0.05$, **$p < 0.01$ indicating significant inhibition of LXJD as compared to model group. Data are shown as mean ± SD. n = 3 mice.

0.18, Caco-2 > -0.4, and AlogP <5. Subsequently, a final list of 125 potential targets for the 144 bioactive compounds was obtained by several integrated approaches, including the WES algorithm, TCMSP database, PharmGkb, Comparative Toxicogenomics database, and Therapeutic Targets database. These potential targets could be classified into the following subgroups: cytokines and chemokines, enzymes, signaling molecules, and transcription factors, and nuclear receptors. Most of these targets exhibited abnormal expression and were designated as the therapeutic targets in psoriasis, such as the cytokines and chemokines (IL-1β, IL-6, TNF, IFN-γ, CXCL8, CCL2). As expected, drugs targeting TNF-α have been applied in the clinic and have shown promising therapeutic effects on psoriasis (Chima and Lebwohl, 2018). Moreover, a total of 125 potential targets were significantly enriched as GO terms (BPs), including inflammatory response, cell proliferation, inflammatory response, NF-κB transcription factor activity, and cytokine production, which are strongly associated with the pathogenesis of psoriasis. Then, the compound-target network was constructed, showing complex interactions between 144 active compounds and 125 targets. Among these, ESR1 was the most common target of 113 compounds, constituting up to 77.1% of the total candidates. Reportedly, *ESR1* is the top-ranked hub gene, which is downregulated in psoriasis and related to anti-apoptotic functions (Zeng et al., 2016), deeming it as a potential therapeutic target for psoriasis. Consistently, our compound-target network indicated that the active compounds from LXJD formula could activate ESR1. Moreover, *IL1B* and *STAT3* were also reported as hub genes in psoriasis (Choudhary et al., 2020) and targets of LXJD formula. In this compound-target network, most of the active compounds were connected to multiple targets and exerted pharmacological effects. For example, quercetin exhibited the highest number of target interactions. Quercetin possesses anti-tumor activity (Xu et al., 2015) and anti-proliferative effects (Delgado et al., 2014); also, it is shown to have appreciable anti-psoriasis effects in IMQ-induced mice. The underlying mechanism might involve the improvement of antioxidant, anti-inflammatory activity, and inhibition on NF-κB signaling pathway activation (Chen et al., 2017). In addition, the anti-psoriasis effects of Paeonol (Meng et al., 2017), Baicalin (Hung et al., 2018), Paeoniflorin (Zhao et al., 2016), and Wogonin (Chi et al., 2003) have been demonstrated in an IMQ-induced psoriasis-like mouse model.

To further elucidate the complex mechanism of LXJD formula in the treatment of psoriasis, we established an integrated map of "psoriasis-related pathways" by integrating the key pathways obtained from the KEGG database using target-pathway network analysis. This map showed that the active compounds in LXJD formula interacting with these predicted targets are associated with the MAPK, calcium, PI3K/AKT, and NF-κB signaling pathways. These interactions regulate inflammation, cell proliferation, metabolism, cell survival, cell cycle, and immune response, and ultimately improve psoriasis.

Different complex diseases caused by the same disease gene exhibit overlapping protein-protein interactions and biological processes. Therefore, when a drug acts on the proteins associated with multiple diseases, it might show multiple therapeutic effects (Li et al., 2012). For example, peroxisome proliferator-activated receptor gamma (PPARG or PPAR-γ), a nuclear receptor, is one of the primary targets of LXJD formula, according to our compound-target network. PPAR-γ can bind to DNA and regulate the transcription of genes involved in lipid and glucose metabolism. Activation of PPAR-γ has favorable effects on adipocyte function, insulin sensitivity, lipoprotein metabolism, and vascular structure and function. PPAR-γ has been recognized as a therapeutic target in cardiovascular disease and diabetes mellitus. In addition, several studies demonstrated that PPAR-γ agonists may have antidepressant properties, open-label administration of the PPAR-γ agonist, pioglitazone, was associated with improvement in depressive symptoms and reduced cardiometabolic risk (Kemp et al., 2014). In the skin, PPAR-γ has a critical role in keratinocyte homeostasis, exhibiting pro-differentiation, antiproliferation, and immunomodulatory functions. The expression of PPAR-γ was reduced in a psoriasis hyperproliferative epidermis (Lima et al., 2013). Reportedly, diabetic patients treated with troglitazone (PPAR-γ agonist) showed substantial improvement in their psoriatic plaques (Pershadsingh et al., 1998). In addition to relieving the symptoms of patients with chronic psoriasis, this drug has modified the abnormal phenotype of transplanted psoriatic skin (Hanley et al., 1999). Furthermore, treatment with thiazolidinediones (PPAR-γ agonist) in patients with plaque psoriasis improved their cutaneous symptoms (Pershadsingh et al., 1998; Ellis et al., 2000). Based on the target-disease network, we could speculate that LXJD formula has potential pharmacological effects on immune system disease, endocrine system disease, skin disease, cardiovascular disease, metabolic disease, and mental disorder. Consistently, a previous study identified that psoriasis is not confined to skin impairment, and an increased morbidity of metabolic syndrome, cardiovascular disease, depression, and anxiety are also associated complications (Lima et al., 2013). Chronic inflammation caused by disorganized immune activation and correlated systemic abnormalities might underpin the common pathogenesis of psoriasis and related diseases. There is evidence that an imbalance between different T cells, e.g., T helper cells 17 (Th17) vs. regulatory T cells (Treg) and abnormal cytokine production are the driving forces in common for the progression and development of mental disorder and immune system disease (Ahmad et al., 2017; Ahmad et al., 2017; Bakheet et al., 2019; Ahmad et al., 2020). Many compounds, which have been shown to have promising effects in multiple immune-mediated inflammatory disorders such as asthma, rheumatoid arthritis, and alcoholic liver disease, have therapeutic potential in psoriatic inflammation as well (Alzahrani et al., 2019; Al-Harbi et al., 2020; Nadeem et al., 2020). Collectively, the herbs in LXJD formula exhibit efficacy in psoriasis treatment and in treating related complications, indicating that multiple diseases may be treated using a common herbal medicine.

Metabolomics data might provide useful information to explore the mechanisms underlying these associated diseases, especially metabolism disorders (Lee et al., 2003). Herein, we employed LC-MS to analyze psoriasis patients' serum metabolomics and investigate the metabolic changes associated with LXJD formula treatment. In concordance with the previous study, the elements of glycerophospholipid metabolism were significantly altered in the plasma of psoriatic patients (Zeng et al., 2017). The current metabolomics results indicated that glycerophospholipid metabolism involving 11 metabolites was significantly influenced in psoriasis patients according to MetPA, and the most influencing targets were related to the therapeutic intervention of LXJD formula against psoriasis. The compound-target network showed that PPAR-γ could be activated by LXJD formula. There is evidence that the PPAR-γ agonist could regulate glycerophospholipid metabolism (Tan et al., 2017), which is consistent with our metabolomics data showing that LXJD formula improved the perturbed metabolic pathways of glycerophospholipid metabolism. Based on this, we inferred that LXJD formula might regulate the glycerophospholipid metabolism through activating PPAR-γ. In addition, abnormalities in glycerophospholipid metabolism are the characteristics of diabetes mellitus (Xu et al., 2013). Dang et al. also revealed that the alteration of glycerophospholipid metabolism pathways is associated with atherosclerosis (Dang et al., 2016). Therefore, glycerophospholipid metabolism might be a drug target for psoriasis and related complications, including diabetes mellitus and atherosclerosis. LXJD formula could treat these associated diseases by regulating the altered metabolism.

Finally, we utilized an IMQ-induced psoriasis-like mouse model to validate the predicted targets and mechanisms of LXJD formula. In line with the current findings from systems pharmacology, LXJD formula could ameliorate psoriasis lesions, inhibit keratinocytes proliferation, improve keratinocytes differentiation, and suppress the infiltration of CD3+ T cells in an IMQ-induced psoriasis-like mouse model. This therapeutic effect was mediated by inhibiting the MAPK, PI3K/AKT, and NF-κB signaling pathways and reducing the subsequent release of inflammatory cytokines.

CONCLUSION AND LIMITATION

In conclusion, our systems pharmacological network identified active compounds and potential target proteins and elucidated the pharmacological mechanism of LXJD formula for the treatment of psoriasis and related diseases. These targets have been validated by our *in vivo* experiments. The metabolic changes associated with LXJD formula treatment adequately complemented the interaction between the Chinese herbal compounds and body metabolism, thereby revealing the underlying mechanism. These studies provided convincing evidence and a biological basis for LXJD formula in the treatment of psoriasis, contributing to its clinical application and generalization.

Certainly, there are still some limitations in our study. Even though LXJD formula has been proven as a safe treatment for psoriasis (Sun et al., 2020) and been used widely in China for decades, it still cause concerns about its toxicity due to different sources of herbs and different types of concoctions. In this animal study, no significant impact on body weight was found after LXJD formula treatment (data not shown). Nonetheless, further toxicity/safety evaluation studies need to be done in future. Components of Chinese herbal medicine are complicated, it is not clarified whether there are new intermediate metabolites or side effects caused by the interaction between compounds. We were not able to validate all of the 144 compounds in this formula by UPLC-MS analysis. Besides, a new intermediate metabolite might have an effect on psoriasis in a pre-clinical *in vivo* psoriasis model and/or human trial testing as well. We investigated the whole formula effect on a psoriasis-like animal model and corresponding predicted targets, but the effect of individual compounds on corresponding predicted targets remains unclear. Despite these potentially interesting associations, cautious interpretation and further validation tests are warranted.

Although further validation tests will be required to support deep assessments, the current study combining systems pharmacology, metabolomics, and experiment evaluation illustrated the correlation among active compounds, targets, and metabolism, contributing to the understanding of the mechanism of LXJD formula in the treatment of psoriasis.

AUTHOR CONTRIBUTIONS

This work includes significant contributions from all authors. JZ, YW, and PL conceived the study and designed the experiments. JZ and YW carried out the systems pharmacology analysis, JF identified the main components in the LXJD formula extract, YW, WC, and ZC performed the clinical study and metabolomics analysis. JZ, YL, TD, and CQ conducted animal experiments. JZ wrote the manuscript. YW and PL edited the manuscript. All authors read and approved the final manuscript.

REFERENCES

Ahmad, S. F., Ansari, M. A., Nadeem, A., Bakheet, S. A., Al-Ayadhi, L. Y., Alsaad, A. M. S., et al. (2020). Upregulation of Interleukin (IL)-31, a Cytokine Producing CXCR1 Peripheral Immune Cells, Contributes to the Immune Abnormalities of Autism Spectrum Disorder. *J. Neuroimmunology* 349, 577430. doi:10.1016/j.jneuroim.2020.577430

Ahmad, S. F., Nadeem, A., Ansari, M. A., Bakheet, S. A., Attia, S. M., Zoheir, K. M. A., et al. (2017). Imbalance between the Anti- and Pro-inflammatory Milieu in Blood Leukocytes of Autistic Children. *Mol. Immunol.* 82, 57–65. doi:10.1016/j.molimm.2016.12.019

Ahmad, S. F., Zoheir, K. M. A., Ansari, M. A., Nadeem, A., Bakheet, S. A., Al-Ayadhi, L. Y., et al. (2017). Dysregulation of Th1, Th2, Th17, and T Regulatory Cell-Related Transcription Factor Signaling in Children with Autism. *Mol. Neurobiol.* 54 (6), 4390–4400. doi:10.1007/s12035-016-9977-0

Al-Harbi, N. O., Nadeem, A., Ahmad, S. F., Bakheet, S. A., El-Sherbeeny, A. M., Ibrahim, K. E., et al. (2020). Therapeutic Treatment with Ibrutinib Attenuates Imiquimod-Induced Psoriasis-like Inflammation in Mice through Downregulation of Oxidative and Inflammatory Mediators in Neutrophils and Dendritic Cells. *Eur. J. Pharmacol.* 877, 173088. doi:10.1016/j.ejphar.2020.173088

Alhosaini, K., Ansari, M. A., Nadeem, A., Attia, S. M., Bakheet, S. A., Al-Ayadhi, L. Y., et al. (2021). Dysregulation of Ki-67 Expression in T Cells of Children with Autism Spectrum Disorder. *Children* 8 (2), 116. doi:10.3390/children8020116

Alzahrani, K. S., Nadeem, A., Ahmad, S. F., Al-Harbi, N. O., Ibrahim, K. E., El-Sherbeeny, A. M., et al. (2019). Inhibition of Spleen Tyrosine Kinase Attenuates Psoriasis-like Inflammation in Mice through Blockade of Dendritic Cell-Th17

Inflammation axis. *Biomed. Pharmacother.* 111, 347–358. doi:10.1016/j.biopha.2018.12.060

Bakheet, S. A., Ansari, M. A., Nadeem, A., Attia, S. M., Alhoshani, A. R., Gul, G., et al. (2019). CXCR3 Antagonist AMG487 Suppresses Rheumatoid Arthritis Pathogenesis and Progression by Shifting the Th17/Treg Cell Balance. *Cell Signal.* 64, 109395. doi:10.1016/j.cellsig.2019.109395

Ben-Arye, E., Ziv, M., Frenkel, M., Lavi, I., and Rosenman, D. (2003). Complementary Medicine and Psoriasis: Linking the Patient's Outlook with Evidence-Based Medicine. *Dermatology* 207 (3), 302–307. doi:10.1159/000073094

Chen, H., Lu, C., Liu, H., Wang, M., Zhao, H., Yan, Y., et al. (2017). Quercetin Ameliorates Imiquimod-Induced Psoriasis-like Skin Inflammation in Mice via the NF-Kb Pathway. *Int. Immunopharmacology* 48, 110–117. doi:10.1016/j.intimp.2017.04.022

Chi, Y. S., Lim, H., Park, H., and Kim, H. P. (2003). Effects of Wogonin, a Plant Flavone from Scutellaria Radix, on Skin Inflammation: *In Vivo* Regulation of Inflammation-Associated Gene Expression. *Biochem. Pharmacol.* 66 (7), 1271–1278. doi:10.1016/s0006-2952(03)00463-5

Chima, M., and Lebwohl, M. (2018). TNF Inhibitors for Psoriasis. *Sem Cutan. Med. Surg.* 37 (3), 134–142. doi:10.12788/j.sder.2018.039

Choudhary, S., Pradhan, D., Khan, N. S., Singh, H., Thomas, G., and Jain, A. K. (2020). Decoding Psoriasis: Integrated Bioinformatics Approach to Understand Hub Genes and Involved Pathways. *Cpd* 26, 3619–3630. doi:10.2174/1381612826666200311130133

Damevska, K., Neloska, L., Nikolovska, S., Gocev, G., and Duma, S. (2014). Complementary and Alternative Medicine Use Among Patients with Psoriasis. *Dermatol. Ther.* 27 (5), 281–283. doi:10.1111/dth.12139

Dang, V. T., Huang, A., Zhong, L. H., Shi, Y, and Werstuck, G. H, (2016). Comprehensive Plasma Metabolomic Analyses of Atherosclerotic Progression Reveal Alterations in Glycerophospholipid and Sphingolipid Metabolism in Apolipoprotein E-Deficient Mice. *Sci. Rep.* 6, 35037. doi:10.1038/srep35037

Delgado, L., Fernandes, I., González-Manzano, S., de Freitas, V., Mateus, N., and Santos-Buelga, C. (2014). Anti-proliferative Effects of Quercetin and Catechin Metabolites. *Food Funct.* 5 (4), 797–803. doi:10.1039/c3fo60441a

Dogra, N. K., Kumar, S., Thakur, K., and Kumar, D. (2018). Antipsoriatic Effect of Fatty Acid Enriched Fraction of Vernonia Anthelmintica Willd. Fruits. *J. Ethnopharmacology* 224, 85–90. doi:10.1016/j.jep.2018.05.038

Ellis, C. N., Varani, J., Fisher, G. J., Zeigler, M. E, Benson, S. C, Chi, Y, et al. (2000). Troglitazone Improves Psoriasis and Normalizes Models of Proliferative Skin Disease: Ligands for Peroxisome Proliferator-Activated Receptor-Gamma Inhibit Keratinocyte Proliferation. *Arch. Dermatol.* 136, 609–616. doi:10.1001/archderm.136.5.609

Gamret, A. C., Price, A., Fertig, R. M., Lev-Tov, H., and Nichols, A. J. (2018). Complementary and Alternative Medicine Therapies for Psoriasis. *JAMA Dermatol.* 154 (11), 1330–1337. doi:10.1001/jamadermatol.2018.2972

Hanley, K., Kömüves, L. G., Bass, N. M., He, S., Jiang, Y., Crumrine, D., et al. (1999). Fetal Epidermal Differentiation and Barrier Development *In Vivo* Is Accelerated by Nuclear Hormone Receptor Activators1. *J. Invest. Dermatol.* 113, 788–795. doi:10.1046/j.1523-1747.1999.00743.x

Heng, M. C. Y., Song, M. K., Harker, J., and Heng, M. K. (2000). Drug-induced Suppression of Phosphorylase Kinase Activity Correlates with Resolution of Psoriasis as Assessed by Clinical, Histological and Immunohistochemical Parameters. *Br. J. Dermatol.* 143 (5), 937–949. doi:10.1046/j.1365-2133.2000.03767.x

Hung, C.-H., Wang, C.-N., Cheng, H.-H., Liao, J.-W., Chen, Y.-T., Chao, Y.-W., et al. (2018). Baicalin Ameliorates Imiquimod-Induced Psoriasis-like Inflammation in Mice. *Planta Med.* 84 (15), 1110–1117. doi:10.1055/a-0622-8242

Kemp, D. E., Schinagle, M., Gao, K., Conroy, C., Ganocy, S. J., Ismail-Beigi, F., et al. (2014). PPAR-γ Agonism as a Modulator of Mood: Proof-Of-Concept for Pioglitazone in Bipolar Depression. *CNS Drugs* 28 (6), 571–581. doi:10.1007/s40263-014-0158-2

Kurd, S. K., Smith, N., VanVoorhees, A., Troxel, A. B., Badmaev, V., Seykora, J. T., et al. (2008). Oral Curcumin in the Treatment of Moderate to Severe Psoriasis Vulgaris: a Prospective Clinical Trial. *J. Am. Acad. Dermatol.* 58 (4), 625–631. doi:10.1016/j.jaad.2007.12.035

Lee, C.-H., Olson, P., and Evans, R. M. (2003). Minireview: Lipid Metabolism, Metabolic Diseases, and Peroxisome Proliferator-Activated Receptors. *Endocrinology* 144, 2201–2207. doi:10.1210/en.2003-0288

Li, X., Xu, X., Wang, J., Yu, H, Wang, X, Yang, H, et al. (2012). A System-Level Investigation into the Mechanisms of Chinese Traditional Medicine: Compound Danshen Formula for Cardiovascular Disease Treatment. *PLoS One* 7 (9), e43918. doi:10.1371/journal.pone.0043918

Lima, E. D. A., Lima, M. M. D. D. A., Marques, C. D. L., Duarte, A. L. B. P., Pita, I. D. R., and Pita, M. G. D. R., (2013). Peroxisome Proliferator-Activated Receptor Agonists (PPARs): a Promising prospect in the Treatment of Psoriasis and Psoriatic Arthritis. *Bras. Dermatol.* 88 (6), 1029–1035. doi:10.1590/abd1806-4841.20132653

Lipinski, C. A., Lombardo, F., Dominy, B. W., and Feeney, P. J, (2001). Experimental and Computational Approaches to Estimate Solubility and Permeability in Drug Discovery and Development Settings. *Adv. Drug Deliv. Rev.* 46 (1-3), 3–26. doi:10.1016/s0169-409x(00)00129-0

Liu, J., Mu, J., Zheng, C., Chen, X, Guo, Z, Huang, C, et al. (2016). Systems-Pharmacology Dissection of Traditional Chinese Medicine Compound Saffron Formula Reveals Multi-Scale Treatment Strategy for Cardiovascular Diseases. *Sci. Rep.* 6, 19809. doi:10.1038/srep19809

Lv, W. J., Liu, C., Li, Y. F., Chen, W-Q, Li, Z-Q, Li, Y, et al. (2019). Systems Pharmacology and Microbiome Dissection of Shen Ling Bai Zhu San Reveal Multiscale Treatment Strategy for IBD. *Oxid Med. Cel Longev* 2019, 8194804. doi:10.1155/2019/8194804

Ma, L., Chen, H., Dong, P., and Lu, X, (2013). Anti-inflammatory and Anticancer Activities of Extracts and Compounds from the Mushroom Inonotus Obliquus. *Food Chem.* 139 (1-4), 503–508. doi:10.1016/j.foodchem.2013.01.030

Meng, Y., Wang, M., Xie, X., Di, T., Zhao, J., Lin, Y., et al. (2017). Paeonol Ameliorates Imiquimod-Induced Psoriasis-like Skin Lesions in BALB/c Mice by Inhibiting the Maturation and Activation of Dendritic Cells. *Int. J. Mol. Med.* 39 (5), 1101–1110. doi:10.3892/ijmm.2017.2930

Mireku, E. A., Kusari, S., Eckelmann, D., Mensah, A. Y., Talontsi, F. M., and Spiteller, M. (2015). Anti-inflammatory Tirucallane Triterpenoids from Anopyxis Klaineana Pierre (Engl.), (Rhizophoraceae). *Fitoterapia* 106, 84–91. doi:10.1016/j.fitote.2015.08.007

Nadeem, A., Ahmad, S. F., Al-Harbi, N. O., El-Sherbeeny, A. M., Alasmari, A. F., Alanazi, W. A., et al. (2020). Bruton's Tyrosine Kinase Inhibitor Suppresses Imiquimod-Induced Psoriasis-like Inflammation in Mice through Regulation of IL-23/IL-17A in Innate Immune Cells. *Int. Immunopharmacology* 80, 106215. doi:10.1016/j.intimp.2020.106215

Pershadsingh, H. A., Sproul, J. A., Benjamin, E., Finnegan, J, and Amin, N. M (1998). Treatment of Psoriasis with Troglitazone Therapy. *Arch. Dermatol.* 134, 1304–1305. doi:10.1001/archderm.134.10.1304

Reiss, F., and Jaimovich, L. (1958). The Influence of Sitosterol upon Psoriasis Vulgaris. *Dermatology* 117 (5), 393–401. doi:10.1159/000255614

Ru, J., Li, P., Wang, J., Zhou, W, Li, B, Huang, C, et al. (2014). TCMSP: a Database of Systems Pharmacology for Drug Discovery from Herbal Medicines. *J. Cheminform* 6, 13. doi:10.1186/1758-2946-6-13

Srivastava, R. (2014). A Review on Phytochemical, Pharmacological, and Pharmacognostical Profile of Wrightia Tinctoria: Adulterant of Kurchi. *Phcog Rev.* 8 (15), 36–44. doi:10.4103/0973-7847.125528

Sun, L., Li, T., Zhou, D., Yang, X., Tian, J., Zhao, J., et al. (2020). "Efficacy and Safety of Liangxue Jiedu Decoction for the Treatment of Progressive Psoriasis Vulgaris: a Multicenter, Randomized, Controlled Study". *J. Tradit Chin. Med.* 40 (2), 296–304.

Talbott, W., and Duffy, N. (2015). Complementary and Alternative Medicine for Psoriasis: what the Dermatologist Needs to Know. *Am. J. Clin. Dermatol.* 16 (3), 147–165. doi:10.1007/s40257-015-0128-6

Tan, J., Wang, Y., Wang, S., Zhang, N., Wu, S., Yuan, Z., et al. (2017). Untargeted Metabolomics Analysis of Adipogenic Transformation in OP9-DL1 Cells Using Liquid Chromatography-Mass Spectrometry: Implications for Thymic Adipogenesis. *Cell Biol Int* 41 (4), 447–456. doi:10.1002/cbin.10740

Tetko, I. V., and Bruneau, P. (2004). Application of ALOGPS to Predict 1-octanol/water Distribution Coefficients, logP, and logD, of AstraZeneca In-house Database. *J. Pharm. Sci.* 93 (12), 3103–3110. doi:10.1002/jps.20217

Tsoukalas, D., Fragoulakis, V., Sarandi, E., Docea, A. O, Tsilimidos, G, Aschner, M, et al. (2019). Targeted Metabolomic Analysis of Serum Fatty Acids for the Prediction of Autoimmune Diseases. *Front. Mol. Biosci.* 6, 120. doi:10.3389/fmolb.2019.00120

World health organization (2016). *Global Report on Psoriasis*, 2016, 7–9.

Xu, F., Tavintharan, S., Sum, C. F., Woon, K., Lim, S. C., and Ong, C. N. (2013). Metabolic Signature Shift in Type 2 Diabetes Mellitus Revealed by Mass Spectrometry-Based Metabolomics. *J. Clin. Endocrinol. Metab.* 98 (6), E1060–E1065. doi:10.1210/jc.2012-4132

Xu, G., Shi, H., Ren, L., Gou, H., Gong, D., Gao, X., et al. (2015). Enhancing the Anti-colon Cancer Activity of Quercetin by Self-Assembled Micelles. *Int. J. Nanomedicine* 10, 2051–2063. doi:10.2147/IJN.S75550

Yalçin, B., Tezel, G. G., Arda, N., Erman, M., and Alli, N. (2007). Vascular Endothelial Growth Factor, Vascular Endothelial Growth Factor Receptor-3 and Cyclooxygenase-2 Expression in Psoriasis. *Anal. Quant Cytol. Histol.* 29 (6), 358–364.

Yuan, N., Gong, L., Tang, K., He, L, Hao, W, Li, X, et al. (2020). An Integrated Pharmacology-Based Analysis for Antidepressant Mechanism of Chinese Herbal Formula Xiao-Yao-San. *Front. Pharmacol.* 11, 284. doi:10.3389/fphar.2020.00284

Zeng, C. W., Wen, B., Hou, G. X., Lei, L, Jia, X, Chen, X, et al. (2017). Lipidomics Profiling Reveals the Role of Glycerophospholipid Metabolism in Psoriasis. *Gigascience* 6 (10), 1–11. doi:10.1093/gigascience/gix087

Zeng, X., Zhao, J., Wu, X., Shi, H., Liu, W., Cui, B., et al. (2016). PageRank Analysis Reveals Topologically Expressed Genes Correspond to Psoriasis and Their Functions Are Associated with Apoptosis Resistance. *Mol. Med. Rep.* 13 (5), 3969–3976. doi:10.3892/mmr.2016.4999

Zhang, G.-z., Wang, J.-S., Wang, P., Jiang, C.-Y., Deng, B.-X., Li, P., et al. (2009). Distribution and Development of the TCM Syndromes in Psoriasis Vulgaris. *J. Traditional Chin. Med.* 29 (3), 195–200. doi:10.1016/s0254-6272(09)60064-9

Zhao, J., Di, T., Wang, Y., Wang, Y., Liu, X., Liang, D., et al. (2016). Paeoniflorin Inhibits Imiquimod-Induced Psoriasis in Mice by Regulating Th17 Cell Response and Cytokine Secretion. *Eur. J. Pharmacol.* 772, 131–143. doi:10.1016/j.ejphar.2015.12.040

5

A Skin Lipidomics Study Reveals the Therapeutic Effects of Tanshinones in a Rat Model of Acne

Tingting Chen[1], Zhaoming Zhu[1], Qunqun Du[1], Zhuxian Wang[1], Wenfeng Wu[1], Yaqi Xue[1], Yuan Wang[1], Yufan Wu[1], Quanfu Zeng[1], Cuiping Jiang[1], Chunyan Shen[1], Li Liu[1], Hongxia Zhu[2] and Qiang Liu[1]**

[1]School of Traditional Chinese Medicine, Southern Medical University, Guangzhou, China, [2]Integrated Hospital of Traditional Chinese Medicine, Southern Medical University, Guangzhou, China

***Correspondence:**
Hongxia Zhu
gzzhx2012@163.com
Qiang Liu
liuqiang@smu.edu.cn

Tanshinone (TAN), a class of bioactive components in traditional Chinese medicinal plant Salvia miltiorrhiza, has antibacterial and anti-inflammatory effects, can enhance blood circulation, remove blood stasis, and promote wound healing. For these reasons it has been developed as a drug to treat acne. The purpose of this study was to evaluate the therapeutic effects of TAN in rats with oleic acid-induced acne and to explore its possible mechanisms of action through the identification of potential lipid biomarkers. In this study, a rat model of acne was established by applying 0.5 ml of 80% oleic acid to rats' back skin. The potential metabolites and targets involved in the anti-acne effects of TAN were predicted using lipidomics. The results indicate that TAN has therapeutic efficacy for acne, as supported by the results of the histological analyses and biochemical index assays for interleukin (IL)-8, IL-6, IL-β and tumor necrosis factor alpha. The orthogonal projection of latent structure discriminant analysis score was used to analyze the lipidomic profiles between control and acne rats. Ninety-six potential biomarkers were identified in the skin samples of the acne rats. These biomarkers were mainly related to glycerophospholipid and sphingolipid metabolism, and the regulation of their dysfunction is thought to be a possible therapeutic mechanism of action of TAN on acne.

Keywords: tanshinone, skin lipidomics, acne, glycerophospholipid metabolism, sphingolipid metabolism

INTRODUCTION

Salvia miltiorrhiza Bunge, a traditional Chinese medicine plant, was first recorded by Zhu Di in "Puji Fang" for acne treatment. Tanshinones (TANs), a class of chemical compounds and the major active component in *Salvia miltiorrhiza* Bunge, has also been reported as a treatment for cardiovascular disease (Weng et al., 2013; Maione et al., 2014; Maione et al., 2015; Jia et al., 2016). TAN has been recently shown to improve the condition of the facial skin by helping to reduce scarring through improving blood circulation and promoting cell metabolism (Li et al., 2016). Pharmacological studies show that cryptotanshinone has anti-acne effects (Yu et al., 2016) and Tanshinone IIA has an inhibitory effect on the growth of *Propionibacterium acnes* (Li and Zhou, 2018). In addition, TANs have exhibited anti-oxidant (Fang et al., 2008; Li et al., 2008; Li et al., 2013), anti-bacterial, anti-inflammatory (Bai et al., 2008; Tang et al., 2011; Chen et al., 2019), and anti-fibrosis (Jiang et al., 2019) effects. Furthermore, a recent report has found TAN to regulate tissue repair (Bernut et al., 2020). Consequently, TAN has been included in the research and development of cosmetic materials (Tao et al., 2013; Natshch et al., 2019).

Acne is one of the most common skin diseases and affects approximately 85% of the population at some point in their lifetimes (Thiboutot et al., 2018). Its pathogenesis is multifactorial and includes an increased level and sensitivity of androgen receptors (Barros and Thiboutot, 2017), excessive sebum secretion (Li et al., 2017), abnormal ductal keratosis of sebaceous glands in hair follicles (Das and Reynolds, 2014), and the colonization of *Propionibacterium acnes*, leading to an inflammatory response in the skin (Zouboulis, 2009). A pivotal factor in the aetiopathogenesis of acne is the quantitative and qualitative modification of skin lipids. Skin lipids play a significant role in the occurrence of acne lesions (Makrantonaki et al., 2011), as they can dramatically influence skin condition via different mechanisms, such as maintaining physical chemistry function, biochemistry function, and microecology function (Jia et al., 2018).

Lipidomics, a branch of metabonomics, is the study of the properties of all lipid molecules in living organisms (Han and Gross, 2003). It enables the analysis of lipids by quantifying changes in individual lipids, subgroups and molecular species. Liquid chromatography-mass spectrometry (LC-MS) is an analysis technique that allows for the comprehensive analysis of lipids and molecular types, including the lipids in lipid cells and keratinocytes (Kofeler et al., 2012; Zhao et al., 2014). In this study, changes in the lipidomic profile of the skin were analyzed using the ultra-performance liquid chromatography (UPLC)-Orbitrap MS system. Similar studies have been performed with respect to cancer, metabolic syndrome and skin diseases (Camera et al., 2016). UPLC-quadruple time-of-flight-MS is a high-resolution MS technique that can analyze the complete structure of a lipid species (van Smeden et al., 2014).

MATERIAL AND METHODS

Chemicals and Reagents

MS-grade methanol, MS-grade acetonitrile and high-performance liquid chromatography (HPLC)-grade 2-propanol were purchased from Thermo Fisher. HPLC-grade formic acid and HPLC-grade ammonium formate were purchased from Sigma. HPLC-grade acetonitrile was purchased from Merck KGaA (Darmstadt, Germany). Analytical-grade pure phosphoric acid was purchased from Guangzhou Chemical Reagent Factory. Reference standards of Tanshinone I, Crytotanshinone, Tanshinone IIA (purity >98%) were purchased from the National Institutes for Food and Drug Control (Beijing, China). Diydrotanshinone I (purity >98%) was purchased from Guangzhou Qiyun Biotechnology Co., Ltd. (Guangdong, China).

TAN and TAN Gel Preparation

TANs are major active components of the dried root of *Salvia miltiorrhiza* Bunge. The *Salvia miltiorrhiza* Bunge pieces were purchased from Guangzhou Weida Chinese Medicine Decoction Pieces Co. Ltd., (Guangdong, China), Batch number: 201909-3. TANs were extracted and isolated from the pieces through solvent extraction. First, the pieces were pulverized into smaller, coarse granules, weighed and refluxed in 95% ethanol (1:10 w/v) for three times, 2 h each time, and filtered (Shen et al., 2017b). The filtrates were combined, with ethanol removed by decompression, resulting in a thick, concentrated filtrate paste with relative density of 1.30–1.35 (60°C). This paste was washed in hot water until colorless, dried at 80°C, and crushed into a fine powder.

The TAN gel was produced by dissolving this powder in ethanol, adding carbomer, water and triethanolamine. The TAN gel (100 mg TAN in 1 g gel) was red-brown in color and transparent.

Qualitative and Quantitative Evaluation of TAN

The qualitative and quantitative analysis of TAN were used UHPLC-Orbitrap-MS instrument and HPLC with an UV detection system, respectively. The specific UHPLC-ESI-MS and HPLC methods used are included in the **Supplementary Material**.

Experimental Animals and Acne Model

All animal were approved by the Animal Care and Use committee of the Southern Medical University (Approval No. L2019036, Guangdong, China). Adult male Sprague Dawley rats (220 ± 20 g) were purchased from the Experimental Animals Center of Southern Medical University. The rats were housed at a humidity of 40–65%, a temperature of 19–23 °C and a 12 h light-dark cycle (Jiang et al., 2007).

The rats were allocated into experimental groups through a randomized block design. All experimental procedures and data analyses were conducted in a blinded fashion. After one week of acclimatization, the rats were randomly selected as control group (C, $n = 8$) or model group. The acne rat model was established by applying oleic acid. Briefly, rats were anesthetized using intraperitoneal injections of 3% sodium pentobarbital (Sigma-Aldrich, United States). Their back hair was depilated about 4 cm^2. 0.5 ml of 80% oleic acid (Aladdin Bio-Chem Technology, Shanghai, China) was applied to the back skin once daily for 14 days. Once the acne model was established, the acne rats were divided into the acne model group (M, $n = 8$) and the TAN gel administration group (T, $n = 8$) according to a random number control table. The rats in the TAN gel group received a dose of 1.0 g d^{-1} for 7 days. The rats in the Control and Model groups received no TAN gel treatment.

Histopathological Examination

Sections of skin tissues from the rats were fixed in 4% formalin, embedded in paraffin, and sliced into 3–5 μm thick sections. The sections were stained with hematoxylin-eosin for histopathological analysis and observed under a light microscope (BX53; Olympus).

Examination of Serum Inflammatory Factors

Serum samples were centrifuged and the supernatants assayed for cytokine release using the Cytokine RAT interleukin (IL)-8, IL-6,

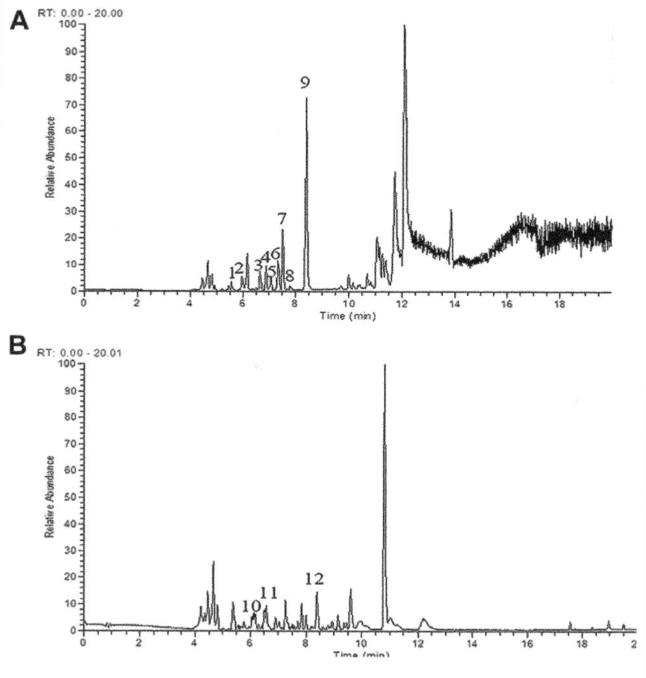

FIGURE 1 | UHPLC-Orbitrap-MS spectrometry of TAN. Positive(A): Salvia miltiorrhiza new quinone B (1), Tanshinaldehyde(2), Dihydrotanshinone I(3), Tanshinone IIB (4), dehydromiltirone (5), Tanshinone I(6), Cryptotanshinone (7), Methylenetanshinquinone (8), Tanshinone IIA (9), Negative(B):Danshin spiroketal lactone (10), Danshenxinkun A (11), Alpha-(3,4-dihydroxyphenyl)lactic acid (12).

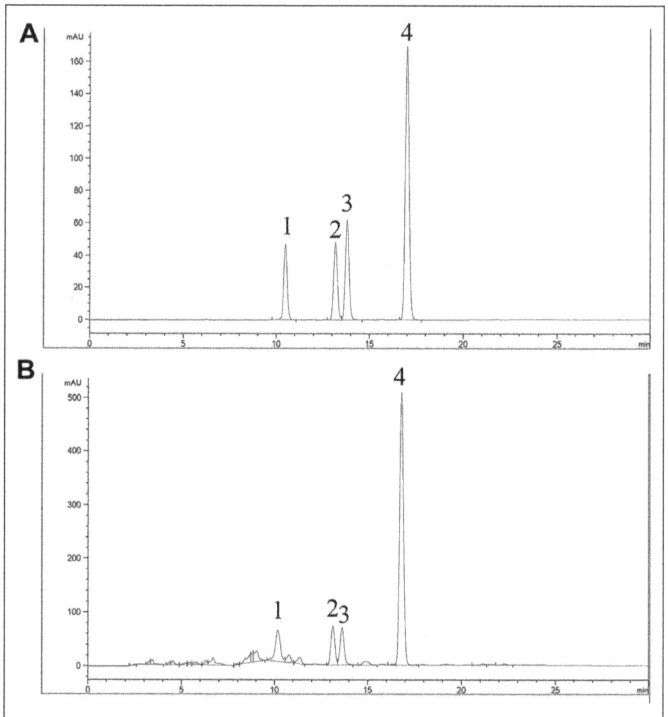

FIGURE 2 | High-performance liquid chromatography chromatogram of A:standard mixture of 1:Diydrotanshinone I, 2:Tanshinone I, 3: Crytotanshinone, 4: Tanshinone IIA, B:TAN sample.

IL-1β, and tumor necrosis factor alpha (TNF-α) Kit. The detection was conducted according to the kit manual (Shen et al., 2017a).

Lipid Extraction and Analysis

Lipids were extracted using the methyl tert-butyl ether (MTBE) method. Briefly, the skin samples were homogenized in 200 μl water and 240 μl methanol. MTBE (800 μl) was added to the homogenized sample, which was then ultrasonicated at 4°C for 20 min and afterward left to stand at room temperature for 30 min. The solution was centrifuged at 14,000 g at 10°C for 15 min, after which the upper layer was collected and dried with nitrogen. The lipid extracts were re-dissolved for analysis using 200 μl of a 90% isopropanol/acetonitrile mixture.

Q-Exactive Plus mass spectrometer (Thermo Fisher Scientific) was connected to an UHPLC Nexera LC-30A (SHIMADZU) via an electrospray ionization ion (ESI) source for the lipid analysis. The chromatographic conditions were shown in **Supplementary Material**.

Data Analysis and Presentation

"LipidSearch" was used to carry out peak recognition, peak extraction, and lipid identification (secondary identification) of the lipid molecules and internal standard lipid molecules. Both the precursor tolerance and product tolerance were set at 5 ppm, and the product ion threshold was set at 5%.

Simca 14.1 software (Umetrics AB, Umea, Sweden) was used for the multivariate analysis, including the principal component analysis (PCA) and orthogonal partial least-squares discrimination analysis (OPLS-DA) (Park et al., 2020). All lipid species and subclasses were found to have equal variances and were analyzed using variation multiple analysis and t-tests.

Statistical Analysis

The experimental data were expressed as mean ± standard deviation (S.D), unless otherwise stated. Statistical analyses were performed using SPSS statistics software version 21.0 (SPSS Inc. Chicago, United States). Comparison of the same parameter among groups was analyzed by one-way ANOVA. A value of $p < 0.05$ was considered to be statistically significant.

RESULTS

Quantitative Analysis and Qualitative Composition of TAN

UHPLC-Orbitrap-MS was used to characterize the chemical TAN composition. The total ion current chromatograms of the TAN are shown in **Figure 1**. Twelve major compounds were identified, including amounts of terpene like Salvia miltiorrhiza new quinone B, tanshinaldehyde, Dihydrotanshinone I, tanshinone IIB, dehydromiltirone, tanshinone I, cryptotanshinone, methylenetanshinquinone,

TABLE 1 | Linear range, regression equation, coefficient of determination (r^2) and amounts of marker compounds in TAN.

Compound	Linear range (μg/ml)	Regression equation	r^2	Amount (mg/g)	
				Mean	RSD (%)
Diydrotanshinone I	1.94–62.00	Y = 38.556X–2.2323	0.9999	33.6	1.08
Tanshinone I	3.13–100.00	Y = 38.377X–16.044	0.9996	27.8	0.06
Crytotanshinone	1.94–62.00	Y = 46.918X+18.035	0.9997	21.8	1.12
Tanshinone IIA	6.25–200.00	Y = 52.32X–16.816	0.9995	141.0	0.08

Y: peak area (mAU) of compounds; X: concentration (μg/ml) of compounds.

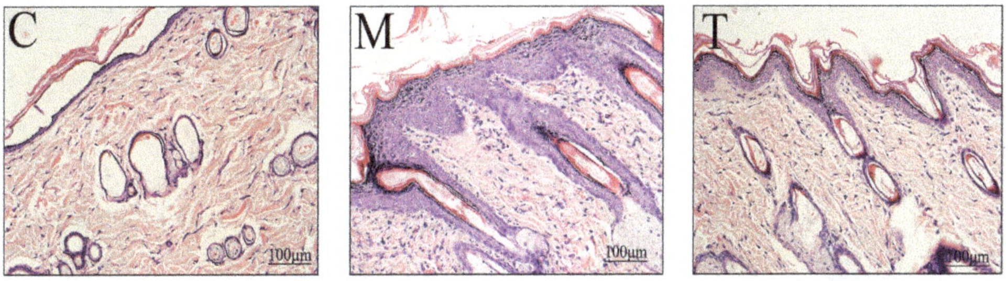

FIGURE 3 | Skin histopathology among the three treatment groups (hematoxylin-eosin, 200 × magnification). C: control rats; M: oleic acid-induced acne rats; T: oleic acid-induced acne + TAN-treated rats.

tanshinone IIA, Danshin spiroketal lactone, Danshenxinkun A and a phenolic acid alpha-(3,4-dihydroxyphenyl)lactic acid. Details of the TAN compounds detected are shown in **Supplementary Table S3**.

The TAN HPLC results are shown in **Figure 2** and **Table 1**. All components were clearly distinguished at the retention time of 30 min. Dihydrotanshinone, Tanshinone I, crytotanshinone, and Tanshinone IIA were marked as markers of TAN, and were defined as 33.6, 27.8, 21.8, and 141.0 mg in 1 g TAN, respectively.

Effect of TAN on Oleic Acid-Induced Acne in Rats

The histological results are presented in **Figure 3**. In the M group, acne-like lesions developed on the back skin. Histological analysis of the skin revealed hyperplasia of the stratified squamous epithelium, which was accompanied by significant thickening of the stratum corneum. In the M group, dermis hyperemia, inflammatory cell infiltration, and sebaceous gland size were significantly increased (**Figure 3A**). Excessive keratinization of hair follicle sebaceous glands, blocking hair follicle pores, and a key pathological mechanism of acne development, was observed. M rats treated with TAN (**Figure 3B**) exhibited skin tissue similar to that of C rats, with improved keratosis, reduced inflammatory cell infiltration, and smaller sebaceous glands (**Figure 3C**).

As illustrated in **Figure 4**, IL-8, IL-6, IL-β, and TNF-α expression were significantly higher in rats from the M group than the C and T groups ($p < 0.05$). The T group had similar serum cytokine levels to that of the C group, suggesting that TAN treatment was able to reverse high cytokine levels, present in the untreated M group, to levels exhibited by the C group ($p < 0.05$).

Effect of TAN on Skin Lipidomics in Rats With Oleic Acid-Induced Acne

According to the International Lipid Classification and Nomenclature Committee, lipid compounds can be divided into eight categories (Fahy et al., 2009). Each category can be sub-divided into different lipid classes based on polarity. Each class, based on differences in saturation or the length of the carbon chain, can be further subdivided into different molecular species (lipid species). Altogether, a three-level classification of lipid compounds is achieved. In this study, 28 lipid classes and 1,197 lipid species were identified. **Figure 5** shows the number of lipid species in each lipid class.

According to the LipidSearch analysis, a visual data matrix was generated and exported to Simca 14.1 software for multivariate data analysis. PCA revealed the lipid changes in the C group compared to the M group. The results are illustrated in the score plots of **Figures 6A,B**. The model parameter (R^2X), which indicates the explanatory power of a model, of **Figures 6A,B**, were 0.746 and 0.606, respectively.

OPLS-DA analysis demonstrated clear differentiation in lipidomic profiles between C and M groups as indicated in **Figure 6C** (R^2X = 0.609, R^2Y = 0.964, Q^2 = 0.924) and **Figure 6D** (R^2X = 0.670, R^2Y = 0.986, Q^2 = 0.895). Permutation testing and cross validation support this finding (**Figure 6**). **Table 2** lists the significantly different lipids.

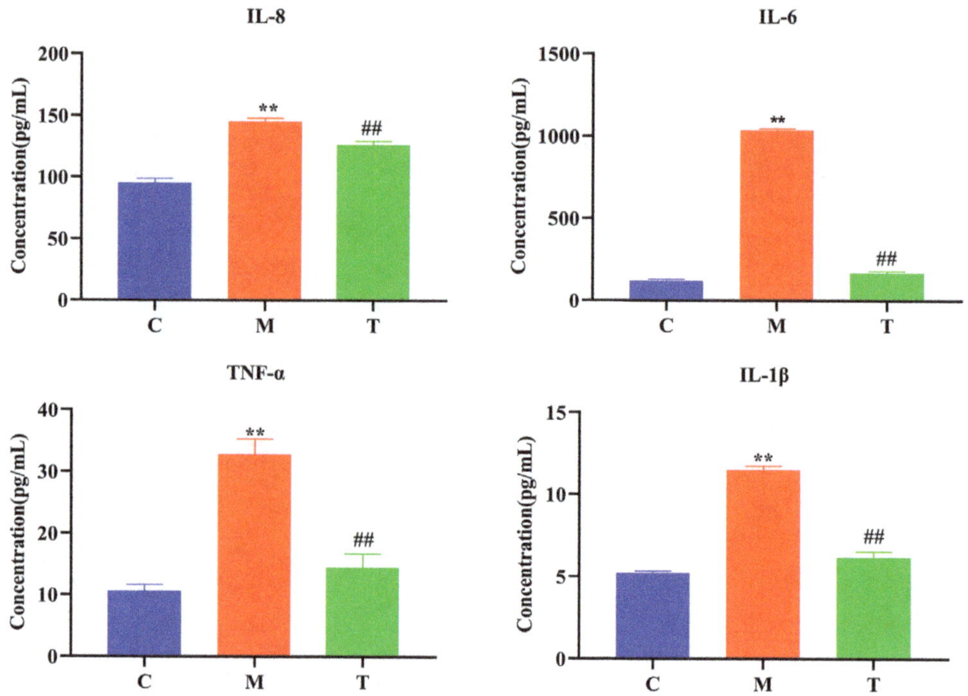

FIGURE 4 | Expression levels of the serum inflammatory factors interleukin (IL)-8, IL-6, IL-β, and tumor necrosis factor alpha (TNF-α) (**, $p < 0.01$ vs. C rats; ##, $p < 0.01$ vs. M rats).

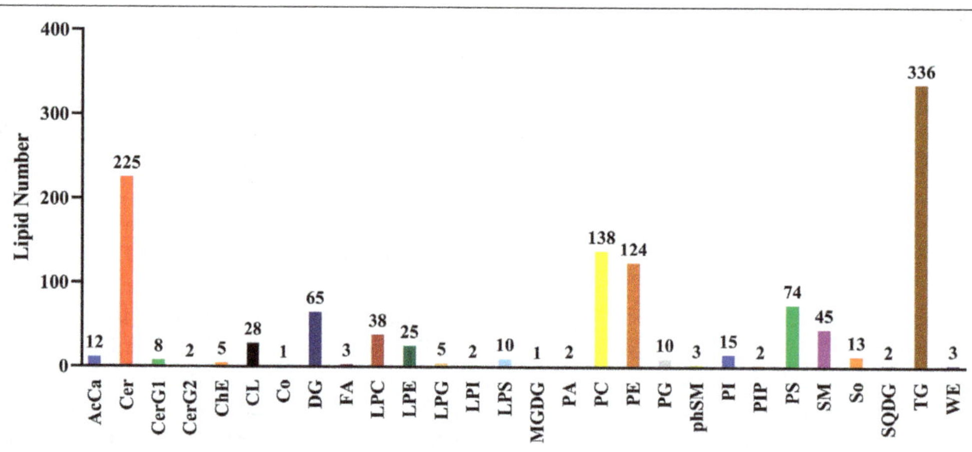

FIGURE 5 | The number of lipid species within each identified lipid class based on. the International Lipid Classification and Nomenclature Committee.

A total of 96 lipid species, 55 and 41 in positive and negative ion mode, respectively, were identified. In negative ion mode, the concentrations of 35 ceramides (Cers), 4 phosphatidylethanolamines (PEs), 1 lysophosphatidyl ethanolamine (LPE), and 1 fatty acid (FA) were significantly increased ($p < 0.05$) in the M group compared to the C group. In positive ion mode, the concentrations of 17 Cers, 2 acyl carnitines (AcCas), 5 diglycerides (DGs), 1 lysophosphatidylcholine (LPC), 1 So, and 9 triglycerides (TGs) were significantly increased, while the concentrations of 12 TGs were significantly decreased ($p < 0.05$), in the M group compared to the C group.

To further elucidate the metabolic differences between the C and M groups, the identified lipids were analyzed using a clustering heatmap. Significantly different lipids between M and C groups were considered to be potential biomarkers (**Figure** 7). The heatmap in **Figure 7** directly expresses the variability of each lipid species, and illustrates their relative increase (red) or decrease (blue) in M rats compared to the

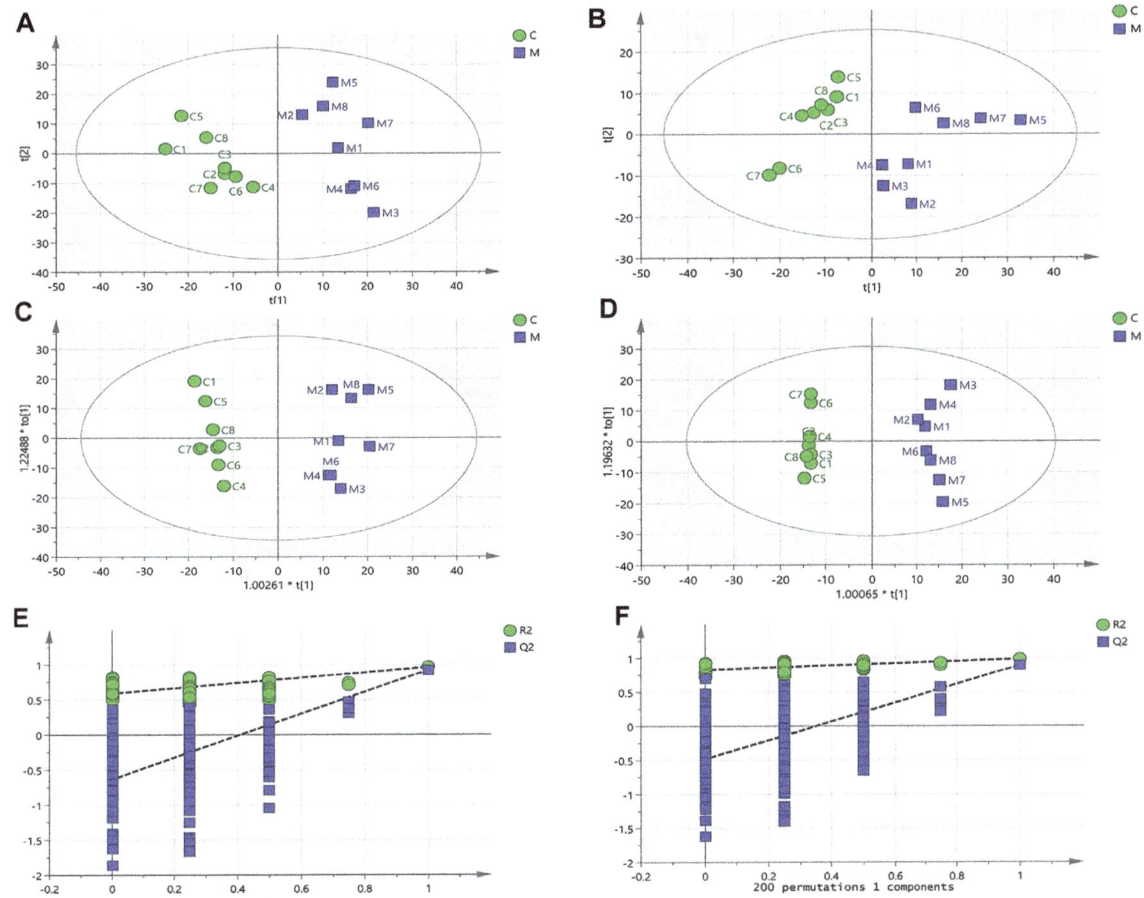

FIGURE 6 | Multivariate data analysis of skin lipidomics. **(A)** The principal component analysis (PCA) score plots from the skin lipid profiles of the C and M experimental groups in positive ion mode ($R^2X = 0.746$, Q2 = 0.531). **(B)** The PCA score plots from the skin lipid profiles of the C and M experimental groups in negative ion mode ($R^2X = 0.606$, Q2 = 0.405). **(C)** The orthogonal partial least-squares discrimination analysis (OPLS-DA) score plots from the skin lipid profiles of the C and M experimental groups in positive ion mode ($R^2X = 0.609$, $R^2Y = 0.964$, Q2 = 0.924). **(D)** The OPLS-DA score plots from the skin lipid profiles of the C and M experimental groups in negative ion mode ($R^2X = 0.670$, $R^2Y = 0.986$, Q2 = 0.895). **(E)** Permutation test of the lipid species from the OPLS-DA model in positive ion mode ($R^2 = 0.576$, Q2 = −0.623). **(F)** Permutation test of the lipid species from the OPLS-DA model in negative ion mode ($R^2 = 0.834$, Q2 = −0.580).

C and T groups, which leads us to postulate that TAN can improve the disease state as shown in **Figure 3**.

The lipid metabolism pathway analysis was performed using Metabolomics Pathway Analysis (MetPA) 5.0. A total of 96 identified metabolites were mapped to the Human Metabolome Database to obtain IDs to perform pathway enrichment analysis. The differential lipid species were analyzed using MetPA, and the results are shown in **Table 3**. Impact values >0.01 and p-values < 0.05 were considered as the screening conditions. **Figure 8** demonstrates that sphingolipid and glycerophospholipid metabolism had the highest impact factors.

DISCUSSION

The therapeutic effects of TAN on acne were observed in a rat model of oleic acid-induced acne. Our results indicated an upregulation of 84 lipid species and a downregulation 12 lipid species in M rats compared to C rats. This is in agreement with previous metabolome database reports of a dysregulation in lipid species, in particular sphingolipid and glycerophospholipid metabolism, as a sign of acne (Camera et al., 2016).

Change of Sphingolipid Metabolism

In this study, we found that Cer concentrations in the M group were increased, suggesting that Cers were more active in the M rats than those in the C group. Among them, concentrations of Cer(d42:1), Cer(34:0), and Cer(34:1), ultra-long chain Cers, were significantly increased. The altered Cer expression profiles may lead to decreased extracellular lipid matrix density and increased risk of exogenous invasion, which in turn stimulates the Th2/Th22 inflammatory response (Li et al., 2020). In addition, disturbed Cer expression profiles, and impaired barrier function, result in ongoing production of cytokines and chemokines, such as IL-1α, TNF-α, and β-defensins, that exacerbate the inflammatory response (Kanoh et al., 2019). In skin, Cers regulate the balance between keratinocyte proliferation

TABLE 2 | 96 identified potential biomarkers among the C, M and T.

Lipid species	m/z	Rt (min)	C VS M		M[a]	T[b]
			P	Log2FC		
Negative						
Cer(d18:1/34:2)	830.7607	19.32406	0.0000	5.0295	↑	↓
Cer(d18:1/24:0)	726.6253	13.20895	0.0000	4.9656	↑	↓
Cer(d18:0/20:0)	670.5627	11.234	0.0000	4.5779	↑	↓
Cer(d42:2)	708.6148	13.82625	0.0000	3.9576	↑	↓
Cer(d18:0/20:0)	656.5835	12.71269	0.0003	3.7028	↑	↓
Cer(d18:0/21:0)	670.5991	12.89282	0.0000	3.6849	↑	↓
Cer(d17:0/25:0)	710.6304	15.03509	0.0000	3.5645	↑	↓
Cer(d54:1)	878.8182	20.47176	0.0014	3.4766	↑	↓
Cer(d18:0/26:0)	740.6774	15.76791	0.0007	3.4186	↑	↓
Cer(d18:0/23:0)	698.6304	13.9686	0.0000	3.3660	↑	↓
Cer(d18:1/30:1)	776.7137	17.99825	0.0000	3.2814	↑	↓
Cer(d52:1)	850.7869	19.29828	0.0000	3.2581	↑	↓
Cer(d18:1/28:1)	748.6824	16.714	0.0000	3.1965	↑	↓
Cer(d72:3)	1157.043	22.55396	0.0000	3.0347	↑	↓
Cer(d18:1/18:0)	642.5314	10.19465	0.0000	3.0183	↑	↓
Cer(d18:0/34:1)	850.7869	19.77001	0.0000	2.9937	↑	↓
Cer(d52:2)	848.7713	19.07259	0.0000	2.9919	↑	↓
Cer(d56:2)	904.8339	21.00001	0.0008	2.7741	↑	↓
Cer(d18:0/36:3)	874.7869	19.13745	0.0003	2.7521	↑	↓
Cer(d18:1/24:1?	708.6148	12.65092	0.0000	2.7243	↑	↓
Cer(d38:1)	654.5678	11.708	0.0000	2.6137	↑	↓
Cer(d50:1)	822.7556	18.55095	0.0000	2.5725	↑	↓
Cer(d18:1/32:1)	804.745	19.2463	0.0000	2.5524	↑	↓
Cer(d18:0/34:2)	848.7713	18.67903	0.0003	2.5181	↑	↓
Cer(d70:3)	1129.011	22.0871	0.0000	2.3984	↑	↓
Cer(d56:2)	904.8339	21.35417	0.0000	2.3947	↑	↓
Cer(d18:1/16:0)	614.5001	9.02884	0.0000	2.3678	↑	↓
Cer(d57:2)	918.8495	21.47109	0.0030	2.3654	↑	↓
Cer(d18:0/34:4)	844.74	16.90961	0.0008	2.3121	↑	↓
Cer(d16:1/26:1)	708.6148	12.9112	0.0000	2.2731	↑	↓
Cer(d18:1/18:0)	626.5365	10.70592	0.0000	2.1982	↑	↓
Cer(d59:3)	944.8652	21.84285	0.0035	2.0980	↑	↓
Cer(d55:2)	890.8182	20.85184	0.0000	2.0728	↑	↓
Cer(d60:4)	956.8652	21.56007	0.0001	2.0672	↑	↓
Cer(d18:0)	820.74	17.66335	0.0003	2.0053	↑	↓
FA (20:5)	301.2173	2.033	0.0049	2.5654	↑	↓
LPE (20:0)	508.3409	5.446,271	0.0000	2.0328	↑	↓
PE (16:1/18:2)	712.4923	7.434,218	0.0001	2.9635	↑	↓
PE (18:0/18:2)	742.5392	9.448,973	0.0004	2.5266	↑	↓
PE (24:2/18:2)	822.6018	12.57836	0.0000	2.0977	↑	↓
PE (36:5)	736.4923	7.194,899	0.0100	2.0491	↑	↓
Positive						
DG (15:0)	348.2745	1.3521	0.0000	6.6497	↑	↓
AcCa(20:4)	448.3421	2.1250	0.0000	2.3769	↑	↓
AcCa(18:2)	424.3421	2.1920	0.0001	2.2946	↑	↓
Cer(d18:1/24:0)	666.6395	14.8970	0.0000	3.7160	↑	↓
Cer(d36:1)	566.5507	13.2694	0.0000	3.5810	↑	↓
Cer(d40:1)	622.6133	15.5625	0.0001	3.3591	↑	↓
Cer(d18:0/24:0)	668.6551	14.7050	0.0016	3.2196	↑	↓
Cer(d18:0/16:0)	572.5249	10.1544	0.0000	3.0980	↑	↓
Cer(d18:1/54:0)	1101.088	24.5525	0.0000	3.0138	↑	↓
Cer(d18:1/16:1)	552.4986	8.8579	0.0000	2.6150	↑	↓
Cer(d50:1)	794.7596	13.5360	0.0000	2.5911	↑	↓
Cer(d18:1/24:0)	666.6395	13.7101	0.0000	2.5894	↑	↓
Cer(d34:1)	538.5194	12.2471	0.0002	2.5210	↑	↓
Cer(d50:2)	776.749	14.0652	0.0000	2.4725	↑	↓
Cer(d18:1/56:0)	1129.12	24.8739	0.0000	2.4222	↑	↓
Cer(d18:0/22:0)	640.6238	13.6112	0.0000	2.3973	↑	↓
Cer(d18:0/17:0)	586.5405	10.6643	0.0015	2.2800	↑	↓
Cer(d18:2/51:2)	1052.994	22.1339	0.0000	2.2269	↑	↓
Cer(d44:1)	678.6759	17.9162	0.0001	2.0399	↑	↓
Cer(d18:1/26:0)	694.6708	14.8389	0.0000	2.0371	↑	↓

(Continued on following page)

TABLE 2 | *(Continued)* 96 identified potential biomarkers among the C, M and T.

Lipid species	m/z	Rt (min)	C VS M		M[a]	T[b]
			P	Log2FC		
DG (36:2p)	622.5769	13.3210	0.0001	2.5883	↑	↓
DG (22:0/18:2)	694.6344	15.5480	0.0000	2.5602	↑	↓
DG (24:0/18:2)	722.6657	16.7877	0.0000	2.4717	↑	↓
DG (24:1/18:2)	720.6501	15.4434	0.0000	2.0170	↑	↓
LPC(24:0)	608.465	9.0185	0.0000	2.2503	↑	↓
So(d18:0)	302.3054	2.6342	0.0000	3.4427	↑	↓
TG (30:1/20:0/22:4)	1151.068	25.0762	0.0001	3.2637	↑	↓
TG (26:1/24:1/24:2)	1181.114	25.6011	0.0001	2.8942	↑	↓
TG (30:1/18:1/22:3)	1123.036	24.7924	0.0000	2.8787	↑	↓
TG (67:4)	1083.005	21.1760	0.0000	2.8079	↑	↓
TG (30:1/22:2/24:1)	1209.146	25.8468	0.0001	2.7197	↑	↓
TG (30:1/18:2/24:1)	1153.083	25.3393	0.0002	2.6218	↑	↓
TG (30:1/24:1/24:2)	1237.177	26.0781	0.0002	2.2441	↑	↓
TG (24:0/20:4/24:1)	1095.005	24.4620	0.0000	2.1535	↑	↓
TG (30:1/18:2/22:1)	1125.052	25.0774	0.0003	2.0958	↑	↓
TG (16:0/12:1/18:2)	790.6919	16.9359	0.0001	−2.0249	↑	↓
TG (15:0/16:0/16:1)	808.7389	19.7909	0.0002	−2.0465	↑	↓
TG (16:0/14:0/18:3)	818.7232	18.1460	0.0001	−2.0516	↑	↓
TG (8:0/8:0/24:1)	710.6293	14.7050	0.0066	−2.0949	↑	↓
TG (4:0/16:0/18:0)	684.6137	15.8794	0.0019	−2.0951	↑	↓
TG (15:0/16:0/16:0)	810.7545	20.7548	0.0001	−2.1094	↑	↓
TG (6:0/16:0/16:0)	684.6137	15.5811	0.0033	−2.1311	↑	↓
TG (16:0/8:0/18:1)	738.6606	16.7619	0.0003	−2.1414	↑	↓
TG (16:0/16:1/18:2)	846.7545	19.3644	0.0001	−2.1634	↓	↑
TG (16:0/14:0/16:0)	796.7389	20.3731	0.0001	−2.1929	↓	↑
TG (16:0/12:1/16:0)	766.6919	18.3072	0.0003	−2.1941	↓	↑
TG (8:0/18:1/18:2)	762.6606	15.7967	0.0019	−2.2486	↓	↑
TG (6:0/18:1/18:2)	734.6293	14.7557	0.0006	−2.2570	↓	↑
TG (16:0/12:1/16:0)	766.6919	17.9574	0.0002	−2.2812	↓	↑
TG (16:0/14:1/16:0)	794.7232	19.1828	0.0002	−2.3662	↓	↑
TG (4:0/16:0/16:0)	656.5824	14.6726	0.0038	−2.4827	↓	↑
TG (16:0/14:0/18:1)	822.7545	20.3946	0.0001	−2.4857	↓	↑
TG (6:0/16:0/16:1)	682.598	14.6957	0.0031	−2.6041	↓	↑
TG (6:0/16:0/18:1)	710.6293	15.6969	0.0024	−2.8806	↓	↑
TG (4:0/16:0/16:1)	654.5667	13.5966	0.0007	−3.6163	↓	↑

(↑):Upregulated ($p < 0.05$, n = 8) (↓): Downregulated ($p < 0.05$, n = 8).
[a]*Trends of the M group compared with the C group of the metabolites.*
[b]*Trends of the T group compared with the M group of the metabolites.*

and differentiation by exerting anti-proliferative and pro-apoptotic effects. Increased Cer synthesis, along with increased rates of keratinocyte differentiation, have been detected *in vitro* and *in vivo* models (Mizutani et al., 2013). We postulate that these increases may lead to corneum thickening in the M group, compared to the C and T groups. The role of Cers and its derivatives in regulating immune responses has been extensively studied. Cers are considered bioactive transmitters that are involved in various inflammatory signaling pathways. Further research is needed to determine whether extracellular Cer accumulating in the lipid matrix of the stratum corneum is also involved in inflammation and the immune response in acne. Notably, Cers can be broken down by ceramidase to produce sphingosine and FAs.

Change of Glyceride Metabolism

DGs are secreted by sebaceous glands and help maintain skin barrier stability. DGs are also second messengers involved in the inflammatory response (Grkovich and Dennis, 2009). TGs are formed by the combination of DGs and FAs by glyceryl diesteryl transferase. TGs on the skin surface can be degraded by resident skin bacteria to generate DGs and free FAs (Camera et al., 2016). DGs result from the hydrolysis of TGs. In this study, variations in DG and TG differential metabolites in M compared to C and T groups indicates their dysregulation, suggesting another area of investigation for acne treatment.

The synthesis of TGs *in vivo* involves two main pathways: monoglycerol and diglycerol synthesis. TGs are hydrolyzed into glycerol and FAs by a series of lipases, which then undergo β-oxidation for absorption and use by the body. TG hydrolysis requires catalysis by hormone-sensitive lipases which exist in two main forms: short- and long-chain forms. The short-chain form is mainly expressed in adipose tissue and catalyzes the hydrolysis of TGs into FAs. The long-chain form is expressed in steroidal tissues, such as the testes, and hydrolyzes cholesterol esters into free cholesterol, which is then converted, by a series of enzymatic reactions, into androgens and estrogens.

In this study, 29 different TG compounds were identified, with 58.6% were found in significantly higher concentrations in C rats compared to M rats. However, according to the TG-

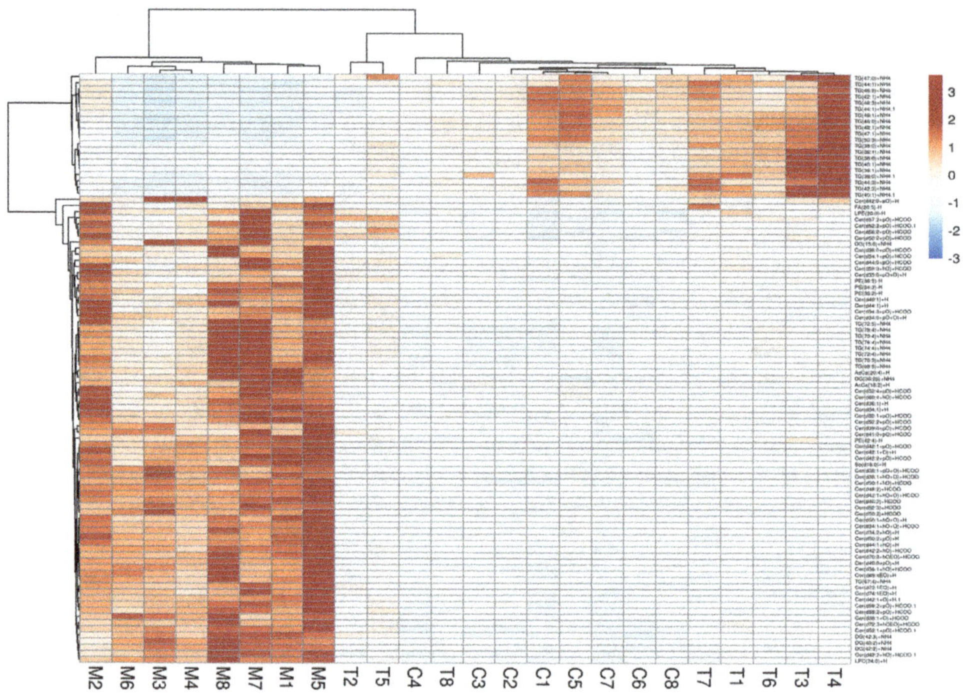

FIGURE 7 | Heatmap of 96 lipid species among the experimental groups. Each line of this graph represents an accurate mass ordered by the retention time and is colored by its abundance intensity. The scale from −3 blue (low) to + 3 red (high) represents the abundance.

TABLE 3 | Ingenuity pathway analysis with MetPA from differential lipid species.

Pathway name	Match status	*P*	−log(p)	Holm p	FDR	Impact	KEGG
Sphingolipid metabolism	2/21	0.0026767	2.5724	0.22484	0.22484	0.42394	00600
Glycerophospholipid metabolism	2/36	0.0078181	2.1069	0.6489	0.32836	0.12185	00564
Glycosylphosphatidylinositol (GPI)-anchor biosynthesis	1/14	0.054479	1.2638	1.0	1.0	0.00399	00563
Glycerolipid metabolism	1/16	0.062056	1.2072	1.0	1.0	0.01402	00561

omics analysis, TGs had fewer differential metabolites, with an inconsistent variation trend, in contrast to the DG results. The enzymes catalyzing TG hydrolysis may therefore be dysfunctional in the M rats. For glycerolipids, TG accumulation in non-adipose tissue is associated with lipid toxicity (Liu et al., 2012). In the M group, abnormal fat infiltration was observed, which could have contributed to increased lipid toxicity and acne initiation in those rats.

Change of Fatty Acid Metabolism

FAs are the most basic unit and metabolite of lipid metabolism; its structure and intracellular concentrations have important implications for lipid metabolism in cells. In our study, it was found that DGs and FAs exhibited a uniform increasing or decreasing trend in model group rats.

In biological systems, carnitine can combine with FAs to form AcCa, which promotes the transport of FAs to the mitochondrial intima for fatty acid β-oxidation.

Change of Glycerylphospholipid Metabolism

Glycerylphospholipids, such as phosphatidylcholine (PC), PE, LPC, lysophosphatidic acid (LPA), and LPE, are components of all cell membranes. Typical phospholipid molecules consist of hydrophilic phosphate heads and two lipophilic (hydrophobic) fatty chains. These lipids induce intracellular signal transduction by activating G-protein-coupled receptors on the cell membrane. Consequently, they play important biological functions in embryogenesis, cell proliferation, lymphocyte homing, and the inflammation-induced immune response. The lipid biomarkers obtained in this study were mainly from the LPC, PE, and LPE subgroups.

LPC is produced by phospholipase A2-mediated hydrolysis of PC, as depicted in **Figure 8**. LPC is a biologically active lipid that can be produced under pathological conditions. It is an amphoteric molecule that functions as both a surfactant and a detergent. LPC content is regulated to maintain proper cellular activity, as it easily damages cells at high concentrations; for example, through weakening the integrity of monocytes and smooth muscle cells. As a member of the stain remover

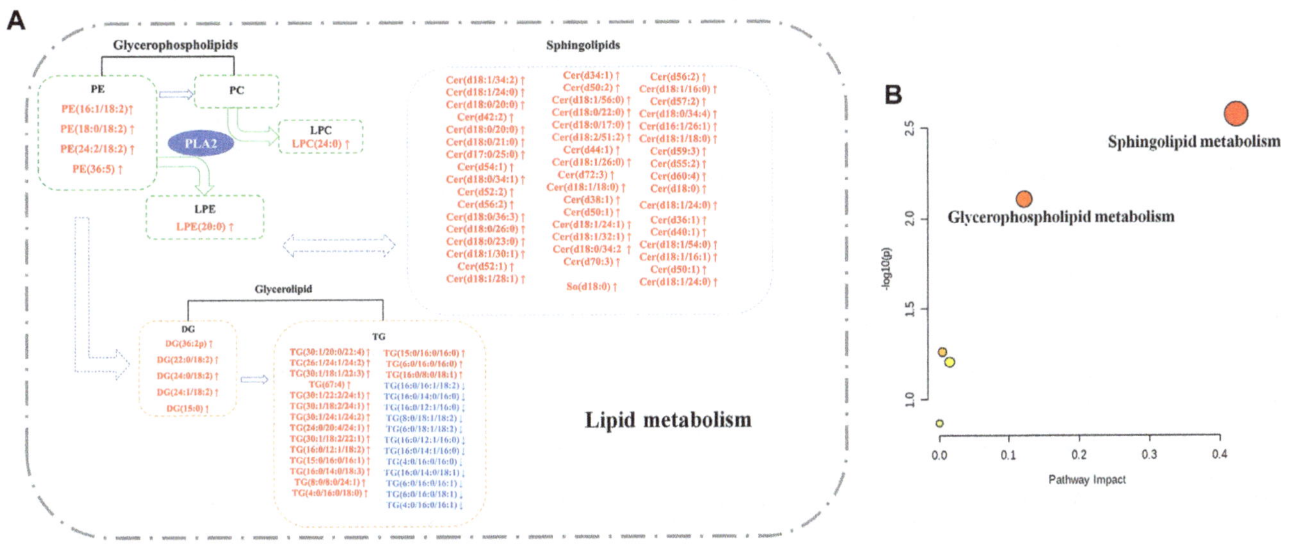

FIGURE 8 | Lipid metabolic pathway analysis of identified differential lipid species. **(A)** The network of potential biomarker variation in M rats compared to C rats in Lipid Metabolism. Red (↑): upregulation; Blue (↓): downregulation. **(B)** The Metabolomics Pathway Analysis identified sphingolipid metabolism, glycerophospholipid metabolism, and linoleic acid metabolism from the significantly differential lipid species. The size and color of each circle are based on pathway impact values and *p*-values, respectively.

family, LPC can cause cell lysis at higher concentrations, while at lower concentrations can change membrane permeability. LPC has been found to injure endothelial cells in the human umbilical vein. Moreover, it has also been reported to be involved in various pathological conditions such as diabetes, obesity, atherosclerosis, and cancer (Kabarowski et al., 2005). We therefore postulate that this would be a new biomarker to promote the occurrence of acne.

In the heathly human body, activated ethanolamine combines with DGs to produce PE. LPE is a metabolite generated by the enzymatic hydrolysis of PE by phospholipase A1. The PE-LPE metabolic pathway is involved in various cellular metabolic pathways (Shirvan et al., 2017). These aforementioned phospholipids play a role in several metabolic pathways in the body, including those involving the metabolism of glycerolipids, arachidonic acids, linoleic acids, α-linoleic acids; integrative metabolism; and the retrograde endocannabinoid signaling pathway. During phospholipid synthesis and metabolism, lipid metabolites are produced *via* the action of enzymes. Under normal physiological conditions, the amount of these lipid metabolites is regulated, but under an inflammatory state, they can aggregate and produce pathological effects. Many lipid metabolites are also biologically active secondary messengers and, in many cases, are associated with the onset of disease. The pathways involved in glycerolipid metabolism imply that LPCs, PEs, and LPEs can be converted into one another, as illustrated in **Figure 8**. In conclusion, we speculate that the uncontrolled lipid species can be a warning signal of acne.

CONCLUSION

To summarize, using lipidomic analysis, this study identified 96 different lipid species from the sphingolipid and glycerophospholipid metabolism pathways in an oleic acid-induced acne model. Our results suggest that TAN may effectively treat acne by regulating the metabolism of lipids, such as phospholipids and sphingolipids. In addition, lipidomics may be useful in investigating the effects, and explaining possible mechanisms of action, of other traditional medicinal plants on skin diseases.

AUTHOR CONTRIBUTIONS

Conceptualization, Funding acquisition, and Supervision: QL, HZ; Data curation: TC, ZZ; tanshinones extract of Salvia miltiorrhiza: YWa, QD; HPLC analysis: YX, ZW; Animal experiment: ZZ, TC, and WW; Investigation: YWu, QZ; Methodology: CJ, CS, and LL; Visualization and Writing—original draft: TC, ZZ; Writing-original draft preparation: ZZ, TC; Writing-review editing: TC, QL, and HZ.

REFERENCES

Bai, A., Lu, N., Guo, Y., and Fan, X. (2008). Tanshinone IIA Ameliorates Trinitrobenzene Sulfonic Acid (TNBS)-induced Murine Colitis. *Dig. Dis. Sci.* 53 (2), 421–428. doi:10.1007/s10620-007-9863-8

Barros, B., and Thiboutot, D. (2017). Hormonal Therapies for Acne. *Clin. Dermatol.* 35 (2), 168–172. doi:10.1016/j.clindermatol.2016.10.009

Bernut, A., Loynes, C. A., Floto, R. A., and Renshaw, S. A. (2020). Deletion ofcftrLeads to an Excessive Neutrophilic Response and Defective Tissue Repair in a Zebrafish Model of Sterile Inflammation. *Front. Immunol.* 11, 1733. doi:10.3389/fimmu.2020.01733

Camera, E., Ludovici, M., Tortorella, S., Sinagra, J.-L., Capitanio, B., Goracci, L., et al. (2016). Use of Lipidomics to Investigate Sebum Dysfunction in Juvenile Acne. *J. Lipid Res.* 57 (6), 1051–1058. doi:10.1194/jlr.M067942

Chen, Z., Gao, X., Jiao, Y., Qiu, Y., Wang, A. L., Yu, M. L., et al. (2019). Tanshinone

IIA Exerts Anti-Inflammatory and Immune-Regulating Effects on Vulnerable Atherosclerotic Plaque Partially via the TLR4/MyD88/NF-Kappa B Signal Pathway. *Front. Pharmacol.* 10, 850. doi:10.3389/fphar.2019.00850

Das, S., and Reynolds, R. V. (2014). Recent Advances in Acne Pathogenesis: Implications for Therapy. *Am. J. Clin. Dermatol.* 15 (6), 479–488. doi:10.1007/s40257-014-0099-z

Fahy, E., Subramaniam, S., Murphy, R. C., Nishijima, M., Raetz, C. R. H., Shimizu, T., et al. (2009). Update of the LIPID MAPS Comprehensive Classification System for Lipids. *J. Lipid Res.* 50, S9–S14. doi:10.1194/jlr.R800095-JLR200

Fang, Z. Y., Lin, R., Yuan, B. X., Yang, G.-D., Liu, Y., and Zhang, H. (2008). Tanshinone IIA Downregulates the CD40 Expression and Decreases MMP-2 Activity on Atherosclerosis Induced by High Fatty Diet in Rabbit. *J. Ethnopharmacol.* 115 (2), 217–222. doi:10.1016/j.jep.2007.09.025

Grkovich, A., and Dennis, E. A. (2009). Phosphatidic Acid Phosphohydrolase in the Regulation of Inflammatory Signaling. *Adv. Enzyme Regul.* 49 (1), 114–120. doi:10.1016/j.advenzreg.2009.01.005

Han, X., and Gross, R. W. (2003). Global Analyses of Cellular Lipidomes Directly from Crude Extracts of Biological Samples by ESI Mass Spectrometry: a Bridge to Lipidomics. *J. Lipid Res.* 44 (6), 1071–1079. doi:10.1194/jlr.R300004-JLR200

Jia, L., Song, N., Yang, G., Ma, Y., Li, X., Lu, R., et al. (2016). Effects of Tanshinone IIA on the Modulation of miR-33a and the SREBP-2/Pcsk9 Signaling Pathway in Hyperlipidemic Rats. *Mol. Med. Rep.* 13 (6), 4627–4635. doi:10.3892/mmr.2016.5133

Jia, Y., Gan, Y., He, C., Chen, Z., and Zhou, C. (2018). The Mechanism of Skin Lipids Influencing Skin Status. *J. Dermatol. Sci.* 89 (2), 112–119. doi:10.1016/j.jdermsci.2017.11.006

Jiang, J.-G., Huang, X.-J., Chen, J., and Lin, Q.-S. (2007). Comparison of the Sedative and Hypnotic Effects of Flavonoids, Saponins, and Polysaccharides Extracted from Semen Ziziphus Jujube. *Nat. Product. Res.* 21 (4), 310–320. doi:10.1080/14786410701192827

Jiang, Y., Hu, F. F., Li, Q., Shen, C., Yang, J., and Li, M. (2019). Tanshinone IIA Ameliorates the Bleomycin-Induced Endothelial-To-Mesenchymal Transition via the Akt/mTOR/p70S6K Pathway in a Murine Model of Systemic Sclerosis. *Int. Immunopharmacol.* 77, 105968. doi:10.1016/j.intimp.2019.105968

Kabarowski, J. H. S., Zhu, K., Le, L. Q., Witte, O. N., and Xu, Y. (2005). Lysophosphatidylcholine as a Ligand for the Immunoregulatory Receptor G2A (Retraction of Vol 293, Pg 702, 2001). *Science* 307 (5707), 206. doi:10.1126/science.307.5707.206b

Kanoh, H., Ishitsuka, A., Fujine, E., Matsuhaba, S., Nakamura, M., Ito, H., et al. (2019). IFN-gamma Reduces Epidermal Barrier Function by Affecting Fatty Acid Composition of Ceramide in a Mouse Atopic Dermatitis Model. *J. Immunol. Res.* 2019, 3030268. doi:10.1155/2019/3030268

Köfeler, H. C., Fauland, A., Rechberger, G. N., and Trötzmüller, M. (2012). Mass Spectrometry Based Lipidomics: an Overview of Technological Platforms. *Metabolites* 2 (1), 19–38. doi:10.3390/metabo2010019

Li, Y. F., and Zhou, Y. L. (2018). The Therapeutic Effect of Tanshinone IIA on Propionibacterium Acnes-Induced Inflammation *In Vitro*. *Dermatol. Ther.* 31 (6), e12716. doi:10.1111/dth.12716

Li, Y. I., Elmer, G., and LeBoeuf, R. C. (2008). Tanshinone IIA Reduces Macrophage Death Induced by Hydrogen Peroxide by Upregulating Glutathione Peroxidase. *Life Sci.* 83 (15-16), 557–562. doi:10.1016/j.lfs.2008.08.003

Li, W.-J., Kong, S.-Z., Luo, H., Jia, Z.-B., and Cheng, Y. (2013). Electrochemical and Spectroelectrochemical Studies of Four Tanshinones from Salvia Miltiorrhiza Bunge. *Chin. Chem. Lett.* 24 (12), 1145–1147. doi:10.1016/j.cclet.2013.08.003

Li, Y., Shi, S., Gao, J., Han, S., Wu, X., Jia, Y., et al. (2016). Cryptotanshinone Downregulates the Profibrotic Activities of Hypertrophic Scar Fibroblasts and Accelerates Wound Healing: A Potential Therapy for the Reduction of Skin Scarring. *Biomed. Pharmacother.* 80, 80–86. doi:10.1016/j.biopha.2016.03.006

Li, X., He, C., Chen, Z., Zhou, C., Gan, Y., and Jia, Y. (2017). A Review of the Role of Sebum in the Mechanism of Acne Pathogenesis. *J. Cosmet. Dermatol.* 16 (2), 168–173. doi:10.1111/jocd.12345

Li, Q., Fang, H., Dang, E., and Wang, G. (2020). The Role of Ceramides in Skin Homeostasis and Inflammatory Skin Diseases. *J. Dermatol. Sci.* 97 (1), 2–8. doi:10.1016/j.jdermsci.2019.12.002

Liu, L., Yu, S., Khan, R. S., Homma, S., Schulze, P. C., Blaner, W. S., et al. (2012). Diacylglycerol Acyl Transferase 1 Overexpression Detoxifies Cardiac Lipids in PPARγ Transgenic Mice. *J. Lipid Res.* 53 (8), 1482–1492. doi:10.1194/jlr.M024208

Maione, F., De Feo, V., Caiazzo, E., De Martino, L., Cicala, C., and Mascolo, N. (2014). Tanshinone IIA, a Major Component of Salvia Milthorriza Bunge, Inhibits Platelet Activation via Erk-2 Signaling Pathway. *J. Ethnopharmacol.* 155 (2), 1236–1242. doi:10.1016/j.jep.2014.07.010

Maione, F., Cantone, V., Chini, M. G., De Feo, V., Mascolo, N., and Bifulco, G. (2015). Molecular Mechanism of Tanshinone IIA and Cryptotanshinone in Platelet Anti-aggregating Effects: an Integrated Study of Pharmacology and Computational Analysis. *Fitoterapia* 100, 174–178. doi:10.1016/j.fitote.2014.11.024

Makrantonaki, E., Ganceviciene, R., and Zouboulis, C. C. (2011). An Update on the Role of the Sebaceous Gland in the Pathogenesis of Acne. *Dermato-Endocrinol.* 3 (1), 41–49. doi:10.4161/derm.3.1.13900

Mizutani, Y., Sun, H., Ohno, Y., Sassa, T., Wakashima, T., Obara, M., et al. (2013). Cooperative Synthesis of Ultra Long-Chain Fatty Acid and Ceramide during Keratinocyte Differentiation. *Plos One* 8 (6), e67317. doi:10.1371/journal.pone.0067317

Natshch, H., Vettorato, E., and Touitou, E. (2019). Ethosomes for Dermal Administration of Natural Active Molecules. *Curr. Pharm. Des.* 25 (21), 2338–2348. doi:10.2174/1381612825666190716095826

Park, S. H., Lee, J. E., Lee, S. M., Lee, J., Seo, C. S., Hwang, G. S., et al. (2020). An Unbiased Lipidomics Approach Identifies Key Lipid Molecules as Potential Therapeutic Targets of Dohongsamul-Tang against Non-alcoholic Fatty Liver Diseases in a Mouse Model of Obesity. *J. Ethnopharmacol.* 260, 112999. doi:10.1016/j.jep.2020.112999

Shen, C. Y., Jiang, J. G., Li, M. Q., Zheng, C. Y., and Zhu, W. (2017a). Structural Characterization and Immunomodulatory Activity of Novel Polysaccharides from Citrus Aurantium Linn. Variant Amara Engl. *J. Funct. Foods* 35, 352–362. doi:10.1016/j.jff.2017.05.055

Shen, C. Y., Zhang, W. L., and Jiang, J. G. (2017b). Immune-enhancing Activity of Polysaccharides from Hibiscus sabdariffa Linn. Via MAPK and NF-kB Signaling Pathways in RAW264.7 Cells. *J. Funct. Foods* 34, 118–129. doi:10.1016/j.jff.2017.03.060

Parande Shirvan, S., Ebrahimby, A., Dousty, A., Maleki, M., Movassaghi, A., Borji, H., et al. (2017). Somatic Extracts of Marshallagia Marshalli Downregulate the Th2 Associated Immune Responses in Ovalbumin-Induced Airway Inflammation in BALB/c Mice. *Parasit. Vectors* 10, 233. doi:10.1186/s13071-017-2159-8

Tang, S., Shen, X.-Y., Huang, H.-Q., Xu, S.-W., Yu, Y., Zhou, C.-H., et al. (2011). Cryptotanshinone Suppressed Inflammatory Cytokines Secretion in RAW264.7 Macrophages through Inhibition of the NF-Kb and MAPK Signaling Pathways. *Inflammation* 34 (2), 111–118. doi:10.1007/s10753-010-9214-3

Tao, S., Justiniano, R., Zhang, D. D., and Wondrak, G. T. (2013). The Nrf2-Inducers Tanshinone I and Dihydrotanshinone Protect Human Skin Cells and Reconstructed Human Skin against Solar Simulated UV. *Redox. Biol.* 1 (1), 532–541. doi:10.1016/j.redox.2013.10.004

Thiboutot, D. M., Dréno, B., Abanmi, A., Alexis, A. F., Araviiskaia, E., Barona Cabal, M. I., et al. (2018). Practical Management of Acne for Clinicians: An International Consensus from the Global Alliance to Improve Outcomes in Acne. *J. Am. Acad. Dermatol.* 78 (2), S1–S23. doi:10.1016/j.jaad.2017.09.078

van Smeden, J., Janssens, M., Kaye, E. C. J., Caspers, P. J., Lavrijsen, A. P., Vreeken, R. J., et al. (2014). The Importance of Free Fatty Acid Chain Length for the Skin Barrier Function in Atopic Eczema Patients. *Exp. Dermatol.* 23 (1), 45–52. doi:10.1111/exd.12293

Weng, Y.-S., Kuo, W.-W., Lin, Y.-M., Kuo, C.-H., Tzang, B.-S., Tsai, F.-J., et al. (2013). Danshen Mediates through Estrogen Receptors to Activate Akt and Inhibit Apoptosis Effect of Leu27IGF-II-Induced IGF-II Receptor Signaling Activation in Cardiomyoblasts. *Food Chem. Toxicol.* 56, 28–39. doi:10.1016/j.fct.2013.01.008

Yu, Z. W., Lv, H. Y., Han, G., and Ma, K. (2016). Ethosomes Loaded with Cryptotanshinone for Acne Treatment through Topical Gel Formulation. *Plos One*, 11, e0159967. doi:10.1371/journal.pone.0159967

Zhao, Y.-Y., Wu, S.-P., Liu, S., Zhang, Y., and Lin, R.-C. (2014). Ultra-performance Liquid Chromatography-Mass Spectrometry as a Sensitive and Powerful Technology in Lipidomic Applications. *Chem. Biol. Interact.* 220, 181–192. doi:10.1016/j.cbi.2014.06.029

Zouboulis, C. C. (2009). Propionibacterium Acnes and Sebaceous Lipogenesis: A Love-Hate Relationship? *J. Invest. Dermatol.* 129 (9), 2093–2096. doi:10.1038/jid.2009.190

6

Hyaluronic Acid-Mediated Drug Delivery System Targeting for Inflammatory Skin Diseases

Kang Nien How[1], Wei Hsum Yap[2], Calvin Lai Hock Lim[2], Bey Hing Goh[3,4] and Zee Wei Lai[2]*

[1] Dermatology Unit, Faculty of Medicine and Health Sciences, Universiti Putra Malaysia, Serdang, Malaysia, [2] Faculty of Medical and Health Sciences, School of Biosciences, Taylor's University, Subang Jaya, Malaysia, [3] College of Pharmaceutical Sciences, Zhejiang University, Hangzhou, China, [4] Biofunctional Molecule Exploratory Research Group (BMEX), School of Pharmacy, Monash University Malaysia, Bandar Sunway, Malaysia

***Correspondence:**
Zee Wei Lai
zeewei.lai@taylors.edu.my

Hyaluronic acid (HA), a major component of extracellular matrix has been widely applied in pharmaceutical and cosmetic industries due to its reported pharmacological properties. Various types of HA drug delivery system including nanoparticles, cryogel-based formulations, microneedle patches, and nano-emulsions were developed. There are studies reporting that several HA-based transdermal delivery systems exhibit excellent biocompatibility, enhanced permeability and efficient localized release of anti-psoriasis drugs and have shown to inhibit psoriasis-associated skin inflammation. Similarly HA is found in abundant at epidermis of atopic dermatitis (AD) suggesting its role in atopic AD pathology. Anti-allergenic effect of atopic eczema can be achieved through the inhibition of CD44 and protein kinase C alpha (PKCα) interaction by HA. Herein, we aim to evaluate the current innovation on HA drug delivery system and the other potential applications of HA in inflammatory skin diseases, focusing on atopic dermatitis and psoriasis. HA is typically integrated into different delivery systems including nanoparticles, liposomes, ethosomes and microneedle patches in supporting drug penetration through the stratum corneum layer of the skin. For instance, ethosomes and microneedle delivery system such as curcumin-loaded HA-modified ethosomes were developed to enhance skin retention and delivery of curcumin to CD44-expressing psoriatic cells whereas methotrexate-loaded HA-based microneedle was shown to enhance skin penetration of methotrexate to alleviate psoriasis-like skin inflammation. HA-based nanoparticles and pluronic F-127 based dual responsive (pH/temperature) hydrogels had been described to enhance drug permeation through and into the intact skin for AD treatment.

Keywords: hyaluronic acid, inflammatory skin diseases, psoriasis, atopic dermatitis, drug delivery, CD44 receptor

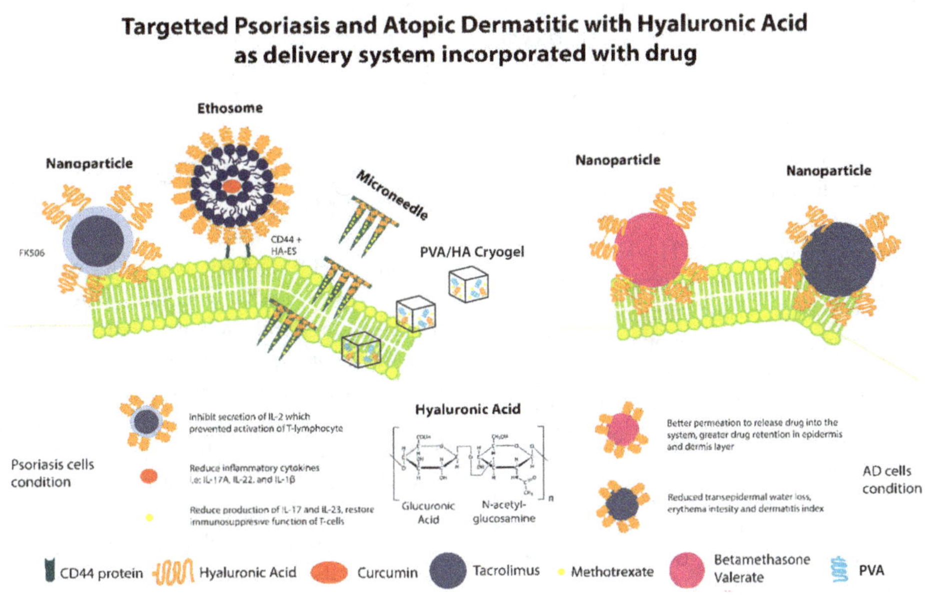

GRAPHICAL ABSTRACT | HA-mediated Drug Delivery System Targeting Inflammatory Skin Diseases (Psoriasis and Atopic Dermatitis).

INTRODUCTION

Skin as the first line of defense against infection is made up of three main layers which vary in functions and anatomy: epidermis (outer layer), dermis (middle layer) and hypodermis (bottom layer) (Prost-Squarcioni, 2006). As it interacts with environment, skin acts as a protector against diseases, excessive water loss, UV damage, mechanical injury, and also helps in regulate body temperature (Logger et al., 2019). Skin and subcutaneous diseases are the 4th leading cause of disability globally in 2013 excluding mortality, with dermatitis being the greatest burden among all costing approximately 9.3 million disability-adjusted life years (Karimkhani et al., 2017). Psoriasis is reported to affect 2% of worldwide population due to genetic and environmental factors (Mohd Affandi et al., 2018). Psoriasis is an inflammatory skin diseases which is chronic with strong genetic predisposition and autoimmune pathogenic traits (Du et al., 2019) that is causing burden to patient either physically or physiologically (Boehncke and Schön, 2015). For mild to moderate psoriasis, topical corticosteroids are the first-line treatment. However, long term application of topical corticosteroids can produce adverse effects such as epidermal thinning, atrophy, ulceration and facial erythema (Coondoo et al., 2014).

Atopic dermatitis (AD), a common chronic inflammatory skin disease poses a significant threat to both patient and the economy. It also affects the quality of individual life as well as their families (Kapur et al., 2018). The disease is believed to arise due to the complex interplay between skin barrier malfunction, immune dysregulation and infectious agents from environment factor (Kapur et al., 2018). In Canada, it was reported that an estimated cost of $1.4 billion annually is incurred to assist AD patient in getting treatment, like emollients application, as well as frequent physician visits which impacted the economy (Barbeau and Lalonde, 2006). AD has significant impact on the patients quality of life as there will be constant itchiness which can lead to skin trauma and sleep deprivation (Kapur et al., 2018).

CD44, a receptor for HA is found to be highly expressed in psoriatic skin. The concentration is negatively correlated with HA distribution (Zhang et al., 2019). It was found that anti-allergenic effect can be achieved through the inhibition of CD44 and PKCα interaction by HA (Kim et al., 2008). Based on the understanding of the characteristic of HA and HA-CD44 pathway, HA is widely used as a nano-drug delivery system to enhance the therapeutic effect of drug at the lesion site (Taetz et al., 2009). HA assisted drug delivery systems that has been described include nanoparticle, ethosomes and microneedle. It is an important vehicle to enhance drug-skin penetration and an important vehicle to retain moisture in AD in view of barrier dysfunction. The objective of this review is to review the role of HA as a drug delivery system in inflammatory skin diseases namely psoriasis and atopic dermatitis.

Abbreviations: HA, hyaluronic acid; AD, atopic dermatitis; LMWHA, low molecular weight hyaluronic acid; HMWHA, high molecular weight hyaluronic acid; IL, interleukin; SC, stratum corneum; PKCα; protein kinase C alpha; HaCat, human keratinocyte cell line.

STRUCTURAL AND FUNCTIONAL CHARACTERISTICS OF HYALURONIC ACID

Hyaluronic acid (HA), a major component of extracellular matrix has been widely applied in pharmaceutical and cosmetic industries due to its reported pharmacological properties which includes anti-aging (Bukhari et al., 2018), anti-inflammatory (Chen, 2018), skin repairing (Narurkar et al., 2016), tissue regeneration (Bukhari et al., 2018) and wound recovery properties (Chen, 2018). HA possess good biocompatibility, high moisture retention, and tuneable viscoelastic properties (Sze et al., 2016). It is a natural unbranched polymer composed of repeating disaccharide units of D-glucuronic acid and N-acetylglucosamine linked by a glucuronidic β (1–3) bond. HA with different molecular weights exhibit distinct properties. For instance, low molecular weight HA (LMW-HA) is reported to be associated with promoting angiogenesis whereas high molecular weight HA (HMW-HA) inhibits angiogenesis. The appropriate balance between synthesis and degradation of HA is vital in the regulation of various biological functions including cell proliferation, migration, differentiation (Bychkov and Kuzmina, 2015), vasculogenesis and angiogenesis (Pardue et al., 2008), as well as regulating cell adhesion and motility (Kouvidi et al., 2011), as determined by their molecular weight. LMW-HA on the other hand exerts opposite effect as compared to HMW-HA where it demonstrates biological activities such as antioxidant properties and pronounced free radical scavenging has been developed in recent years (Ke et al., 2011). In addition, LMW-HA has also shown to induce inflammatory genes in T-24 carcinoma cells, in eosinophils (Ohkawara et al., 2000) as well as dendritic cells (Termeer et al., 2000). Both sizes of HA are safe and efficacious, and the market is expecting a continuing emergence of HA-based products in the coming years (Tabassum and Hamdani, 2014).

PSORIASIS

Psoriasis is a chronic inflammatory autoimmune skin disease characterized by marked epidermal proliferation and abnormal differentiation with activation of both innate and acquired immunity (Rendon and Schäkel, 2019). This autoimmune disorder is multifactorial, and inflammation is known to play a major role in its development. Research have showed that activated Th1 and Th17 T cells (CD4+ T cells), CD8+ T cells, as well as increased levels of cytokines such as IL-17, IL-23, TNF-α and IL-27, have been directly implicated in psoriasis immunopathogenesis (Luger and Loser, 2018). The immunology and genetics studies of psoriasis have provided insights into the heterogeneity and regulatory pathways that govern psoriasis, and assist in the development of therapy based on patients biogenetic markers and identify new avenues for treatment based on a more complete understanding of the immunological mechanisms. Topical administration is one of the important approaches to treat psoriasis. Drugs are applied directly to the affected skin lesions to inhibit inflammatory symptoms of psoriasis. Topical administration of drugs with narrow therapeutic window can reduce systemic absorption compared to drugs delivered through oral and intravenous routes which help to reduce adverse systemic effects. Though topically applied drugs provide prolonged duration of action, the stratum corneum limits the amount of drugs being percutaneously absorbed, resulting in poor clinical efficacy. Hence, novel and improved percutaneous delivery system to overcome the stratum corneum barrier of psoriatic skin is vital to antipsoriatic drug for topical therapy.

HA AS A DRUG DELIVERY SYSTEM IN PSORIASIS

Currently, HA is widely incorporated as part of the transdermal delivery system to enhance drug penetration in psoriasis treatment. Various forms of drug delivery systems including HA-based nanoparticles, ethosomes, cryogels, and microneedle patches have been developed to enhance drug permeation through and into the intact skin for psoriasis treatment. The excellent solubility properties of HA resulted in its development as one of the most important topical carriers for the localized delivery of drugs to the skin and also as a drug delivery agent for ophthalmic, nasal, pulmonary, parenteral and topical routes of administration (Brown and Jones, 2005). HA acts as mucoadhesive, retaining the drug at specific site of action/absorption. It also can modify the *in vivo* release and absorption rate of the therapeutic agent and it is able to localize delivery of drug to the epidermis. The types of psoriasis drugs that have been incorporated into these HA-based delivery systems include methotrexate, tacrolimus, and corticosteroids, all which are first-line treatments for moderate to severe psoriasis.

One of the novel nano-topical drug delivery system developed using HA-modified ethosomes target CD44 in the inflamed epidermis (Zhang et al., 2019). Ethosomes are novel deformable liposomes derived from dispersing liposomes in small-chain biocompatible alcohols and they are demonstrated to be more superior than classic liposomes which significantly increase skin retention of drugs (Touitou et al., 2000). The incorporation of curcumin in HA-modified ethosomes target CD44 in the inflamed epidermis (Zhang et al., 2019). Recent studies have found that CD44 protein is highly expressed in the epidermis of psoriatic inflamed skin, suggesting that CD44 can serve as a potential target of novel active-targeting nanocarriers for topical administration to increase skin drug retention and enhance drug efficacy (Lindqvist et al., 2012). The HA-modified ethosomes showed specific adhesion CD44 in imiquimod-induced psoriasis-like inflamed skin, and that the increased topical drug delivery of curcumin reduced TNF-α, IL-17A, IL-17F, IL-22, and IL-1β mRNA levels; and lower CCR6 protein expression.

Another formulated hybrid nanoparticle system based on the combination of amphiphilic conjugations of HA–Cholesterol-self-assembled nanoparticles and hydrotropic nicotinamide was developed to enhance the permeation of tacrolimus (FK506) in the treatment of psoriasis (Wan et al., 2017). Commercial FK506 is an ointment formulation use to treat atopic dermatitis, but it is applied to other skin diseases like psoriasis (Malecic and Young, 2016). FK506 is a type of macrolide immunosuppressive drug which prevents activation of T-lymphocyte through inhibition of IL-2, a cytokine that is responsible for the development and persistence of psoriasis lesions (Goebel et al., 2011). However, topical treatment of tacrolimus ointment on hyperkeratotic psoriatic plaques did not promote FK506 deposition due to its high hydrophobicity and high molecular weight (Zonnevdd et al., 1998). The combination of HA–Cholesterol nanoparticles exhibited a significant synergistic effect on the permeation of FK506 ointment and that it presented a synergistic effect on antipsoriasis which might increase the therapeutic effect and minimize systemic side effects (Wan et al., 2017).

Synthetic biodegradable polymers have significant versatility and diverse biomedical applications owing to their tailorable designs or modifications. Poly(vinyl alcohol) (PVA) is a water soluble biodegradable synthetic polymer with good biocompatibility, and it can be physically cross-linked by the freeze-thaw method (Stauffer and Peppast, 1992) to form hydrogels useful in pharmaceutical formulations. The development of PVA/HA cryogels loaded with methotrexate showed good *in vivo* biocompatibility after systemic and topical administration in laboratory animals. The pH-responsive swelling and releasing abilities of these PVA/HA cryogels allow these systems to be developed as topical formulations for psoriasis therapy.

Meanwhile, development of pH-responsive biodegradable poly-L-glutamic acid (PGA)-fluocinolone acetonide (FLUO) conjugate allows the controlled release of the FLUO to reduce skin inflammation (Dolz-Pérez et al., 2020). However, PGA-FLUO showed limitations in the release of drug in the epidermis which bring about the application of PGA-FLUO within hyaluronic acid (HA)-poly-L-glutamate cross polymer (HA-CP) resulted in slower and sustained drug transfer in the epidermis allowing sufficient residence time for drug activity (Dolz-Pérez et al., 2020).

Microneedle patch is a highly efficient and versatile device which attracted extensive scientific and industrial interests in the past decades due to prominent properties including painless penetration, low cost, excellent therapeutic efficacy, and relative safety. The robust microneedle enabling transdermal delivery has a paramount potential to create advanced functional devices with superior nature for biomedical applications. Methotrexate, an analogue of folic acid has been used as a drug to treat psoriasis skin condition (Czarnecka-Operacz and Sadowska-Przytocka, 2014). Methotrexate has been shown to down-regulate interleukin-17 and interferon-c, inhibit proliferation of effector T cells and restore the immunosuppressive function of regulatory T cells (Chen, 2018). Nevertheless, its high molecular weight, hydrophilicity and inability to maintain a stable form at physiological pH restricted the permeability of methotrexate by passive diffusion through the stratum corneum (Alvarez-Figueroa et al., 2001). The development of methotrexate-loaded HA-based microneedle patch successfully penetrated imiquimod (IMQ)-induced thickened epidermis in mice and alleviated the psoriasis-like skin inflammation (Du et al., 2019). In addition, the methotrexate-loaded HA-based microneedle patches were significantly more efficacious than taking the same dose of drug orally. This significantly reduced the amount of methotrexate required for the microneedle patch delivery system required for a comparable amelioration, which in turn lowered its systemic toxicity (Du et al., 2019).

HA AS A BIOMARKER IN PSORIASIS

Serum HA had been utilized as a biomarker for psoriasis as studies reported that concentration of serum HA increases significantly in patients with serious cutaneous psoriasis (Yamamoto et al., 1997). This is due to the ability of low molecular weight HA (LMWHA) in inducing inflammatory cytokine gene expression and serving as a ligand for toll-like receptors (TLRs). In addition, presence of IL-1β, tumor necrosis factor-α (TNF-α) and degradative enzymes such as metalloproteinases will lead to an increase in hyaluronan synthetases (HAS) 1–3 and hyaluronidases that synthesize LMWHA by degrading HMWHA (Mehta et al., 2011; Hellman et al., 2019). In psoriasis, TLRs play a vital role as innate immune responses through activation of TLR7 and TLR9 and also the secretion of interleukin-23 (IL-23) *via* autoimmune plasmacytoid dendritic cell activation which releases interferon-a, that further signals Tip-DC (tumor necrosis factor-a and inducible nitric oxide synthase-producing dendritic cell) activation (Yamamoto, 2015). Other TLRs including TLR2 and TLR4 contribute to the pathogenesis of psoriasis plaque, guttate (Garcia-Rodriguez et al., 2013) and also psoriatic arthritis (Carrasco et al., 2011). HA is highly abundant in psoriatic skin, and it signals through TLR4 and TLR2. Meanwhile the binding of HA on CD44 also induces secretion of IL-6 and inflammation in T cells and neutrophils (Jiang et al., 2011).

ATOPIC DERMATITIS

Atopic dermatitis (AD) is the most common chronic inflammatory skin disease affecting infants and children (Siegfried and Hebert, 2015). Factors causing AD includes defect in terminal epithelial differentiation, immune dysregulation, altered skin microbiome and altered composition of stratum corneum (SC) intracellular lipids leading to barrier dysfunction (Bieber et al., 2017; Nakatsuji et al., 2017). Impairment of the SC permeability barrier functions cause dehydration due to an increase of transepidermal water loss, followed by inflammation due to the increasing release of cytokines, chemokines and interleukines (Damiani et al., 2019). Skin hydration, anti-bacterial measures and topical immunosuppressant therapy using topical corticosteroids calcineurin inhibitors are the common approaches in the management of AD (Sathishkumar and Moss, 2016).

HA'S ROLE IN ATOPIC DERMATITIS

HA is found to be related to inflammatory skin dermatoses (Ohtani et al., 2009; Barnes et al., 2012) The synthesis of HA is regulated by hyaluronan synthases (HAS). In normal circumstances, HAS1 is found to be regulating epidermal differentiation. However, role of HAS3 becomes apparent during pathological condition (Malaisse et al., 2014). The earlier studies provide conflicting evidences on HA role in epidermal differentiation (Maytin et al., 2004; Passi et al., 2004; Bourguignon et al., 2006; Farwick et al., 2011). Latest evidence by Malaisse et al. (2014) acknowledge the fact that though HA present at high level, it is not necessary for homeostatic epidermal differentiation (Malaisse et al., 2014). However, HA become important in pathological condition. During inflammation, HAS3 is upregulated while HAS1 is downregulated. Heparin binding-epidermal growth factor. (HB-EGF) is found to be possibly linked to HAS expression in AD lesions. However, how HAS involved in the pathomechanism of keratinocyte inflammation is still unclear and thus requiring further studies (Malaisse et al., 2014).

HA IN MEDICAL DEVICE MOISTURIZERS

The basic principle AD treatment is optimal skin care that address the skin barrier defect. Moisturizers restore the ability of lipid bilayer to restore, retain and redistribute water. They penetrate and contribute to the reorganization of the structure of the skin layers. Thus, moisturizers play an important role in AD management (Giam et al., 2016). Moisturizers can be categorized into three main groups, namely humectant, occlusive and emollients. These products are formulated in various delivery system including gel, foam, cream, ointment and lotion. They also contain various composition to enhance its efficacy. Humectants work by attracting fluids from the deeper epidermis to SC and has a biological similarities to the natural moisturizing factors of the corneocytes (Giam et al., 2016). HA being a natural component of the skin, has been one of the most favorite humectant used in almost all nutricosmetic products with moisturizing properties (Bukhari et al., 2018). It helps in attracting and retaining fluid, and skin barrier repair (Maytin et al., 2004; Goh et al., 2019). However it is rarely used primarily as a sole ingredient, but rather working synergistically with other category of moisturizer to achieve its role in skin repair (Draelos, 2011; Frankel et al., 2011; Pacha and Hebert, 2012; Micali et al., 2018). The molecular weight of HA shall be considered, as HA with a molecular weight higher than 50 kDa may reduce skin penetration. Thus, HMWHA is used to form a film to impede epidermal water loss, while LMWHA is utilized to improve skin penetration to restore a sustained physiological and hydrated microenvironment for optimize skin rejuvenation and tissue repair (Symonette et al., 2014).

HA AS A DRUG DELIVERY SYSTEM IN ATOPIC DERMATITIS

Similar to psoriasis, various forms of drug delivery systems including HA-based nanoparticles and pluronic F-127 based dual responsive (pH/temperature) hydrogels have been described to enhance drug permeation through and into the intact skin for AD treatment. The types of drugs that have been incorporated into these HA-based delivery systems include tacrolimus, bethamethasone valerate and gallic acid, a principal component of traditional Chinese medicine Cortex Moutan.

Topical calcineurin inhibitor, namely tacrolimus ointment (Protropic®) and pimecrolimus cream (Elidel®) are steroid sparing agents for the treatment of atopic dermatitis. However the potency of tacrolimus 0.1% was only found to be equivalent to medium potency topical steroid(Eichenfield et al., 2014), possibly due to the limited skin penetration due to its large molecular size. A novel HA-coated tacrolimus-loaded nanoparticles (HA-TCS-CS-NPs) was described (Zhuo et al., 2018). It was noted that the physiochemical properties had been optimized, *in vivo* drug release was more sustained, drug permeation and retention had been improvised, and anti-AD efficacy in AD mice model was found to be superior in comparison with tacrolimus solution (Zhuo et al., 2018). However, this study did not compare their nanoparticles with the marketed Protropic®. Similar technology had been used to encapsulate betamethasone valerate (BMV), a medium potency topical corticosteroid. It was found that (HA-BMV-CS-NP) demonstrated optimum physicochemical characteristics, including fine particle size, high zeta potential, high entrapment efficacy and loading capacity. It also demonstrated higher drug permeation and drug retention(Pandey et al., 2019).

Pluronic F-127 (PF127) is a non-ionic triblock copolymer of poly(ethylene oxide)-b-poly(propylene oxide)-b-poly(ethylene oxide), thermo-responsive polymer capable to form gel from its aqueous solution. Chitosan is a cationic pH-responsive biopolymer that swells in acidic pH and shrinks in basic pH, while HA is an anionic pH-responsive biopolymer that can swell in basic pH and shrink in acidic pH (Chatterjee et al., 2019). The conjugation of these polymers formed a dual-responsive hydrogels [PF127/HA-Ala-Chito(oligo)]. It had been used to incorporate gallic acid, the principal component of traditional Chinese medicine Cortex Moutan, recommended in the treatment of atopic dermatitis. This anti-inflammatory and anti-allergic herbal medicine is claimed to have similar effect like corticosteroids without their side effects. PF127/HA-Ala-chito(oligo) drug delivery system was found to have improve rheological properties, mechanical stability and pH responsiveness. This drug delivery system was found to exhibit better gallic acid release under neutral pH condition. The mechanical stability and sustain drug release property despite increasing acidity in the external environment. However, further modification of this drug delivery system is required to involve non-toxic biomaterials (Chatterjee et al., 2019).

CONCLUSION

HA is widely utilized in dermatology as it is a natural, non-immunogenic polysaccharide with good biocompatibility and degradability (Huang and Huang, 2018). The moisturizing properties of HA made it exist in almost all moisturizing and antiaging cosmetics. The identification of CD44 receptors and HA on both psoriasis and AD epidermis had led to many researchers exploring this component as a possible new way for drug delivery Research on this field flourishes further even more with the improve understanding of nanomedicine. However, the current research are mainly in the pre-clinical phase. There are still large gaps in terms of best material to be utilized to improve the safety and efficacy of drug delivery. The mechanism of HA based drug delivery system is still unclear. The role of HA and its receptor on both AD and psoriasis is also yet to be well defined. Thus, more work needs to be done on all aspect of HA and its receptors on patho-mechanism of inflammatory skin diseases and its potential role in improvising future drug delivery.

AUTHOR CONTRIBUTIONS

KNH, ZWL, and WHY conceived the idea and wrote the manuscript. All authors contributed to the article and approved the submitted version.

REFERENCES

Alvarez-Figueroa, M. J., Delgado-Charro, M. B., and Blanco-Méndez, J. (2001). Passive and iontophoretic transdermal penetration of methotrexate. *Int. J. Pharm.* 212, 101–107. doi: 10.1016/s0378-5173(00)00599-8

Barbeau, M., and Lalonde, H. (2006). Burden of atopic dermatitis in Canada. *Int. J. Dermatol.* 45, 31–36. doi: 10.1111/j.1365-4632.2004.02345.x

Barnes, L., Carraux, P., Saurat, J. H., and Kaya, G. (2012). Increased expression of CD44 and hyaluronate synthase 3 is associated with accumulation of hyaluronate in spongiotic epidermis. *J. Invest. Dermatol.* 132 (3), 736. doi: 10.1038/jid.2011.384

Bieber, T., D'Erme, A. M., Akdis, C. A., Traidl-Hoffmann, C., Lauener, R., Schäppi, G., et al. (2017). Clinical phenotypes and endophenotypes of atopic dermatitis: Where are we, and where should we go? *J. Allergy Clin. Immunol.* 139, S58–S64. doi: 10.1016/j.jaci.2017.01.008

Boehncke, W. H., and Schön, M. P. (2015). Psoriasis. *Lancet* 386, 983–994. doi: 10.1016/S0140-6736(14)61909-7

Bourguignon, L. Y., Ramez, M., Gilad, E., Singleton, P. A., Man, M. Q., Crumrine, D. A., et al. (2006). Hyaluronan-CD44 interaction stimulates keratinocyte differentiation, lamellar body formation/secretion, and permeability barrier homeostasis. *J. Invest. Dermatol.* 126 (6), 1356–1365. doi: 10.1038/sj.jid.5700260

Brown, M. B., and Jones, S. A. (2005). Hyaluronic acid: a unique topical vehicle for the localized delivery of drugs to the skin. *J. Eur. Acad. Dermatol. Venereology JEADV* 19 (3), 308–318. doi: 10.1111/j.1468-3083.2004.01180.x

Bukhari, S. N. A., Roswandi, N. L., Waqas, M., Habib, H., Hussain, F., Khan, S., et al. (2018). Hyaluronic acid, a promising skin rejuvenating biomedicine: A review of recent updates and pre-clinical and clinical investigations on cosmetic and nutricosmetic effects. *Int. J. Biol. Macromol.* 120, 1682–1695. doi: 10.1016/j.ijbiomac.2018.09.188

Bychkov, S. M., and Kuzmina, S. A. (2015). "The Biological Role of Hyaluronic Acid," in *Hyaluronic Acid* (Chichester, UK: John Wiley & Sons, Ltd), 9–75. doi:10.1002/9781118695920.ch2.

Carrasco, S., Neves, F., Fonseca, M., Gonçalves, C., Saad, C., Sampaio-Barros, P., et al. (2011). Toll-like receptor (TLR) 2 is upregulated on peripheral blood monocytes of patients with psoriatic arthritis: a role for a gram-positive inflammatory Trigger. *Clin. Exp. Rheumatol.* 29, 958–962.

Chatterjee, S., Hui, P. C., Kan, C., and Wang, W. (2019). Dual-responsive (pH/temperature) Pluronic F-127 hydrogel drug delivery system for textile-based transdermal therapy. *Sci. Rep.* 9 (1), 1–13. doi: 10.1038/s41598-019-48254-6

Chen, Z. (2018). What's new about the mechanism of methotrexate action in psoriasis? *Br. J. Dermatol.* 179, 818–819. doi: 10.1111/bjd.16908

Coondoo, A., Phiske, M., Verma, S., and Lahiri, K. (2014). Side-effects of topical steroids: A long overdue revisit. *Indian Dermatol. Online J.* 5, 425. doi: 10.4103/2229-5178.142483

Czarnecka-Operacz, M., and Sadowska-Przytocka, A. (2014). The possibilities and principles of methotrexate treatment of psoriasis - The updated knowledge. *Postep. Dermatologii i Alergol.* 31, 392–400. doi: 10.5114/pdia.2014.47121

Damiani, G., Eggenhöffner, R., Pigatto, P. D. M., and Bragazzi, N. L. (2019). Nanotechnology meets atopic dermatitis: Current solutions, challenges and future prospects. Insights and implications from a systematic review of the literature. *Bioact. Mater.* 4, 380–386. doi: 10.1016/j.bioactmat.2019.11.003

Dolz-Pérez, I., Sallam, M. A., Masiá, E., Morelló-Bolumar, D., Pérez del Caz, M. D., Graff, P., et al. (2020). Polypeptide-corticosteroid conjugates as a topical treatment approach to psoriasis. *J. Control. Release.* 318, 210–222. doi: 10.1016/j.jconrel.2019.12.016

Draelos, Z. D. (2011). A clinical evaluation of the comparable efficacy of hyaluronic acid-based foam and ceramide-containing emulsion cream in the treatment of mild-to-moderate atopic dermatitis. *J. Cosmet. Dermatol.* 10 (3), 185–188. doi: 10.1111/j.1473-2165.2011.00568.x

Du, H., Liu, P., Zhu, J., Lan, J., Li, Y., Zhang, L., et al. (2019). Hyaluronic Acid-Based Dissolving Microneedle Patch Loaded with Methotrexate for Improved Treatment of Psoriasis. *ACS Appl. Mater. Interfaces.* 11 (46), 43588–43598. doi: 10.1021/acsami.9b15668

Eichenfield, L. F., Tom, W. L., Berger, T. G., Krol, A., Paller, A. S., Schwarzenberger, K., et al. (2014). Guidelines of care for the management of atopic dermatitis: Section 2. Management and treatment of atopic dermatitis with topical therapies. *J. Am. Acad. Dermatol.* 71 (1), 116–132. doi: 10.1016/j.jaad.2014.03.023

Farwick, M., Gauglitz, G., Pavicic, T., Köhler, T., Wegmann, M., Schwach-Abdellaoui, K., et al. (2011). Fifty-kDa hyaluronic acid upregulates some epidermal genes without changing TNF-α expression in reconstituted epidermis. *Skin Pharmacol. Physiol.* 24 (4), 210–217. doi: 10.1159/000324296

Frankel, A., Sohn, A., Patel, R. V., and Lebwohl, M. (2011). Bilateral comparison study of pimecrolimus cream 1% and a ceramide-hyaluronic acid emollient foam in the treatment of patients with atopic dermatitis. *J. Drugs Dermatol.* 10 (6), 666. doi: 10.1016/j.jaad.2010.09.266

Garcia-Rodriguez, S., Arias-Santiago, S., Perandrés-López, R., Castellote, L., Zumaquero, E., Navarro, P., et al. (2013). Increased gene expression of Toll-like receptor 4 on peripheral blood mononuclear cells in patients with psoriasis. *J. Eur. Acad. Dermatol. Venereol.* 27, 242–250. doi: 10.1111/j.1468-3083.2011.04372.x

Giam, Y. C., Hebert, A. A., Dizon, M. V., Van Bever, H., Tiongco-Recto, M., Kim, K.-H., et al. (2016). A review on the role of moisturizers for atopic dermatitis. *Asia Pac. Allergy* 6 (2), 120–128. doi: 10.5415/apallergy.2016.6.2.120

Goebel, A. S. B., Neubert, R. H. H., and Wohlrab, J. (2011). Dermal targeting of tacrolimus using colloidal carrier systems. *Int. J. Pharm.* 404, 159–168. doi: 10.1016/j.ijpharm.2010.11.029

Goh, J. X. H., Tan, L. T.-H., Yew, H. C., Pusparajah, P., Lingham, P., Long, C. M., et al. (2019). Hydration effects of moisturizing gel on normal skin: A pilot study. *Prog. Drug Discovery Biomed. Sci.* 2 (1), a0000023. doi: 10.36877/pddbs.a0000023

Hellman, U., Engström-Laurent, A., Larsson, A., and Lindqvist, U. (2019). Hyaluronan concentration and molecular mass in psoriatic arthritis: biomarkers of disease severity, resistance to treatment, and outcome. *Scand. J. Rheumatol.* 48, 284–293. doi: 10.1080/03009742.2019.1577490

Huang, G., and Huang, H. (2018). Hyaluronic acid-based biopharmaceutical delivery and tumor-targeted drug delivery system. *J. Control. Release.* 278, 122–126. doi: 10.1016/j.jconrel.2018.04.015

Jiang, D., Liang, J., and Noble, P. W. (2011). Hyaluronan as an immune regulator in human diseases. *Physiol. Rev.* 91, 221–264. doi: 10.1152/physrev.00052.2009

Kapur, S., Watson, W., and Carr, S. (2018). Atopic dermatitis. *Allergy Asthma Clin. Immunol.* 14 (suppl 2), 44–52. doi: 10.1186/s13223-018-0281-6

Karimkhani, C., Dellavalle, R. P., Coffeng, L. E., Flohr, C., Hay, R. J., Langan, S. M., et al. (2017). Global skin disease morbidity and mortality an update from the global burden of disease study 2013. *JAMA Dermatol.* 153, 406–412. doi: 10.1001/jamadermatol.2016.5538

Ke, C., Sun, L., Qiao, D., Wang, D., and Zeng, X. (2011). Antioxidant acitivity of low molecular weight hyaluronic acid. *Food Chem. Toxicol.* 49 (10), 2670–2675. doi: 10.1016/j.fct.2011.07.020

Kim, Y., Lee, Y. S., Hahn, J. H., Choe, J., Kwon, H. J., Ro, J. Y., et al. (2008). Hyaluronic acid targets CD44 and inhibits FcεRI signaling involving PKCδ, Rac1, ROS, and MAPK to exert anti-allergic effect. *Mol. Immunol.* 45, 2537–2547. doi: 10.1016/j.molimm.2008.01.008

Kouvidi, K., Berdiaki, A., Nikitovic, D., Katonis, P., Afratis, N., Hascall, V. C., et al. (2011). Role of receptor for hyaluronic acid-mediated motility (RHAMM) in low molecular weight hyaluronan (LMWHA)-mediated fibrosarcoma cell adhesion. *J. Biol. Chem.* 286 (44), 38509–38520. doi: 10.1074/jbc.M111.275875

Lindqvist, U., Pihl-Lundin, I., and Engström-Laurent, A. (2012). Dermal distribution of hyaluronan in psoriatic arthritis: Coexistence of CD44, MMP3 and MMP9. *Acta Derm. Venereol.* 92 (4), 372–377. doi: 10.2340/00015555-1286

Logger, J., Olydam, J., Woliner-van der Weg, W., and van Erp, P. (2019). Noninvasive Skin Barrier Assessment: Multiparametric Approach and Pilot Study. *Cosmetics* 6:20. doi: 10.3390/cosmetics6010020

Luger, T. A., and Loser, K. (2018). Novel insights into the pathogenesis of psoriasis. *Clin. Immunol. (Orlando Fla.)* 186, 43–45. doi: 10.1016/j.clim.2017.07.014

Malaisse, J., Bourguignon, V., De Vuyst, E., Lambert De Rouvroit, C., Nikkels, A. F., Flamion, B., et al. (2014). Hyaluronan metabolism in human keratinocytes and atopic dermatitis skin is driven by a balance of hyaluronan synthases 1 and 3. *J. Invest. Dermatol.* 134, 2174–2182. doi: 10.1038/jid.2014.147

Malecic, N., and Young, H. (2016). Tacrolimus for the management of psoriasis: Clinical utility and place in therapy. *Psoriasis Targets Ther.* 6, 153–163. doi: 10.2147/PTT.S101233

Maytin, E. V., Chung, H. H., and Seetharaman, V. M. (2004). Hyaluronan participates in the epidermal response to disruption of the permeability barrier in vivo. *Am. J. Pathol.* 165, 1331–1341. doi: 10.1016/S0002-9440(10)63391-3

Mehta, N. N., Yu, Y. D., Saboury, B., Foroughi, N., Krishnamoorthy, P., Raper, A., et al. (2011). Systemic and vascular inflammation in patients with moderate to severe psoriasis as measured by [18F]-fluorodeoxyglucose positron emission tomography-computed tomography (FDG-PET/CT): A pilot study. *Arch. Dermatol.* 147, 1031–1039. doi: 10.1001/archdermatol.2011.119

Micali, G., Paternò, V., Cannarella, R., Dinotta, F., and Lacarrubba, F. (2018). Evidence-based treatment of atopic dermatitis with topical moisturizers. *G. Ital. di Dermatologia e Venereol.* 153, 396–402. doi: 10.23736/S0392-0488.18.05898-4

Mohd Affandi, A., Khan, I., and Ngah Saaya, N. (2018). Epidemiology and Clinical Features of Adult Patients with Psoriasis in Malaysia: 10-Year Review from the Malaysian Psoriasis Registry, (2007-2016). *Dermatol. Res. Pract.* 2018, 1–8. doi: 10.1155/2018/4371471

Nakatsuji, T., Chen, T. H., Narala, S., Chun, K. A., Two, A. M., Yun, T., et al. (2017). Antimicrobials from human skin commensal bacteria protect against Staphylococcus aureus and are deficient in atopic dermatitis. *Sci. Transl. Med.* 9 eaah4680. doi: 10.1126/scitranslmed.aah4680

Narurkar, V. A., Cohen, J. L., Dayan, S., Kaminer, M. S., Rivkin, A., Shamban, A., et al. (2016). A Comprehensive Approach to Multimodal Facial Aesthetic Treatment: Injection Techniques and Treatment Characteristics From the HARMONY Study. *Dermatologic Surg.* 42 (Suppl 2), S177–S191. doi: 10.1097/DSS.0000000000000743

Ohkawara, Y., Tamura, G., Iwasaki, T., Tanaka, A., Kikuchi, T., and Shirato, K. (2000). Activation and transforming growth factor-β production in eosinophils by hyaluronan. *Am. J. Respir. Cell Mol. Biol.* 23, 444–451. doi: 10.1165/ajrcmb.23.4.3875

Ohtani, T., Memezawa, A., Okuyama, R., Sayo, T., Sugiyama, Y., Inoue, S., et al. (2009). Increased hyaluronan production and decreased E-cadherin expression by cytokine-stimulated keratinocytes lead to spongiosis formation. *J. Invest. Dermatol.* 129 (6), 1412–1420. doi: 10.1038/jid.2008.394

Pacha, O., and Hebert, A. A. (2012). Treating atopic dermatitis: Safety, efficacy, and patient acceptability of a ceramide hyaluronic acid emollient foam. *Clin. Cosmet. Investig. Dermatol.* 5, 39. doi: 10.2147/CCID.S23269

Pandey, M., Choudhury, H., Gunasegaran, T. A. P., Nathan, S. S., Md, S., Gorain, B., et al. (2019). Hyaluronic acid-modified betamethasone encapsulated polymeric nanoparticles: fabrication, characterisation, in vitro release kinetics, and dermal targeting. *Drug Deliv. Transl. Res.* 9, 520–533. doi: 10.1007/s13346-018-0480-1

Pardue, E. L., Ibrahim, S., and Ramamurthi, A. (2008). Role of hyaluronan in angiogenesis and its utility to angiogenic tissue engineering. *Organogenesis* 4 (4), 203–214. doi: 10.4161/org.4.4.6926

Passi, A., Sadeghi, P., Kawamura, H., Anand, S., Sato, N., White, L. E., et al. (2004). Hyaluronan suppresses epidermal differentiation in organotypic cultures of rat keratinocytes. *Exp. Cell Res.* 296 (2), 123–134. doi: 10.1016/j.yexcr.2004.01.031

Prost-Squarcioni, C. (2006). Histologie de la peau et des follicules pileux. *Medecine/Sciences* 22, 131–137. doi: 10.1051/medsci/2006222131

Rendon, A., and Schäkel, K. (2019). Psoriasis pathogenesis and treatment. *Int. J. Mol. Sci.* 20 (6), 1475. doi: 10.3390/ijms20061475

Sathishkumar, D., and Moss, C. (2016). Topical therapy in atopic dermatitis in children. *Indian J. Dermatol.* 61, 656–661. doi: 10.4103/0019-5154.193677

Siegfried, E., and Hebert, A. (2015). Diagnosis of Atopic Dermatitis: Mimics, Overlaps, and Complications. *J. Clin. Med.* 4, 884–917. doi: 10.3390/jcm4050884

Stauffer, S. R., and Peppast, N. A. (1992). Poly(vinyl alcohol) hydrogels prepared by freezing-thawing cyclic processing. *Polymer* 33 (18), 3932–3936. doi: 10.1016/0032-3861(92)90385-A

Symonette, C. J., Kaur Mann, A., Tan, X. C., Tolg, C., Ma, J., Perera, F., et al. (2014). Hyaluronan-Phosphatidylethanolamine Polymers Form Pericellular Coats on Keratinocytes and Promote Basal Keratinocyte Proliferation. *BioMed. Res. Int.* 2014. doi: 10.1155/2014/727459

Sze, J. H., Brownlie, J. C., and Love, C. A. (2016). Biotechnological production of hyaluronic acid: a mini review. *3 Biotech.* 6, 1–9. doi: 10.1007/s13205-016-0379-9

Tabassum, N., and Hamdani, M. (2014). Plants used to treat skin diseases. *Pharmacogn. Rev.* 8, 52–60. doi: 10.4103/0973-7847.125531

Taetz, S., Bochot, A., Surace, C., Arpicco, S., Renoir, J. M., Schaefer, U. F., et al. (2009). Hyaluronic acid-modified DOTAP/DOPE liposomes for the targeted delivery of anti-telomerase siRNA to CD44-expressing lung cancer cells. *Oligonucleotides* 19, 103–115. doi: 10.1089/oli.2008.0168

Termeer, C. C., Hennies, J., Voith, U., Ahrens, T., M. Weiss, J., Prehm, P., et al. (2000). Oligosaccharides of Hyaluronan Are Potent Activators of Dendritic Cells. *J. Immunol.* 165, 1863–1870. doi: 10.4049/jimmunol.165.4.1863

Touitou, E., Dayan, N., Bergelson, L., Godin, B., and Eliaz, M. (2000). Ethosomes - novel vesicular carriers for enhanced delivery: characterization and skin penetration properties. *J. Controlled release* 65 (3), 403–418. doi: 10.1016/s0168-3659(99)00222-9

Wan, T., Pan, W., Long, Y., Yu, K., Liu, S., Ruan, W., et al. (2017). Effects of nanoparticles with hydrotropic nicotinamide on tacrolimus: Permeability through psoriatic skin and antipsoriatic and antiproliferative activities. *Int. J. Nanomedicine.* 12, 1485. doi: 10.2147/IJN.S126210

Yamamoto, T., Matsuuchi, M., Irimajiri, J., Katayama, I., and Nishioka, K. (1997). John Libbey Eurotext - European Journal of Dermatology - Elevated circulating hyaluronan in patients with generalized pustular psoriasis. *Eur. J. Dermatol.* 7 (6), 409–411.

Yamamoto, T. (2015). Hyaluronic acid in psoriasis. *J. Eur. Acad. Dermatol. Venereol.* 29, 2487–2487. doi: 10.1111/jdv.12581

Zhang, Y., Xia, Q., Li, Y., He, Z., Li, Z., Guo, T., et al. (2019). CD44 assists the topical anti-psoriatic efficacy of curcumin-loaded hyaluronan-modified ethosomes: A new strategy for clustering drug in inflammatory skin. *Theranostics* 9 (1), 48. doi: 10.7150/thno.29715

Zhuo, F., Abourehab, M. A. S., and Hussain, Z. (2018). Hyaluronic acid decorated tacrolimus-loaded nanoparticles: Efficient approach to maximize dermal targeting and anti-dermatitis efficacy. *Carbohydr. Polym.* 197, 478–489. doi: 10.1016/j.carbpol.2018.06.023

7

Astragalus mongholicus Bunge Water Extract Exhibits Anti-Inflammatory Effects in Human Neutrophils and Alleviates Imiquimod-Induced Psoriasis-Like Skin Inflammation in Mice

Wei-Jen Cheng[1,2,3], *Chih-Chao Chiang*[1,4], *Cheng-Yu Lin*[5], *Yu-Li Chen*[6], *Yann-Lii Leu*[5], *Jia-Yu Sie*[5], *Wen-Ling Chen*[5], *Chung-Yuan Hsu*[3], *Jong-Jen Kuo*[2,3,7]* and *Tsong-Long Hwang*[5,6,8,9]*

[1]*Graduate Institute of Clinical Medical Sciences, College of Medicine, Chang Gung University, Taoyuan, Taiwan,* [2]*School of Traditional Chinese Medicine, College of Medicine, Chang Gung University, Taoyuan, Taiwan,* [3]*Center for Traditional Chinese Medicine, Chang Gung Memorial Hospital, Taoyuan, Taiwan,* [4]*Puxin Fengze Chinese Medicine Clinic, Taoyuan, Taiwan,* [5]*Graduate Institute of Natural Products, College of Medicine, Chang Gung University, Taoyuan, Taiwan,* [6]*Research Center for Chinese Herbal Medicine, Research Center for Food and Cosmetic Safety, Graduate Institute of Health Industry Technology, College of Human Ecology, Chang Gung University of Science and Technology, Taoyuan, Taiwan,* [7]*Graduate Institute of Traditional Chinese Medicine, School of Traditional Chinese Medicine, College of Medicine, Chang Gung University, Taoyuan, Taiwan,* [8]*Department of Anesthesiology, Chang Gung Memorial Hospital, Taoyuan, Taiwan,* [9]*Department of Chemical Engineering, Ming Chi University of Technology, New Taipei City, Taiwan*

***Correspondence:**
Jong-Jen Kuo
kjj308@gmail.com
Tsong-Long Hwang
htl@mail.cgu.edu.tw

Neutrophils are the primary immune cells in innate immunity, which are related to various inflammatory diseases. *Astragalus mongholicus Bunge* is a Chinese medicinal herb used to treat various oxidative stress-related inflammatory diseases. However, there are limited studies that elucidate the effects of *Astragalus mongholicus Bunge* in human neutrophils. In this study, we used isolated human neutrophils activated by various stimulants to investigate the anti-inflammatory effects of *Astragalus mongholicus Bunge* water extract (AWE). Cell-free assays were used to examine free radicals scavenging capabilities on superoxide anion, reactive oxygen species (ROS), and nitrogen-centered radicals. Imiquimod (IMQ) induced psoriasis-like skin inflammation mouse model was used for investigating anti-psoriatic effects. We found that AWE inhibited superoxide anion production, ROS generation, and elastase release in human neutrophils, which exhibiting a direct anti-neutrophil effect. Moreover, AWE exerted a ROS scavenging ability in the 2,2'-Azobis (2-amidinopropane) dihydrochloride assay, but not superoxide anion in the xanthine/xanthine oxidase assay, suggesting that AWE exhibited anti-oxidation and anti-inflammatory capabilities by both scavenging ROS and by directly inhibiting neutrophil activation. AWE also reduced CD11b expression and adhesion to endothelial cells in activated human neutrophils. Meanwhile, in mice with psoriasis-like skin inflammation, administration of topical AWE reduced both the affected area and the severity index score. It inhibited neutrophil infiltration, myeloperoxidase release, ROS-induced damage, and skin proliferation. In summary,

AWE exhibited direct anti-inflammatory effects by inhibiting neutrophil activation and anti-psoriatic effects in mice with IMQ-induced psoriasis-like skin inflammation. Therefore, AWE could potentially be a pharmaceutical Chinese herbal medicine to inhibit neutrophilic inflammation for anti-psoriasis.

Keywords: neutrophil, inflammation, psoriasis, traditional Chinese medicine, *astragalus mongholicus bunge*

1 INTRODUCTION

Astragalus mongholicus Bunge (AM; "Huang Qi" in Chinese) is one of the most important and widely used traditional Chinese medicines, having anti-inflammatory effects and multiple bioactivities such as protecting viral myocarditis injury, regulating blood sugar, and promoting wound healing (Chen et al., 2012; Agyemang et al., 2013; Piao and Liang, 2014; Qi et al., 2017). Furthermore, AM is also an antioxidant with a mitochondrial protective effect that contributes to anti-aging and anti-cancer effects (Li XT. et al., 2012). AM contains several bioactive ingredients, such as polysaccharides, flavonoids, and saponins (Fu J. et al., 2014), that are reported to provide anti-inflammatory effects and other benefits against many diseases or pathological conditions in various models (Shahzad et al., 2016).

Neutrophils are the most abundant leukocytes for innate immunity in the human body. In the process of respiratory burst, activated neutrophils generate abundant superoxide anion via reduced nicotinamide adenine dinucleotide phosphate (NADPH) oxidase (Dahlgren and Karlsson, 1999; Jaquet et al., 2011; Wang et al., 2012; Ruhnau et al., 2014), which are converted to reactive oxygen species (ROS), such as OH^-, HOCl, and H_2O_2, by catalase, myeloperoxidase (MPO), and superoxide dismutase (SOD) (Thannickal and Fanburg, 2000; Dupre-Crochet et al., 2013; Reczek and Chandel, 2015). As such, neutrophils tend to produce an enormous amount of ROS against microorganisms, including bacteria, fungi, and viruses. However, excessive production of ROS from neutrophils may cause tissue damage (Glennon-Alty et al., 2018). Aside from that, activated neutrophils also release granules containing proteolytic enzymes, such as neutrophil elastases, MPO, and cathelicidin (Faurschou and Borregaard, 2003), that contribute to tissue damage. Overproduction of ROS, proteolytic enzymes, and cytokines by neutrophils can also cause several pathological conditions, which could aggravate many clinical diseases (Papayannopoulos, 2018).

One such condition is psoriasis, an inflammatory skin disease with complicated etiology. Psoriasis reportedly affects approximately 3% of the population worldwide (Gupta et al., 2014). However, the prevalence of this disease varies with race and geographic location. For example, in a review of epidemiological data of psoriasis, the overall prevalence of psoriasis was estimated to be 3.7% in the US National Health Survey. However, studies in Asians revealed a prevalence ranging from 0.05 to 0.47% (Kaufman and Alexis, 2018). In Europe, the prevalence of psoriasis is approximately 2% according to a previous study (Boehncke and Schön, 2015). Moreover, psoriasis has been reported to affect 1.9–3.5% of people in eastern Africa, but only 0.025–0.9% in western Africa. This difference has been attribute to the genetic difference among different races and ethnicities (Kaufman and Alexis, 2018). Its classical manifestations include raised plaques and scales on the skin, and these psoriasis skin lesions are attributed to the over-proliferation and abnormal differentiation of keratinocytes, which is related to tissue damage by ROS and the release of cytokines by the infiltration of adaptive and innate immune cells (Rendon and Schäkel, 2019). Moreover, psoriatic lesions also usually exhibit neutrophil accumulation (Schön et al., 2017). Previous studies showed that neutrophils play a role in amplifying immune reaction, and neutrophil extracellular traps correlate with disease severity in patients with psoriasis (Lowes et al., 2014; Chiang et al., 2019). Oxidative stress is also involved in disease severity in clinical psoriasis patients (Cannavò et al., 2019). It influences the pathogenesis of psoriasis via several signaling pathways, such as nuclear factor-κB (NF-κB) and mitogen-activated protein kinase (MAPK) (Zhou et al., 2009). In the mouse model of imiquimod (IMQ)-induced psoriasis-like skin inflammation, excess ROS production contributed to histopathological changes in skin lesions (Baek et al., 2012).

Currently, T cells and dendritic cells are considered as the primary immune cells that release cytokines associated with psoriasis, such as interleukin (IL)-17A, IL-22, tumor necrosis factor (TNF)-α, and interferon (IFN)-γ, which affect keratinocyte proliferation (Nadeem et al., 2020b). Developing drugs that target these inflammatory mediators is one of the therapeutic strategies for psoriasis. For example, ibrutinib, a Bruton's tyrosine kinase inhibitor, suppresses IMQ-induced psoriasis-like skin inflammation in mice by downregulating IL-17A and IL-23 expression (Nadeem et al., 2020a). It can also decrease oxidative stress and inflammatory mediator levels in neutrophils and dendritic cells (Al-Harbi et al., 2020). However, emerging evidence has demonstrated that neutrophils may play a crucial role in psoriasis (Wang and Jin, 2020). Neutrophils produce many inflammatory mediators, forming neutrophil extracellular traps (NETs) and secreting IL-17, contributing to psoriasis skin inflammation (Schön et al., 2017). It is well-known that the interaction between IL-17A and keratinocyte causes the pathogenesis of psoriasis (Furue et al., 2020). Nevertheless, neutrophils are the primary source of IL-17A expression observed in psoriatic skin lesions, and interactions between infiltrated neutrophils and keratinocytes strengthen the IL-23/Th17 axis (Katayama, 2018). Moreover, neutrophils and mast cells, not T cells, are the dominant immune cells that release IL-17 in psoriatic skin, and neutrophils release abundant IL-17 during NET formation (Lin et al., 2011). A study demonstrated that NETs generated by neutrophils could establish self-amplifying inflammation reactions in psoriasis (Herster et al., 2020). In summary, neutrophils could secrete IL-17A, which affects keratinocytes, after infiltrating into the epidermis. NET formation by neutrophils also amplifies the inflammatory reactions in innate and adaptive immune cells, leading to the pathogenesis of psoriasis (Chiang et al., 2019).

Despite reports that AM can exhibit anti-inflammatory and anti-oxidation effects against various conditions, whether it could offer the same benefits against psoriasis and ROS overproduction by neutrophils remains unknown. Herein, we investigate *Astragalus mongholicus Bunge* water extract (AWE) and its anti-inflammatory effect on human neutrophils. We also examined the potential therapeutic effect of topical AWE against psoriasis in mice.

2 MATERIALS AND METHODS

2.1 Reagents

The herbal materials used in this study were the dried roots of *Astragalus mongholicus Bunge* which were purchased from Chang Gung Memorial Hospital, Taoyuan, Taiwan. Astragaloside IV was purchased from Sunhank technology Co. Ltd., Tainan, Taiwan. Calycosin-7-O-β-D-glucoside was purchased from Wuhan ChemFaces Biochemical Co., Ltd. (Wuhan, China). Ononin and calycosin were purchased from Sigma-Aldrich (St. Louis, MO, United States). Ficoll-paque PLUS was purchased from GE Healthcare (Little Chalfont, Buckinghamshire, United Kingdom). Hank's balanced salts solution (HBSS) was purchased from Gibco (Grand Island, NY, United States). Meo-Sac-Ala-Ala-Pro-Val-*p*-nitroanilide was purchased from Calbiochem (La Jolla, CA, United States). Lactate dehydrogenase (LDH) assay kits were purchased from Promega (Madison, WI, United States). Leukotriene B4 (LTB_4) and Leu-Glu-Ser-Ile-Phe-Arg-Ser-Leu-Leu-Phe-Arg-Val-Met (trifluoroacetate salt, MMK-1) were purchased from Tocris Bioscience (Ellisville, MO, United States). Xanthine was purchased from Santa Cruz Biotechnology (Santa Cruz, CA, United States). Water-soluble tetrazolium-1 (WST-1) was obtained from Dojindo (Kumamoto, Japan). Dihydroethidine (HE) was purchased from Invitrogen (Carlsbad, CA, United States). Fluorescein isothiocyanate (FITC)-labeled anti-cluster of differentiation molecule 11b (CD11b) was purchased from eBioscience (San Diego, CA, United States). Anti-lymphocyte antigen 6 complex locus G6D (Ly6G) antibody was purchased from BioLegend (San Diego, CA, United States). Anti-myeloperoxidase (MPO) antibody was obtained from Abcam (Cambridge, United Kingdom). Anti-Ki67 antibody was procured from GeneTex International Corporation (Hsinchu, Taiwan). Anti-4-Hydroxynonenal (HNE) antibody was purchased from Bioss Antibodies Inc. (Woburn, MA, United States). The rabbit anti-rat immunoglobulin G (IgG) was from ImmunoReagent Inc. (Beijing, China). Other bioassay and reagents were purchased from Sigma-Aldrich (St. Louis, MO, United States).

2.2 Astragalus mongholicus Bunge Water Extract Preparation

AWE was prepared in boiling water. Briefly, 131.25 g (35 Taiwan mace) of herbal materials was soaked in 600 ml of sterile double distilled water (ddH_2O) for 30 min and then boiled at 100°C for another 30 min. The extracts were filtered through a sterile 0.45 μm filter and then concentrated and powdered with an oil-pumping freeze dryer (LABCONCO, Kansas City, MO, United States). The AWE powder was stored at −20°C until further use and was dissolved in ddH_2O before use in the subsequent experiments. A voucher specimen (CGU_AM-01) was deposited in the Graduate Institute of Natural Products, Chang Gung University, Taoyuan, Taiwan.

2.3 High-Performance Liquid Chromatography Analysis

A Hitachi chromatography system (Hitachi, Tokyo, Japan) was used to analyze the composition of AWE. A previous study described the setting of the HPLC machine, standard solution preparation, and AWE solution preparation in detail (Matkowski et al., 2003). Ononin, calycosin, and calycosin-7-O-β-D-glucoside were used as standard references. AWE fingerprinting was performed under the detection wavelength at 260 nm.

2.4 Ultra-Performance Liquid Chromatography-Tandem Mass Spectrometry Condition

A Shimazu UPLC-MS/MS system coupled with Nexera X2 UPLC and LCMS-8045 (Shimazu, Kyoto, Japan) was used to analyze Astragaloside IV, the marker constituent of AWE according to government guidelines of Taiwan Herbal Pharmacopeia. Liquid chromatography was carried out using a YMC-Triart C18 column (2.1 × 50 mm, 1.9 μm particle size) (YMC, Kyoto, Japan). The mobile phase was 34% MeCN aqueous solution with 0.1% formic acid. The injection volume was 5 μL. The flow rate was 0.5 ml/min. The column temperature was maintained at 40°C. For the sample preparation, 110 mg AWE was dissolved in 10 ml of ddH_2O and partitioned with 10 ml of *n*-Butanol three times. Before analysis, the organic layer (18.4 mg) was collected and dissolved in MeOH at a 1 mg/ml concentration (Kafle et al., 2020).

2.5 Human Neutrophil Isolation

This study was approved by the institutional review board of Chang Gung Memorial Hospital (Registration number: IRB 100 1278C). All healthy volunteers aged 20–32 years old provided written consent prior to blood donation. Human neutrophils were prepared and isolated from healthy individuals using the Ficoll-Hypaque density gradient centrifugation method (Paoliello-Paschoalato et al., 2014). The isolated human neutrophils were suspended at 4°C in Ca^{2+}-free Hanks' balanced salt solution (HBSS) before further experiments (Tsai et al., 2015).

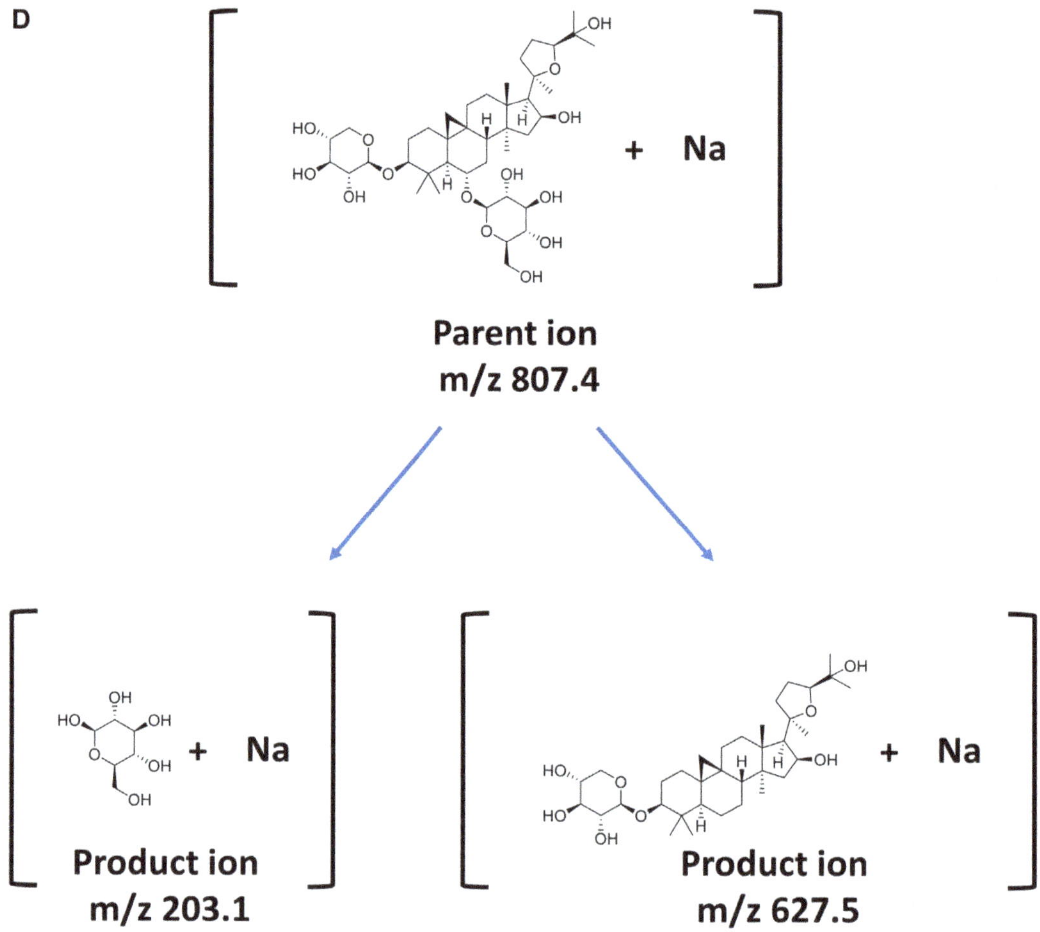

FIGURE 1 | Continued.

Another nitrogen-centered free radical compound, 2,2'-azino-bis(3-ethylbenzothiazolin-6-sulfonic acid) diammonium salt (ABTS), which has a blue color when dissolved in a potassium persulfate solution, was used in this study. ABTS (7 mM) was mixed with potassium persulfate (2.45 mM) in ddH_2O, and then ddH_2O (as the control), L-ascorbic acid (vitamin C (10, 15, and 30 μM), as the positive control), or AWE (10, 30, or 100 μg/ml) was added, then the assay was incubated at 25°C for 15 min. The change in light absorbance was determined spectrophotometrically at 734 nm (Rajendran et al., 2004).

2.10 Assessment CD11b Expression in Activated Neutrophils

Integrins, a kind of membrane protein, which promotes neutrophils to adhere to endothelial cells and then migrate to the inflammatory site, were expressed in activated neutrophils. In this study, we evaluated the effect of AWE on CD11b expression in fMLF-activated neutrophils. Human neutrophils (2.5×10^6 cells/ml) were incubated with ddH_2O (as the control) or AWE (10, 30, or 100 μg/ml) at 37°C for 5 min, and then neutrophils were stimulated by fMLF (0.1 μM) for another 5 min (pre-treated with 1 μg/ml CB for 3 min). The supernatant was removed after centrifugation (200 g, for 8 min) at 4°C, then neutrophils in the pallet were resuspended in HBSS, which contained 0.5% bovine serum albumin (BSA) and FITC-labeled anti-CD11b (1 μg/ml) and incubated at 4°C for 90 min in the dark. Immunofluorescence was measured using flow cytometry (Chiang et al., 2020).

2.11 Functional Study of Neutrophil Adhesion

Since neutrophil adhesion to endothelial cells plays a key role in the inflammatory response, the inhibition of adhesion will influence the recruitment of neutrophils to the inflammatory site. To assess the effect of AWE on neutrophil adhesion function *in vitro*, we used the mouse brain-derived endothelial cell 3 (bEnd.3). Human neutrophils (4×10^6 cells/mL) were pre-treated with Hoechst 3,342 (1 ng/ml) at 37°C for 10 min. After washing out the dye by centrifugation (200 × g, for 8 min) and removing the supernatant, neutrophils were resuspended and incubated with ddH_2O or AWE (100 μg/ml) for 5 min, then were activated with fMLF (0.1 μM) for 10 min, with pre-treatment with CB (1 μg/ml) for 2 min. Activated neutrophils were transferred to

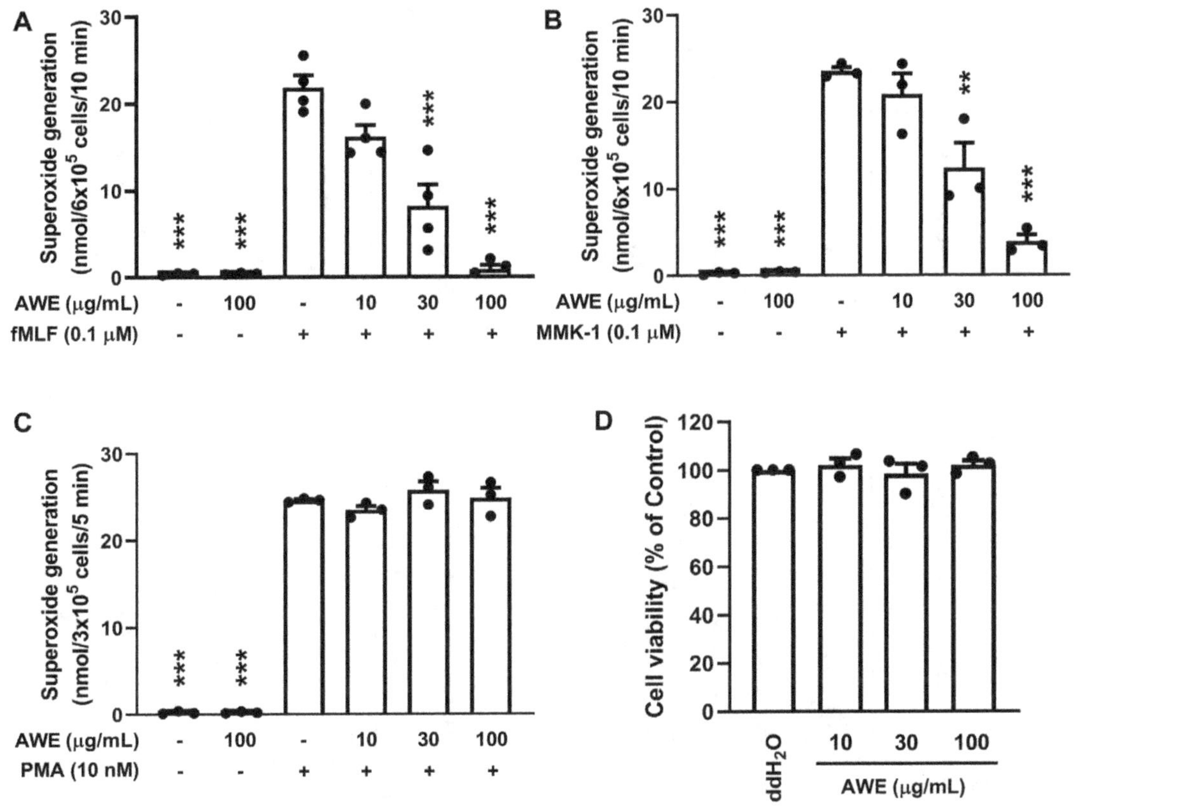

FIGURE 2 | AWE inhibited superoxide anion generation in activated human neutrophils. Human neutrophils (3×10^5 or 6×10^5 cells/mL) were incubated with ddH_2O (as the control) or AWE (10, 30, or 100 μg/ml) for 5 min, and then were activated by **(A)** fMLF, **(B)** MMK-1 for 10 min, or **(C)** PMA for 5 min. Superoxide anion production was monitored using ferricytochrome c reduction at 550 nm. **(D)** Human neutrophils were incubated with ddH_2O (as the control) or different concentrations of AWE for 15 min. Cytotoxicity was represented by LDH release as a percentage of the total. The Total LDH release was determined by lysing cells with 0.1% of Triton X-100 at 37°C for 30 min. The cell viability was calculated as one minus percent of LDH release. Data are expressed as mean ± S.E.M. ($n = 3$ or 4). Statistical analysis was conducted using the one-way analysis of variance (ANOVA), followed by Tukey's multiple comparison test if there were statistical differences in the results of ANOVA. Adjusted p-values of Tukey's multiple comparison tests were defined as $^{***}p < 0.001$ and $^{**}p < 0.01$ compared with the control.

wells containing bEnd.3 cells and incubated for 15 min at 37°C. After incubation, the medium and non-adherent neutrophils were washed with HBSS, and the adherent neutrophils were fixed with 4% paraformaldehyde in HBSS. Cells were observed and counted using a fluorescence microscope (IX81; Olympus, Center Valley, PA, United States) (Chen et al., 2016).

2.12 Imiquimod-Induced Psoriasis-like Skin Inflammation in Mice

All animal experiments in this study were approved and regulated by the Institutional Animal Care and Use Committee of Chang Gung University, Taoyuan, Taiwan (IACUC approval No. CGU14-150).

Eight-to ten-week-old BALB/C male mice that weighed approximately 20 g each were obtained from BioLasco Co., Ltd., Yilan, Taiwan. Aldara (3M Health Care Limited, United Kingdom), which contains 5% imiquimod (IMQ), was used to induce psoriasis-like skin inflammation. AWE was dissolved in the vehicle with 40% ethanol and 60% ddH_2O before application on the skin. The mice were divided into three groups: mice in the control group received no treatment; mice in the IMQ plus vehicle group were treated with IMQ (62.5 mg/day) and vehicle (100 μL/day); mice in the IMQ plus AWE group received equal doses of IMQ and AWE (10 mg/day), which were dissolved in vehicle (Chiang et al., 2020).

Before experiments, mice were given 1 week to adapt to the environment in 12-h light/12-h dark cycles with adequate food and water supply. The backs of mice were shaved with a depilatory machine and hair removal cream before the study. From days 1–5, 100 μL AWE or vehicle was topically applied to each mouse, followed by treatment with IMQ cream. Each day, we used pipette tips to drop 50 μL of AWE (100 mg/ml) or vehicle slowly and homogeneously on the back of the mice under anesthesia. After the solution had dried (approximately 10 min), we applied another 50 μL of solution on the back of the mice, that is, a total of 100 μL per day. We applied the IMQ cream approximately 30 min later while the solution had dried. Subsequently, we returned the mice to the cages and waited for them to awaken from anesthesia. A hand-held microscope and camera were used to obtain photos before the application of drugs every day. The severity of psoriatic lesions was assessed according

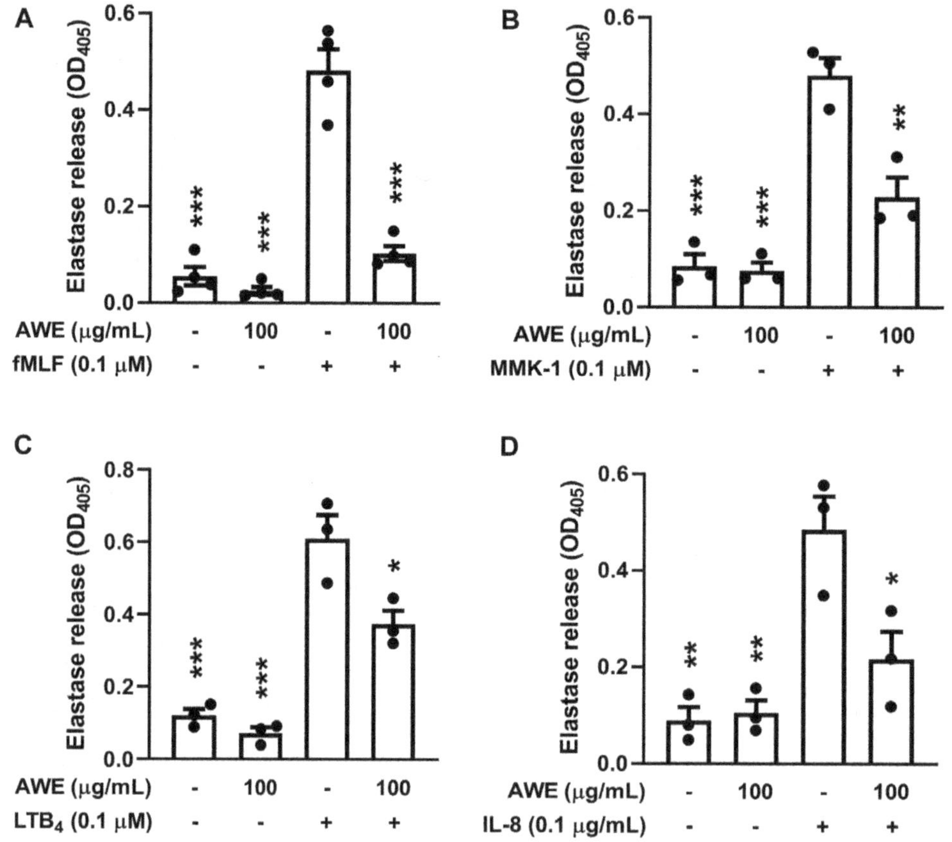

FIGURE 3 | AWE inhibited elastase release in activated human neutrophils by different stimulants. Human neutrophils (6 × 10^5 cells/mL) were incubated with ddH_2O (as the control) or AWE (100 μg/ml) for 5 min, and then activated by **(A)** fMLF, **(B)** MMK-1, **(C)** LTB_4, or **(D)** IL-8 and CB (0.5 μg/ml for fMLF and MMK-1 and 2 μg/ml for IL-8 and LTB_4) for another 10 min. Elastase release was measured by spectrophotometrically at 405 nm. Data are expressed as mean ± S.E.M. (n = 3 or 4). Statistical analysis was conducted using the one-way analysis of variance (ANOVA), followed by Tukey's multiple comparison test if there were statistical differences in the results of ANOVA. Adjusted p-values of Tukey's multiple comparison tests were defined as $^{***}p < 0.001$, $^{**}p < 0.01$, and $^{*}p < 0.05$ compared with the control.

to the human psoriasis area and severity index (PASI) score. The PASI score evaluates lesions including erythema, scaling, and thickness independently according to severity as: 0 for normal; one for mild; two for moderate; three for severe; four for very severe condition in psoriasis lesions. The images of psoriatic lesions were scored by two investigators, Dr. Cheng and Dr. Chiang. The image files were renamed for blinding purpose. The final scores of each image were the average score of the two investigators.

On day 6, mice were sacrificed by deep anesthesia, and then the skin samples were collected from their backs then fixed in 10% paraformaldehyde. The skin sections were subjected to hematoxylin-eosin (H&E) and immunohistochemical (IHC) staining including Ly6G (a neutrophil marker), MPO (an ROS catalyzer released by neutrophils), ki67 (a skin proliferation marker), and 4-HNE (an ROS-induced damage marker from lipid peroxidation chain reaction) following a standard protocol (Baek et al., 2012; El Malki et al., 2013). Images were quantified using ImageJ 1.53e (Wayne Rasband and contributors, Research Services Branch, National Institute of Health, Bethesda, Maryland, United States) (Schneider et al., 2012). The intensity and area of staining in IHC images were calculated. In HE images, epidermal area and average thickness were calculated.

2.13 Immunohistochemistry

The formalin-fixed paraffin-embedded skin samples were dewaxed and rehydrated before IHC. IHC was performed using an automatic immunohistochemistry staining device according to the manufacturer's instructions (Bond, Leica BioSystems). The tissue sections were retrieved using Bond Epitope Retrieval Solution 1 (Ly6G, MPO, and 4-HNE) or 2 (Ki67) at 100°C for 20 min (Ly6G, MPO, and 4-HNE) or 30 min (Ki67) on the Bond-max automated immunostainer (Leica BioSystems) and stained with antibodies for Ly6G (mouse monoclonal antibody, 1:500 dilution; incubated for 60 min; BioLegend, category no. 127602), MPO (rabbit polyclonal antibody, 1:50 dilution; incubated for 60 min; Abcam, category no. ab9535), Ki67 (rabbit polyclonal antibody, 1:200 dilution; incubated for 30 min; GeneTex, category no.: GTX16667), and 4-HNE (rabbit polyclonal antibody, 1:600 dilution; incubated for 60 min; Bioss, category no.: bs-6313R). For Ly6G staining, secondary antibody staining with 5 μg/ml rabbit anti-rat IgG (ImmunoReagent, category no.: RbxRt-003-DHRPX) for 30 min

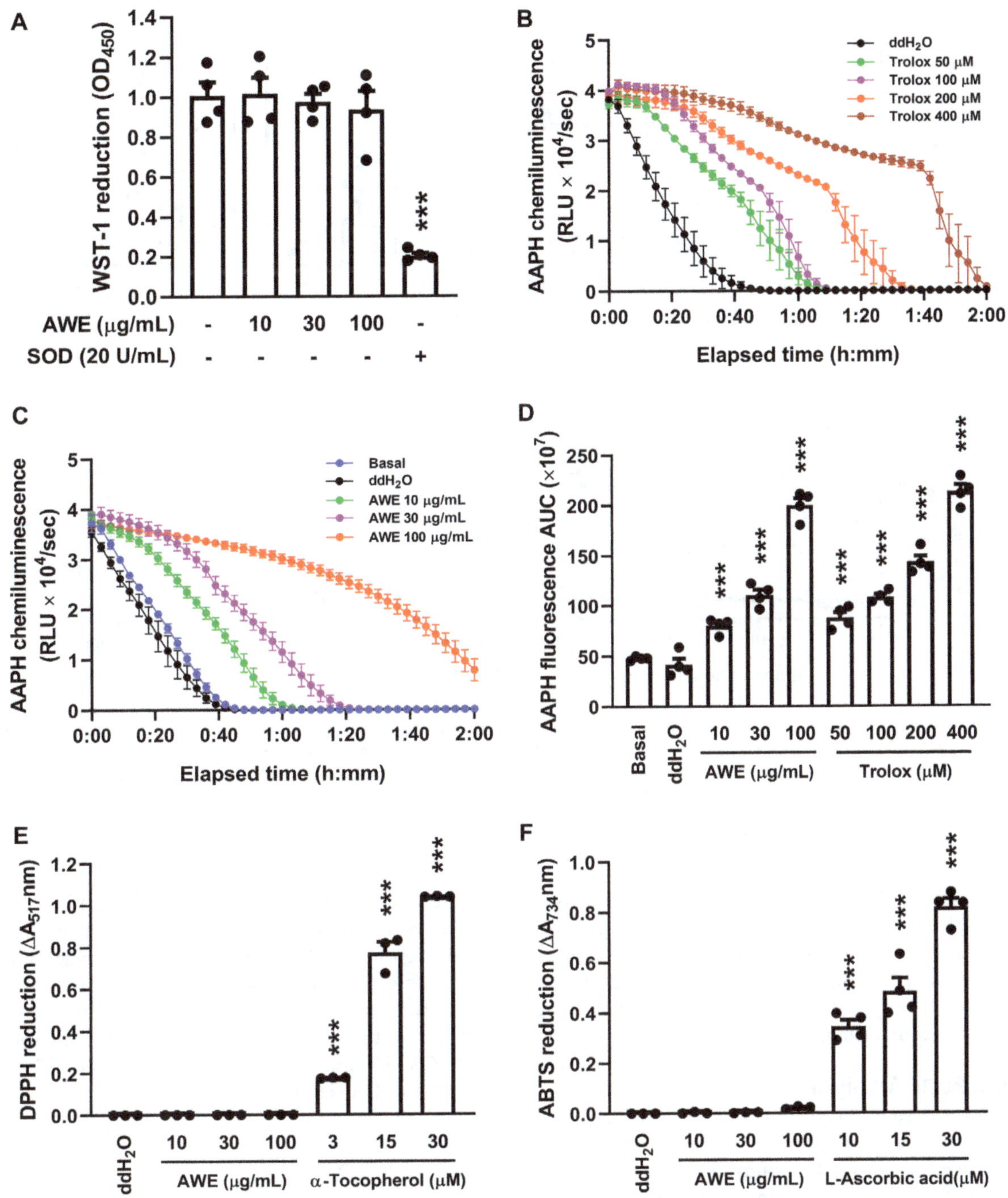

FIGURE 4 | AWE has a significant ROS scavenging effect but neither superoxide anion nor nitrogen-centered radicals. **(A)** 1 mM $CaCl_2$ in HBSS and xanthine oxidase were incubated with ddH_2O (as the control). AWE (10, 30, and 100 μg/ml) was added for 3 min and then xanthine (0.1 mM) for another 10 min. Reduction of WST-1 by superoxide anion was measured spectrophotometrically at 450 nm. Superoxide dismutase (SOD) 20 U/ml was used as the positive control. Fluorescein decay curve induced by AAPH and cleared by **(B)** Trolox and **(C)** AWE in different concentrations. **(D)** The area under the curve of AWE and Trolox. **(E)** DPPH (100 μM in 99% EtOH) was incubated with ddH_2O (as the control), AWE (10, 30, and 100 μg/ml) or α-tocopherol (3, 15, and 30 μM). The reduction of DPPH was measured spectrophotometrically at 517 nm. **(F)** ABTS (7 mM in ddH_2O) was incubated with ddH_2O (as the control), AWE (10, 30, and 100 μg/ml) or L-ascorbic acid (10, 15, and 30 μM). The reduction of ABTS was measured spectrophotometrically at 734 nm. Data are expressed as the mean ± S.E.M. ($n = 3$ or 4). Statistical analysis was conducted using the one-way analysis of variance (ANOVA), followed by Tukey's multiple comparison test if there were statistical differences in the results of ANOVA. Adjusted p-values of Tukey's multiple comparison tests were defined as $^{***}p < 0.001$ compared with ddH_2O alone.

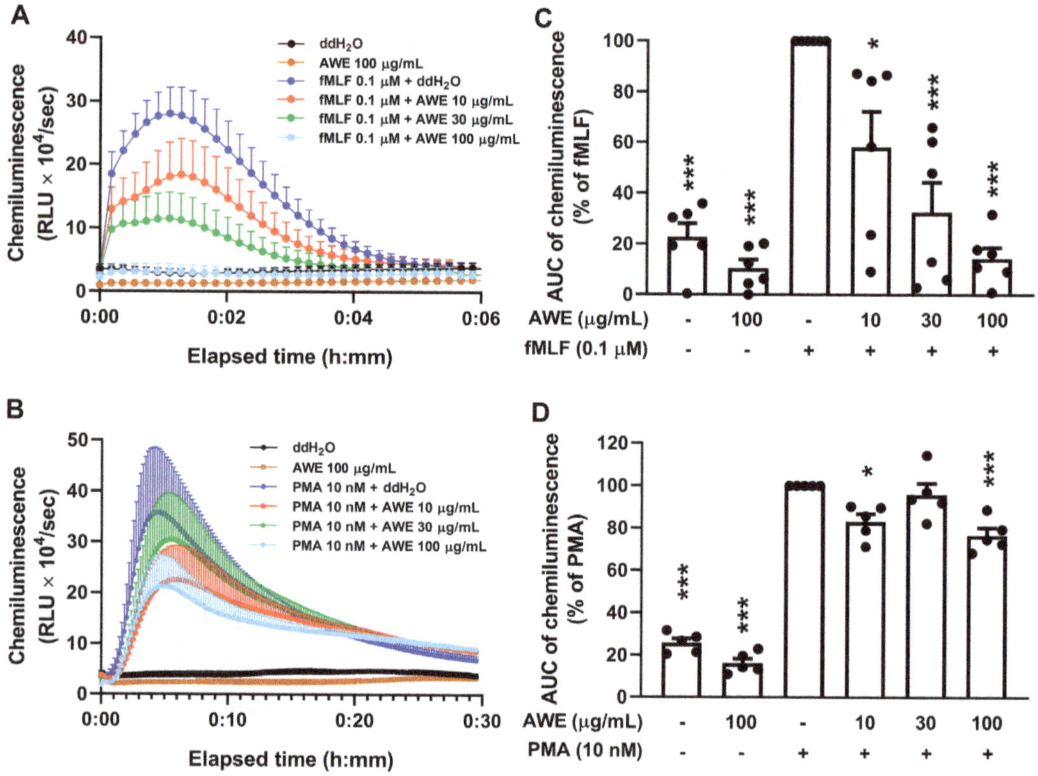

FIGURE 5 | AWE both inhibited neutrophil activation and scavenged ROS generation in fMLF-activated human neutrophils in luminol-enhanced chemiluminescence assay. Human neutrophil (7 × 10^5 cells/mL) were incubated with ddH$_2$O (as the control) or AWE (10, 30, and 100 μg/ml) for 5 min and stimulated with **(A)** fMLF (0.1 μM) for another 6 min or **(B)** PMA (10 nM) for 30 min. The area under curve (AUC) of chemiluminescence in **(C)** fMLF or **(D)** PMA are shown as the mean ± S.E.M. (n = 5 or 6). Statistical analysis was conducted using the one-way analysis of variance (ANOVA), followed by Tukey's multiple comparison test if there were statistical differences in the results of ANOVA. Adjusted p-values of Tukey's multiple comparison tests were defined as $^{***}p < 0.001$ and $^{*}p < 0.05$ compared with the control.

was performed after primary staining. A polymer detection system (Bond Polymer Refine Detection, Leia BioSystems) was used to reduce nonspecific staining. The tissue sections were treated with liquid 3,3′-diaminobenzidine reagent using 3′-diaminobenzidine tetrahydrochloride as the chromogen and hematoxylin as the counterstain.

2.14 Statistical Analysis

All data were expressed as mean ± standard error of the mean (S.E.M.). One-way analysis of variance (ANOVA) was used for comparison between groups in this study. A two-tailed p-value < 0.05 represented a statistically significant difference. Post-hoc analyses were performed using Tukey's multiple comparisons tests for each two-group comparison if the results of the one-way ANOVA indicated significant differences. Results with an adjusted p-value < 0.05 in Tukey's multiple comparisons tests represented a statistically significant difference. For ordinal scale data analysis (PASI scores), a nonparametric analysis method of Kruskal–Wallis test was used in the ANOVA. Post-hoc multiple comparison analyses were performed using the two-stage linear step-up procedure of Benjamini, Krieger, and Yekutieli for every two-group comparison if the results of the Kruskal–Wallis test indicated significant differences. Results with an adjusted q-value < 0.05 using the two-stage linear step-up procedure of Benjamini, Krieger, and Yekutieli for multiple comparison tests represented a statistically significant difference. Data processing and analysis were conducted by using Sigmaplot 14.0 (Systat Software, San Jose, CA, United States) and Prism 9 (GraphPad Software, San Diego, CA, United States).

3 RESULTS

3.1 Identification and Quantification of AWE Using HPLC and UPLC-MS/MS

The fingerprint of the AWE using HPLC is shown in **Figure 1A**. Calycosin-7-*O*-beta-D-glucoside, ononin, and calycosin were identified in the AWE sample using HPLC retention times compared with standard references (**Figure 1B**). The multiple reaction monitoring (MRM) scan in a positive model was utilized to detect Astragaloside IV by acquiring the sodium adduct parent ion $(M + Na)^+$ to product ion transitions of m/z 807.4 → 627.5 and m/z 807.4 → 203.15 with collision voltage of 53 and 59 eV, respectively (Kafle et al., 2020). Product ion of m/z 627.5 was used

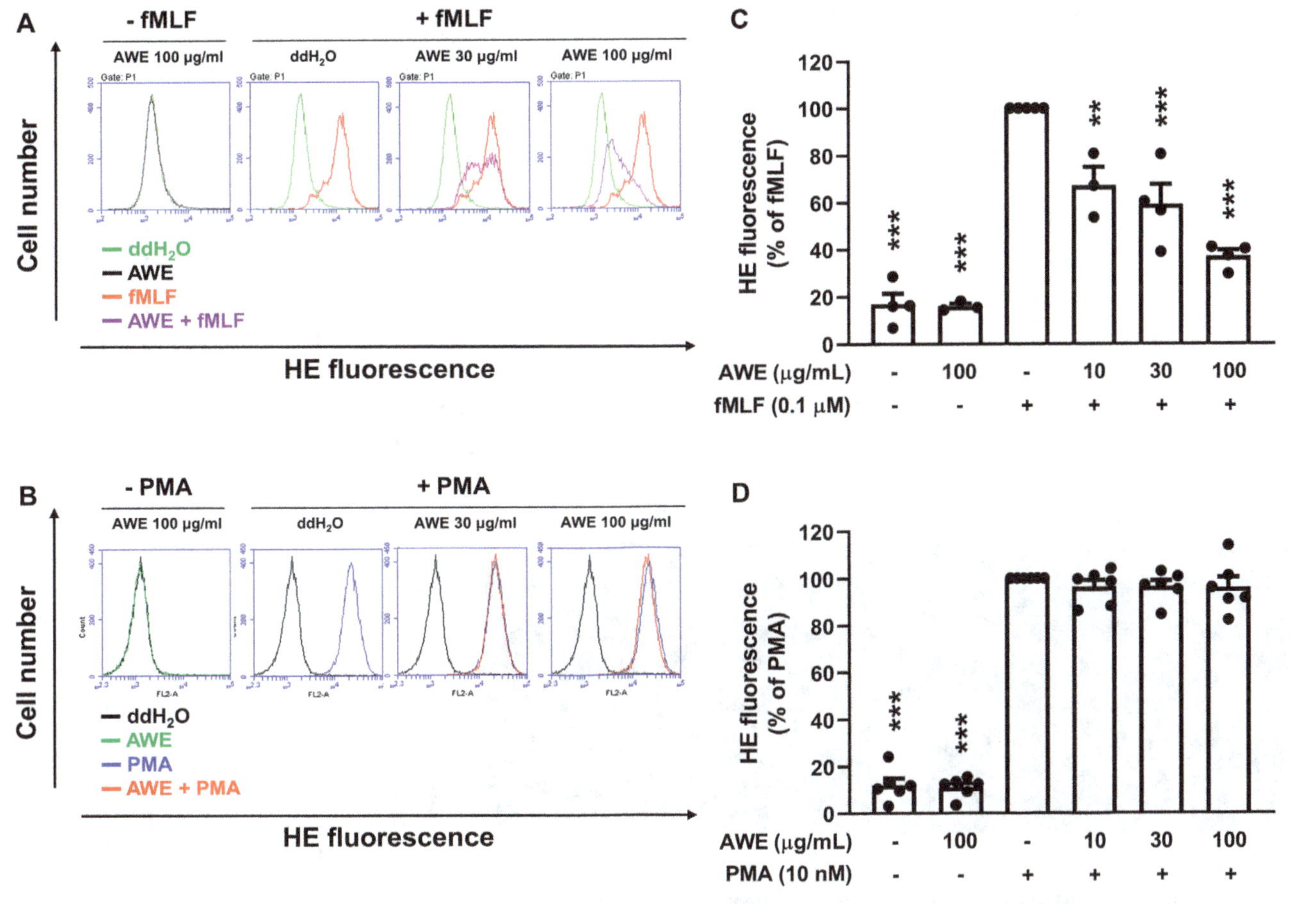

FIGURE 6 | AWE inhibits intracellular superoxide anion generation in fMLF-activated human neutrophils. Human neutrophils labeled with HE were incubated with ddH_2O (as the control) or AWE (10, 30, and 100 μg/ml) for 5 min and then stimulated with **(A)** fMLF (0.1 μM) or **(B)** PMA (10 nM) for an additional 5 min. The representative histograms demonstrating typical fluorescence-activated cell sorting profiles are shown. Mean fluorescence intensities are shown as **(C)** and **(D)**. Data are expressed as the mean ±S.E.M. (n = 3–6). Statistical analysis was conducted using the one-way analysis of variance (ANOVA), followed by Tukey's multiple comparison test if there were statistical differences in the results of ANOVA. Adjusted p-values of Tukey's multiple comparison tests were defined as $^{***}p < 0.001$ and $^{**}p < 0.01$ compared with the control.

for quantification. A linear calibration curve (y = 31083x + 18200, $R^2 = 0.9932$) was produced using 0.625, 1.25, 2.5, 5, 10 ng/ml of Astragaloside IV. Astragaloside IV in AWE was identified according to the peak retention time and two product ion fragments in MRM channels (**Figure 1C**). The quantification of Astragaloside IV in the AWE was 0.048%. The structure of calycosin-7-*O*-beta-D-glucoside, ononin, calycosin, and astragaloside IV is shown in **Figures 1A,D**.

3.2 AWE Inhibits Superoxide Anion Generation and Elastase Release in Activated Human Neutrophils

Neutrophils generate a large amount of superoxide anion by activating NADPH oxidase, further creating abundant ROS by various enzymes. AWE (100 μg/ml) significantly reduced superoxide anion generation in fMLF- and MMK-1-activated human neutrophils in a dose-dependent manner (**Figures 2A,B**), both $p < 0.001$. Nevertheless, AWE was unable to attenuate PMA, a PKC activator, stimulated human neutrophils (**Figure 2C**). Moreover, we found that at 100 μg/ml concentration, AWE did not affect cell viability in the LDH releasing assay (**Figure 2D**).

Human neutrophils create abundant granules into the cytosome, which contain numerous proteolytic and ROS-producing enzymes, including neutrophil elastase, MPO, and cathelicidin (Faurschou and Borregaard, 2003). We observed that AWE (100 μg/ml) significantly inhibited the release of neutrophil elastase in activated human neutrophils with various stimulants such as fMLF ($p <$ 0.001), MMK-1 (p = 0.002), IL-8 (p = 0.0197), and LTB_4 (p = 0.0121) (**Figure 3**). Taken together, these results indicate that AWE inhibits granule releasing and superoxide anion generation, which contributes to oxidative stress production; thus, these data supported the earlier finding that AWE reduced oxidative stress production.

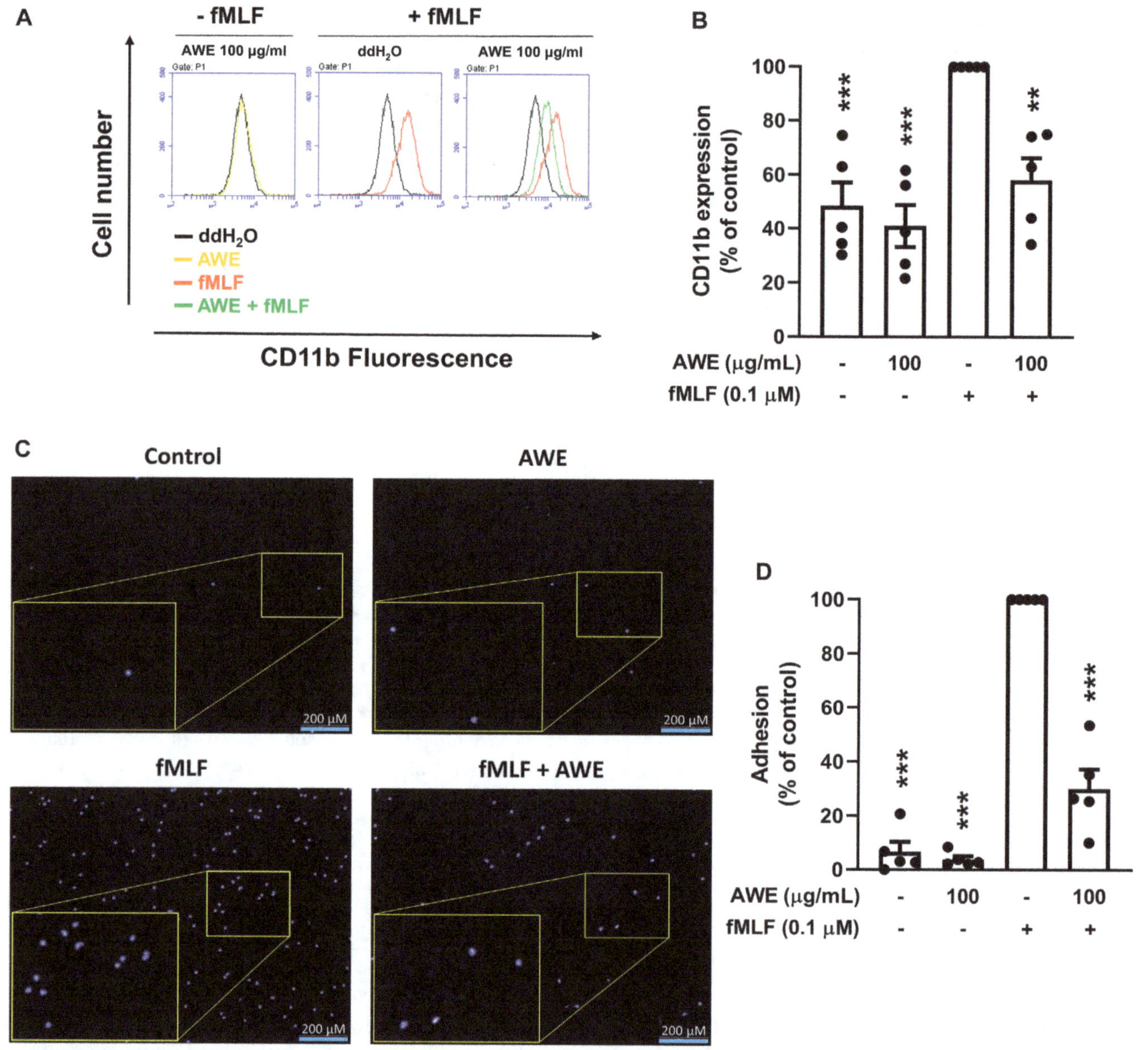

FIGURE 7 | AWE suppressed the adhesion of fMLF-activated human neutrophils to bEnd.3 cells by inhibiting CD11b expression. **(A)** Human neutrophils were incubated with ddH_2O (as the control) or AWE (100 μg/ml) for 5 min and then activated by fMLF (0.1 μM)/CB (1 μg/ml) for an additional 5 min. Representative histograms demonstrating typical fluorescence in the absence or presence of FITC-labeled anti-CD11b. **(B)** Mean fluorescence intensities are shown. **(C)** Hoechst 33342-labeled human neutrophils (4×10^6 cells/mL) were incubated with ddH_2O or AWE (100 μg/ml) for 5 min, then fMLF (0.1 μM) was used as the stimulant. The activated human neutrophils were added into bEnd.3 cells for 15 min. Adherent neutrophils on bEnd.3 cells were detected using a fluorescence microscope. Scale bar represented 200 μm. Representative histograms for fluorescent microscopy are shown. **(D)** Adherent human neutrophils were counted and quantified. Data are expressed as the mean ± S.E.M. (n = 5). Statistical analysis was conducted using the one-way analysis of variance (ANOVA), followed by Tukey's multiple comparison test if there were statistical differences in the results of ANOVA. Adjusted p-values of Tukey's multiple comparison tests were defined as $^{***}p < 0.001$ and $^{**}p < 0.01$ compared with the control.

3.3 AWE has a Substantially ROS Scavenging Effect but Neither Superoxide Anion nor Nitrogen-Centered Radicals

Previous studies demonstrated that AM has abundant anti-oxidative stress activity (Shahzad et al., 2016). Therefore, we used various cell-free oxidative stress generation assays to clarify the ROS scavenging ability of AWE. **Figure 4A** shows that AWE failed to inhibit the superoxide anion produced by the xanthine/xanthine oxidase system, with superoxide dismutase as the positive control ($p < 0.001$). This result implied that while AWE was not able to remove the superoxide anion directly, it may regulate the production of the superoxide anion in activated human neutrophils.

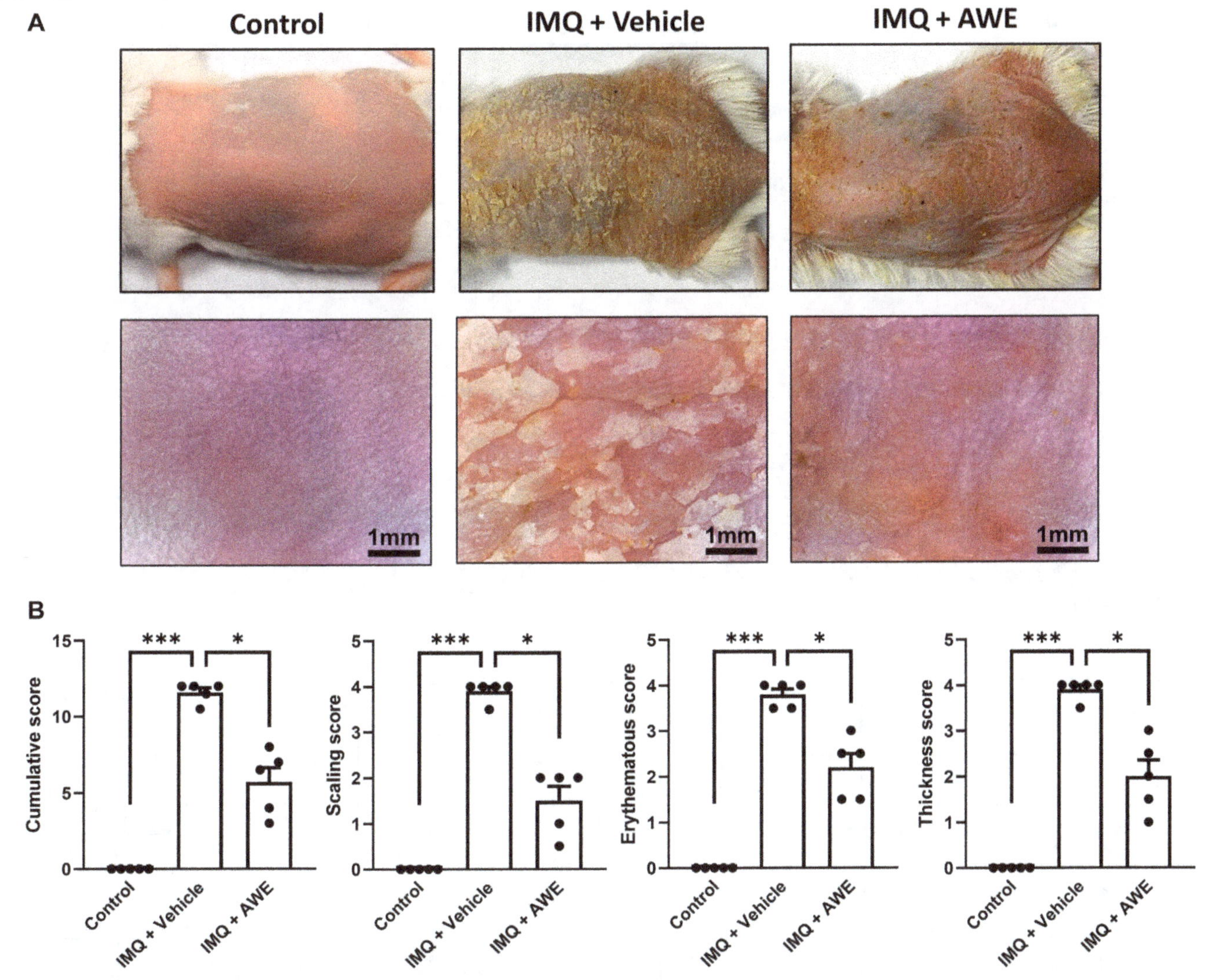

FIGURE 8 | AWE ameliorated the severity of IMQ-induced psoriasis-like skin inflammation. (A) The skin change of IMQ-induced psoriasis-like skin inflammation was observed using a digital camera and a hand-held digital microscope. The scale bar of the picture in a hand-held digital microscope was 1 mm. **(B)** PASI scores, including erythema, thickness, scaling, and cumulative scores in study groups, are shown. Data are expressed as mean S.E.M. ($n = 5$). Statistical analysis was conducted using the Kruskal–Wallis test, followed by multiple comparison test with the two-stage linear step-up procedure of Benjamini, Krieger, and Yekutieli if there were statistical differences in the results of the Kruskal–Wallis test. Adjusted q-values of multiple comparison tests using the two-stage linear step-up procedure of Benjamini, Krieger, and Yekutieli were defined as $^{***}q < 0.001$ and $^{*}q < 0.05$ compared with the IMQ plus vehicle group.

The clearance ability of AWE against ROS and nitrogen-centered radicals was further examined with oxygen-radical absorbance capacity assays, ABTS, and DPPH radical assays, and we observed that AWE and Trolox both had significant antioxidant effects (**Figures 4B–D**), as the APPH-produced ROS was cleared by AWE and Trolox to avoid the degeneration of fluorescein. However, there was no scavenging ability of nitrogen-centered radicals observed in AWE in the ABTS and DPPH assays (**Figures 4E,F**), in which vitamins C and E were the respective positive controls. These results suggested that AWE had a substantially better ROS scavenging ability than superoxide anion and nitrogen-centered radicals.

Taken together, our results revealed that AWE significantly reduced the oxidative stress generated by fMLF-activated human neutrophils, and this effect might have resulted from regulating the activation of human neutrophils and directly scavenging ROS by AWE.

3.4 AWE Reduced Neutrophil-Generated Oxidative Stress by Inhibiting Neutrophil Activation and by Scavenging ROS

Intracellular and extracellular ROS were detected using luminol-enhanced chemiluminescence. AWE significantly inhibited ROS production in fMLF-activated human neutrophils at different concentrations (**Figures 5A,C**). The p-values were 0.0115, <0.001, and <0.001 for 10, 30, and 100 μg/ml. Moreover, our work revealed that AWE had a superior inhibitory effect on ROS production than on

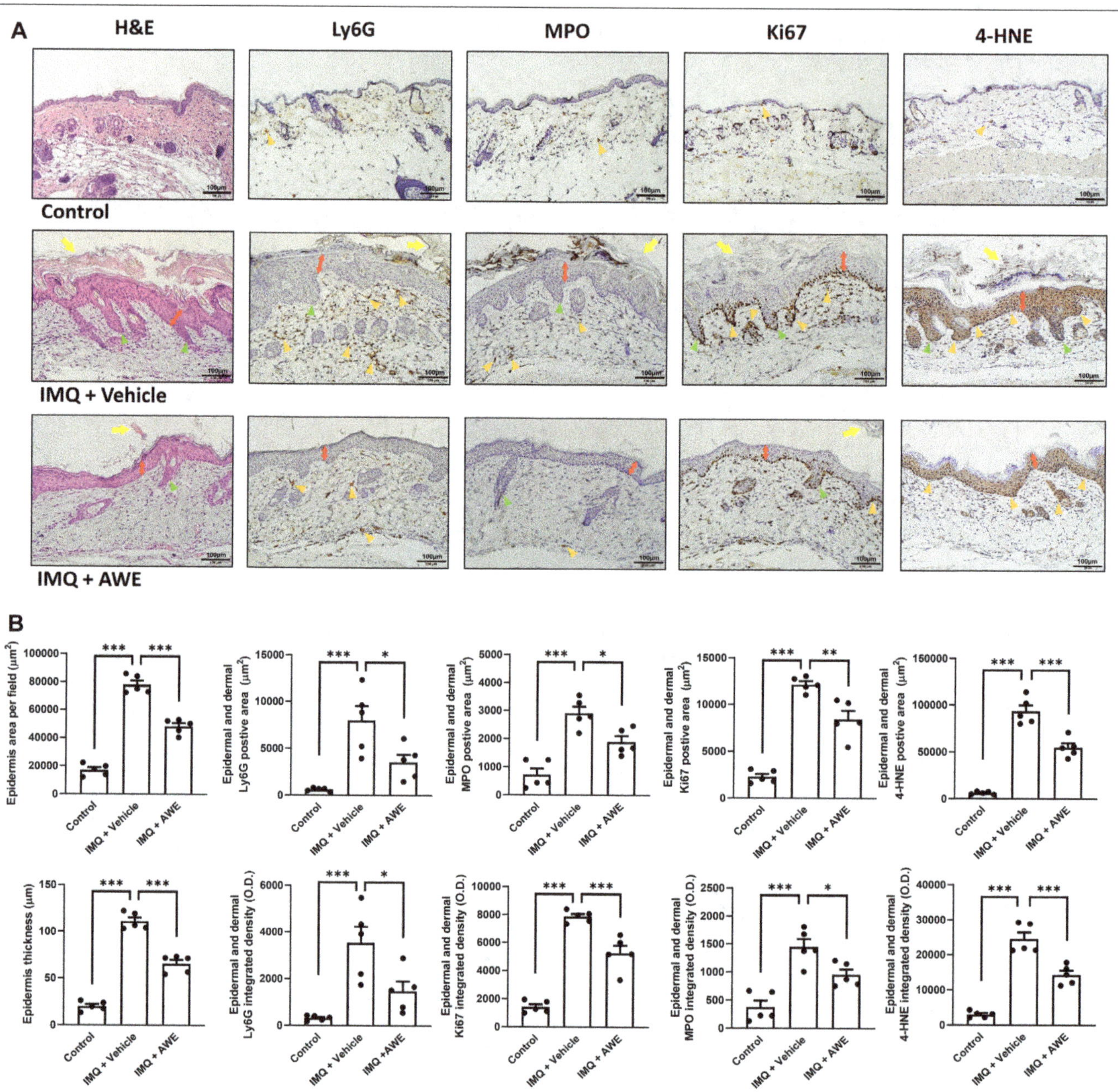

FIGURE 9 | AWE reduced the epidermal thickness and neutrophil infiltration in IMQ-induced psoriasis-like skin inflammation in mice. The mice were sacrificed by deep anesthesia on day 6 after topical IMQ and AWE or vehicle treatment for 5 days. Their back skins were collected and stored in 4% formaldehyde. Hematoxylin-eosin (H&E) staining and immunohistochemical (IHC) staining for Ly6G, MPO (the neutrophil infiltration and activation marker), Ki67 (the epidermal proliferation marker), and 4-HNE (the ROS marker) were performed for all samples (marked as orange triangles). The representative images **(A)** were observed under a microscope. The scale bar was 100 μm. The IMQ plus vehicle group exhibited psoriasis-like skin inflammation. The typical histological manifestations are marked as yellow arrows (hyperkeratosis), double-sided red arrows (acanthosis), and green triangles (elongation of rete-like ridges). AWE significantly decreased neutrophil infiltration and epidermal thickness in IMQ-induced psoriasis-like skin inflammation in mice. **(B)** The quantified image data using ImageJ. Epidermal area and average epidermal thickness were calculated in H&E staining. Ly6G-, MPO-, Ki67-, and 4-HNE-positive area and integrated density were calculated in IHC staining. Data are expressed as mean S.E.M. ($n = 5$). Statistical analysis was conducted using the one-way analysis of variance (ANOVA), followed by Tukey's multiple comparison test if there were statistical differences in the results of ANOVA. Adjusted p-values of Tukey's multiple comparison tests were defined as ***$p < 0.001$, **$p < 0.01$, and *$p < 0.05$ compared with the IMQ plus vehicle group.

superoxide anion generation; the IC_{50} were 17.894 μg/ml and 29.539 μg/ml, respectively. Interestingly, AWE only had a minor inhibitory effect on ROS production in PMA-stimulated human neutrophils (**Figures 5B,D**). The p-values were 0.0136, 0.9461, and <0.001 for 10, 30, and 100 μg/ml. We also noted that AWE was able to reduce ROS production in resting human neutrophils without any stimulant. Taken together, these results indicate that AWE might have a direct antioxidant effect on ROS generation in activated human neutrophils.

Since AWE showed a significantly stronger inhibitory effect on superoxide anion generation in fMLF-activated human neutrophils rather than in PMA-stimulated neutrophils, we used HE as an intracellular superoxide anion probe to clarify AWE's inhibitory effects on human neutrophils (Laurindo et al., 2008). The result suggests that AWE significantly reduced the fluorescein in HE-labelled and fMLF-activated human neutrophils (**Figures 6A,C**). Consistent with our previous findings, AWE failed to inhibit the intracellular superoxide anion generation in PMA-activated human neutrophils (**Figures 6B,D**). Together, these findings suggest that AWE had a substantial inhibitory effect in fMLF-activated human neutrophils.

3.5 AWE Inhibited Activated Neutrophils From Expressing CD11b Integrin and Adhering to Endothelial Cells

The neutrophil surface adhesion molecules, CD11b, were labeled with FITC and detected using flow cytometry. Human neutrophils increased the expression of CD11b following stimulation by fMLP. In contrast, AWE significantly inhibited CD11b expression in the cell membrane of activated human neutrophils (**Figures 7A,B**), $p < 0.001$, suggesting that AWE could decrease cell adhesion and migration in activated human neutrophils.

To ascertain whether the effects of AWE on reduction of adhesion protein can further decrease cell adhesion in activated human neutrophils, we used bEnd.3 cells to mimic the endothelial environment with fMLF-activated neutrophils. We found that AWE significantly reduced the adhesion of activated human neutrophils to bEnd.3 endothelial cells (**Figures 7C,D**), $p = 0.0037$. Taken together, AWE in 100 μg/ml had a significant inhibitory effect on CD11b expression and on cell adhesion in fMLF-activated human neutrophils.

3.6 AWE Reduces Neutrophil Infiltration and Ameliorates IMQ-Induced Psoriasis-like Skin Inflammation in Mice

IMQ is a toll-like (TLR-7/8) receptor agonist. Application of IMQ on mice skin causes immune cell infiltration and skin inflammatory changes, such as erythema, scaling, hyperkeratosis formation, similar to those of human psoriasis (Baek et al., 2012; El Malki et al., 2013). Compared with that of the control group (without IMQ), mice treated with IMQ cream for 5 days exhibited gross skin appearance that showed psoriasis-like skin inflammation (**Figure 8A**). However, the topical administration of AWE alleviated psoriasis-like skin inflammation symptoms in the IMQ plus AWE group compared to that in the IMQ plus vehicle group, in which severe scaling and skin thickening were found. In addition, AWE significantly reduced the PASI score based on skin thickness ($p = 0.0484$), erythema ($p = 0.0490$), and scaling ($p = 0.0477$) in this mouse model (**Figure 8B**).

In the IMQ plus vehicle group, the IMQ-induced skin inflammation resulted in the thickened epidermis (also called acanthosis) in the H&E staining, while IHC staining revealed increased levels of Ki67, the epidermal proliferation marker. Moreover, increased Ly6G and MPO expression were observed in the IHC, indicating that neutrophils were activated and recruited from peripheral tissues. Increased 4-HNE level from lipid peroxidation implied cell damage by ROS generated by infiltrated immune cells, leading to the pathogenesis of psoriasis (**Figure 9A**). Aside from that, severe neutrophil infiltration was also observed in the epidermis and dermis area, which is a typical psoriasis manifestation (Munro's microabscess). Increased thickness of the epidermis represented skin edema of psoriatic skin lesions. Hyperkeratosis and parakeratosis were also found in the epidermis area. In the IMQ plus AWE group, topical AWE (10 mg/day) significantly reduced epidermal thickness (skin edema) and hyperkeratosis compared to IMQ plus vehicle group. The IHC staining revealed a lower Ki67 positive area and integrated density (**Figure 9B**). In addition, lower Ly6G and MPO demonstrated that AWE inhibited neutrophil recruitment and infiltration. Reduced 4-HNE level represented decreased ROS-induced damage in the epidermis. Meanwhile, the control group had a normal epidermis and did not display neutrophil infiltration.

In summary, these results show that topical AWE administration significantly inhibited neutrophil recruitment and infiltration, thereby reducing ROS-induced damage in the epidermis and skin proliferation in the IMQ-induced psoriasis-like skin inflammation mouse model.

4 DISCUSSION

Oxidative stress is caused by free radicals, such as ROS or reactive nitrogen species. Excessive ROS production, which leads to an imbalance between oxidative stress and antioxidants, causes cell and tissue damage (Xie et al., 2019). Plant polysaccharides are antioxidant constituents and abundant in natural herbal products (Jiao et al., 2016). Astragalus polysaccharides (APS), the primary components of AM, can inhibit neutrophils infiltration in the lipopolysaccharide (LPS)-induced acute lung injury rat model and reduce MPO activity and ROS level in the bronchoalveolar lavage fluid (Fang et al., 2017). A murine asthma model induced by ovalbumin-LPS demonstrated that APS inhibits neutrophil-dominant airway inflammation and how this could relate to the modulation of endoplasmic reticulum stress (Lu et al., 2016). The mechanisms underlying APS improvement of cell and tissue damage are also associated with NF-κB and p38-MAPK signaling pathways (Lu et al., 2016; Fan et al., 2019).

AM contains several bioactive flavonoids, including calycosin, calycosin-7-*O*-β-D-glucoside, ononin, and formononetin. Formononetin and calycosin, which are the non-glycoside forms of ononin and calycosin-7-*O*-β-D-glucoside, respectively (Yang et al., 2013), have a protective effect in LPS-induced cell injury and in H_2O_2-induced liver injury (Jiang et al., 2015; Li et al., 2015). Calycosin-7-*O*-β-D-glucoside and calycosin can scavenge nitro-oxide, resulting in tissue damage in the cerebral I/R injury rat model (Fu S. et al., 2014). Moreover, studies have shown that these isoflavones have neuroprotective effects that may involve the phosphatidylinositol 3-kinase-Akt signaling pathway (Jiang et al., 2015; Gu et al., 2021).

Astragaloside IV, an essential and influential saponin in AM, is known to have protective effects against organ and tissue injury (Li L. et al., 2017; Zhang et al., 2020). It has also been reported to exhibit ROS scavenging activity against oxidative stress, protecting ischemia/reperfusion (I/R) injury in the hearts and brain (Li H. et al., 2018; Jiang et al., 2019). Cycloastragenol, another triterpenoid saponin, is a hydrolysis product of Astragaloside IV that also has significant anti-inflammatory and antioxidant capabilities (Yu Y. et al., 2018), and is reported to play an inhibitory role in ROS-associated endoplasmic reticulum stress via NLRP3 inflammasome (Zhao et al., 2015).

These anti-oxidation components make AM an effective antioxidant that protects cells and tissues against ROS damage. Herein, AWE exhibited significant ROS scavenging capability in the AAPH cell-free system, which was compatible with other studies that showed that AM could clear ROS in H_2O_2 assay (Han et al., 2017; Adesso et al., 2018). Interestingly, we also found that AWE cleared neither the superoxide anion generated by xanthine oxidase nor the nitrogen-centered radicals, including DPPH and ABTS.

Neutrophils, the most plentiful leukocyte in blood, contained NADPH oxidase, which is the primary source of ROS production in the human body (Dahlgren and Karlsson, 1999; Jaquet et al., 2011; Wang et al., 2012; Ruhnau et al., 2014). Activated human neutrophils generate abundant ROS by respiratory burst, degranulation, and release neutrophil extracellular traps, causing tissue damage and aggravating many clinical diseases (Papayannopoulos, 2018).

Our study showed that AWE significantly reduced superoxide generation in fMLF-activated human neutrophils. However, even if AWE revealed a substantial ROS scavenging capability in the AAPH assay, it only showed a minor effect on clearing ROS while using luminol-enhanced chemiluminescence with or without stimulating neutrophils. Moreover, AWE did not directly scavenge superoxide anion in the cell-free xanthine/xanthine oxidase system. These results demonstrate that AWE had a significant inhibitory effect on superoxide anion generation in fMLF-activated human neutrophils.

When neutrophils are activated, granules inside the cytoplasm containing abundant proteolytic enzymes such as elastase and MPO, which contribute to a large ROS production, are released against microorganisms (Faurschou and Borregaard, 2003). Our study showed that AWE's inhibitory effect on neutrophil activation also inhibited elastase release when neutrophils were activated by various stimulants.

Neutrophils in the peripheral blood respond to chemoattractants to infiltrate infectious or inflammatory tissues. The expression of surface adhesive molecular CD11b/CD18 and β2 integrins are well known to regulate neutrophil adhesion and transmigration (Sekheri et al., 2021). Our results also showed that AWE inhibited fMLF-activated human neutrophils by inhibiting the expression of CD11b on the cell membrane. Further, there was decreased neutrophil adherence to the vascular endothelial cell. Consistent with previous Astragaloside IV studies, we also found the same inhibitory effects on neutrophil infiltration to the inflammatory site by LPS-induced inflammatory or infectious murine model (Zhang and Frei, 2015; Huang et al., 2016), which may have resulted from the inhibition of neutrophil that express surface adherence proteins CD11b/CD18 and the downregulation of intercellular adhesion molecule-1 (ICAM-1) via NF-κB pathway (Li M. et al., 2012). In contrast, another study analyzing APS using human neutrophils and human umbilical vein endothelial cells (HUVECs) demonstrated that APS promotes the adhesion of human neutrophils to HUVECs and the upregulation of ICAM-1 on the surface of IL-1 treated endothelial cells; no effect on CD18 expression in human neutrophils treated with APS was observed (Hao et al., 2004).

Psoriasis is a chronic immune-mediated disease with erythematous, scaling, and thickening in the skin. Neutrophil infiltration causes neutrophilic inflammation, which can worsen the symptoms (Lowes et al., 2014; Chiang et al., 2019). Topical application of IMQ, a toll-like receptor 7/8 agonist, on mouse skin causes immune cell accumulation, releasing cytokine and ROS, which damages dermal and epidermal tissues, leading to psoriasis-like skin changes (Baek et al., 2012; El Malki et al., 2013). This change is due to cell proliferation in the epidermis. Ki67, a marker for cell proliferation, is overexpressed in proliferating keratinocytes in psoriatic skin, which can be regulated by T cells (Alhosaini et al., 2021). Increased IL-17-related immune responses contribute to skin cell proliferation observed in a psoriasis animal model (Nadeem et al., 2018). Although T cell and antigen-presenting cells have been known to be involved in the pathogenesis of psoriasis, neutrophils play a critical role by infiltrating the epidermis and secreting copious amounts of IL-17A, thus affecting keratinocytes and leading to skin proliferation (Katayama, 2018). In this study, we found that in the IMQ-induced psoriasis-like skin inflammation model, the topical application of AWE significantly improved skin inflammation and both the individual and cumulative PASI scores. Moreover, AWE reduced dermal thickness, neutrophil infiltration, MPO release, ROS-induced damage, and skin proliferation, as observed in microscopic IHC-stained slides. These results are consistent with a recent study of cycloastragenol on IMQ-induced psoriasis-like skin lesions, which regulate macrophage via inhibiting NLRP3 inflammasome-mediated pyroptosis (Deng et al., 2019).

In the pathogenesis of psoriasis, multiple immune cell interactions lead to skin proliferation and hyperkeratosis. Resident macrophages also play an important role in releasing chemoattractants to recruit neutrophils from peripheral blood to the inflammatory site. It is not clear whether the inhibitory effect of AWE on neutrophil recruitment in this animal model is associated with the inhibition of macrophage activation or not. However, studies have found that APS and astragaloside IV could activate isolated mouse peritoneal macrophages and RAW 264.7 through the NF-κB pathway (Lee and Jeon, 2005; Li Y. et al., 2017; Wang et al., 2017; Li ZP. et al., 2018). In different cancer cell lines, such as breast cancer (Li et al., 2019), lung cancer (Bamodu et al., 2019), and liver cancer (Yu J. et al., 2018), APS exerts anti-tumor effects by activating macrophages (Liu et al., 2017; Li et al., 2020). Moreover, APS has been found to promote alveolar macrophage phagocytosis and decrease lung inflammation in a chronic obstructive pulmonary disease animal model (Chu et al., 2016). Interestingly, the flavonoids and saponin in *Astragalus* also exerted an inhibitory effect on LPS-stimulated RAW 264.7 macrophages and mouse peritoneal macrophages via the NF-κB pathway (Wang et al., 2002; Lee DY. et al., 2013; Li J. et al., 2018). The inhibitory effect of astragaloside IV on macrophages via the NF-κB pathway has also been reported in a mouse abdominal aortic aneurysm model (Wang et al., 2018). Another rat dialysis peritoneal fibrosis model demonstrated that *Astragalus* extract inhibited macrophage recruitment and activation (Li et al., 2014).

Some studies on astragaloside IV have reported that it promotes macrophages M2 polarization to reduce the inflammatory state and increase tissue healing in cerebral ischemia–reperfusion injury and inflammatory bowel disease animal models (Li et al., 2021; Tian et al., 2021). Nevertheless, another study on the effect of astragaloside IV in lung cancer showed a decrease in M2 macrophages to reduce tumor growth and metastasis (Xu et al., 2018).

Despite the inconsistent results of studies on the effect of *Astragalus* on the macrophages, we focused on the effect of AWE on neutrophils and found the inhibitory effect on neutrophil recruitment and activation in psoriasis animal models. However, our limited results could not rule out the possible effect of AWE on macrophages in psoriasis. Further studies are needed to determine the promoting or inhibitory effect of the different components in AWE on macrophages.

In this study, AWE showed its antioxidant capability of ROS scavenge and directly inhibited neutrophil activation, further ameliorating neutrophilic inflammation in IMQ-induced psoriasis-like skin lesions in mice. We also identified active components in AWE, including calycosin, ononin, calycosin-7-*O*-β-D-glucoside, and Astragaloside IV. Since APS, flavonoids, and saponins in AM have anti-inflammatory bioactivities, further research is warranted to clarify whether the anti-inflammatory effects observed were attributed to individual components or combination effects. Furthermore, research targeting the signaling pathway on inhibiting activation of neutrophils by AWE could promote developing anti-neutrophilic inflammation drugs.

5 CONCLUSION

In summary, our work demonstrated the direct inhibitory effect of AWE on fMLF-activated human neutrophils, which also inhibited superoxide generation and elastase release. Moreover, AWE effectively scavenged ROS in the AAPH assay and directly inhibited neutrophil activation, further reducing CD11b expression and adhesion to vascular endothelial cells. AWE also ameliorated skin lesions in IMQ-induced psoriasis-like skin inflammation and inhibited neutrophil infiltration, MPO release, ROS-induced damage, and skin proliferation. Our results suggest that AWE can potentially inhibit neutrophil activation and alleviate neutrophilic inflammation in psoriasis.

AUTHOR CONTRIBUTIONS

Conceptualization, W-JC and C-CC; Methodology, W-JC, C-CC, Y-LC, and Y-LL; Validation, Y-LC and W-JC; Investigation, W-JC, C-CC, C-YL, J-YS, and W-LC; Data curation, W-JC; Writing—original draft preparation, W-JC and C-CC; Writing—review and editing, W-JC, C-CC, C-YH, and J-JK; Visualization, W-JC; Supervision, J-JK and T-LH; All authors have read and agreed to the published version of the manuscript.

ACKNOWLEDGMENTS

We thank Yu-Chia Chang for the analysis of the chemical structure. We also thank Ya-Xuan Wang and the Pathology Core of the Molecular Medicine Research Center at Chang Gung University for technical assistance. We thank Chueh-Yung Tsao at Chang Gung University for the statistical analysis. We thank BioRender.com for image assistance. The graphical abstract was adapted from "The IL-23/IL-17 Axis in Psoriasis" by BioRender.com (2020). Retrieved from https://app.biorender.com/biorender-templates

REFERENCES

Adesso, S., Russo, R., Quaroni, A., Autore, G., and Marzocco, S. (2018). Astragalus Membranaceus Extract Attenuates Inflammation and Oxidative Stress in Intestinal Epithelial Cells via NF-κB Activation and Nrf2 Response. *Int. J. Mol. Sci.* 19 (3), 800. doi:10.3390/ijms19030800

Agyemang, K., Han, L., Liu, E., Zhang, Y., Wang, T., and Gao, X. (2013). Recent Advances inAstragalus membranaceusAnti-Diabetic Research: Pharmacological Effects of its Phytochemical Constituents. *Evid. Based Complement. Altern. Med.* 2013, 1–9. doi:10.1155/2013/654643

Al-Harbi, N. O., Nadeem, A., Ahmad, S. F., Bakheet, S. A., El-Sherbeeny, A. M., Ibrahim, K. E., et al. (2020). Therapeutic Treatment with Ibrutinib Attenuates Imiquimod-Induced Psoriasis-like Inflammation in Mice through Downregulation of Oxidative and Inflammatory Mediators in Neutrophils and Dendritic Cells. *Eur. J. Pharmacol.* 877, 173088. doi:10.1016/j.ejphar.2020.173088

Alhosaini, K., Ansari, M. A., Nadeem, A., Attia, S. M., Bakheet, S. A., Al-Ayadhi, L. Y., et al. (2021). Dysregulation of Ki-67 Expression in T Cells of Children with Autism Spectrum Disorder. *Children* 8 (2), 116. doi:10.3390/children8020116

Baek, J. O., Byamba, D., Wu, W. H., Kim, T. G., and Lee, M. G. (2012). Assessment of an Imiquimod-Induced Psoriatic Mouse Model in Relation to Oxidative Stress. *Arch. Dermatol. Res.* 304 (9), 699–706. doi:10.1007/s00403-012-1272-y

Bamodu, O. A., Kuo, K. T., Wang, C. H., Huang, W. C., Wu, A. T. H., Tsai, J. T., et al. (2019). Astragalus Polysaccharides (PG2) Enhances the M1 Polarization of Macrophages, Functional Maturation of Dendritic Cells, and T Cell-Mediated Anticancer Immune Responses in Patients with Lung Cancer. *Nutrients* 11 (10), 2264. doi:10.3390/nu11102264

Betigeri, S., Thakur, A., and Raghavan, K. (2005). Use of 2,2'-Azobis(2-Amidinopropane) Dihydrochloride as a Reagent Tool for Evaluation of Oxidative Stability of Drugs. *Pharm. Res.* 22 (2), 310–317. doi:10.1007/s11095-004-1199-x

Boehncke, W. H., and Schön, M. P. (2015). Psoriasis. *Lancet* 386 (9997), 983–994. doi:10.1016/S0140-6736(14)61909-7

Cannavò, S. P., Riso, G., Casciaro, M., Di Salvo, E., and Gangemi, S. (2019). Oxidative Stress Involvement in Psoriasis: a Systematic Review. *Free Radic. Res.* 53 (8), 829–840. doi:10.1080/10715762.2019.1648800

Chang, H. L., Chang, F. R., Chen, J. S., Wang, H. P., Wu, Y. H., Wang, C. C., et al. (2008). Inhibitory Effects of 16-Hydroxycleroda-3,13(14)e-Dien-15-Oic Acid on Superoxide Anion and Elastase Release in Human Neutrophils through Multiple Mechanisms. *Eur. J. Pharmacol.* 586 (1-3), 332–339. doi:10.1016/j.ejphar.2008.02.041

Chen, X., Peng, L. H., Li, N., Li, Q. M., Li, P., Fung, K. P., et al. (2012). The Healing and Anti-scar Effects of Astragaloside IV on the Wound Repair *In Vitro* and *In Vivo*. *J. Ethnopharmacol.* 139 (3), 721–727. doi:10.1016/j.jep.2011.11.035

Chen, P. J., Wang, Y. L., Kuo, L. M., Lin, C. F., Chen, C. Y., Tsai, Y. F., et al. (2016). Honokiol Suppresses TNF-α-Induced Neutrophil Adhesion on Cerebral Endothelial Cells by Disrupting Polyubiquitination and Degradation of IκBα. *Sci. Rep.* 6, 26554. doi:10.1038/srep26554

Chen, T., Zou, H., Wu, X., Liu, C., Situ, B., Zheng, L., et al. (2018). Nanozymatic Antioxidant System Based on MoS2 Nanosheets. *ACS Appl. Mater. Inter.* 10 (15), 12453–12462. doi:10.1021/acsami.8b01245

Chiang, C. C., Cheng, W. J., Korinek, M., Lin, C. Y., and Hwang, T. L. (2019). Neutrophils in Psoriasis. *Front. Immunol.* 10, 2376. doi:10.3389/fimmu.2019.02376

Chiang, C. C., Cheng, W. J., Lin, C. Y., Lai, K. H., Ju, S. C., Lee, C., et al. (2020). Kan-Lu-Hsiao-Tu-Tan, a Traditional Chinese Medicine Formula, Inhibits Human Neutrophil Activation and Ameliorates Imiquimod-Induced Psoriasis-like Skin Inflammation. *J. Ethnopharmacol.* 246, 112246. doi:10.1016/j.jep.2019.112246

Chu, X., Liu, X. J., Qiu, J. M., Zeng, X. L., Bao, H. R., and Shu, J. (2016). Effects of Astragalus and Codonopsis Pilosula Polysaccharides on Alveolar Macrophage Phagocytosis and Inflammation in Chronic Obstructive Pulmonary Disease Mice Exposed to PM2.5. *Environ. Toxicol. Pharmacol.* 48, 76–84. doi:10.1016/j.etap.2016.10.006

Dahlgren, C., and Karlsson, A. (1999). Respiratory Burst in Human Neutrophils. *J. Immunol. Methods* 232 (1-2), 3–14. doi:10.1016/s0022-1759(99)00146-5

Deng, G., Chen, W., Wang, P., Zhan, T., Zheng, W., Gu, Z., et al. (2019). Inhibition of NLRP3 Inflammasome-Mediated Pyroptosis in Macrophage by Cycloastragenol Contributes to Amelioration of Imiquimod-Induced Psoriasis-like Skin Inflammation in Mice. *Int. Immunopharmacol.* 74, 105682. doi:10.1016/j.intimp.2019.105682

Dupré-Crochet, S., Erard, M., and Nüβe, O. (2013). ROS Production in Phagocytes: Why, when, and where? *J. Leukoc. Biol.* 94 (4), 657–670. doi:10.1189/jlb.1012544

El Malki, K., Karbach, S. H., Huppert, J., Zayoud, M., Reissig, S., Schüler, R., et al. (2013). An Alternative Pathway of Imiquimod-Induced Psoriasis-like Skin Inflammation in the Absence of Interleukin-17 Receptor a Signaling. *J. Invest. Dermatol.* 133 (2), 441–451. doi:10.1038/jid.2012.318

Fan, L., Li, M., Cao, F. Y., Zeng, Z. W., Li, X. B., Ma, C., et al. (2019). Astragalus Polysaccharide Ameliorates Lipopolysaccharide-Induced Cell Injury in ATDC5 Cells via miR-92a/KLF4 Mediation. *Biomed. Pharmacother.* 118, 109180. doi:10.1016/j.biopha.2019.109180

Fang, J., Yang, Y., Liu, J., Song, W., and Xu, S. (2017). Astragalus Polysaccharide Alleviates Lipopolysaccharide-Induced Lung Injury in Rats by Inhibiting Neutrophil Activation. *Xi Bao Yu Fen Zi Mian Yi Xue Za Zhi* 33 (8), 1020–1023.

Faurschou, M., and Borregaard, N. (2003). Neutrophil Granules and Secretory Vesicles in Inflammation. *Microbes Infect.* 5 (14), 1317–1327. doi:10.1016/j.micinf.2003.09.008

Fu, J., Wang, Z., Huang, L., Zheng, S., Wang, D., Chen, S., et al. (2014a). Review of the Botanical Characteristics, Phytochemistry, and Pharmacology of Astragalus Membranaceus (Huangqi). *Phytother Res.* 28 (9), 1275–1283. doi:10.1002/ptr.5188

Fu, S., Gu, Y., Jiang, J. Q., Chen, X., Xu, M., Chen, X., et al. (2014b). Calycosin-7-O-β-D-glucoside Regulates Nitric Oxide /caveolin-1/matrix Metalloproteinases Pathway and Protects Blood-Brain Barrier Integrity in Experimental Cerebral Ischemia-Reperfusion Injury. *J. Ethnopharmacol.* 155 (1), 692–701. doi:10.1016/j.jep.2014.06.015

Furue, M., Furue, K., Tsuji, G., and Nakahara, T. (2020). Interleukin-17A and Keratinocytes in Psoriasis. *Int. J. Mol. Sci.* 21 (4), 1275. doi:10.3390/ijms21041275

Glennon-Alty, L., Hackett, A. P., Chapman, E. A., and Wright, H. L. (2018). Neutrophils and Redox Stress in the Pathogenesis of Autoimmune Disease. *Free Radic. Biol. Med.* 125, 25–35. doi:10.1016/j.freeradbiomed.2018.03.049

Gu, Y., Chen, X., Fu, S., Liu, W., Wang, Q., Liu, K. J., et al. (2021). Astragali Radix Isoflavones Synergistically Alleviate Cerebral Ischemia and Reperfusion Injury via Activating Estrogen Receptor-PI3K-Akt Signaling Pathway. *Front. Pharmacol.* 12, 533028. doi:10.3389/fphar.2021.533028

Gupta, R., Debbaneh, M. G., and Liao, W. (2014). Genetic Epidemiology of Psoriasis. *Curr. Dermatol. Rep.* 3 (1), 61–78. doi:10.1007/s13671-013-0066-6

Han, R., Tang, F., Lu, M., Xu, C., Hu, J., Mei, M., et al. (2017). Astragalus Polysaccharide Ameliorates H2O2-Induced Human Umbilical Vein Endothelial Cell Injury. *Mol. Med. Rep.* 15 (6), 4027–4034. doi:10.3892/mmr.2017.6515

Hao, Y., Qiu, Q. Y., and Wu, J. (2004). Effect of Astragalus Polysaccharides in Promoting Neutrophil-Vascular Endothelial Cell Adhesion and Expression of Related Adhesive Molecules. *Zhongguo Zhong Xi Yi Jie He Za Zhi* 24 (5), 427–430.

Herster, F., Bittner, Z., Archer, N. K., Dickhöfer, S., Eisel, D., Eigenbrod, T., et al. (2020). Neutrophil Extracellular Trap-Associated RNA and LL37 Enable Self-Amplifying Inflammation in Psoriasis. *Nat. Commun.* 11 (1), 105. doi:10.1038/s41467-019-13756-4

Huang, P., Lu, X., Yuan, B., Liu, T., Dai, L., Liu, Y., et al. (2016). Astragaloside IV Alleviates E. Coli-Caused Peritonitis via Upregulation of Neutrophil Influx to the Site of Infection. *Int. Immunopharmacol.* 39, 377–382. doi:10.1016/j.intimp.2016.08.011

Jaquet, V., Marcoux, J., Forest, E., Leidal, K. G., McCormick, S., Westermaier, Y., et al. (2011). NADPH Oxidase (NOX) Isoforms Are Inhibited by Celastrol with a Dual Mode of Action. *Br. J. Pharmacol.* 164 (2b), 507–520. doi:10.1111/j.1476-5381.2011.01439.x

Jiang, Y. H., Sun, W., Li, W., Hu, H. Z., Zhou, L., Jiang, H. H., et al. (2015). Calycosin-7-O-β-D-glucoside Promotes Oxidative Stress-Induced Cytoskeleton Reorganization through Integrin-Linked Kinase Signaling Pathway in Vascular Endothelial Cells. *BMC Complement. Altern. Med.* 15, 315. doi:10.1186/s12906-015-0839-5

Jiang, M., Ni, J., Cao, Y., Xing, X., Wu, Q., and Fan, G. (2019). Astragaloside IV Attenuates Myocardial Ischemia-Reperfusion Injury from Oxidative Stress by Regulating Succinate, Lysophospholipid Metabolism, and ROS Scavenging System. *Oxid. Med. Cel Longev.* 2019, 9137654. doi:10.1155/2019/9137654

Jiao, R., Liu, Y., Gao, H., Xiao, J., and So, K. F. (2016). The Anti-oxidant and Antitumor Properties of Plant Polysaccharides. *Am. J. Chin. Med.* 44 (3), 463–488. doi:10.1142/S0192415X16500269

Kafle, B., Baak, J., and Brede, C. (2020). Quantification by LC-MS/MS of Astragaloside IV and Isoflavones in Astragali Radix Can Be More Accurate by Using Standard Addition. *Phytochem. Anal.* 32, 466–473. doi:10.1002/pca.2994

Katayama, H. (2018). Development of Psoriasis by Continuous Neutrophil Infiltration into the Epidermis. *Exp. Dermatol.* 27 (10), 1084–1091. doi:10.1111/exd.13746

Kaufman, B. P., and Alexis, A. F. (2018). Psoriasis in Skin of Color: Insights into the Epidemiology, Clinical Presentation, Genetics, Quality-Of-Life Impact, and Treatment of Psoriasis in Non-White Racial/Ethnic Groups. *Am. J. Clin. Dermatol.* 19 (3), 405–423. doi:10.1007/s40257-017-0332-7

Laurindo, F. R., Fernandes, D. C., and Santos, C. X. (2008). Assessment of Superoxide Production and NADPH Oxidase Activity by HPLC Analysis of Dihydroethidium Oxidation Products. *Methods Enzymol.* 441, 237–260. doi:10.1016/S0076-6879(08)01213-5

Lee, K. Y., and Jeon, Y. J. (2005). Macrophage Activation by Polysaccharide Isolated from Astragalus Membranaceus. *Int. Immunopharmacol.* 5 (7-8), 1225–1233. doi:10.1016/j.intimp.2005.02.020

Lee, C. L., Hwang, T. L., He, W. J., Tsai, Y. H., Yen, C. T., Yen, H. F., et al. (2013a). Anti-neutrophilic Inflammatory Steroidal Glycosides from Solanum Torvum. *Phytochemistry* 95, 315–321. doi:10.1016/j.phytochem.2013.06.015

Lee, D. Y., Noh, H. J., Choi, J., Lee, K. H., Lee, M. H., Lee, J. H., et al. (2013b). Anti-inflammatory Cycloartane-type Saponins of Astragalus Membranaceus. *Molecules* 18 (4), 3725–3732. doi:10.3390/molecules18043725

Li, M., Qu, Y. Z., Zhao, Z. W., Wu, S. X., Liu, Y. Y., Wei, X. Y., et al. (2012a). Astragaloside IV Protects against Focal Cerebral Ischemia/reperfusion Injury Correlating to Suppression of Neutrophils Adhesion-Related Molecules. *Neurochem. Int.* 60 (5), 458–465. doi:10.1016/j.neuint.2012.01.026

Li, X. T., Zhang, Y. K., Kuang, H. X., Jin, F. X., Liu, D. W., Gao, M. B., et al. (2012b). Mitochondrial protection and Anti-aging Activity of Astragalus Polysaccharides and Their Potential Mechanism. *Int. J. Mol. Sci.* 13 (2), 1747–1761. doi:10.3390/ijms13021747

Li, Z., Zhang, L., He, W., Zhu, C., Yang, J., and Sheng, M. (2014). Astragalus Membranaceus Inhibits Peritoneal Fibrosis via Monocyte Chemoattractant Protein (MCP)-1 and the Transforming Growth Factor-β1 (TGF-β1) Pathway in Rats Submitted to Peritoneal Dialysis. *Int. J. Mol. Sci.* 15 (7), 12959–12971. doi:10.3390/ijms150712959

Li, J., Han, L., Ma, Y. F., and Huang, Y. F. (2015). Inhibiting Effects of Three Components of Astragalus Membranaceus on Oxidative Stress in Chang Liver Cells. *Zhongguo Zhong Yao Za Zhi* 40 (2), 318–323.

Li, L., Hou, X., Xu, R., Liu, C., and Tu, M. (2017a). Research Review on the Pharmacological Effects of Astragaloside IV. *Fundam. Clin. Pharmacol.* 31 (1), 17–36. doi:10.1111/fcp.12232

Li, Y., Meng, T., Hao, N., Tao, H., Zou, S., Li, M., et al. (2017b). Immune Regulation Mechanism of Astragaloside IV on RAW264.7 Cells through Activating the NF-κB/MAPK Signaling Pathway. *Int. Immunopharmacol.* 49, 38–49. doi:10.1016/j.intimp.2017.05.017

Li, H., Wang, P., Huang, F., Jin, J., Wu, H., Zhang, B., et al. (2018a). Astragaloside IV Protects Blood-Brain Barrier Integrity from LPS-Induced Disruption via Activating Nrf2 Antioxidant Signaling Pathway in Mice. *Toxicol. Appl. Pharmacol.* 340, 58–66. doi:10.1016/j.taap.2017.12.019

Li, J., Xu, L., Sang, R., Yu, Y., Ge, B., and Zhang, X. (2018b). Immunomodulatory and Anti-inflammatory Effects of Total Flavonoids of Astragalus by Regulating NF-KB and MAPK Signalling Pathways in RAW 264.7 Macrophages. *Pharmazie* 73 (10), 589–593. doi:10.1691/ph.2018.8633

Li, Z. P., Liu, H. B., Zhang, Q. W., Li, L. F., Bao, W. R., Ma, D. L., et al. (2018c). Interference of Quercetin on Astragalus Polysaccharide-Induced Macrophage Activation. *Molecules* 23 (7), 1563. doi:10.3390/molecules23071563

Li, W., Song, K., Wang, S., Zhang, C., Zhuang, M., Wang, Y., et al. (2019). Anti-tumor Potential of astragalus Polysaccharides on Breast Cancer Cell Line Mediated by Macrophage Activation. *Mater. Sci. Eng. C Mater. Biol. Appl.* 98, 685–695. doi:10.1016/j.msec.2019.01.025

Li, S., Sun, Y., Huang, J., Wang, B., Gong, Y., Fang, Y., et al. (2020). Anti-tumor Effects and Mechanisms of Astragalus Membranaceus (AM) and its Specific Immunopotentiation: Status and prospect. *J. Ethnopharmacol.* 258, 112797. doi:10.1016/j.jep.2020.112797

Li, L., Gan, H., Jin, H., Fang, Y., Yang, Y., Zhang, J., et al. (2021). Astragaloside IV Promotes Microglia/macrophages M2 Polarization and Enhances Neurogenesis and Angiogenesis through PPARγ Pathway after Cerebral Ischemia/reperfusion Injury in Rats. *Int. Immunopharmacol.* 92, 107335. doi:10.1016/j.intimp.2020.107335

Lin, Y. K., Leu, Y. L., Huang, T. H., Wu, Y. H., Chung, P. J., Su Pang, J. H., et al. (2009). Anti-inflammatory Effects of the Extract of Indigo Naturalis in Human Neutrophils. *J. Ethnopharmacol.* 125 (1), 51–58. doi:10.1016/j.jep.2009.06.014

Lin, A. M., Rubin, C. J., Khandpur, R., Wang, J. Y., Riblett, M., Yalavarthi, S., et al. (2011). Mast Cells and Neutrophils Release IL-17 through Extracellular Trap Formation in Psoriasis. *J. Immunol.* 187 (1), 490–500. doi:10.4049/jimmunol.1100123

Liu, A. J., Yu, J., Ji, H. Y., Zhang, H. C., Zhang, Y., and Liu, H. P. (2017). Extraction of a Novel Cold-Water-Soluble Polysaccharide from Astragalus Membranaceus and its Antitumor and Immunological Activities. *Molecules* 23 (1), 62. doi:10.3390/molecules23010062

Lowes, M. A., Suárez-Fariñas, M., and Krueger, J. G. (2014). Immunology of Psoriasis. *Annu. Rev. Immunol.* 32, 227–255. doi:10.1146/annurev-immunol-032713-120225

Lu, Y., Xing, Q. Q., Xu, J. Y., Ding, D., and Zhao, X. (2016). Astragalus Polysaccharide Modulates ER Stress Response in an OVA-LPS Induced Murine Model of Severe Asthma. *Int. J. Biol. Macromol.* 93 (Pt), 995–1006. doi:10.1016/j.ijbiomac.2016.09.058

Matkowski, A., Woźniak, D., Lamer-Zarawska, E., Oszmiański, J., and Leszczyńska, A. (2003). Flavonoids and Phenol Carboxylic Acids in the oriental Medicinal Plant Astragalus Membranaceus Acclimated in Poland. *Z. Naturforsch C J. Biosci.* 58 (7-8), 602–604. doi:10.1515/znc-2003-7-826

Nadeem, A., Ahmad, S. F., El-Sherbeeny, A. M., Al-Harbi, N. O., Bakheet, S. A., and Attia, S. M. (2018). Systemic Inflammation in Asocial BTBR T+ Tf/J Mice Predisposes Them to Increased Psoriatic Inflammation. *Prog. Neuropsychopharmacol. Biol. Psychiatry* 83, 8–17. doi:10.1016/j.pnpbp.2017.12.015

Nadeem, A., Ahmad, S. F., Al-Harbi, N. O., El-Sherbeeny, A. M., Alasmari, A. F., Alanazi, W. A., et al. (2020a). Bruton's Tyrosine Kinase Inhibitor Suppresses Imiquimod-Induced Psoriasis-like Inflammation in Mice through Regulation of IL-23/IL-17A in Innate Immune Cells. *Int. Immunopharmacol.* 80, 106215. doi:10.1016/j.intimp.2020.106215

Nadeem, A., Ahmad, S. F., Al-Harbi, N. O., Ibrahim, K. E., Alqahtani, F., As Sobeai, H. M., et al. (2020b). Inhibition of Interleukin-2-Inducible T-Cell Kinase Causes Reduction in Imiquimod-Induced Psoriasiform Inflammation through Reduction of Th17 Cells and Enhancement of Treg Cells in Mice. *Biochimie* 179, 146–156. doi:10.1016/j.biochi.2020.09.023

Paoliello-Paschoalato, A. B., Azzolini, A. E., Cruz, M. F., Marchi, L. F., Kabeya, L. M., Donadi, E. A., et al. (2014). Isolation of Healthy Individuals' and Rheumatoid Arthritis Patients' Peripheral Blood Neutrophils by the Gelatin and Ficoll-Hypaque Methods: Comparative Efficiency and Impact on the Neutrophil Oxidative Metabolism and Fcγ Receptor Expression. *J. Immunol. Methods* 412, 70–77. doi:10.1016/j.jim.2014.07.001

Papayannopoulos, V. (2018). Neutrophil Extracellular Traps in Immunity and Disease. *Nat. Rev. Immunol.* 18 (2), 134–147. doi:10.1038/nri.2017.105

Piao, Y. L., and Liang, X. C. (2014). Astragalus Membranaceus Injection Combined with Conventional Treatment for Viral Myocarditis: a Systematic Review of Randomized Controlled Trials. *Chin. J. Integr. Med.* 20 (10), 787–791. doi:10.1007/s11655-014-1825-3

Qi, Y., Gao, F., Hou, L., and Wan, C. (2017). Anti-Inflammatory and Immunostimulatory Activities of Astragalosides. *Am. J. Chin. Med.* 45 (6), 1157–1167. doi:10.1142/S0192415X1750063X

Rajendran, M., Manisankar, P., Gandhidasan, R., and Murugesan, R. (2004). Free Radicals Scavenging Efficiency of a Few Naturally Occurring Flavonoids: a Comparative Study. *J. Agric. Food Chem.* 52 (24), 7389–7394. doi:10.1021/jf0400718

Reczek, C. R., and Chandel, N. S. (2015). ROS-dependent Signal Transduction. *Curr. Opin. Cel Biol.* 33, 8–13. doi:10.1016/j.ceb.2014.09.010

Rendon, A., and Schäkel, K. (2019). Psoriasis Pathogenesis and Treatment. *Int. J. Mol. Sci.* 20 (6), 1475. doi:10.3390/ijms20061475

Ruhnau, J., Schulze, K., Gaida, B., Langner, S., Kessler, C., Bröker, B., et al. (2014). Stroke Alters Respiratory Burst in Neutrophils and Monocytes. *Stroke* 45 (3), 794–800. doi:10.1161/STROKEAHA.113.003342

Schneider, C. A., Rasband, W. S., and Eliceiri, K. W. (2012). NIH Image to ImageJ: 25 Years of Image Analysis. *Nat. Methods* 9 (7), 671–675. doi:10.1038/nmeth.2089

Schön, M. P., Broekaert, S. M. C., and Erpenbeck, L. (2017). Sexy Again: the Renaissance of Neutrophils in Psoriasis. *Exp. Dermatol.* 26 (4), 305–311. doi:10.1111/exd.13067

Sekheri, M., Othman, A., and Filep, J. G. (2021). β2 Integrin Regulation of Neutrophil Functional Plasticity and Fate in the Resolution of Inflammation. *Front. Immunol.* 12, 660760. doi:10.3389/fimmu.2021.660760

Shahzad, M., Shabbir, A., Wojcikowski, K., Wohlmuth, H., and Gobe, G. C. (2016). The Antioxidant Effects of Radix Astragali (Astragalus Membranaceus and Related Species) in Protecting Tissues from Injury and Disease. *Curr. Drug Targets* 17 (12), 1331–1340. doi:10.2174/1389450116666150907104742

Thannickal, V. J., and Fanburg, B. L. (2000). Reactive Oxygen Species in Cell Signaling. *Am. J. Physiol. Lung Cel Mol. Physiol.* 279 (6), L1005–L1028. doi:10.1152/ajplung.2000.279.6.L1005

Tian, L., Zhao, J. L., Kang, J. Q., Guo, S. B., Zhang, N., Shang, L., et al. (2021). Astragaloside IV Alleviates the Experimental DSS-Induced Colitis by Remodeling Macrophage Polarization through STAT Signaling. *Front. Immunol.* 12, 740565. doi:10.3389/fimmu.2021.740565

Tsai, Y. F., Yu, H. P., Chung, P. J., Leu, Y. L., Kuo, L. M., Chen, C. Y., et al. (2015). Osthol Attenuates Neutrophilic Oxidative Stress and Hemorrhagic Shock-Induced Lung Injury via Inhibition of Phosphodiesterase 4. *Free Radic. Biol. Med.* 89, 387–400. doi:10.1016/j.freeradbiomed.2015.08.008

Wang, W. M., and Jin, H. Z. (2020). Role of Neutrophils in Psoriasis. *J. Immunol. Res.* 2020, 3709749. doi:10.1155/2020/3709749

Wang, Y. P., Li, X. Y., Song, C. Q., and Hu, Z. B. (2002). Effect of Astragaloside IV on T, B Lymphocyte Proliferation and Peritoneal Macrophage Function in Mice. *Acta Pharmacol. Sin* 23 (3), 263–266.

Wang, Q., Zhou, H., Gao, H., Chen, S. H., Chu, C. H., Wilson, B., et al. (2012). Naloxone Inhibits Immune Cell Function by Suppressing Superoxide Production through a Direct Interaction with Gp91phox Subunit of NADPH Oxidase. *J. Neuroinflammation* 9, 32. doi:10.1186/1742-2094-9-32

Wang, Z., Liu, Z., Zhou, L., Long, T., Zhou, X., and Bao, Y. (2017). Immunomodulatory Effect of APS and PSP Is Mediated by Ca2+-cAMP and TLR4/NF-κB Signaling Pathway in Macrophage. *Int. J. Biol. Macromol.* 94, 283–289. doi:10.1016/j.ijbiomac.2016.10.018

Wang, J., Zhou, Y., Wu, S., Huang, K., Thapa, S., Tao, L., et al. (2018). Astragaloside IV Attenuated 3,4-Benzopyrene-Induced Abdominal Aortic Aneurysm by

Ameliorating Macrophage-Mediated Inflammation. *Front. Pharmacol.* 9, 496. doi:10.3389/fphar.2018.00496

Xie, X., He, Z., Chen, N., Tang, Z., Wang, Q., and Cai, Y. (2019). The Roles of Environmental Factors in Regulation of Oxidative Stress in Plant. *Biomed. Res. Int.* 2019, 9732325. doi:10.1155/2019/9732325

Xu, F., Cui, W. Q., Wei, Y., Cui, J., Qiu, J., Hu, L. L., et al. (2018). Astragaloside IV Inhibits Lung Cancer Progression and Metastasis by Modulating Macrophage Polarization through AMPK Signaling. *J. Exp. Clin. Cancer Res.* 37 (1), 207. doi:10.1186/s13046-018-0878-0

Yang, L. P., Shen, J. G., Xu, W. C., Li, J., and Jiang, J. Q. (2013). Secondary Metabolites of the Genus Astragalus: Structure and Biological-Activity Update. *Chem. Biodivers* 10 (6), 1004–1054. doi:10.1002/cbdv.201100444

Yang, S. C., Chen, P. J., Chang, S. H., Weng, Y. T., Chang, F. R., Chang, K. Y., et al. (2018). Luteolin Attenuates Neutrophilic Oxidative Stress and Inflammatory Arthritis by Inhibiting Raf1 Activity. *Biochem. Pharmacol.* 154, 384–396. doi:10.1016/j.bcp.2018.06.003

Yu, J., Ji, H. Y., and Liu, A. J. (2018a). Alcohol-soluble Polysaccharide from Astragalus Membranaceus: Preparation, Characteristics and Antitumor Activity. *Int. J. Biol. Macromol.* 118 (Pt B), 2057–2064. doi:10.1016/j.ijbiomac.2018.07.073

Yu, Y., Zhou, L., Yang, Y., and Liu, Y. (2018b). Cycloastragenol: An Exciting Novel Candidate for Age-Associated Diseases. *Exp. Ther. Med.* 16 (3), 2175–2182. doi:10.3892/etm.2018.6501

Zhang, W. J., and Frei, B. (2015). Astragaloside IV Inhibits NF- κ B Activation and Inflammatory Gene Expression in LPS-Treated Mice. *Mediators Inflamm.* 2015, 274314. doi:10.1155/2015/274314

Zhang, J., Wu, C., Gao, L., Du, G., and Qin, X. (2020). Astragaloside IV Derived from Astragalus Membranaceus: A Research Review on the Pharmacological Effects. *Adv. Pharmacol.* 87, 89–112. doi:10.1016/bs.apha.2019.08.002

Zhao, Y., Li, Q., Zhao, W., Li, J., Sun, Y., Liu, K., et al. (2015). Astragaloside IV and Cycloastragenol Are Equally Effective in Inhibition of Endoplasmic Reticulum Stress-Associated TXNIP/NLRP3 Inflammasome Activation in the Endothelium. *J. Ethnopharmacol.* 169, 210–218. doi:10.1016/j.jep.2015.04.030

Zhou, Q., Mrowietz, U., and Rostami-Yazdi, M. (2009). Oxidative Stress in the Pathogenesis of Psoriasis. *Free Radic. Biol. Med.* 47 (7), 891–905. doi:10.1016/j.freeradbiomed.2009.06.033

8

Punicalagin Alleviates Psoriasis by Inhibiting NF-κB-Mediated IL-1β Transcription and Caspase-1-Regulated IL-1β Secretion

Lipeng Tang[1,2,3†], Tong Li[1,2,3,4†], Bowen Zhang[3†], Zihao Zhang[5], Xiaoyi Sun[5], Ying Zhu[1,2,3], Bing Feng[1,2,3], Zuqing Su[1,2,3], Laijun Yang[3], Hongxia Li[3], Huazhen Liu[6], Yuchao Chen[6], Zhenhua Dai[6], Xirun Zheng[7], Mingxian Li[7], Chutian Li[7], Jie Zhao[7], Xinmin Qiu[8], Shuyan Ye[9], Han Liu[7], Guangjuan Zheng[1,2,3,7*], Ben Li[4*] and Chuanjian Lu[1,2,9,10*]*

[1]State Key Laboratory of Dampness Syndrome of Chinese Medicine, The Second Clinical College of Guangzhou University of Chinese Medicine, Guangzhou, China, [2]Guangdong-Hong Kong-Macau Joint Lab on Chinese Medicine and Immune Disease Research, The Second Clinical College of Guangzhou University of Chinese Medicine, Guangzhou, China, [3]Department of Pharmacology of Traditional Chinese Medicine, The Second Clinical College of Guangzhou University of Chinese Medicine, Guangzhou, China, [4]Department of Pharmacy, The Second Clinical College of Guangzhou University of Chinese Medicine, Guangzhou, China, [5]School of Life Sciences and Biopharmaceutics, Guangdong Pharmaceutical University, Guangzhou, China, [6]Section of Immunology, Guangdong Provincial Academy of Chinese Medical Sciences, Guangzhou, China, [7]Department of Pathology, The Second Clinical College of Guangzhou University of Chinese Medicine, Guangzhou, China, [8]Genetic Testing Lab, The Second Clinical College of Guangzhou University of Chinese Medicine, Guangzhou, China, [9]Department of Dermatology, The Second Clinical College of Guangzhou University of Chinese Medicine, Guangzhou, China, [10]Guangdong Provincial Key Laboratory of Clinical Research on Traditional Chinese Medicine Syndrome, The Second Clinical College of Guangzhou University of Chinese Medicine, Guangzhou, China

***Correspondence:**
Lipeng Tang
tanglp@gzucm.edu.cn
Guangjuan Zheng
zhengguangjuan@gzucm.edu.cn
Ben Li
lcyxlb@126.com
Chuanjian Lu
lcj@gzucm.edu.cn

†These authors have contributed equally to this work

Psoriasis is a chronic and inflammatory skin disorder characterized by inflammation and epidermal hyperplasia. Punicalagin (PUN) is a main active ingredient of pomegranate (*Punica granatum* L.) peel with multiple biological activities, such as antibacterial, antioxidant and anti-tumor effects. However, the potential effect of PUN on psoriasis remains unknown. In this study, we want to investigate the pharmacological effect of PUN on psoriasis by using imiquimod (IMQ)-induced psoriatic mice model *in vivo* and tumor necrosis factor *a* (TNF-α) and interleukin-17A (IL-17A)-stimulated HaCaT cells *in vitro*. Our results showed that PUN can effectively alleviate the severity of psoriasis-like symptoms. Mechanistically, PUN potently suppresses the aberrant upregulation of interleukin-1β (IL-1β) and subsequent IL-1β-mediated inflammatory cascade in keratinocytes by inhibiting the nuclear factor kappa B (NF-κB) activation and cleaved caspase-1 expression *in vitro* and *in vivo*. Taken together, our findings indicate that PUN can relieve psoriasis by repressing NF-κB-mediated IL-1β transcription and caspase-1-regulated IL-1β secretion, which provide evidence that PUN might represent a novel and promising candidate for the treatment of psoriasis.

Keywords: psoriasis, punicalagin, NF-κB, caspase-1, IL-1β

INTRODUCTION

Psoriasis is a chronic, recurrent, inflammatory skin disease affecting more than 60 million people worldwide (Parisi et al., 2013). The typical clinical manifestations of psoriasis are abnormal papules, erythema, thickened scaly spots, local dull pain and skin itching (Nestle et al., 2009), which seriously affect the patient's quality of life. Despite the newly developed biologics, such as adalimumab, guselkumab and mirikizumab (Armstrong and Read, 2020; Ghoreschi et al., 2021), have revolutionized moderate-to-severe plaque psoriasis, the biologics are too expensive for ordinary patients. Additionally, the long-term use of the biologics may lead to serious side effects (Scherer et al., 2010; Reich et al., 2015), including tumors. In addition, mild-to-moderate plaque psoriatic patients are usually treated with topical therapies (glucocorticoids and vitamin D derivatives) or systemic medications (methotrexate, acitretin, and cyclosporine) (Armstrong and Read, 2020). However, topical therapies or systemic medications have many contraindications or side effects (Boehncke and Schön, 2015; Reich et al., 2015). Therefore, seeking an economical, safe and effective treatment is extremely urgent for psoriasis.

Although most psoriasis-related researches have mainly focused on the interleukin-23 (IL-23)/interleukin-17 (IL-17) axis, emerging evidence indicates that interleukin-1β (IL-1β) also plays a critical role in psoriasis. Moorchung et al. (2015) identified a strong association of IL-1β *511C/T* (the C/T base transitions at positions -511 in the transcription initiation site) polymorphism with the genotypes and alleles in psoriasis. Moreover, Hébert et al. (2014) showed that the polymorphism of IL-1β *gene* could help to discriminate the early or late onset of psoriasis. Additionally, several studies indicated that IL-1β expression was significantly increased in both psoriatic plasma and skin lesion (Cai et al., 2019b; Verma et al., 2021). Furthermore, upregulated IL-1β could further amplify the skin inflammation by enhancing IL-17 production in dermal γδ T-cell and promoting chemokines [such as C-X-C motif chemokine ligand 1 (CXCL-1) and C-C motif chemokine ligand 20 (CCL-20)] secretion in keratinocytes (Cai et al., 2011; Cai et al., 2019b). Interestingly, IL-1β has also been pointed to be involved in the recurrence of psoriasis. Naik et al. (2017) showed that epithelial stem cells (EpSCs) in the psoriatic skin lesions can release numerous IL-1β upon a secondary stimulation, ultimately leading to inflammation recollection and psoriasis recurrence. Taken together, these findings suggest that IL-1β might be a promising therapeutic target for psoriasis intervention.

Punicalagin (PUN, **Supplementary Figure S1**), which is the main active ingredient of pomegranate (*Punica granatum* L.) peel, possesses multiple bioactivities, such as antioxidant (Chen et al., 2012), antibacterial (Sun Q. et al., 2019) and anti-tumor (Morsy et al., 2019; Huang et al., 2020; Pan et al., 2020) activities. Intriguingly, the regulatory effects of punicalagin on suppressing inflammation have attracted the researcher's attention. Punicalagin is proved to be able to alleviate various inflammatory diseases, including inflammatory bowel disease (Shah et al., 2016), ankylosing spondylitis (Feng et al., 2020) and rheumatoid arthritis (Huang et al., 2021). However, it is still unknown whether PUN exert a possible therapeutic effect on inflammatory skin disease, in particular psoriasis.

To evaluate the potential pharmacological effect of PUN on psoriasis, we made use of imiquimod (IMQ)-induced psoriasis-like mice model and tumor necrosis factor α (TNF-α) and IL-17A-stimulated HaCaT cells. We found that PUN can relieve psoriasis-like symptoms by suppressing the nuclear factor kappa B (NF-κB)-mediated IL-1β transcription and caspase-1-regulated IL-1β secretion *in vivo* and *in vitro*. Our findings suggest that PUN may represent a promising lead compound for developing newly anti-psoriatic drugs.

MATERIALS AND METHODS

Experimental Reagents

Punicalagin (P0023, purity ≥98%) was purchased from Sigma-Aldrich (St. Louis, MO, United States). IMQ cream was obtained from Sichuan Med-Shine Pharmaceutical Co., Ltd. (Sichuan, China). IL-17A (12047-HNAE), TNF-α (10602-HNAE), IL-1β (10139-HNAE) were purchased from Sino Biological Inc. (Beijing, China).

Mice and its Experiments

Male BALB/c mice (6–8 weeks of age), which were purchased from Animal Research Laboratory of Guangdong Province (Guangzhou, China), were maintained under specific pathogen-free conditions. After quarantine, mice were divided into five groups: Control group, IMQ group, IMQ + DEX group (DEX, dexamethasone cream, positive drug for psoriasis), IMQ + Vehicle group, IMQ + PUN group (25 mg/kg PUN). The shaved back of mice was applied with a daily topical dose of 62.5 mg of IMQ cream (5%) at 9:00 am for 7 consecutive days. In addition, control mice were treated with the same dose of Vaseline. Moreover, mice in IMQ + DEX group were topically administrated with DEX once a day (at 12:00 am) for 7 consecutive days. Furthermore, mice in IMQ + Vehicle group or IMQ + PUN group were topically administrated with vehicle gel (Sun et al., 2013) (0.3 g carbomer 940, 0.15 g azone, 4.5 g 96% ethanol and distilled water to 15 g) or PUN gel (0.3 g carbomer 940, 0.15 g azone, 4.5 g 96% ethanol, 78.125 mg PUN powder and distilled water to 15 g) twice a day (at 12:00 am and 4:00 pm) for 7 consecutive days. This experiment is finished on the eighth day, and follow-up verification is carried out. All procedures were approved and supervised by Guangzhou University of Chinese Medicine Animal Care and Use Committee (Approval No. 2020082, Guangdong, China).

Hematoxylin and Eosin Staining

The experiment was terminated on the eighth day. The skin collected from mice was fixed in neutral formalin for 48 h, then dehydrated and embedded in paraffin. Slicing the cross-section of the skin, the morphological characteristics of different groups mice were observed under a microscope (Olympus) after H&E staining. Acanthosis hyperplasia is evaluated by Photoshop 2021 software, the cortical direction of all pictures is adjusted to the level and the size of 1,000 pixels * 1,000 pixels is intercepted, finally the lasso tool is used to determine the pixels of the acanthosis layer in this size. Acanthosis (in^2) = width pixels * height pixels/horizontal resolution * vertical resolution.

Immunohistochemical Staining

Immunohistochemical staining was performed using paraffin-embedded mouse back skin sections. Experiment was operated in the following order: baking slices, dewaxing, antigen retrieval and membrane rupture. After this, the samples were stained with 5% bovine serum albumin (BSA) for 1 h at room temperature, Ki67 antibody (16667, Abcam) or phospho-NF-κB (Ser536) p65 (AF2006, Affinity) incubation for overnight, and further incubated with the anti-rabbit antibody. Using diaminobenzidine (DAB) staining solution to color development and hematoxylin to counterstain the nucleic acids. Dehydrated to wax before observed under the Olympus microscope. Ki67 positive cells per 10 cm are the number of Ki67 positive staining cells in the area of 10 * 10 cm at random, and three areas are selected for each picture. Expression of phosphorylated p65 per 10 cm is the number of cells expressed phosphorylated p65 (Ser536) in the area of 10 * 10 cm at random, and three areas are selected for each picture.

Cell Culture and Stimulation

Human HaCaT cells (human keratinocytes) were purchased from China Center for Type Culture Collection (GDC106) and examined without pollution. HaCaT cells were cultured in MEM α Nucleosides Medium (C12571500BT, Gibco) containing 10% fetal bovine serum (FBS) (10,099-141C, Gibco), 1% Sodium Pyruvate (100X) (11360070, Gibco) and 1% MEM Non-Essential Amino Acids Solution (100X) (11140050, Gibco) in 37° and 5% CO_2 incubator.

Quantitative real-Time PCR

The whole operations were performed in an RNA-free environment and used RNA-free tools. First, total RNA was extracted from cell or skin samples using TRIzol™ reagent (15596018, Life Technologies). Then, 1 μg RNA was used for reverse transcription by using a cDNA Reverse transcriptase kit (K1622, Thermo Scientific). The qPCR was performed in triplicate using SYBR green master mix (FP205-02, Tiangen) on Real-Time PCR System (Applied Biosystem 7,500, Life Technologies). *GAPDH* was used as the reference gene for normalization.

Western Blotting

Total protein was extracted from samples using RIPA buffer (P0013C, Beyotime) containing 1% phosphatase and protease inhibitors (P1206, Applygen) following the instructions. The nuclear and cytoplasm protein fractions were isolated using the NE-PER Nuclear and Cytoplasmic Extraction Reagents (78,835, Thermo Scientific) following the instructions. Using BCA Protein Assay Kit (9S8K-29538-413, Thermo Scientific) normalized the total protein for the follow-up experiments. Quantified samples were separated by sodium dodecyl sulfate-polyacrylamide gel electrophoresis (SDS-PAGE) and transferred to polyvinylidene fluoride (PVDF) membranes (IPYH00010, Merck Millipore). 5% skimmed milk is slowly shaken at room temperature to block the membrane for 1 h and then primary antibodies incubate these membranes overnight at 4°C. The next day membranes were incubated by the species-specific secondary antibody at room temperature for 1 h and exposed by Immobilon Western Chemiluminescent HRP Substrate (WBKLS0500, Merck Millipore). The antibodies used in the experiment are as follows: GAPDH (1:2,000; 60004-1-Ig, Proteintech), ß-Tubulin (1:2,000; 10094-1-AP, Proteintech), Lamin B1 (1:2,000; 12987-1-AP, Proteintech), IL-1β (1:1,000; 216,995, Abcam), cleaved IL-1β (1:1,000; 83,186, CST), NF-κB p65 (1:1,000; 8,242, CST), phospho-NF-κB p65 (Ser536) (1:1,000; 3,033, CST), cleaved caspase-1 (1:1,000; 4,199, CST) and caspase-1 (1:1,000; 179,515, Abcam) for HaCaT cells samples; IL-1β (1:1,000; 234,437, Abcam), cleaved IL-1β (1:1,000; 63,124, CST), caspase-1 (1:1,000; 24,232, CST) and cleaved caspase-1 (1: 1,000; 89,332, CST) for mice samples. GAPDH and ß-Tubulin were shown as housekeeping proteins for the normalization of total protein or cytoplasmic protein; Lamin B1 as the loading control for nuclear protein.

Immunofluorescence Staining

HaCaT cells were seeded and treated in the 96-well plates. After being fixed in 4% paraformaldehyde, the HaCaT cells were permeabilized with phosphate buffer solution (PBS) containing 0.5% Triton X-100 for 10 min, and subsequently were blocked with 5% BSA for 1 h. Next, the primary antibody against p65 (1: 1,200; 8,242, CST) incubated the cells overnight at 4°C. Then anti-rabbit IgG (H + L), F(ab')2 fragment secondary antibody (1:500; 4,413, CST) was used to incubate cells for 60 min at room temperature. After counterstaining with 4′, 6-diamidino-2-phenylindole (DAPI), the cell in the 96-well plates were observed and imaged under the Nikon microscope.

Statistical Analysis

Statistical analysis was performed using SPSS and Sigmaplot software. The whole statistics were presented as mean ± standard error of mean (S.E.M.). Analysis of one-way ANOVA with Student-Newman-Keuls method or non-parametric datasets with Kruskal–Wallis test was used for multiple comparisons. Probability values <0.05 were considered significant. $^*p < 0.05$; $^{**}p < 0.01$; $^{***}p < 0.001$; *N.S.*, non-significant. Error bars depict S.E.M.

RESULTS

Punicalagin Alleviates Psoriasis-Like Symptoms in IMQ-Induced Mice

To evaluate whether PUN has potential pharmacological effects on psoriasis, we conducted an IMQ-induced psoriatic *in vivo* model and then topically applied with DEX cream, vehicle gel or PUN gel on the shaven back skin of IMQ-treated mice for consecutive 7 days (**Figure 1A**). We found that IMQ treatment can cause severe psoriasis-like phenotypes, including erythema and severe plaque. In addition, mice with vehicle gel treatment also developed psoriasis-like manifestations. However, these

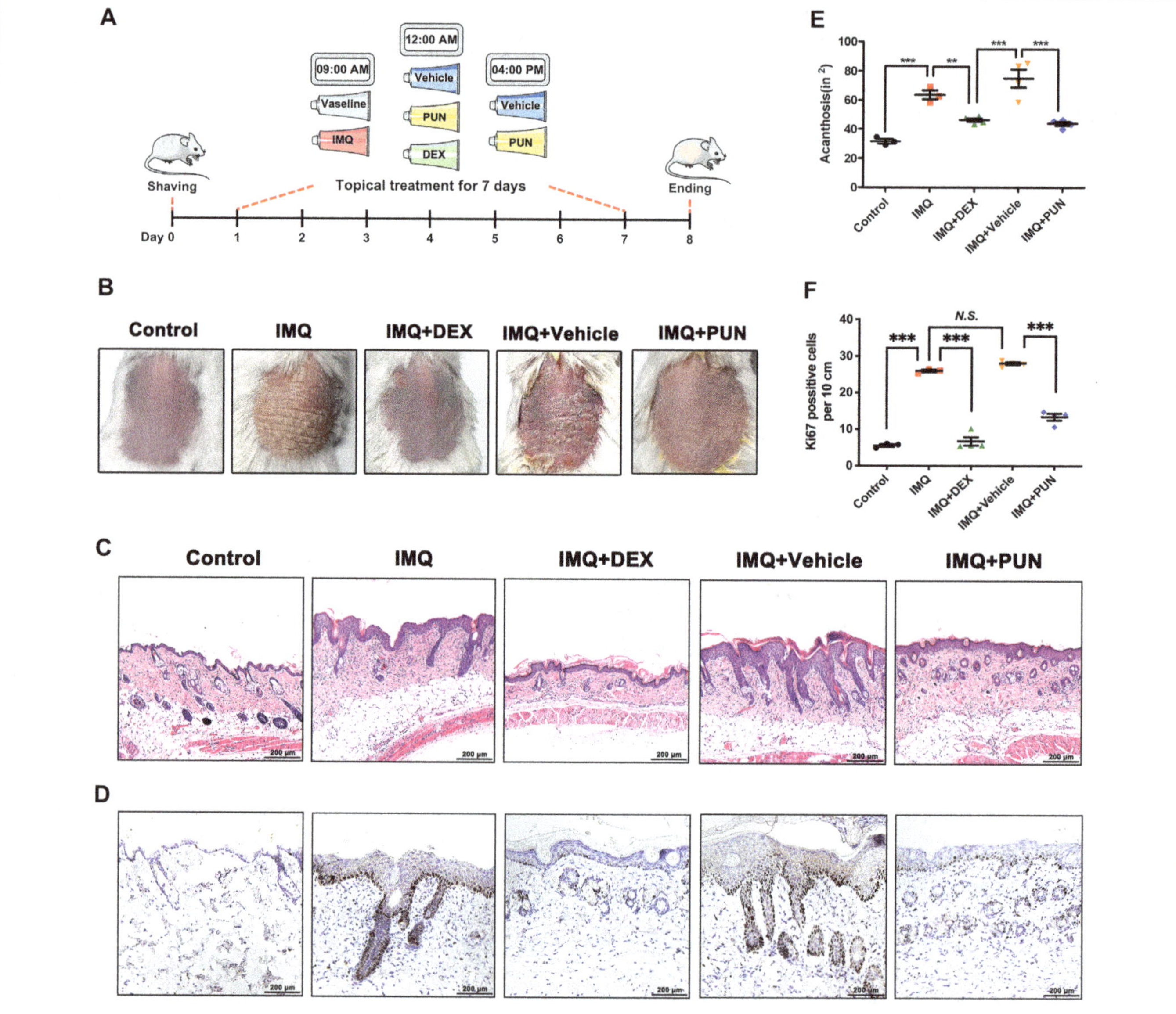

FIGURE 1 | Punicalagin significantly ameliorates IMQ-induced psoriasis-like symptoms *in vivo*. **(A)** A schematic showing the experimental design. **(B)** Phenotypic appearances of mice back skin in Control/IMQ/IMQ + DEX/IMQ + Vehicle/IMQ + PUN groups on day 8. **(C)** Histological changes of mice back skin in Control/IMQ/IMQ + DEX/IMQ + Vehicle/IMQ + PUN groups. Scale bar, 200 μm. **(D)** Ki67 staining of mice back skin in Control/IMQ/IMQ + DEX/IMQ + Vehicle/IMQ + PUN groups. Scale bar, 200 μm. **(E)** Histological analysis of acanthosis in Control/IMQ/IMQ + DEX/IMQ + Vehicle/IMQ + PUN groups. **(F)** The numbers of Ki67 positive cells in lesion skin derived from mice treated with Vaseline/IMQ/IMQ + DEX/IMQ + Vehicle/IMQ + PUN. $^{**}p < 0.01$, $^{***}p < 0.001$, *N.S.*, non-significant. One-way ANOVA with Student-Newman-Keuls method for **(E, F)**. Data represent the mean ± S.E.M.

psoriatic-related phenotypes can be improved by application of DEX or PUN (25 mg/kg) (**Figure 1B**). The results of H&E staining and histological analysis were in line with the macroscopic appearance. Mice treating with IMQ or IMQ + Vehicle gel became severe epidermal hyperplasia and acanthosis. As expected, topical administration of DEX attenuated IMQ-induced epidermal thickening and acanthosis. Similarly, topical treatment with 25 mg/kg PUN also ameliorated the above-mentioned manifestations (**Figures 1C,E**). Moreover, we also detected the expression of Ki67. We found that Ki67-positive cells were significantly reduced in the skin lesions after application of DEX or PUN gel (**Figures 1D,F**). Taken together, these results indicate that PUN can effectively relieve the severity of IMQ-induced psoriatic-like symptoms.

Punicalagin Reduces TNF-α and IL-17A-Induced IL-1β Upregulation *via* Inhibiting the Activation of NF-κB and the Expression of Caspase-1 *in Vitro*

To further explore the underlying mechanism by which PUN ameliorates psoriasis, we tested the anti-inflammatory

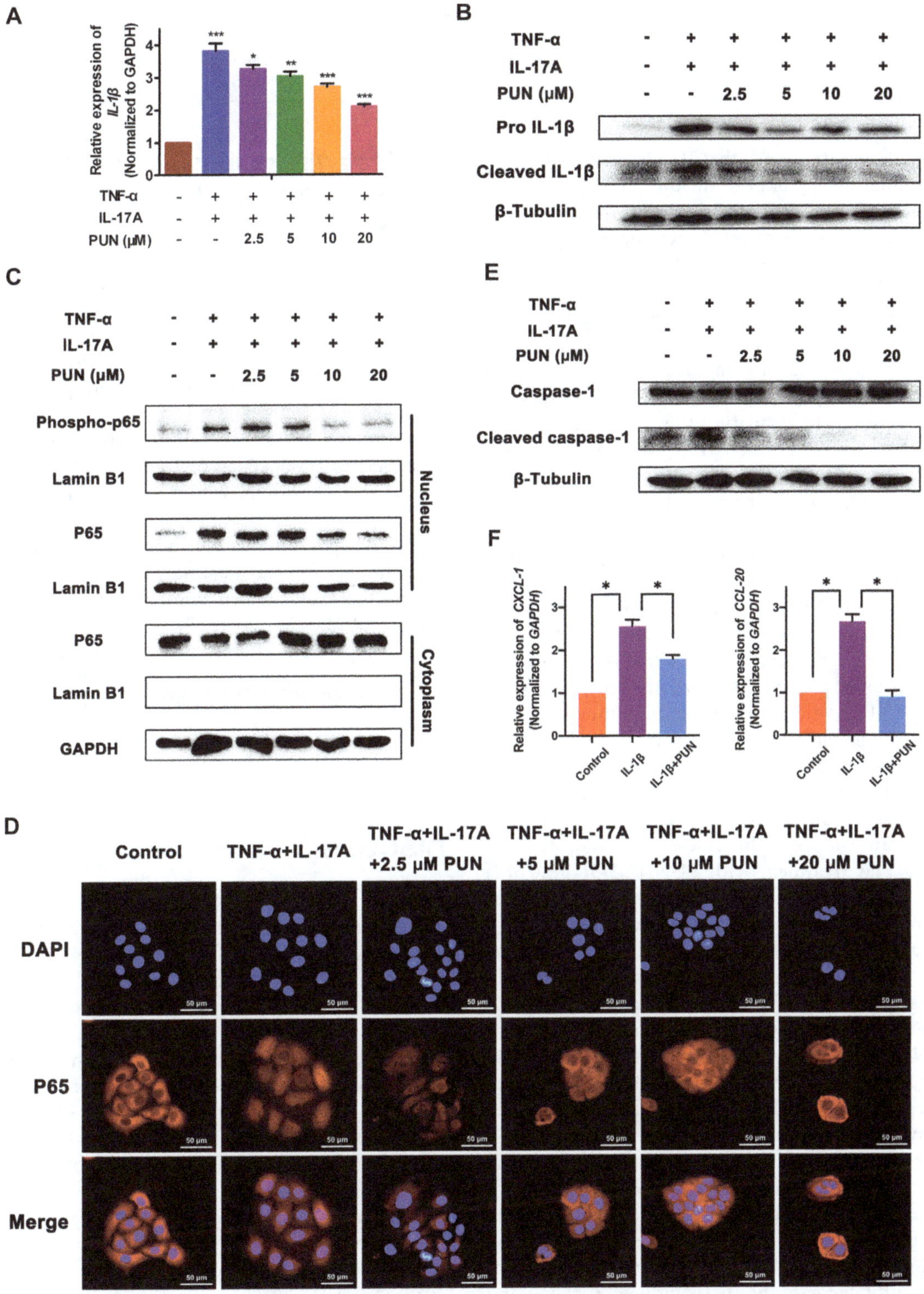

FIGURE 2 | Punicalagin suppresses the TNF-α and IL-17A-induced IL-1β upregulation *via* inhibiting NF-κB activation and cleaved caspase-1 expression *in vitro*. **(A)** The relative mRNA level of *IL-1β* in different groups. Here we used IL-17A (25 ng/ml) and TNF-α (25 ng/ml) to stimulate HaCaT cells. Simultaneously, we also added 2.5/5/10/20 μM PUN into these IL-17A and TNF-α-stimulated HaCaT cells. The total RNA was subsequently extracted after treatment with IL-17A (25 ng/ml) + TNF-α (25 ng/ml) and 2.5/5/10/20 μM PUN for 24 h. **(B)** The pro- and mature expression of IL-1β in different groups. The total protein was collected after treatment with IL-17A (25 ng/ml) + TNF-α (25 ng/ml) and 2.5/5/10/20 μM PUN for 48 h. **(C)** The expression of phosphorylation (Ser536) and total p65 in the cytoplasm and nucleus after exposure of IL-17A (25 ng/ml) + TNF-α (25 ng/ml) and 2.5/5/10/20 μM PUN for 24 h. **(D)** Immunostaining with an anti-p65 antibody showed that 2.5/5/10/20 μM

(Continued)

FIGURE 2 | PUN functionally blocks TNF-α and IL-17A-induced nuclear translocation of p65. Scale bar, 50 μm. **(E)** The expression of cleaved and total caspase-1 after exposure of IL-17A (25 ng/ml) + TNF-α (25 ng/ml) and 2.5/5/10/20 μM PUN for 48 h. **(F)** The relative mRNA level of *CXCL-1* (left) and *CCL-20* (right) in HaCaT cells after treatment with IL-1β and IL-1β + PUN for 48 h $^{*}p < 0.05$, $^{**}p < 0.01$, $^{***}p < 0.001$. One-way ANOVA with Student-Newman-Keuls method for **(A, F)**. Data represent the mean ± S.E.M.

properties of PUN *in vitro*. Since that IL-17A and TNF-α are the key inflammatory cytokines in the pathogenesis of psoriasis, we used IL-17A and TNF-α to stimulate HaCaT cells and conducted an inflammatory psoriatic *in vitro* model. We found that the mRNA and pro-/mature protein levels of IL-1β, another important cytokine in psoriasis, were significantly increased after stimulation with IL-17A and TNF-α. Intriguingly, PUN can reduce the upregulated IL-1β gene and pro-/mature protein expression in a dose-dependent way (**Figures 2A,B**). Given the pivotal role of NF-κB pathway in regulating the gene transcription (Xia et al., 2018; Sun P. et al., 2019), we next examined whether PUN can modulate the activation of NF-κB signaling pathway. Our preliminary work found that NF-κB undergoes activation through phosphorylation of p65 (Ser536) and nuclear translocation of p65 (**Supplementary Figure S2**), which is consistent with the previous studies (Christian et al., 2016; Varshney et al., 2016; Huang et al., 2021). Firstly, we detected the modulatory effects of PUN on the phosphorylation of p65 (Ser536) *in vitro*. We found that the phosphorylation of p65 (Ser536) was markedly enhanced by IL-17A and TNF-α, whereas PUN can functionally reduce the expression of phosphorylation of p65 (Ser536) in a dose-dependent way (**Figure 2C**). Since activated p65 will perform nuclear translocation and subsequently promote downstream IL-1β gene transcription, therefore, we further examined whether PUN can suppress the nuclear translocation of p65. We found that treatment with PUN (2.5/5/10/20 μM) could effectively block TNF-α and IL-17A-induced nuclear translocation of p65, respectively (**Figure 2D**). Moreover, pro IL-1β can be cleaved by cleaved caspase-1 and then become mature form of IL-1β. Here we showed that PUN could decrease the enhancement of pro- and mature IL-1β by IL-17A and TNF-α, therefore, we also detected the regulatory effects of PUN on cleaved caspase-1. As shown in **Figure 2E**, we found that PUN potently reduced the IL-17A and TNF-α-induced upregulation of cleaved caspase-1 in a dose-dependent way. As we all known, excessive IL-1β secretion will fuel psoriatic inflammatory processes by stimulating keratinocytes to secrete multiple chemokines, such as CXCL-1 and CCL-20. Hence, we also detected whether PUN can regulate the IL-1β-mediated secretion of CXCL-1 and CCL-20 in HaCaT cells. The qPCR results revealed that PUN can efficiently decrease the IL-1β-induced *CXCL-1* and *CCL-20* production (**Figure 2F**). Taken together, our findings suggest that PUN can inhibit the TNF-α and IL-17A-mediated IL-1β upregulation *via* suppressing p65 activation and cleaved caspase-1 expression *in vitro*, finally resulting in the repression of the subsequent IL-1β-mediated chemokines secretion.

Punicalagin Inhibits NF-κB-Mediated IL-1β Transcription and Caspase-1-Regulated IL-1β Secretion *in Vivo*

To determine whether PUN also reduced the IL-1β expression *in vivo*, we measured the gene and protein levels of IL-1β in skin lesion derived from Control/IMQ/IMQ + DEX/IMQ + Vehicle/IMQ + PUN group. As shown in **Figures 3A,B**, topical application of IMQ or IMQ + Vehicle caused a significant upregulation of IL-1β in both gene and protein level, whereas treatment with PUN potently decreased the upregulated level of IL-1β in IMQ-applied groups. Furthermore, we also examined the potential regulatory effects of PUN on the Ser536 phosphorylated p65 *in vivo*. Consistent with the *in vitro* results, we found that topical administration with IMQ can significantly enhance the levels of phosphorylation of p65 in the keratinocytes. Nonetheless, topical treatment with PUN can remarkably repress the expression of phosphorylated p65 in keratinocytes (**Figures 3C,D**). Moreover, PUN can also potently suppress the protein expression of cleaved caspase-1 and the mRNA level of *CXCL-1* and *CCL-20 in vivo* (**Figures 3E,F**). Together, these *in vivo* results also confirm that PUN can functionally attenuate the IL-1β expression and its subsequent inflammatory cascade by repressing the NF-κB activation and the cleaved caspase-1 expression.

DISCUSSION

PUN, the most abundant polyphenol in pomegranate (*Punica granatum L.*) peel, is often used in health care products or cosmetics because of its excellent antioxidant effects. Recently, PUN is proven to be capable of treating various diseases, including cervical cancer (Zhang et al., 2020), non-small cell lung malignancies (Fang et al., 2021), osteoarthritis (Liu F. et al., 2021) and diabetic cardiomyopathy (Fu et al., 2021). However, its effects on psoriasis remain unknown so far. Here, we gave the first evidence that PUN can alleviate the severity of psoriasis by downregulating IL-1β expression and subsequent IL-1β-mediated inflammatory responses *in vitro* and *in vivo* (**Figure 4**).

Previous studies demonstrated the key pathogenetic role of IL-1β in aggravating psoriatic inflammatory cascade and recalling psoriasis recurrent-related inflammatory memory (Naik et al., 2017; Cai et al., 2019b). Therefore, targeting IL-1β might be a promising strategy for treating psoriasis. Recently, Mansouri et al. (2015) and Skendros et al. (2017) independently showed that using IL-1β antagonists, such as canakinumab and gevokizumab, can successfully reduce the area and severity index scores of generalized pustular psoriasis. In this study, we present another evidence that targeting IL-1β by PUN could ameliorate psoriasis.

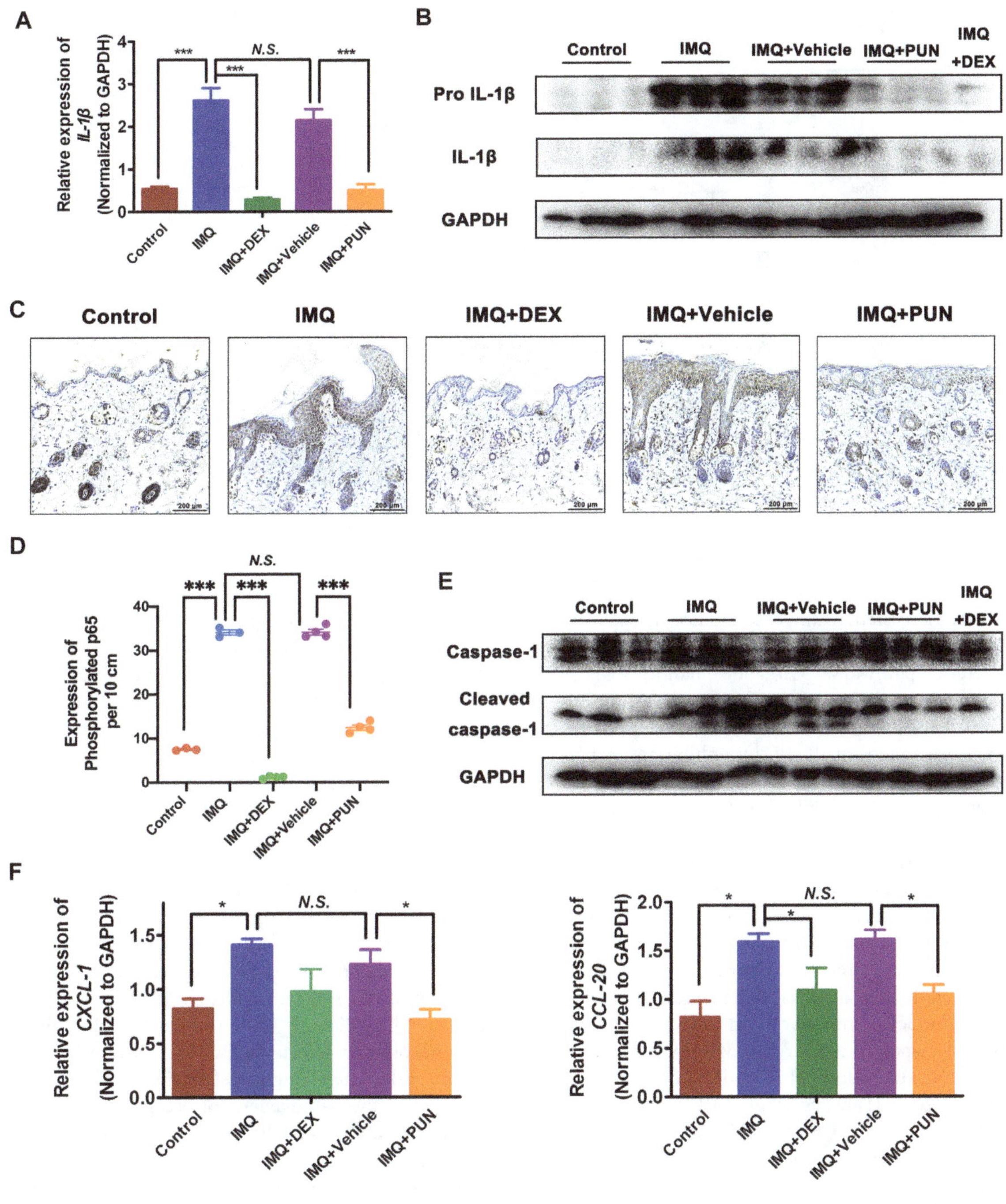

FIGURE 3 | Punicalagin attenuates the enhancement of IL-1β by suppressing NF-κB activation and caspase-1 expression *in vivo*. **(A)** The relative mRNA level of *IL-1β* in Control/IMQ/IMQ + DEX/IMQ + Vehicle/IMQ + PUN groups. **(B)** The protein expression of IL-1β in Control/IMQ/IMQ + DEX/IMQ + Vehicle/IMQ + PUN groups. **(C, D)** Immunohistochemical staining and statistical analysis of phosphorylated p65 (Ser536) in skin sections derived from the Control/IMQ/IMQ + DEX/IMQ + Vehicle/IMQ + PUN group. Scale bars: 200 μm. **(E)** The expression of cleaved and total caspase-1 in skin sections derived from the Control/IMQ/IMQ + DEX/IMQ + Vehicle/IMQ + PUN group. **(F)** The relative mRNA level of *CXCL-1* (left) and *CCL-20* (right) in the skin lesions from Control/IMQ/IMQ + DEX/IMQ + Vehicle/IMQ + PUN groups. *$p < 0.05$, ***$p < 0.001$, *N.S.*, non-significant. One-way ANOVA with Student-Newman-Keuls method for **(A, D, F)**. Data represent the mean ± S.E.M.

These studies suggest that IL-1β inhibitors might open a novel therapeutic avenue for psoriasis.

Formerly, Shah et al. (2016) showed that PUN significantly decreased the gene expression of IL-1β. Besides the regulatory of PUN on the IL-1β gene expression, Huang et al. (2021) showed that PUN also reduces the protein level of IL-1β. Moreover, Martín-Sánchez et al. (2016) and Saeki et al. (2020) found that PUN affects the release of IL-1β by changing the membrane

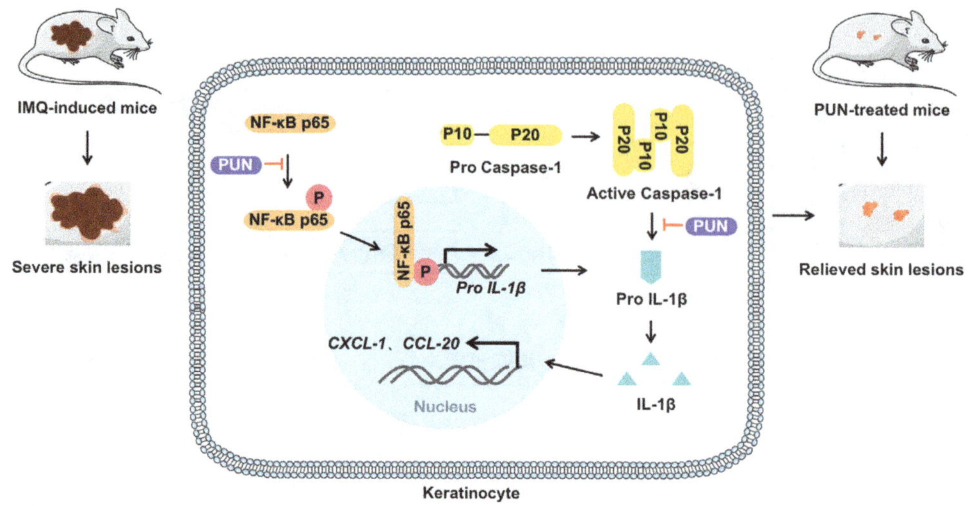

FIGURE 4 | Punicalagin alleviates psoriasis by inhibiting NF-κB-mediated IL-1β transcription and caspase-1-regulated IL-1β secretion. Punicalagin relieves psoriasis by inhibiting NF-κB activation and cleaved caspase-1 expression, which ultimately suppresses the transcription and secretion of IL-1β and consequently represses IL-1β-mediated inflammatory cascade *in vitro* and *in vivo*.

permeabilization. Consistent with these studies, we also found that PUN can regulate the expression and secretion of IL-1β through different pathways. On one hand, PUN can downregulate the transcription of IL-1β *via* suppressing NF-κB activation. On the other hand, PUN can also repress the maturation and secretion of IL-1β by inhibiting caspase-1-mediated pro-IL-1β cleavage. These studies indicate that PUN can function as a potent IL-1β inhibitor to treat various IL-1β-related diseases.

Although most psoriasis-associated studies have mainly focused on the imbalance of T helper 17 cells (Th17) and regulatory T cells (Treg), emerging studies indicate that keratinocytes also play a pivotal role in the initiation and the amplification of psoriasis (Greb et al., 2016). For example, Lande et al. (2014) showed that the antimicrobial peptide LL37, which is released from keratinocyte, can serve as an autoantigen to trigger the initial immune responses in psoriasis. Moreover, Hawkes and others proposed a feedback loop of "Dendritic cell—Th17 cell - Keratinocytes" in 2017 (Hawkes et al., 2017). In this "feed-forward" model, the activated myeloid dendritic cells produce IL-23 and IL-23 acts on Th17 cells to produce IL-17 cytokines. Then, these IL-17 cytokines (such as IL-17A) can stimulate keratinocytes to release a variety of cytokines, chemokines and antimicrobial peptides. These newly released antimicrobial peptides can further trigger the onset of psoriasis. In addition, the cytokines (such as IL-1β) and chemokines (such as CCL-20), which are released from keratinocytes upon IL-17A stimulation, can further amplify local inflammatory responses by increasing dermal IL-17 producing γδ T17 cell expansion. Taken together, these studies suggest that keratinocyte is a critical player in the pathogenesis of psoriasis (Ni and Lai, 2020). Given the important pathogenetic roles of keratinocytes in psoriasis, targeting keratinocyte might be a new therapeutic way for the treatment of psoriasis. Our studies showed that PUN can block this feedback loop of "Dendritic cell—Th17 cell—Keratinocytes" by downregulating the excessive expression of IL-1β and repressing the subsequent IL-1β-triggered inflammatory cascade in keratinocytes. Ultimately, this inhibition of "Dendritic cell—Th17 cell—Keratinocytes" feedback loop contributes to the pharmacological effects of PUN on psoriasis.

Recently, An et al. (2020) and Ge et al. (2021) reported that PUN can ameliorate diabetic nephropathy and collagen-induced arthritis by attenuating nucleotide-binding oligomerization domain, leucine-rich repeat and pyrin domain containing protein 3 (NLRP3)/caspase-1/gasdermin D (GSDMD)-mediated pyroptosis, respectively. Since that pyroptosis is a form of programmed cell death characterized by gasdermin family protein-mediated pore formation, cellular lysis and the release of IL-1β, Broz et al. (2020) and Liu X. et al. (2021) propose an idea that PUN is also a pyroptosis inhibitor. Given the pharmacological effects of PUN on psoriasis in our study, it will be really interesting to determine whether pyroptosis is also involved in the pathogenesis of psoriasis. The relation between pyroptosis and psoriasis may expand our understanding of pathogenesis of psoriasis.

In summary, we demonstrated that PUN alleviates psoriasis by suppressing excessive IL-1β expression and secretion. Mechanistically, functional inhibition of the NF-κB activation and cleaved caspase-1 expression contributes to the anti-psoriatic effects of PUN (**Figure 4**). Our findings suggest that punicalagin might be a promising therapeutic agent for the treatment of psoriasis in future.

AUTHOR CONTRIBUTIONS

CLu, GZ, BL, and LT designed the research; LT, TL, BZ, ZZ, XS, YZ, BF, ZS, LY, HoL, HuL, YC, ZD, XZ, ML, CLi, JZ, XQ, SY, and

HaL performed the research; LT, TL, and BZ analyzed the data; LT, TL, and BZ wrote the paper.

FUNDING

This study was supported by the Joint Funding Project of Municipal Schools (Colleges) of Science and Technology Program of Guangzhou under Grant (No. 202102010192); Innovative and Enhancement Research Program of Guangdong Province under Grant (No. 2019KTSCX025); the Specific Fund of State Key Laboratory of Dampness Syndrome of Chinese Medicine under Grant (SZ2021ZZ23); The 2020 Guangdong Provincial Science and Technology Innovation Strategy Special Fund (Guangdong-Hong Kong-Macau Joint Lab) (2020B1212030006); the Science and Technology Planning Project of Guangzhou under Grant (201807010051); Guangdong Provincial Clinical Research Center for Chinese Medicine Dermatology under Grant (2020B1111170012); Science and Technology Planning Project of Guangzhou under Grant (202102021001); The Specific Research Fund for TCM Science and Technology of Guangdong Provincial Hospital of Chinese Medicine under Grant (YN2018QJ03, YN2019QJ07); The Specific Fund for the Administration of Traditional Chinese Medicine of Guangdong Province under Grant (20222066).

ACKNOWLEDGMENTS

We thank Wenhui Zhang and Junhong Zhang for assistances in animal models.

REFERENCES

An, X., Zhang, Y., Cao, Y., Chen, J., Qin, H., and Yang, L. (2020). Punicalagin Protects Diabetic Nephropathy by Inhibiting Pyroptosis Based on TXNIP/NLRP3 Pathway. *Nutrients* 12 (05), 1516. doi:10.3390/nu12051516

Armstrong, A. W., and Read, C. (2020). Pathophysiology, Clinical Presentation, and Treatment of Psoriasis: A Review. *JAMA* 323 (19), 1945–1960. doi:10.1001/jama.2020.4006

Boehncke, W. H., and Schön, M. P. (2015). Psoriasis. *Lancet* 386 (9997), 983–994. doi:10.1016/s0140-6736(14)61909-7

Broz, P., Pelegrín, P., and Shao, F. (2020). The Gasdermins, a Protein Family Executing Cell Death and Inflammation. *Nat. Rev. Immunol.* 20 (3), 143–157. doi:10.1038/s41577-019-0228-2

Cai, Y., Shen, X., Ding, C., Qi, C., Li, K., Li, X., et al. (2011). Pivotal Role of Dermal IL-17-producing γδ T Cells in Skin Inflammation. *Immunity* 35 (4), 596–610. doi:10.1016/j.immuni.2011.08.001

Cai, Y., Xue, F., Quan, C., Qu, M., Liu, N., Zhang, Y., et al. (2019b). A Critical Role of the IL-1β-IL-1R Signaling Pathway in Skin Inflammation and Psoriasis Pathogenesis. *J. Invest. Dermatol.* 139 (1), 146–156. doi:10.1016/j.jid.2018.07.025

Chen, B., Tuuli, M. G., Longtine, M. S., Shin, J. S., Lawrence, R., Inder, T., et al. (2012). *Pomegranate* Juice and Punicalagin Attenuate Oxidative Stress and Apoptosis in Human Placenta and in Human Placental Trophoblasts. *Am. J. Physiol. Endocrinol. Metab.* 302 (9), E1142–E1152. doi:10.1152/ajpendo.00003.2012

Christian, F., Smith, E. L., and Carmody, R. J. (2016). The Regulation of NF-κB Subunits by Phosphorylation. *Cells* 5 (1), 12. doi:10.3390/cells5010012

Fang, L., Wang, H., Zhang, J., and Fang, X. (2021). Punicalagin Induces ROS-mediated Apoptotic Cell Death through Inhibiting STAT3 Translocation in Lung Cancer A549 Cells. *J. Biochem. Mol. Toxicol.* 35 (6), 1–10. doi:10.1002/jbt.22771

Feng, X., Yang, Q., Wang, C., Tong, W., and Xu, W. (2020). Punicalagin Exerts Protective Effects against Ankylosing Spondylitis by Regulating NF-κB-TH17/JAK2/STAT3 Signaling and Oxidative Stress. *Biomed. Res. Int.* 2020, 4918239. doi:10.1155/2020/4918239

Fu, F., Liu, C., Shi, R., Li, M., Zhang, M., Du, Y., et al. (2021). Punicalagin Protects against Diabetic Cardiomyopathy by Promoting Opa1-Mediated Mitochondrial Fusion via Regulating PTP1B-Stat3 Pathway. *Antioxid. Redox Signaling* 35, 618–641. doi:10.1089/ars.2020.8248

Ge, G., Bai, J., Wang, Q., Liang, X., Tao, H., Chen, H., et al. (2021). Punicalagin Ameliorates Collagen-Induced Arthritis by Downregulating M1 Macrophage and Pyroptosis via NF-κB Signaling Pathway. *Sci. China Life Sci.* [Epub ahead of print]. doi:10.1007/s11427-020-1939-1

Ghoreschi, K., Balato, A., Enerbäck, C., and Sabat, R. (2021). Therapeutics Targeting the IL-23 and IL-17 Pathway in Psoriasis. *Lancet* 397 (10275), 754–766. doi:10.1016/s0140-6736(21)00184-7

Greb, J. E., Goldminz, A. M., Elder, J. T., Lebwohl, M. G., Gladman, D. D., Wu, J. J., et al. (2016). Psoriasis. *Nat. Rev. Dis. Primersnat. Rev. Dis. Primers.* 2, 16082. doi:10.1038/nrdp.2016.82

Hawkes, J. E., Chan, T. C., and Krueger, J. G. (2017). Psoriasis Pathogenesis and the Development of Novel Targeted Immune Therapies. *J. Allergy Clin. Immunol.* 140 (3), 645–653. doi:10.1016/j.jaci.2017.07.004

Hébert, H. L., Bowes, J., Smith, R. L., Mchugh, N. J., Barker, J. N. W. N., Griffiths, C. E. M., et al. (2014). Polymorphisms in IL-1B Distinguish between Psoriasis of Early and Late Onset. *J. Invest. Dermatol.* 134 (5), 1459–1462. doi:10.1038/jid.2013.485

Huang, M., Wu, K., Zeng, S., Liu, W., Cui, T., Chen, Z., et al. (2021). Punicalagin Inhibited Inflammation and Migration of Fibroblast-Like Synoviocytes through NF-κB Pathway in the Experimental Study of Rheumatoid Arthritis. *J. Inflamm. Res.* 14, 1901–1913. doi:10.2147/jir.S302929

Huang, T., Zhang, X., and Wang, H. (2020). Punicalagin Inhibited Proliferation, Invasion and Angiogenesis of Osteosarcoma through Suppression of NF-κB S-ignaling. *Mol. Med. Rep.* 22 (3), 2386–2394. doi:10.3892/mmr.2020.11304

Lande, R., Botti, E., Jandus, C., Dojcinovic, D., Fanelli, G., Conrad, C., et al. (2014). The Antimicrobial Peptide LL37 Is a T-Cell Autoantigen in Psoriasis. *Nat. Commun.* 5, 5621. doi:10.1038/ncomms6621

Liu, F., Yang, H., Li, D., Wu, X., and Han, Q. (2021). Punicalagin Attenuates Osteoarthritis Progression via Regulating Foxo1/Prg4/HIF3α axis. *Bone* 152, 116070. doi:10.1016/j.bone.2021.116070

Liu, X., Xia, S., Zhang, Z., Wu, H., and Lieberman, J. (2021). Channelling Inflammation: Gasdermins in Physiology and Disease. *Nat. Rev. Drug Discov.* 20 (5), 384–405. doi:10.1038/s41573-021-00154-z

Mansouri, B., Richards, L., and Menter, A. (2015). Treatment of Two Patients with Generalized Pustular Psoriasis with the Interleukin-1β Inhibitor Gevokizumab. *Br. J. Dermatol.* 173 (1), 239–241. doi:10.1111/bjd.13614

Martín-Sánchez, F., Diamond, C., Zeitler, M., Gomez, A. I., Baroja-Mazo, A., Bagnall, J., et al. (2016). Inflammasome-dependent IL-1β Release Depends upon Membrane Permeabilisation. *Cell Death Differ* 23 (7), 1219–1231. doi:10.1038/cdd.2015.176

Moorchung, N., Vasudevan, B., Chatterjee, M., Mani, N. S., and Grewal, R. S. (2015). Interleukin-1 Gene Polymorphisms and Their Relation with NFκB Expression and Histopathological Features in Psoriasis. *Indian J. Dermatol.* 60 (5), 432–438. doi:10.4103/0019-5154.159630

Morsy, R. A. A., Abbass, E. A., Hager, E. A. A., Farid, M. H., Ellithy, M. M., and Azmy, A. (2019). Assessment of Anti-carcinogenic Effect of *Pomegranate* in Oral Squamous Cell Carcinoma (Pre-clinical Study). *Pak J. Biol. Sci.* 22 (12), 580–584. doi:10.3923/pjbs.2019.580.584

Naik, S., Larsen, S. B., Gomez, N. C., Alaverdyan, K., Sendoel, A., Yuan, S., et al. (2017). Inflammatory Memory Sensitizes Skin Epithelial Stem Cells to Tissue Damage. *Nature* 550 (7677), 475–480. doi:10.1038/nature24271

Nestle, F. O., Kaplan, D. H., and Barker, J. (2009). Psoriasis. *N. Engl. J. Med.* 361 (5), 496–509. doi:10.1056/NEJMra0804595

Ni, X., and Lai, Y. (2020). Keratinocyte: A Trigger or an Executor of Psoriasis? *J. Leukoc. Biol.* 108 (2), 485–491. doi:10.1002/jlb.5mr0120-439r

Pan, L., Duan, Y., Ma, F., and Lou, L. (2020). Punicalagin Inhibits the Viability, Migration, Invasion, and EMT by Regulating GOLPH3 in Breast Cancer Cells. *J. Recept. Signal. Transduct. Res.* 40 (2), 173–180. doi:10.1080/10799893.2020.1719152

Parisi, R., Symmons, D. P., Griffiths, C. E., and Ashcroft, D. M. (2013). Global Epidemiology of Psoriasis: a Systematic Review of Incidence and Prevalence. *J. Invest. Dermatol.* 133 (2), 377–385. doi:10.1038/jid.2012.339

Reich, K., Mrowietz, U., Radtke, M. A., Thaci, D., Rustenbach, S. J., Spehr, C., et al. (2015). Drug Safety of Systemic Treatments for Psoriasis: Results from the German Psoriasis Registry PsoBest. *Arch. Dermatol. Res.* 307 (10), 875–883. doi:10.1007/s00403-015-1593-8

Saeki, A., Tsuchiya, K., Suda, T., Into, T., Hasebe, A., Suzuki, T., et al. (2020). Gasdermin D-independent Release of Interleukin-1β by Living Macrophages in Response to Mycoplasmal Lipoproteins and Lipopeptides. *Immunology* 161 (2), 114–122. doi:10.1111/imm.13230

Scherer, K., Spoerl, D., and Bircher, A. J. (2010). Adverse Drug Reactions to Biologics. *J. Dtsch Dermatol. Ges* 8 (6), 411–426. doi:10.1111/j.1610-0387.2010.07339.x

Shah, T. A., Parikh, M., Patel, K. V., Patel, K. G., Joshi, C. G., and Gandhi, T. R. (2016). Evaluation of the Effect of Punica Granatum Juice and Punicalagin on NFκB Modulation in Inflammatory Bowel Disease. *Mol. Cel Biochem.* 419, 65–74. doi:10.1007/s11010-016-2750-x

Skendros, P., Papagoras, C., Lefaki, I., Giatromanolaki, A., Kotsianidis, I., Speletas, M., et al. (2017). Successful Response in a Case of Severe Pustular Psoriasis after Interleukin-1β Inhibition. *Br. J. Dermatol.* 176 (1), 212–215. doi:10.1111/bjd.14685

Sun, J., Zhao, Y., and Hu, J. (2013). Curcumin Inhibits Imiquimod-Induced Psoriasis-Like Inflammation by Inhibiting IL-1beta and IL-6 Production in Mice. *PloS one* 8 (6), e67078. doi:10.1371/journal.pone.0067078

Sun, P., Sun, N., Yin, W., Sun, Y., Fan, K., Guo, J., et al. (2019). Matrine Inhibits IL-1β Secretion in Primary Porcine Alveolar Macrophages through the MyD88/NF-κB Pathway and NLRP3 Inflammasome. *Vet. Res.* 50 (1), 53. doi:10.1186/s13567-019-0671-x

Sun, Q., Li, C., Lin, J., Peng, X., Wang, Q., Jiang, N., et al. (2019). Celastrol Ameliorates *Aspergillus Fumigatus* Keratitis via Inhibiting LOX-1. *Int. Immunopharmacol.* 70, 101–109. doi:10.1016/j.intimp.2019.02.017

Varshney, P., Narasimhan, A., Mittal, S., Malik, G., Sardana, K., and Saini, N. (2016). Transcriptome Profiling Unveils the Role of Cholesterol in IL-17A Signaling in Psoriasis. *Sci. Rep.* 6, 19295. doi:10.1038/srep19295

Verma, D., Fekri, S. Z., Sigurdardottir, G., Bivik Eding, C., Sandin, C., and Enerbäck, C. (2021). Enhanced Inflammasome Activity in Patients with Psoriasis Promotes Systemic Inflammation. *J. Invest. Dermatol.* 141 (3), 586–e5. e585. doi:10.1016/j.jid.2020.07.012

Xia, Y., Chen, S., Zhu, G., Huang, R., Yin, Y., and Ren, W. (2018). Betaine Inhibits Interleukin-1β Production and Release: Potential Mechanisms. *Front. Immunol.* 9, 2670. doi:10.3389/fimmu.2018.02670

Zhang, L., Chinnathambi, A., Alharbi, S. A., Veeraraghavan, V. P., Mohan, S. K., and Zhang, G. (2020). Punicalagin Promotes the Apoptosis in Human Cervical Cancer (ME-180) Cells through Mitochondrial Pathway and by Inhibiting the NF-kB Signaling Pathway. *Saudi. J. Biol. Sci.* 27 (4), 1100–1106. doi:10.1016/j.sjbs.2020.02.015

9

Chijabyukpi-Tang Inhibits Pro-Inflammatory Cytokines and Chemokines *via* the Nrf2/HO-1 Signaling Pathway in TNF-α/IFN-γ-Stimulated HaCaT Cells and Ameliorates 2,4-Dinitrochlorobenzene-Induced Atopic Dermatitis-Like Skin Lesions in Mice

Ji-Hyun Lee[1], Ji-Ye Lim[1], Eun Hee Jo[2,3], Hyeon Min Noh[4], Sunggu Park[5], Min Cheol Park[2,5] and Dae-Ki Kim[1]**

[1] Department of Immunology and Institute of Medical Sciences, Medical School, Chonbuk National University, Jeonju, South Korea, [2] Research Center of Traditional Korean Medicine, Wonkwang University, Iksan, South Korea, [3] Department of Acupuncture and Moxibustion, College of Korean Medicine, Wonkwang University, Iksan, South Korea, [4] Korean Traditional Medicine Institute, Wonkwang University, Iksan, South Korea, [5] Department of Korean Medical Ophthalmology & Otolaryngology & Dermatology, College of Korean Medicine, Wonkwang University, Iksan, South Korea

Correspondence:
Min Cheol Park
spinx11@wonkwang.ac.kr
Dae-Ki Kim
daekim@jbnu.ac.kr

Chijabyukpi-tang (CBT) is an oriental herbal formula consisting of three herbs (Gardeniae Fructus (*Gardenia jasminoides* J.Ellis.), Phellodendri Cortex (*Phellodendron amurense* Rupr.), Glycyrrhizae Radix (*Glycyrrhiza uralensis* Fisch. ex DC.) at the ratio of 2: 2: 1. CBT has traditionally been used to treat eczema with inflammation in Northeast Asia. The components of CBT have been shown to have anti-inflammatory and anti-oxidant properties, but the exact role and mechanism of CBT on atopic dermatitis (AD) remain unclear. In this study, we investigated the anti-inflammatory effect and mechanism of CBT in the HaCaT human keratinocyte cell line and investigated the anti-atopic effect in mice models of atopic dermatitis-like skin lesions. In the tumor necrosis factor alpha (TNF)-α/ interferon (IFN)-γ-stimulated HaCaT cells, CBT inhibited the production of pro-inflammatory cytokines and chemokines and elevated the nuclear translocation of NF-E2 p45 related factors 2 (Nrf2) and subsequent production of heme oxygenase-1 (HO-1). CBT improved the symptoms of atopic dermatitis-like lesions in 2,4-dinitrochlorobenzene (DNCB)-treated mice by suppressing the levels of serum immunoglobulin E (IgE), and various pro-inflammatory cytokines and chemokines. The improvement effect of CBT on atopic dermatitis-like lesions can be predicted to be due to increased Nrf2 and HO-1 gene expression. These results suggest that CBT is an herbal medicine with the potential for use as a therapeutic agent for inflammatory skin diseases such as atopic dermatitis.

Keywords: *Chijabyukpi-tang*, atopic dermatitis, keratinocytes, cytokine, chemokine, inflammation

INTRODUCTION

Atopic dermatitis (AD) is a chronic relapsing inflammatory skin disease, and the incidence of AD worldwide has been increasing rapidly over the past 30 years (Kapoor et al., 2008). AD occurs most often during childhood and occurs equally in both females and males. In developed countries, about 2–4% of adults and 15–20% of children suffer from AD, and most AD patients are known to have symptoms that last approximately five years (Shaw et al., 2011). AD is characterized by severe skin lesions such as pruritus, erythema, rash, edema, dryness, and skin hypersensitivity (Guttman-Yassky et al., 2011). Because of these features, AD patients often suffer from sleep deprivation, anxiety, and stress, which can lower their quality of life (Kiebert et al., 2002). Many sufferers of AD are also prone to developing other chronic inflammatory diseases including asthma and allergic reactions.

AD is caused by a complex interaction between extrinsic and intrinsic factors. The main risk factor of AD is not yet known, but it is known that mostly immune system dysfunction and environmental factors impair the skin's barrier and exacerbate immunoglobulin E (IgE)-mediated sensitization, severe skin inflammation and immune responses (Darlenski et al., 2014).

AD skin inflammation is orchestrated by the production of pro-inflammatory cytokines and chemokines by keratinocytes that subsequently induces the invasion of immune cells. The immune cells create inflammatory skin lesions following the production of further pro-inflammatory cytokines and chemokines (Homey et al., 2006). According to previous studies, AD patients are known to have increased levels of chemokines (such as IL-8, CCL17, and CXCL10) and cytokines (such as IL-4, IL-6, and IL-13), compared to healthy individuals (Yamanaka and Mizutani, 2011). It is also known that the activation of several oxidative stress-related inflammatory signaling pathways, such as NF-E2 p45 related factors 2 (Nrf2) and heme oxygenase-1 (HO-1), is related to inflammation in AD (Choi et al., 2014; Akram et al., 2016).

Currently, topical ointments and oral medications such as corticosteroids, antihistamines, and immunosuppressive drugs are used to treat AD inflammation and reduce itching (Cury Martins et al., 2015). However, these drugs have serious side effects when repeatedly administered over a long period of time. Therefore, in order to minimize the adverse effects of the long-term use of AD drugs, there is a need for the development of new alternative drugs derived from natural resources with fewer side effects.

Chijabyukpi-tang (CBT) is an oriental herbal formula consisting of three herbs (Gardeniae Fructus, Phellodendri Cortex, Glycyrrhizae Radix), in a 2:2:1 ratio. CBT is a traditional medicine first reported thousands of years ago in the ancient Chinese medicine book "Sang han-lun". CBT has long been used as a treatment for eczema with inflammation (Mie et al., 2009). In addition, it is an oriental herbal formula that is known to eliminate heat in the body, cure humid, jaundice and epidemic diseases. It has also been used to treat severe pain in the lower abdomen, burns, and various infectious symptoms (Chen et al., 2009). The various effects of each herb that constitutes CBT are well known; previous studies have shown that Gardeniae Fructus and Phellodendri Cortex have anti-inflammatory and anti-allergic effects (Hon et al., 2011; Debnath et al., 2018). In addition, Glycyrrhizae Radix has been previously shown to relieve inflammation (Yang et al., 2013). However, there is few scientific research on the CBT in which these herbs are combined. Previous studies have reported that CBT relieves fever and dizziness, and pruritic skin disease (Higashi and Kanzaki, 2006; Choi and Lee, 2017).

Since AD is characterized by inflammation and pruritus, eczema, we first studied the effect of CBT on AD and its mechanism of action. Therefore, the aim of this study was to investigate the anti-inflammatory effect and action mechanism of CBT on TNF-α/IFN-γ-stimulated HaCaT cells (human keratinocyte cell line) and 2,4-dinitrochlorobenzene (DNCB)-induced AD-like skin lesions in mice.

MATERIALS AND METHODS

Cell Culture and Reagents

The HaCaT cell line was obtained from the laboratory of Wonkwang university (Prof. Min Cheol Park). The HaCaT cells were incubated in Dulbecco's modified Eagle's medium (DMEM) supplemented with 10% fetal bovine serum (FBS), 100 units/ml of penicillin, and streptomycin (Welgene, Seoul, Korea). The HaCaT cells were cultured at 37°C in an incubator with a humidified atmosphere of 5% CO_2 and 95% air. DMEM and FBS were purchased from GIBCO BRL (Grand Island, NY, USA). Penicillin and streptomycin were purchased from Welgene (Seoul, Korea). Recombinant human TNF-α, IFN-γ, and IgE mouse ELISA kit were obtained from BioLegend (San Diego, CA, USA). Primary antibodies for Nrf2, Lamin B, HO-1, β-actin, and secondary antibodies used in the western blot analysis were purchased from Santa Cruz Biotechnology (Santa Cruz, CA, USA). 3-(4,5-Dimethyl-2-thiazolyl)-2,5-diphenyl-2H-tetrazolium bromide (MTT), dexamethasone (#D2915), and DNCB were purchased from Sigma-Aldrich. (St. Louis, Mo., USA).

Preparation of CBT

The herb components used in CBT were obtained from the K-herb Research Center, Nong-Lim and Ja-Dam. The identity of the herbs was confirmed by Prof. Min-Chel Park from Wonkwang University of traditional korean medicine. Voucher specimens of Gardeniae Fructus (NLGF-1803) and Phellodendri

Abbreviations: AD, atopic dermatitis; CBT, *Chijabyukpi-tang*; Dexa, dexamethasone; DMSO, dimethyl sulfoxide; DNCB, 2,4-dinitrochlorobenzene; ECL, enhanced chemi-luminescence; ELISA, Enzyme-linked immunosorbent assay; FBS, fetal bovine serum; HO-1, heme oxygenase-1; HPLC, high performance liquid chromatography; H&E, Hematoxylin and eosin; IFN-γ, interferon-γ; IgE, immunoglobulin E; KIOM, Korea Institute of Oriental Medicine; MTT, 3-(4,5-Dimethyl-2-thiazolyl)-2,5-diphenyl-2H-tetrazolium bromide; Nrf2, NF-E2 p45 related factors 2; PDA, photodiode array; qPCR, Quantitative real-time polymerase chain reaction; SDS-PAGE, sodium dodecyl sulfate-polyacrylamide; SEM, standard error of the mean; Th2, T helper 2; TNF-α, tumor necrosis factor-α.

Cortex (NLPC-1801) have been deposited at Nong-Lim. Voucher specimen of Glycyrrhizae Radix (JD8KZ-1902) has been deposited at Ja-Dam. CBT was constructed by mixing the herbs in accordance with each component composition in **Table 1** (www.theplantlist.org). 18 g of CBT was boiled at 100° C in 1,000 ml water for 30 min. Then the extract was collected, and as above, the residue was twice boiled in water. The extracted CBT was filtered and freeze-dried, and the weight of the dried extract was measured, and kept at 4°C until use.

Analysis of High Performance Liquid Chromatography (HPLC)

To perform the HPLC analysis of CBT, the Waters e2695 separation module, 2998 photodiode array (PDA) detector (Waters Corporation, USA) was used. The analytical column used was Phenomenex Luna C18 (250× 4.6 mm). The column temperature was at 40°C, the samples temperature was at 25°C, and the injection volume was 10 µl. The mobile phases were composed of solvent (A) = 0.1% trifluoroacetic acid in water, and solvent (B) = Acetonitrile. The total run time was 120 min and the mobile phase process gradient flow was as follows: (A)/(B) = 80/20 (0-10 min) → (A)/(B) = 80/20 (10-90 min) → (A)/(B) = 40/60 (90-91 min) → (A)/(B) = 0/100 (91-111 min) → (A)/(B) = 80/20 (111-120 min). The mobile phase flow rate was 1.0 ml/min. Samples were detected with a UV detector at a wavelength of 260 nm.

MTT Assay

The viability of HaCaT cells was evaluated using the MTT assay. The MTT assay was carried out as previously described (Lee et al., 2018). Briefly, cells were seeded into a 96-well plate at 1×10^4 cells/well, and treated with various concentrations of CBT (0, 12.5, 25, 50, 100 µg/ml) for 24 h in a 37°C incubator. MTT reagents were added to each well, and the plate was incubated for a further 4 h. After removing the supernatant, the crystallized formazan was dissolved in dimethyl sulfoxide (DMSO), and the absorbance was read at 570 nm using an ELISA plate reader.

Preparation of the HaCaT Nuclear and Cytosol Fractions

The nuclear and cytosol fractions of the HaCaT cells were isolated using the Nuclear/Cytosol Fractionation Kit (BioVision, Inc., CA, USA), according to the manufacturer's instructions. The nuclear and cytosol fractions were stored at -80°C until use.

Quantitative Real-Time Polymerase Chain Reaction (qPCR)

qPCR was carried out to confirm the expression levels of several genes *in vitro* and *in vivo*. Total RNA was isolated from *dorsal skin tissues* and HaCaT cells using 1 ml Trizol *reagent* (Invitrogen, Carlsbad, CA, USA). After the RNA was extracted, cDNA was synthesized using the Prime Script ™ II 1st strand cDNA synthesis kit (Takara Bio, Inc. USA), according to the *manufacturer's protocols*. The cDNA was amplified with SYBR Green PCR Master Mix (Applied Biosystem, CA, USA) using an ABI Real-Time PCR system (Applied Biosystems, Inc., CA, USA). *The primer sequences are shown in* **Table 2**. The RNA gene expression levels of each sample were analyzed three times and normalized to the internal control gene, GAPDH.

Western Blot Analysis

The protein production levels of cells were evaluated using western blot analysis. HaCaT cells were pretreated with various concentrations of CBT (0, 12.5, 25, 50, and 100 µg/ml) for 2 h, and treated with TNF-α/IFN-γ (10 ng/ml each) for 3 h. The cells were harvested, and proteins were extracted using cell lysis buffer (Millipore, Bedford, MA, USA) supplemented with a protease and phosphatase inhibitor cocktail (Thermo Fisher Scientific, Waltham, MA, USA). Proteins (25 µg) were separated *via* electrophoresis in 10% sodium dodecyl sulfate-polyacrylamide (SDS-PAGE) gels, and transferred to PVDF membranes.

TABLE 2 | *Primer sequences for* quantitative real-time polymerase chain reaction (qPCR).

Gene	Forward	Reverse
hIL-6	CTCCACAAGCGCCTTCGGTC	TGTGTGGGGCGGCTACATCT
hIL-13	ACCACGGTCATTGCTCTCACT	GTCAGGTTGATGCTCCATAC
hIL-8	ACCGGAGCACTCCATAAGGCA	AGGCTGCCAAGAGAGCCACG
hCCL17	CCATTCCCCTTAGAAAGCTG	CTCTCAAGGCTTTGCAGGTA
hCXCL10	TTGCTGCCTTATCTTTCTGACTC	ATGGCCTTCGATTCTGGATT
mIL-4	ATGGGTCTCAACCCCCAGCTA	TGCATGGCGTCCCTTCTCCT
mIL-6	GACAACCACGGCCTTCCCTA	GGTACTCCAGAAGACCAGAGG
mIL-8	TTTGGGAGACCTGAGAACAAG	TGCCTGTCAAGCTGACTTCA
mCXCL10	CTGAGTGGGACTCAAGGGAT	TCGTGGCAATGATCTCAACAC
mHO-1	CAGAACCAGCCTGAACTAGC	TGGATGTGTACCTCCTTGGT
mNrf2	ACCAAGGGGCAC CATATAAAAG	CTTCGCCGAGTTGCACTCA
GAPDH	GAAGGTGAAGGTCGGAGT	GAAGATGGTGATGGGATTTC

IL-, Interleukin-; CCL17, Chemokine (C-C motif) ligand 17; CXCL10, C-X-C motif chemokine 10; HO-1, heme oxygenase-1; Nrf2, NF-E2 p45-related factor 2; GAPDH, glyceraldehyde 3-phosphate dehydrogenase.

TABLE 1 | The composition of *Chijabyukpi-tang* (CBT).

Herb medicine	Latin scientific name	Family	Source	Weight (g)/Ratio (%)
Gardeniae Fructus	*Gardenia jasminoides* J.Ellis.	Rubiaceae	Korea	6/40
Phellodendri Cortex	*Phellodendron amurense* Rupr.	Rutaceae	Korea	6/40
Glycyrrhizae Radix	*Glycyrrhiza uralensis* Fisch. ex DC.	Fabaceae	Korea	3/20
Total Amount				**15/100**

Membranes were blocked with 5% BSA in TBS-T at room temperature for 1 h, and incubated with primary antibodies (Nrf2, Lamin B, HO-1, and β-actin; 1:1,000 dilution in 5% BSA) overnight at 4°C. Then, the membranes were washed several times with TBS-T, and incubated with horseradish peroxidase (HRP)-conjugated secondary antibody (1:5,000 dilution in 5% BSA) at room temperature for 1 h. The proteins were detected with enhanced chemi-luminescence (ECL) detection kit (Millipore, Billerica, MA, USA) using the Fusion Fx gel documentation system (Davinch-Invivo^{TM} Imaging System, USA).

Animals

Four-week-old male BALB/c mice were purchased from Samtako Bio Korea (Osan, Korea). All mice (22 ± 2 g) were randomly housed in a controlled environment with 50–60% humidity and a temperature of 21–23°C, under a 12-h dark/light cycle. Mice were allowed free access to standard laboratory chow and tap water. After a one-week period of new environment acclimation, mice were randomly divided into five groups of six mice. This research was performed in accordance with the guidelines of the Animal Experiment Ethics Committee of Chonbuk National University (CBNU-IACUC) (Confirmation No. CBNU 2016-0011).

Experimental Protocols of the Mouse Study

Thirty mice were divided into five groups (n=6) as follows: (1) control (vehicle treatment), (2) DNCB, (3) DNCB + CBT-low dose (CBT-150 mg/kg), (4) DNCB + CBT-high dose (CBT-300 mg/kg) and (5) positive control (dexamethasone (Dexa)-1 mg/kg). Except for the control group, AD-like skin lesions were induced using DNCB as described previously. Briefly, the dorsal skin hairs of all mice were removed. After 24 h, DNCB was dissolved in an acetone and olive oil mixture (4:1 v/v), and the dorsal skin was treated with 1% DNCB solution once a day for three days. Furthermore, 0.5% DNCB solution was treated to the dorsal skin once every two days for ten days to promote AD-like skin lesions. CBT samples and dexamethasone were dissolved in water and orally administered once a day for 11 days (days 4–14) (**Figure 4A**). The experimental animals were anesthetized by ether and euthanized by cervical dislocation for collecting skin tissues and blood serum.

Measurement of Dorsal Skin Moisture Content, Atopic Dermatitis Score, and Dorsal Skin Thickness

On the last day of the experiment, the dorsal skin moisture content (%) was measured using a TS-skin diagnostic system (Aram Huvis Co., Seongnam, Korea), according to the manufacturer's protocol. We assessed the severity of erythema, edema, and stretches on AD-like skin lesions on the dorsal skin five times according to Fan's criteria (Fan et al., 2018). After the dorsal skin tissues of mice were isolated, the thicknesses of the dorsal skin were gauged three times using a micrometer.

Hematoxylin and Eosin (H&E) Staining

After the mice were sacrificed, their dorsal skin tissue specimens (100 μm^2) were fixed in 10% formalin solution at room temperature for 24 h, and then embedded in paraffin wax. The paraffin blocks were sectioned serially into a thickness of 6-μm (n=6), and stained with hematoxylin and eosin (H&E; hematoxylin, 1 min and eosin, 3 min) to examine skin histological changes. Histological changes were observed using a microscope (Olympus CX21, Olympus Corporation, Tokyo, Japan). All images were observed at ×100 magnification.

Enzyme-Linked Immunosorbent Assay (ELISA)

After the mice were anesthetized, blood samples were collected. Blood samples were allowed to clot by incubation at room temperature for 30 min. Then, bloods were centrifuged at 3,000 rpm for 10 min and serum samples were obtained. IgE in serum was analyzed using a total IgE mouse ELISA kit, according to the manufacturer's instructions.

Statistical Analysis

Graph Pad Prism software 5.0 was used for data statistical analysis. All data are represented as means ± standard error of the mean (SEM) of triplicate experiment, and evaluated using one-way ANOVA (analysis of variance) with Tukey's *post-hoc* test to locate differences between groups. A value of $p < 0.05$ was defined as statistically significant.

RESULTS

HPLC Analysis of CBT

The final extraction yield (%) of CBT was 37.77%. The CBT indicator ingredient compounds (crocin, berberine hydrochloride, and glycyrrhizic acid) were analyzed using HPLC. We confirmed the peak of three compounds in the CBT extract by comparison with the standard ingredients' peak. As shown in **Figure 1**, the CBT used in our experiments contains these three components. The content of crocin, berberine hydrochloride, and glycyrrhizic acid in CBT was 28.671 mg/g, 6.255 mg/g, and 6.249 mg/g, respectively.

CBT Reduces the mRNA Expression of Pro-Inflammatory Cytokines and Chemokines in TNF-α/IFN-γ-Stimulated HaCaT Cells

The cytotoxicity of HaCaT cells was examined at various concentrations (12.5, 25, 50, and 100 μg/ml) of CBT for 24 h. As shown in **Figure 2A**, CBT did not show cytotoxicity at all concentration ranges. To evaluate the anti-inflammatory effects of CBT, the production of pro-inflammatory cytokines and chemokines was measured in TNF-α/IFN-γ-treated HaCaT cells. HaCaT cells were pretreated with CBT (0, 12.5, 25, 50, and 100 μg/ml) for 2 h, and stimulated with TNF-α/IFN-γ (10 ng/ml each) for 3 h. Then, the mRNA expression levels of cytokines (IL-6 and IL-13), and chemokines (IL-8, CCL17, and CXCL10) were analyzed using qPCR. CBT was shown to significantly inhibit the

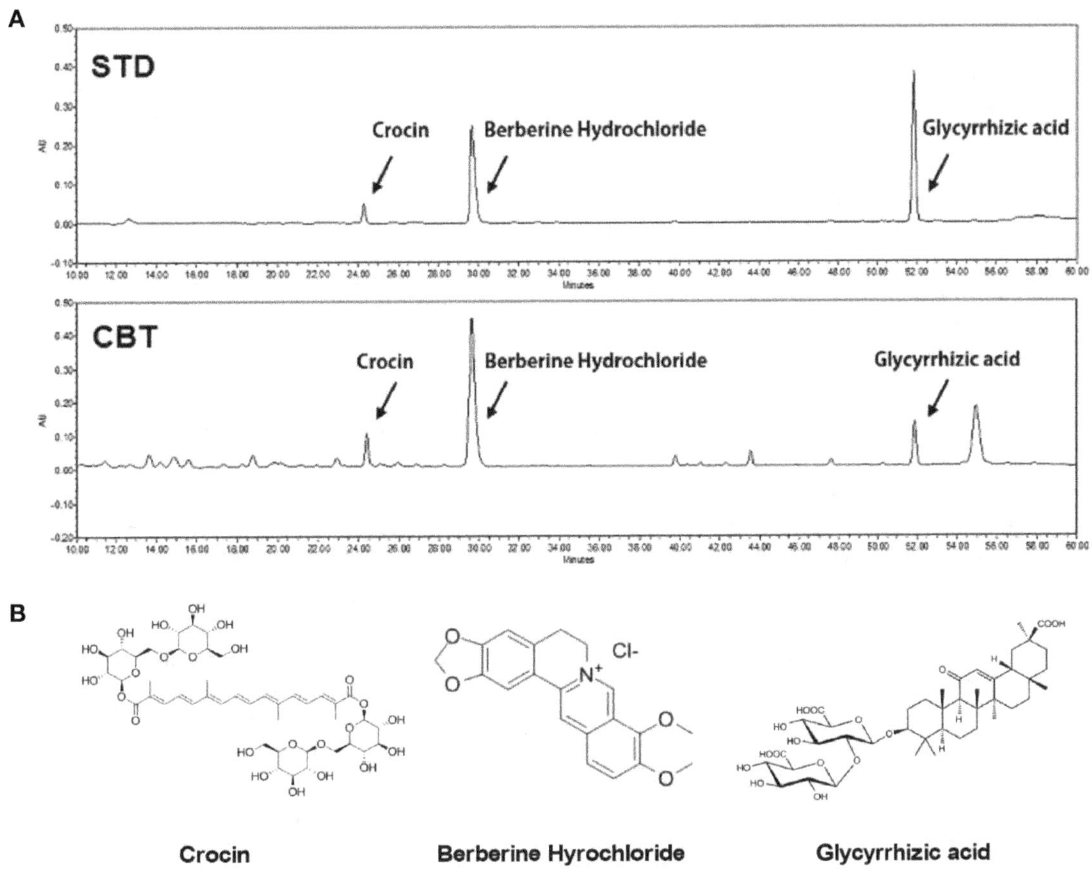

FIGURE 1 | High performance liquid chromatography (HPLC) analysis of *Chijabyukpi-tang* (CBT). HPLC chromatograms of standard compound mixtures (STD) and CBT samples **(A)**. Chemical structures of crocin, berberine hydrochloride, and glycyrrhizic acid **(B)**.

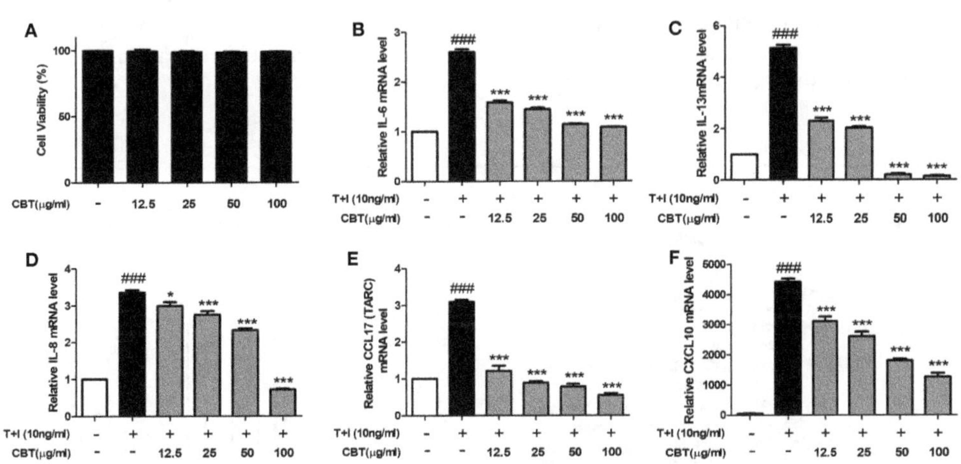

FIGURE 2 | Effects of *Chijabyukpi-tang* (CBT) on the mRNA expression levels of pro-inflammatory cytokines and chemokines in TNF-α/IFN-γ-stimulated HaCaT cells. Cell viability of CBT was measured using MTT assay. The group that did not treatment anything was set as negative control **(A)**. Cells were incubated for 24 h in the presence of CBT (12.5 to 100 μg/ml) or in the absence of CBT (media only). HaCaT cells were pretreated with several concentrations of CBT (12.5, 25, 50, and 100 μg/ml) for 2 h and then stimulated with TNF-α/IFN-γ (each 10 ng/ml) for 3 h. The mRNA expression levels of IL-6 **(B)**, IL-13 **(C)**, IL-8 **(D)**, CCL17 **(E)**, and CXCL10 **(F)** were determined using quantitative real-time polymerase chain reaction (qPCR). Data are shown as mean ± SEM of the three independent experiments. ###$p < 0.001$ compared with the no-treatment condition, *$p < 0.05$, and ***$p < 0.001$ compared with the only TNF-α/IFN-γ treatment condition.

production of TNF-α/IFN-γ-induced cytokines and chemokines in a dose-dependent manner (**Figures 2B–F**).

CBT Up-Regulates Nuclear Nrf2 and HO-1 Protein Levels in TNF-α/IFN-γ-Stimulated HaCaT Cells

The Nrf2/HO-1 signaling pathway plays a crucial mediator role in cell protection from oxidative stress (Loboda et al., 2016). To evaluate whether CBT affects the Nrf2/HO-1 signaling pathway, we investigated the levels of nuclear Nrf2 and HO-1 proteins using western blot. As shown in **Figure 3**, protein levels of nuclear Nrf2 and HO-1 were decreased following cellular stimulation with TNF-α/IFN-γ, however in the groups pretreated with CBT, the nuclear Nrf2 and HO-1 activation was increased in a dose-dependent manner.

CBT Improves DNCB-Induced AD-Like Skin Lesions and Suppresses the Secretion of Serum IgE in Mice

AD-like skin lesions were induced by repeated exposure of the dorsal skin regions of BALB/c mice to DNCB. A significant improvement in dorsal skin condition was observed in mice administrated CBT orally compared to the only DNCB-induced group (n=6) (**Figure 4B**). There were no mouse deaths by CBT (150 and 300 mg/kg) oral administration. We examined H&E staining slides to study the therapeutic effects of CBT on epidermal hyperplasia and the infiltration of inflammatory cells in AD-like dorsal skin tissue. As a result, we found that the dorsal skin thickness of DNCB-induced mice was increased, and that oral administration of CBT reduced the dorsal skin thickness and relieved AD-like lesions in a dose dependent manner (**Figures 4C, D**). The severity scores of the dorsal skin lesions were evaluated with reference to known criteria. We observed that AD-severity scores were suppressed in the CBT-orally administrated mice groups in a dose-dependent manner (**Figure 4E**). We observed a significant decrease in dorsal skin moisture content (%) of approximately 60.9% in the DNCB-treated mice group compared to the non-DNCB-treated mice group. When orally administered with CBT, the DNCB-treated mice group's skin moisture content was elevated. However, no significant difference was observed (**Figure 4F**). IgE is associated with the T helper 2 (Th2) immune response and is known to play an important role in the pathogenesis and progression of AD (Liu et al., 2011). Thus, total IgE measurements have been used to confirm the severity of AD. We analyzed the effect of CBT on serum IgE levels using ELISA. As a result, serum total IgE was increased in the DNCB-treated mice group compared with the control mice group (control mice group: 267.81 ± 84.81 ng/ml; DNCB-treated mice group: 1,932.53 ± 79.57 ng/ml), and it was reduced by oral administration of CBT (CBT 300 mg/kg administered group: 1,503.92 ± 181.21 ng/ml). In particular, the CBT 300 mg/kg and dexamethasone 1 mg/kg mice groups were significantly inhibited (dexamethasone administered group: 1,500.47 ± 236.26 ng/ml) (**Figure 4G**).

CBT Inhibits the mRNA Expression of Pro-Inflammatory Cytokines and Chemokines in DNCB-Treated Mice

Dorsal skin tissues were collected from each mouse, and the effect of CBT on pro-inflammatory cytokines and chemokines was analyzed using qPCR. In dorsal skin tissues, the expression levels of pro-inflammatory cytokines (IL-4 and IL-6), and chemokines (IL-8 and CXCL10) were remarkably increased in the DNCB-treated mice group compared with the control mice group. Expression levels of pro-inflammatory cytokines and chemokines in the CBT-orally administered mice groups were reduced compared to the DNCB-treated mice group in a dose-dependent manner (**Figure 5**).

CBT Elevates the mRNA Expression of Nrf2 and HO-1 in DNCB-Treated Mice

The mRNA expression levels of Nrf2 and HO-1 were measured using qPCR. We observed that the mRNA expression levels of Nrf2 and HO-1 decreased by treatment with DNCB were increased by oral administration of CBT in a dose-dependent manner (**Figure 6**).

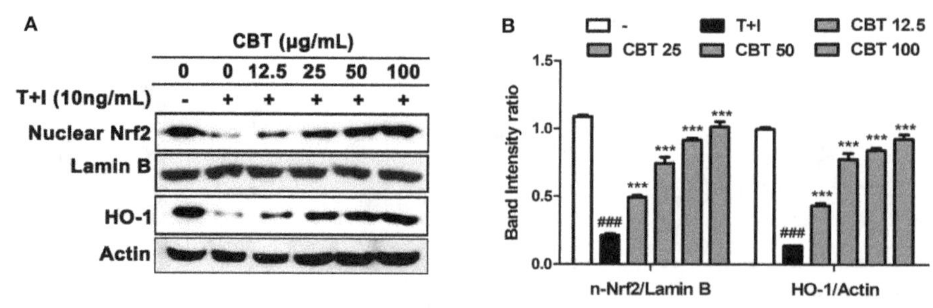

FIGURE 3 | Effects of *Chijabyukpi-tang* (CBT) on the nuclear Nrf2 and HO-1 proteins in TNF-α/IFN-γ-stimulated HaCaT cells. HaCaT cells were pretreated with several concentrations of CBT (12.5, 25, 50, and 100 μg/ml) for 2 h and then stimulated with TNF-α/IFN-γ (each 10 ng/ml) for 3 h. The proteins of nuclear Nrf2, lamin B, HO-1, and actin **(A)** were analyzed using western blotting. The bar graphs represent quantitative density of the bands; nuclear Nrf2/Lamin B, and HO-1/Actin **(B)**. Data are shown as mean ± SEM of the three independent experiments. ###$p < 0.001$ compared with the no-treatment condition, ***$p < 0.001$ compared with the only TNF-α/IFN-γ treatment condition.

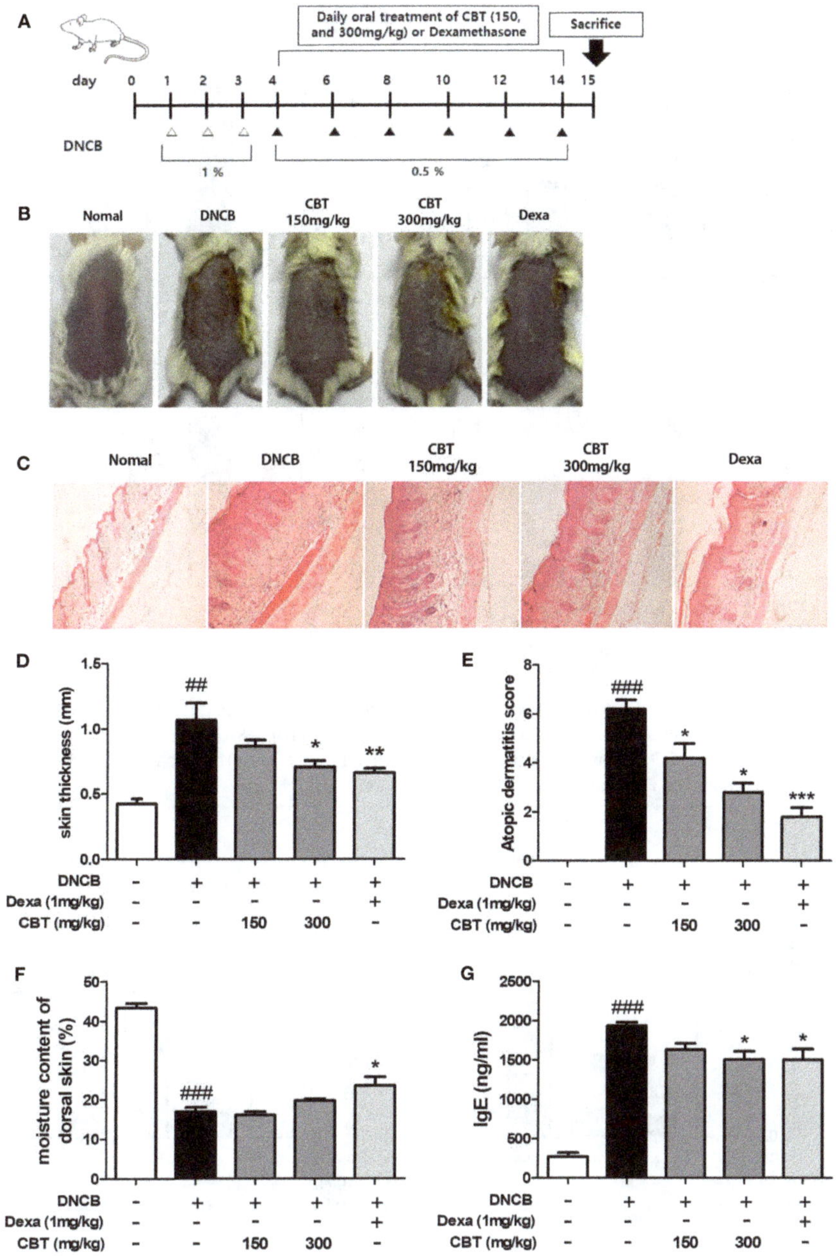

FIGURE 4 | Effects of *Chijabyukpi-tang* (CBT) on clinical signs in 2,4-dinitrochlorobenzene (DNCB)-treated mice skin tissues. The DNCB treatment and oral administration (CBT 150 and 300 mg/kg, and Dexa) schedule used in this experiment **(A)**. On the last day of the experiment, photographs were taken for comparison of skin lesions before the mice were sacrificed. Each dorsal skin picture is representative of each group **(B)**. The histological status of the dorsal skin tissues was observed using hematoxylin and eosin (H&E) staining **(C)**. Images were taken at 100x magnification. The dorsal skin tissue thickness of mice was measured using a micrometer **(D)**. The atopic dermatitis score of mouse dorsal skin lesion was evaluated using the standard evaluation criteria **(E)**. The moisture content of mouse dorsal skin was measured using a Tewameter TM 210 device **(F)**. Serum IgE level was analyzed using enzyme-linked immunosorbent assay (ELISA) **(G)**. Data are shown as mean ± SEM of the three independent experiments. $^{###}p < 0.001$ compared with the control group, $^{*}p < 0.05$, $^{**}p < 0.01$, and $^{***}p < 0.001$ compared with the DNCB-induced group. The Dexa group was set as positive control.

DISCUSSION

AD is a chronic inflammatory skin disease that occurs frequently in infancy and has a high rate of both recurrence and persistence. AD is characterized by severe itching, eczema, erythema, dry skin, and skin hyperplasia, and is also closely related to other inflammatory diseases (Peng and Novak, 2015). In inflammatory AD skin lesions, the levels of serum IgE, cytokines and chemokines are increased, and there is infiltration of Th cells (Leung and Bieber, 2003). Although these factors causing AD

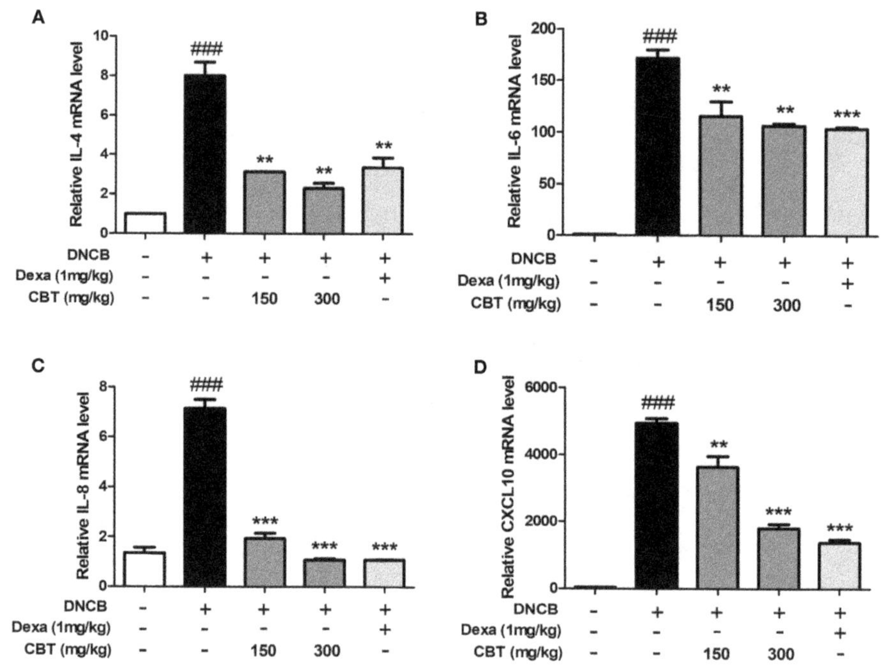

FIGURE 5 | Effects of *Chijabyukpi-tang* (CBT) on the mRNA expression levels of pro-inflammatory cytokines and chemokines in 2,4-dinitrochlorobenzene (DNCB)-treated mice skin tissues. The mRNA expression levels of IL-4 **(A)**, IL-6 **(B)**, IL-8 **(C)**, and CXCL10 **(D)** were analyzed using the quantitative real-time polymerase chain reaction (qPCR). Data are shown as mean ± SEM of the three independent experiments. $^{###}p < 0.001$ compared with the control group, $^{**}p < 0.01$, and $^{***}p < 0.001$ compared with the DNCB-induced group. The Dexa group was set as positive control.

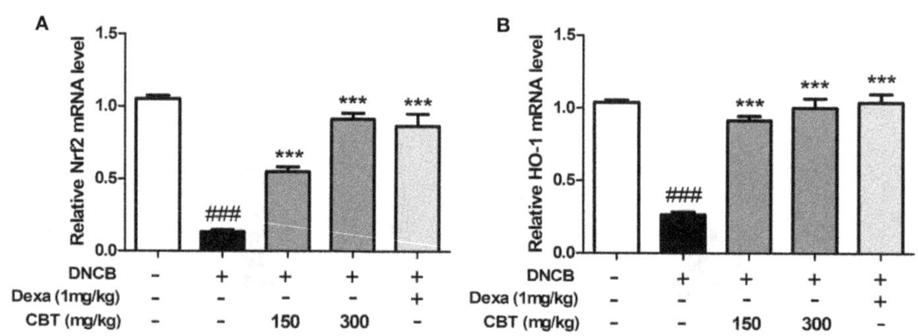

FIGURE 6 | Effects of *Chijabyukpi-tang* (CBT) on the mRNA expression level of HO-1 in DNCB-treated mice skin tissues. The mRNA expression levels of Nrf2 **(A)** and HO-1 **(B)** were analyzed using the quantitative real-time polymerase chain reaction (qPCR). Data are shown as mean ± SEM of the three independent experiments. $^{###}p < 0.001$ compared with the normal group, $^{***}p < 0.001$ compared with the DNCB-treated group. The Dexa group was set as positive control.

progression have been outlined, the exact causes of AD and treatments without side effects have yet to be clarified (Dupuy, 1994). Therefore, there is a need to develop safe and effective therapies for AD, using natural extracts and herbal medicines.

For thousands of years, Northeast Asia (Korea, China, and Japan) has used traditional medicinal herb formulas to treat many diseases. However, since there is no scientific evidence for the efficacy and safety of these medicinal herb formulas, consumers have doubts concerning their use. CBT has been used as a treatment for eczema accompanied with inflammation, but there is still no definitive evidence for the efficacy of CBT treatment on AD. Therefore, we conducted this study to investigate the anti-inflammatory effects of CBT on AD and its mechanism of action.

Keratinocytes are the main cells that compose the stratum corneum and play a key role in AD pathogenesis. When keratinocytes are damaged by repetitive mechanical stimulations such as scratching behavior, various keratinocyte-derived cytokines and chemokines are secreted to promote inflammatory skin disease progression (Asahina and Maeda, 2017). These secreted factors also cause additional responses by recruiting immune cells such as neutrophils, monocytes, and T cells to AD inflammatory skin lesions (Giustizieri et al., 2001). T cells recruited to AD inflammatory skin lesions secrete various cytokines such as IL-4, IL-5, IL-6, and IL-13, and chemokines such as IL-8, CCL17, and CXCL10 (Leung and Sorter, 2001). This secretion of pro-inflammatory cytokines and chemokines is known to be caused by the activation of various signaling pathways. Oxidative stress is one of the factors that drive the progression of AD. Since anti-oxidant enzymes play a major role in protecting cells from oxidative stress, increasing anti-oxidant enzymes is an important strategy for treating AD. As a defense against oxidative stress in cells, Nrf2, a transcription factor, moves from the cytosol to the nucleus and increases the expression of anti-oxidant enzyme genes including HO-1. The increased level of HO-1 protein induces cell protection (Ahmed et al., 2017). The Nrf2/HO-1 signaling pathway is involved in the recruitment of various inflammatory cells into inflammatory lesions and is known to contribute to the anti-inflammatory process (Chen et al., 2006; Ryter et al., 2006). In addition, previous studies have indicated that increased HO-1 gene expression attenuates the development of AD skin lesions (Kirino et al., 2008).

Based on these mechanisms, we investigated the anti-inflammatory effect of CBT on TNF-α/IFN-γ-stimulated keratinocytes, and on DNCB-induced AD-like skin lesions in mice.

Firstly, the major compounds of CBT were identified by HPLC, and it was confirmed that it contains crocin (28.671 mg/g), berberine hydrochloride (6.255 mg/g), and glycyrrhizic acid (6.249 mg/g). Previous studies have reported these compounds have anti-inflammatory and anti-oxidant effects (Fagot et al., 2018; Wang et al., 2018).

HaCaT cells are used in many skin disease studies as they can mimic the symptoms of AD in response to inflammatory stimuli such as TNF-α/IFN-γ. In this study, we observed that CBT induces no toxicity in HaCaT cells, and significantly inhibits the increase in mRNA levels of pro-inflammatory cytokines and chemokines in TNF-α/IFN-γ-stimulated HaCaT cells. To further understand the mechanisms of the regulation of the immune response by CBT, we investigated the effects of CBT on the Nrf2/HO-1 signaling pathway. As a result, we confirmed that CBT promoted the migration of Nrf2 into the nucleus and increased the expression levels of the HO-1 gene in a dose-dependent manner. These results suggest that CBT has anti-inflammatory and protective effects on cells by inhibiting the production of pro-inflammatory cytokines and chemokines *via* the Nrf2/HO-1 signaling pathway.

To establish the AD experimental animal model, DNCB was repeatedly applied to the hairless dorsal skin of BALB/c mice (Matsumoto et al., 2004). The mice treated with DNCB were found to exhibit general AD symptoms such as increasing skin thickness, keratinization, and skin dryness. CBT attenuated the symptoms of mice with AD-like skin lesions in a dose-dependent manner. CBT

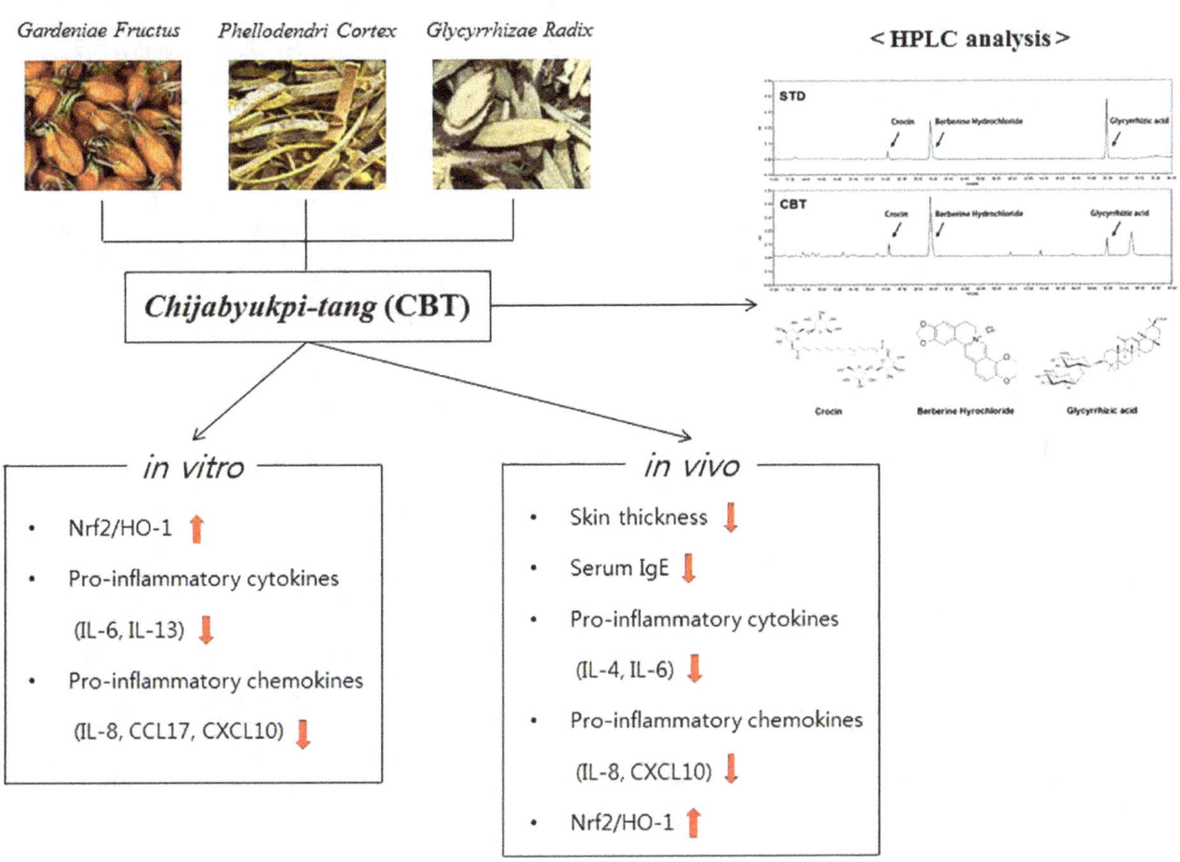

FIGURE 7 | A graphic summary of atopic dermatitis (AD)-like symptoms and related genes regulated by *Chijabyukpi-tang* (CBT).

improved the external condition of the dorsal skin and reduced its thickness. In addition, it has also been observed that the reduction in the moisture content of dorsal skin induced by DNCB-treatment is reversed by oral administration of CBT. DNCB-induced dorsal skin damage leads to AD-like inflammatory skin disease characterized by secretion of a variety of pro-inflammatory cytokines and chemokines by damaged keratinocytes resulting in Th cell activation. In this experiment, serum IgE levels, and expression levels of various cytokines and chemokines in skin tissues were increased by DNCB stimulation. These increased serum IgE and gene expression levels in skin tissues were significantly inhibited by the oral administration of CBT. These data provide experimental evidence for the anti-atopic effect of CBT in AD animal models. In these animal models, we also observed expression levels of Nrf2 and HO-1 in tissues to investigate whether the anti-inflammatory response was mediated through the Nrf2/HO-1 signaling pathway. As a result, we found that the expression levels of the Nrf2 and HO-1 gene were increased in a dose-dependent manner by CBT, similar to the result seen in the HaCaT cells.

In conclusion, CBT induces anti-inflammatory effects by up-regulating Nrf2/HO-1 signaling in TNF-α/IFN-γ-stimulated HaCaT cells. In addition, CBT improves AD-like skin lesions and inhibits inflammatory cytokines and chemokines in DNCB-treated mice models (**Figure 7**). These results suggest that CBT is a potential therapeutic candidate for the treatment of AD. However, the effects of dexamethasone or the individual herbal components (crocin, berberine hydrochloride and glycyrrhizic acid) vs CBT are not yet known, and further studies are required.

AUTHOR CONTRIBUTIONS

D-KK, MP, J-HL, and J-YL designed the study. J-HL and J-YL performed the experiments, analyzed the date. J-YL wrote the draft manuscript. J-HL rewrote and revised the manuscript. EJ, HN, and SP read the manuscript. All authors contributed to the article and approved the submitted version.

ACKNOWLEDGMENTS

This work was supported by the National Research Foundation of Korea (NRF) grants funded by the Korean government (MSIP) (2008-0062484)(2015M3A9E3051054).

REFERENCES

Ahmed, S. M., Luo, L., Namani, A., Wang, X. J., and Tanga, X. (2017). Nrf2 signaling pathway: Pivotal roles in inflammation. *Biochim. Biophys. Acta Mol. Basis Dis.* 1863 (2), 585–597. doi: 10.1016/j.bbadis.2016.11.005

Akram, M., Shin, I., Kim, K. A., Noh, D., Baek, S. H., Chang, S. Y., et al. (2016). A newly synthesized macakurzin C-derivative attenuates acute and chronic skin inflammation: The Nrf2/heme oxygenase signaling as a potential target. *Toxicol. Appl. Pharmacol.* 307, 62–71. doi: 10.1016/j.taap.2016.07.013

Asahina, R., and Maeda, S. (2017). A review of the roles of keratinocyte-derived cytokines and chemokines in the pathogenesis of atopic dermatitis in humans and dogs. *Vet. Dermatol.* 28 , (1) 16–(1) e5. doi: 10.1111/vde.12351

Chen, X. L., Dodd, G., Thomas, S., Zhang, X., Wasserman, M. A., Rovin, B. H., et al. (2006). Activation of Nrf2/ARE pathway protects endothelial cells from oxidant injury and inhibits inflammatory gene expression. *Am. J. Physiol. Heart. Circ. Physiol.* 290 (5), 1862–1870. doi: 10.1152/ajpheart.00651.2005

Chen, F. P., Chen, F. J., Jong, M. S., Tsai, H. L., Wang, J. R., and Hwang, S. J. (2009). Modern use of Chinese herbal formulae from Shang-Han Lun. *Chin. Med. J.* 122 (16), 1889–1894. doi: 10.3760/cma.j.issn.0366-6999.2009.16.010

Choi, W. Y., and Lee, S. J. (2017). Two Case Reports treated with Chijabackpi-tang based on Shanghanlun provisions. *J. Kor. Med. Assoc. Clin. Sanghan-Geumgwe.* 9 (1), 101–113. doi: 10.22891/kmedia.2017.9.1.101

Choi, J. H., Jin, S. W., Han, E. H., Park, B. H., Kim, H. G., Khanal, T., et al. (2014). Platycodon grandiflorum root-derived saponins attenuate atopic dermatitis-like skin lesions via suppression of NF-kappaB and STAT1 and activation of Nrf2/ARE-mediated heme oxygenase-1. *Phytomedicine* 21 (8-9), 1053–1061. doi: 10.1016/j.phymed.2014.04.011

Cury Martins, J., Martins, C., Aoki, V., Gois, A. F., Ishii, H. A., and da Silva, E. M. (2015). Topical tacrolimus for atopic dermatitis. *Cochrane Database Syst. Rev.* 1 (7), CD009864. doi: 10.1002/14651858.CD009864.pub2

Darlenski, R., Kazandjieva, J., Hristakieva, E., and Fluhr, J. W. (2014). Atopic dermatitis as a systemic disease. *Clin. Dermatol.* 32 (3), 409–413. doi: 10.1016/j.clindermatol.2013.11.007

Debnath, T., Lee, Y. M., Lim, J. H., and Lim, B. O. (2018). Anti-allergic and anti-atopic dermatitis effects of Gardenia Fructus extract. *Food. Agr. Immunol.* 29 (1), 665–674. doi: 10.1080/09540105.2018.1436523

Dupuy, P. (1994). Does atopic dermatitis result from cytokine dysregulation? *J. Invest. Dermatol.* 102 (5), 741. doi: 10.1111/1523-1747.ep12398629

Fagot, D., Pham, D. M., Laboureau, J., Planel, E., Guerin, L., Nègre, C., et al. (2018). Crocin, a natural molecule with potentially beneficial effects against skin ageing. *Int. J. Cosmet. Sci.* 40 (4), 388–400. doi: 10.1111/ics.12472

Fan, H. J., Xie, Z. P., Lu, Z. W., Tan, Z. B., Bi, Y. M., Xie, L. P., et al. (2018). Anti-inflammatory and immune response regulation of Si-Ni-San in 2,4-dinitrochlorobenzene-induced atopic dermatitis-like skin dysfunction. *J. Ethnopharmacol.* 222, 1–10. doi: 10.1016/j.jep.2018.04.032

Giustizieri, M. L., Mascia, F., Frezzolini, A., Pità, O. D., Chinni, L. M., Giannetti, A., et al. (2001). Keratinocytes from patients with atopic dermatitis and psoriasis show a distinct chemokine production profile in response to T cell–derived cytokines. *J. Allergy Clin. Immunol.* 107 (5), 871–877. doi: 10.1067/mai.2001.114707

Guttman-Yassky, E., Nograles, K. E., and Krueger, J. G. (2011). Contrasting pathogenesis of atopic dermatitis and psoriasis-part I: clinical and pathologic concepts. *J. Allergy Clin. Immunol.* 127 (5), 1110–1118. doi: 10.1016/j.jaci.2011.01.053

Higashi, Y., and Kanzaki, T. (2006). Effects of Kampo Medicine, Shishi-hakuhi-to, on Elderly Patients with Pruritic Skin Diseases Measured Using a Patient Diary with an Itching Visual Analog Scale. *Nishi. Nihon. Hifuka.* 68 (4), 408–412. doi: 10.2336/nishinihonhifu.68.408

Homey, B., Steinhoff, M., Ruzicka, T., and Leung, D. Y. (2006). Cytokines and chemokines orchestrate atopic skin inflammation. *J. Allergy Clin. Immunol.* 118 (1), 178–189. doi: 10.1016/j.jaci.2006.03.047

Hon, K. L., Chan, B. C., and Leung, P. C. (2011). Chinese herbal medicine research in eczema treatment. *Chin. Med.* 6, 17. doi: 10.1186/1749-8546-6-17

Kapoor, R., Menon, C., Hoffstad, O., Bilker, W., Leclerc, P., and Margolis, D. J. (2008). The prevalence of atopic triad in children with physician-confirmed atopic dermatitis. *J. Am. Acad. Dermatol.* 58 (1), 68–73. doi: 10.1016/j.jaad.2007.06.041

Kiebert, G., Sorensen, S. V., Revicki, D., Fagan, S. C., Doyle, J. J., Cohen, J., et al. (2002). Atopic dermatitis is associated with a decrement in health-related quality of life. *Int. J. Dermatol.* 41 (3), 151–158. doi: 10.1046/j.1365-4362.2002.01436.x

Kirino, M., Kirino, Y., Takeno, M., Nagashima, Y., Takahashi, K., Kobayashi, M., et al. (2008). Heme oxygenase 1 attenuates the development of atopic dermatitis-like lesions in mice: implications for human disease. *J. Allergy Clin. Immunol.* 122 , (2) 290–297. doi: 10.1016/j.jaci.2008.05.031

Lee, J. H., Ki, H. H., Kim, D. K., and Lee, Y. M. (2018). Triticum aestivum sprout extract attenuates 2,4–dinitrochlorobenzene–induced atopic dermatitis–like skin lesions in mice and the expression of chemokines in human keratinocytes. *Mol. Med. Rep.* 18 , (3) 3461–3468. doi: 10.3892/mmr.2018.9339

Leung, D. Y., and Bieber, T. (2003). Atopic dermatitis. *Lancet* 361 (9352), 151–160. doi: 10.1016/S0140-6736(03)12193-9

Leung, D. Y., and Sorter, N. A. (2001). Cellular and immunologic mechanisms in atopic dermatitis. *J. Am. Acad. Dermatol.* 44 (1 Suppl), S1–S12. doi: 10.1067/mjd.2001.109815

Liu, F. T., Goodarzi, H., and Chen, H. Y. (2011). IgE, mast cells, and eosinophils in atopic dermatitis. *Clin. Rev. Allergy Immunol.* 41 (3), 298–310. doi: 10.1007/s12016-011-8252-4

Loboda, A., Damulewicz, M., Pyza, E., Jozkowicz, A., and Dulak, J. (2016). Role of Nrf2/HO-1 system in development, oxidative stress response and diseases: an evolutionarily conserved mechanism. *Cell Mol. Life Sci.* 73 (1), 3221–3247. doi: 10.1007/s00018-016-2223-0

Matsumoto, K., Mizukoshi, K., Oyobikawa, M., Ohshima, H., and Tagami, H. (2004). Establishment of an atopic dermatitis-like skin model in a hairless mouse by repeated elicitation of contact hypersensitivity that enables to conduct functional analyses of the stratum corneum with various non-invasive biophysical instruments. *Skin Res. Technol.* 10 (2), 122–129. doi: 10.1111/j.1600-0846.2004.00062.x

Mie, W., Eiko, S., Kazuhiko, Y., Kazuhiko, U., Masaaki, Y., Yasushi, O., et al. (2009). Shishihakuhito, a traditional Chinese medicine for atopic dermatitis, inhibits IgE-mediated histamine release from rat RBL-2H3 basophilic leukocyte cells. *J. Trad. Med.* 26 (1), 44–49. doi: 10.11339/jtm.26.44

Peng, W., and Novak, N. (2015). Pathogenesis of atopic dermatitis. *Clin. Exp. Allergy* 45 , (3) 566–574. doi: 10.1111/cea.12495

Ryter, S. W., Alam, J., and Choi, A. M. (2006). Heme oxygenase-1/carbon monoxide: from basic science to therapeutic applications. *Physiol. Rev.* 86 (2), 583–650. doi: 10.1152/physrev.00011.2005

Shaw, T. E., Currie, G. P., Koudelka, C. W., and Simpson, E. L. (2011). Eczema prevalence in the United States: data from the 2003 National Survey of Children's Health. *J. Invest. Dermatol.* 131 (1), 67–73. doi: 10.1038/jid.2010.251

Wang, X., Feng, S., Ding, N., He, Y., Li, C., Li, M., et al. (2018). Anti-Inflammatory Effects of Berberine Hydrochloride in an LPS-Induced Murine Model of Mastitis. *Evid. Based Compl. Alternat. Med.* 2018, 5164314. doi: 10.1155/2018/5164314

Yamanaka, K., and Mizutani, H. (2011). The role of cytokines/chemokines in the pathogenesis of atopic dermatitis. *Curr. Probl. Dermatol.* 41, 80–92. doi: 10.1159/000323299

Yang, X. L., Liu, D., Bian, K., and Zhang, D. D. (2013). Study on in vitro anti-inflammatory activity of total flavonoids from Glycyrrhizae Radix et Rhizoma and its ingredients. *Zhongguo Zhong Yao Za Zhi.* 38 (1), 99–104. doi: 10.4268/cjcmm20130120

10

Modulation of the Gut Microbiota by *Sihocheonggan-Tang* Shapes the Immune Responses of Atopic Dermatitis

Jaemoo Chun[1†], So Min Lee[2†], You Mee Ahn[1], Min-Gyung Baek[3,4], Hana Yi[5], Sarah Shin[1] and Jeeyoun Jung[1]*

[1]KM Science Research Division, Korea Institute of Oriental Medicine, Daejeon, South Korea, [2]KM Convergence Research Division, Korea Institute of Oriental Medicine, Daejeon, South Korea, [3]Interdisciplinary Program in Precision Public Health, Korea University, Seoul, South Korea, [4]Department of Public Health Sciences, Korea University, Seoul, South Korea, [5]School of Biosystems and Biomedical Sciences, Korea University, Seoul, South Korea

***Correspondence:**
Jeeyoun Jung
jjy0918@kiom.re.kr

[†]These authors have contributed equally to this work

Atopic dermatitis (AD) is a chronic inflammatory skin disease characterized by complex immune dysregulation and closely related to the gut microbiome. The present study investigated the microbiome-mediated effect of *Sihocheonggan-Tang* (SHCGT) on AD-like symptoms induced by 2,4-dinitrochlorobenzene (DNCB) in BALB/c mice. DNCB was applied regularly to the ear and dorsal skin of BALB/c mice, and SHCGT was administered orally daily for 2 weeks. The composition of the gut microbiota was analyzed using 16S rRNA sequencing, and the effect of gut microbiome-derived metabolites, specifically short-chain fatty acids (SCFAs), was evaluated in tumor necrosis factor-alpha (TNF-α)- and interferon-gamma (IFN-γ)-treated HaCaT cells. SHCGT alleviated DNCB-induced symptoms of AD and the immune response to AD by decreasing the plasma immunoglobulin E level and splenic interleukin-4, interleukin-10, TNF-α, and IFN-γ levels. The gut microbiome composition and the damaged gut epithelial barrier in mice with AD were also significantly altered by SHCGT, and the reduced SCFA levels therein were elevated. We found that SFCAs directly inhibited the mRNA expression of IL-6 and ICAM-1 in TNF-α- and INF-γ-treated HaCaT cells. The finding that SHCGT regulates the gut microbiome and improves DNCB-induced AD in mice suggests that this herbal medicine has therapeutic potential in patients with AD.

Keywords: Sihocheonggan-Tang, atopic dermatitis, gut microbiome, short-chain fatty acids, immune response

INTRODUCTION

Atopic dermatitis (AD) is a chronic inflammatory skin disease caused by immune system dysfunction and environmental stress (Akdis et al., 2000). It is typically characterized by increases in T helper (Th) 2 cell-mediated inflammatory responses, including the release of immunoglobulin E (IgE), interleukin (IL)-4, IL-5, and IL-13 in the acute phase, whereas an increasing proportion of Th1 cells accounts for the chronic phase of the immune response (Biedermann et al., 2015; Moreno et al., 2016). AD is usually treated with topical anti-inflammatory or immunosuppressive agents, such as antihistamines and steroids. However, many of the treatments available focus on reducing the frequency and severity of symptoms and may have severe adverse effects. Therefore, a new approach is needed to treat AD effectively (Paller et al., 2017).

The microbiome is a complex collection of microorganisms that colonize the gut and play a crucial role in the health of the host, including digestion of dietary fiber, production of metabolites, and regulation of the immune response (Makki et al., 2018). Maintaining a correctly balanced microbiota in the gut is important for homeostasis in the host immune response, and disruption of the balance of the gut microbiota could cause various diseases, including allergic and inflammatory disorders (Kamada et al., 2013). Therefore, modulating the composition of the gut microbiome is a promising way of overcoming the adverse effects or limitations of current treatments for these diseases. The gut microbiome could directly or indirectly communicate with the skin as one of the important modulators in the gut-skin axis. The beneficial effects of gut microbiota by probiotics on skin diseases have been demonstrated in animal studies (Salem et al., 2018) Moreover, emerging clinical evidence suggests that AD is associated with an imbalance in bacterial species in the gut (Song et al., 2016) and that treatment with probiotics or prebiotics prevents the development of AD or reduces its severity (Isolauri et al., 2000; Grüber et al., 2010; Foolad et al., 2013; Lin et al., 2019). Thus, regulation of gut microbiome balance could be promising strategy for the treatment and prevention of AD.

Herbal medicines can also restore the composition and beneficial effects of the gut microbiota, thereby improving immune-related diseases, including autoimmune disorders, allergies, and asthma (Richards et al., 2016; An et al., 2017). *Sihocheonggan-Tang* (SHCGT) consists of 15 herbs (*Bupleurum falcatum* L., *Angelica gigas* Nakai, *Paeonia lactiflora* Pall., *Ligusticum striatum* DC., *Rehmannia glutinosa* (Gaertn.) DC., Coptis chinensis Franch., *Scutellaria baicalensis* Georgi, *Phellodendron chinense* C.K.Schneid., *Gardenia jasminoides* J.Ellis, *Forsythia suspensa* (Thunb.) Vahl, *Platycodon grandiflorus* A. DC., *Arctium lappa* L., *Trichosanthes kirilowii* Maxim., *Mentha arvensis* L., and *Glycyrrhiza uralensis* Fisch.). It originates from Yizong Jinjian and has been used to treat inflammatory skin diseases, including AD, in clinical settings in Korea (An et al., 2017). However, the mechanism by which this drug exerts its therapeutic effect in skin diseases such as AD remains to be elucidated.

This study assessed the effects of SHCGT on symptoms of AD, infiltration of immune cells into the dermis and epidermis, and cytokine expression levels in plasma and the spleen in a mouse model of AD. In addition, we investigated changes in the composition of the gut microbiome and gut microbiome-derived metabolites. This study aimed to clarify the gut microbiome-mediated effect involved in the pathogenesis of AD and provide effective AD treatment with SHCGT. This is the first study to demonstrate the relationship between gut microbiome, their producing metabolites, and AD symptoms.

MATERIALS AND METHODS

Analysis of SHCGT by UPLC/Q-TOF MS

SHCGT was purchased from GMP (Good Manufacturing Practice) pharmaceutical factory of Hanpoong Pharm & Foods Co. Ltd. (Jeonju, Republic of Korea). The voucher number of SHCGT in this study is #17083 and stored in Korea institute of Oriental Medicine. According to the manufacturer, one dose of SHCGT consists of Bupleuri radix (0.67 g), Forsythiae Fructus (0.5 g), Cnidii Rhizoma (0.5 g), Trichosanthis Radix (0.5 g), Scutellariae Radix (0.5 g), Gardeniae Fructus (0.5 g), Paeoniae Radix (0.5 g), Arctii Fructus (0.5 g), Coptidis Rhizoma (0.5 g), Angelicae Gigantis Radix (0.5 g), Platycodi Radix (0.5 g), Rehmanniae Radix Preparata (0.5 g), Menthae Herba (0.5 g), Phellodendri Cortex (0.5 g), Glycyrrhizae Radix (0.5 g) (Korea pharmaceutical information center, 2000; **Supplementary Table S1**). Details about preparation of SHCGT and species of fifteen herbal medicines are given in the Supplementary Methods.

In this study, we further verified the chemical characteristics of SHCGT using ultra-performance liquid chromatography (UPLC; Waters Corp., Milford, MA, United States) combined with quadrupole time-of-flight mass spectrometry (Q-TOF MS; Impact HD; Bruker, Bremen, Germany; **Supplementary Figure S1**).

Ten milligrams of SHCGT was mixed with 1 ml of methanol-water solution (50:50, v/v). The sample was vortexed for 1 min and then centrifuged at 12,500 ×*g* and 25°C for 20 min. The supernatant was collected and filtered using a Millex®-LG filter with a 0.20-μm pore size (Millipore, Billerica, MA, United States). A UPLC BEH C18 column (100 × 2.1 mm, 1.7-μm particle size; Waters Corp.) was used to separate the SHCGT at 40°C.

The UPLC/Q-TOF MS data were processed using MS-Dial. The chemical components of SHCGT were identified based on the retention time, m/z, and MS fragment pattern using all publicly available mass spectral databases obtained from RIKEN (http://prime.psc.riken.jp/Metabolomics_Software/MS-DIAL/), which include the MS/MS records of MassBank, ReSpect, GNP, Fiehn HILIC, CASMI2016, RIKEN PlaSMA authentic standards, and RIKEN PlaSMA bio-MS/MS (Tsugawa et al., 2015). Details of the analysis of chemical components using UPLC-Q-TOF MS are given in the Supplementary Methods.

Animal Studies

Animal experiments were executed in accordance with the guidelines of the Institutional Animal Care and Use Committee of the Korea Institute of Oriental Medicine (Approval number #18-021). Six-week-old BALB/c mice were purchased from Saeron Bio Co. (Gyeonggi-do, Republic of Korea) and housed at 20–22°C with a relative humidity of 40–60% on a 12:12-h light/dark cycle in a specific pathogen-free animal facility at the Korea Institute of Oriental Medicine.

After acclimatization for 1 week, the mice were randomized to a sham (control) group ($n = 9$), an AD group ($n = 10$), or an AD + SHCGT group ($n = 10$). All mice were shaved, and AD was induced by DNCB (Sigma-Aldrich, St Louis, MO, United States). During the first week of the AD induction period, 1% DNCB in acetone/olive oil (3:1) was applied to the ear and dorsal skin daily, followed by 0.5% DNCB in acetone/olive oil (3:1) on alternate days for the next 2 weeks (**Figure 1A**). SHCGT or phosphate-buffered saline (100 μL) was administered to the mice by intragastric gavage once daily (**Figure 1A**). The severity of atopic symptoms was evaluated based on a previous method

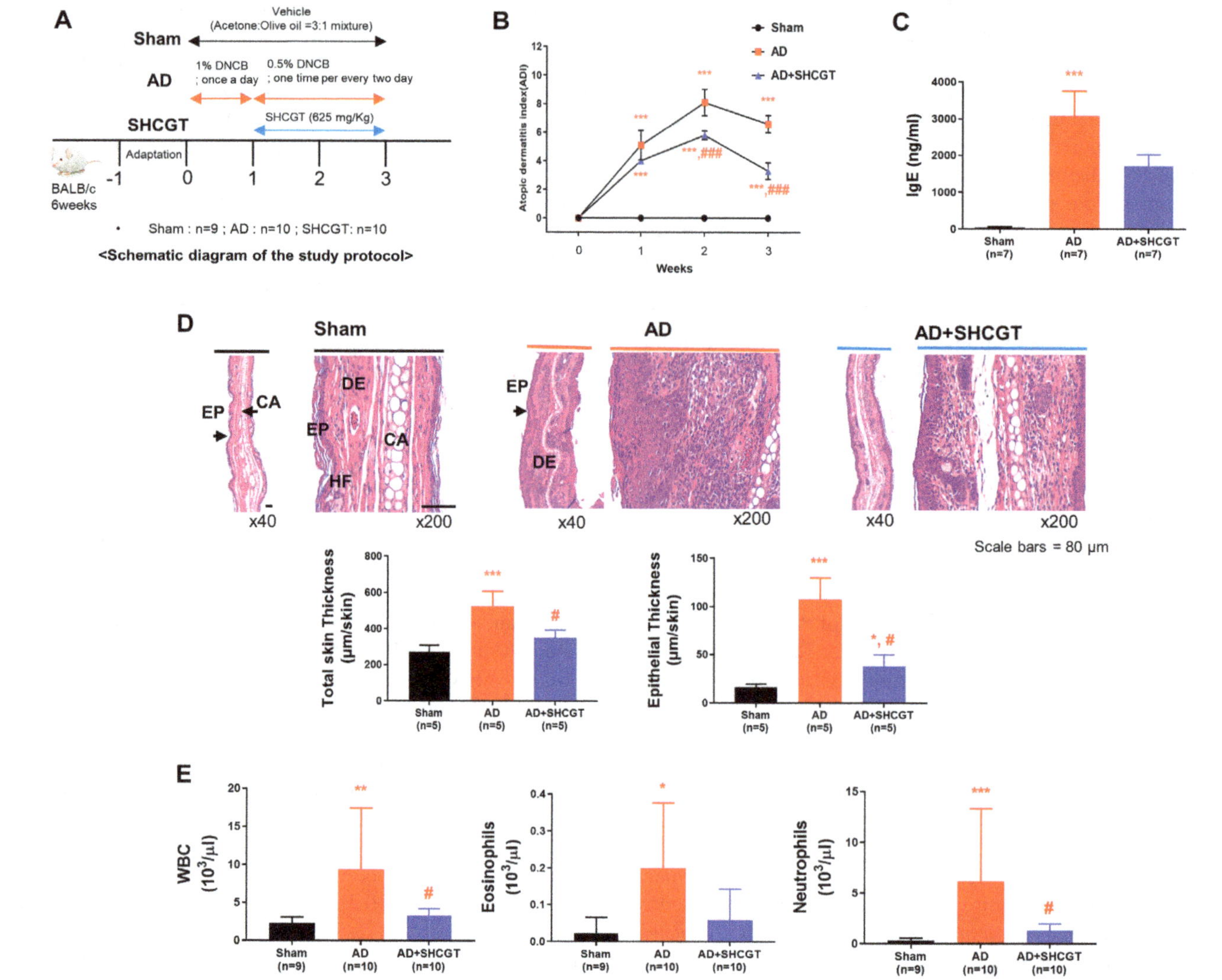

FIGURE 1 | Oral administration of SHCGT suppresses DNCB-induced AD. **(A)** Timeline for induction of AD and treatment with SHCGT. **(B)** The severity of DNCB-induced AD was evaluated based on four symptoms (erythema/edema, pruritus/dryness, erosion, and lichenification) and scored as 0 (none), 1 (mild), 2 (moderate), or 3 (severe). **(C)** Plasma IgE. **(D)** Ear skin specimens stained with hematoxylin. Total skin and epithelial thickness were evaluated by histological analysis. **(E)** Total WBC, eosinophil, and neutrophil levels. $^{*}p < 0.05$, $^{**}p < 0.01$, $^{***}p < 0.001$ vs. sham; $^{\#}p < 0.05$, $^{\#\#\#}p < 0.001$ vs. AD. AD, atopic dermatitis; DNBC, 2,4-dinitrochlorobenzene; IgE, immunoglobulin E; SHCGT, *Sihocheonggan-Tang*; WBC, white blood cell.

(Suto et al., 1999). Briefly, the AD score was measured as the sum of five symptoms, including erythema/edema, pruritus/dryness, erosion, and lichenification (0, none; 1, mild; 2, moderate; 3, severe).

The dose of SHCGT in this study is determined based on the clinical usage. The Ministry of Food and Drug Safety of Korea has approved the efficacy of SHCGT for the treatment of eczema by taking 3,000 mg/day for adult (reference body weight, 60 kg), which can be converted to 625 mg/kg for mouse when applied proportional constant of 0.08 (Nair and Jacob, 2006). Thus, we administrated 625 mg/kg of SHCGT in this study, and confirmed dose-dependent effect in additional experiments (**Supplementary Figure S2**). Details about additional experiments were described in Supplementary Results and **Supplementary Figure S2**.

Measurement of IgE

Blood samples were drawn from the sham, AD and AD+SHCGT groups, and plasma was collected by centrifugation at 2,000 ×*g* for 15 min at 4°C. It was stored at −80°C until the test. Plasma concentrations of total IgE were measured using an enzyme-linked immunosorbent assay kit (Bethyl Laboratories Inc., Montgomery, TX, United States) according to the manufacturer's instructions.

Isolation of Splenocytes and Measurement of Cytokines

The abdominal area was sterilized with 70% ethanol. The spleen was removed aseptically via an incision, and the connective tissues were removed. The spleen was then rinsed in RPMI-1640 medium (Gibco; Thermo Fisher Scientific, San Jose, CA, United States) and placed in a Petri dish containing fresh RPMI-1640 medium. The spleen cells were teased out using forceps and forced through a 22-G needle and then through a 26-G needle three times each. The cells were then transferred to a tube and centrifuged at 200 ×*g* for 10 min to pellet the cells. The spleens were pressed through a sterile Falcon cell strainer (BD Biosciences, Franklin Lakes, NJ, United States). Red blood cell lysis buffer (BioLegend, San Diego, CA, United States) was added to the cell suspension to remove the red blood cells. The spleen cells were centrifuged, suspended in complete RPMI-1640 medium with 10% fetal bovine serum and 1% antibiotics (penicillin, streptomycin, gentamicin; Gibco), and maintained at 37°C in a humidified incubator with 5% CO_2. After incubation for 24 h in a CO_2 incubator, the culture supernatants were assayed for cytokines. IL-4, IL-10, tumor necrosis factor-alpha (TNF-α), and interferon-gamma (IFN-γ) levels were analyzed using the Bio-Plex Pro Mouse Cytokine Th1/Th2 Assay kit (Bio-Rad Laboratories, Hercules, CA, United States).

Immunohistochemical Staining

Samples of equal size were taken from the ear skin, lymph nodes, and small intestine and fixed in 10% neutral buffered formalin for 24 h at 4°C. Paraffin-embedded tissue sections (3–4-μm thick) were stained with hematoxylin and eosin. The sections were stained with toluidine blue for detection of mast cells in the skin and periodic acid-Schiff (PAS) for detection of goblet cells in the small intestine. Intercellular adhesion molecule-1 (ICAM-1; ab119871, Abcam, Cambridge, MA, United States) and thymic stromal lymphopoietin (TSLP; ab115700, Abcam) in the epidermis and dermis of skin, Foxp3 (FJK-16s, Thermo Fisher) in lymph nodes, and tight junction markers, such as claudin-5 (4C3C2, Thermo Fisher), occludin (OC-3F10, Thermo Fisher), and zonula occludens (ZO)-1 (61–7,300, Thermo Fisher), in the tissues of the small intestine were observed by avidin-biotin-peroxidase complex-based immunohistochemical staining. The histological profiles of individual cross-sections of ear skin were observed under a light microscope (Eclipse 80i, Nikon, Tokyo, Japan).

Analysis of the Gut Microbiota

Immediately before the mice were euthanized, fresh fecal samples were collected and stored at −80°C until processing. A FastDNA Spin Kit for Soil (MP Biomedicals, Santa Ana, CA, United States) was used to isolate the fecal DNA. Fecal microbial profiles were determined by analysis of the V3–V4 region of the bacterial 16S rRNA gene using the 250-bp paired-end read strategy on the MiSeq sequencing system (Illumina, San Diego, CA, United States).

Analysis of Short-Chain Fatty Acids

Forty milligrams of stool was diluted in 900 μL of 0.2 M phosphate buffer solution (0.2 M Na_2HPO_4, 0.2 M NaH_2PO_4 in D_2O, pH 7.0). After homogenization at 14,000 ×*g* for 10 min, the extract (700 μL) was transferred to 5-mm nuclear magnetic resonance (NMR) tubes for analysis. One-dimensional 1H NMR spectra were acquired using an Ascend 800-MHz AVANCE III HD Bruker spectrometer (Bruker BioSpin AG) with a triple-resonance 5-mm CPTIC cryogenic probe. Bruker standard 1D nuclear Overhauser enhancement spectroscopy (NOESY)-presat (noesypr1d) pulse sequences were used as follows: relaxation delay, 90° – short delay, 90° – mixing, 90°–Acq, with a relaxation delay of 4.0 s, short delay = 11.3 μs, n = 128, dummy scans = 4, acquisition time = 2.0 s, and mixing time = 10 ms. The 800-MHz Chenomx library (ver. 7.1, Chenomx, Edmonton, AB, Canada) was used to identify short-chain fatty acids (SCFAs), and two-dimensional total correlation spectroscopy and heteronuclear single quantum correlation spectroscopy were also used to assign the individual compounds. In addition, ambiguous peaks due to peak overlap were confirmed by spiking with standard compounds. SCFA metabolites were quantified using Chenomx, which uses the concentration of trimethylsilylpropanoic acid to determine the concentrations of individual compounds (**Supplementary Table S3**).

Culture of HaCaT Cells and Treatment With Short-Chain Fatty Acids

HaCaT cells (human keratinocytes) were obtained from the American Type Culture Collection (Rockville, MD, United States). The cells were cultured in Dulbecco's modified Eagle's medium containing 10% heat-inactivated fetal bovine serum, 100 μg/ml streptomycin, and 100 U/mL penicillin in an incubator with a humidified atmosphere of 5% CO_2 at 37°C. Albiflorin, baicalin, geniposide, glycyrrhizic acid, and paeoniflorin were purchased from Wako Pure Chemical Industries (Osaka, Japan). Apigenin and luteolin purchased from Chengdu Biopurify Phytochemicals Ltd. (Chengdu, China). Berberine hydrochloride was purchased from Shanghai Sunny Biotech Co., Ltd. (Shanghai, China). Physcion was purchased from ChemNorm Biotech Co., Ltd. (Wuhan, China). The purity of compounds used in this study was higher than 98%. A cell counting kit-8 assay (CCK-8, Dojindo, Kumamoto, Japan) was performed to determine the effect of noncytotoxic concentrations of SHCGT, SCFAs and compounds on the viability of HaCaT cells. Briefly, HaCaT cells were treated with SHCGT (125–1,000 μg/ml), compounds (12.5–100 μM), and SCFAs (isobutyrate, propionate, and valerate in the range of 1.25–10 mM) for 24 h. Next, 10 μL of CCK-8 reagent was added to each well and incubated for 2 h. The absorbance of each well was detected at 450 nm using a Benchmark Plus microplate reader (Bio-Rad), and determined the proper concentrations of isobutyrate, propionate, and valerate.

To evaluate the anti-inflammatory effect on keratinocytes, HaCaT cells were pretreated with SHCGT, compounds, and SCFAs at predetermined concentrations in the CCK-8 assay (SHCGT, 125–1,000 μg/ml; Albiflorin, 100 μM; baicalin, 50 μM; geniposide, 100 μM; glycyrrhizic acid, 100 μM; paeoniflorin, 100 μM; apigenin, 25 μM; luteolin, 25 μM; berberine hydrochloride, 50 μM; physcion, 100 μM; isobutyrate, 2.5 mM; propionate, 2.5 mM; and valerate, 2.5 mM) for 6 h and then stimulated with TNF-α (20 ng/ml) and IFN-γ (20 ng/ml) for an additional 18 h.

Quantitative Reverse Transcription-Polymerase Chain Reaction

Total RNA was isolated from HaCaT cells using the RNeasy Kit (Qiagen, Hilden, Germany). Total RNA (1 μg) was converted into cDNA using the High-Capacity cDNA Reverse Transcription Kit (Applied Biosystems, Foster City, CA, United States). Quantitative polymerase chain reaction (PCR) was performed on a CFX Connect Real-Time PCR Detection System (Bio-Rad) using iTaq Universal SYBR Green Supermix (Bio-Rad). The forward primer used for IL-6 was 5-TAC CCC CAG GAG AAG ATT CC-3, and the reverse was 5-GCC ATC TTT GGA AGG TTC AG-3′. The forward primer used for ICAM-1 was 5-GCT GGT GAC ATG CAG CAC C-3, and the reverse was 5-CTC CTC ACC AGC ACC GTG G G-3′. All reactions were performed in triplicate. All gene levels were calculated by comparative delta Ct and normalized using the GAPDH gene level.

Analysis of Gut Microbiome Data

QIIME (Caporaso et al., 2010) with the EzBioCloud 16S rRNA gene sequence database was utilized to analyze the sequencing data (Yoon et al., 2017). The threshold of operational taxonomic units was 97%. OTU data were imported to Microbiomeanalyst (https://www.microbiomeanalyst.ca/; Chong et al., 2020) and subjected to following data analysis. The Shannon index was calculated to determine the alpha diversity, and principal coordinates analysis was performed using weighted normalized UniFrac distances. In addition, linear discriminant analysis effect size (LEfSe) (Segata et al., 2011), a biomarker discovery method, was used to determine the microbiota that best characterized each study group based on the *p*-value (<0.05) and linear discriminant analysis score (>3). Pattern search analysis was also performed to identify the microbiota that were correlated with a particular pattern in abundance (Sham-AD-AD+SHCGT; 1-2-1). We, then, executed the parametric and non-parametric ANOVA tests with post-hoc test to compare the microbiota among groups. Details about the parametric and non-parametric ANOVA tests were in 2.11 Statistical Analysis part.

Statistical Analysis

All the experimental data are presented as the mean ± standard deviation and were analyze differences among the three groups using one-way analysis of variance (ANOVA) followed by Tukey's post hoc test. However, nonparametric analysis was performed using and the Kruskal-Wallis test followed by Dunn's multiple comparison test, when normality and homogeneity of variance was not satisfied through the normality and homogeneity of variance test. The statistical analyses were performed using GraphPad Prism (version 9.0.2, GraphPad Software, San Diego, CA). A p-value < 0.05 was considered statistically significant.

RESULTS

Chemical Components in SHCGT

According to the manufacturer, SHCGT contains five chemical ingredients (10 mg of paeoniflorin, 25 mg of berberine, 22.5 mg of geniposide, 50 mg of baicalin, and 12.5 mg of glycyrrhizic acid in 3 g of SHCGT) as marker compounds (Korea pharmaceutical information center, 2000). In this study, we further identified the chemical components of SHCGT based on UPLC-Q-TOF MS analysis. A total of 2,221 features were detected, and 49 metabolites were putatively matched with reference peaks of primary and secondary metabolites (**Supplementary Figure S1**). In particular, quercetin-3-O-robinoside, ferulic acid, luteolin, hesperidin, albiflorin, apigenin, liquiritigenin, ammonium glycyrrhizinate, rheochrysidin, casticin, and enoxolone were identified according to relative retention time, exact MS, and MS/MS fragments (**Figure 2**). Furthermore, we confirmed the existence and concentration of eight bio-compounds, such as ferulic acid, luteolin, hesperidin, albiflorin, apigenin, ammonium glycyrrhizinate, rheochrysidin, and casticin, with standard compounds (Data not shown).

Effect of SHCGT on DNCB-Induced AD in Mice

To investigate the effect of SHCGT on AD, DNCB was regularly applied to the ear and dorsal skin of BALB/c mice, and SHCGT was administered orally daily for 2 weeks. On days 7–21, atopic dermatitis index (ADI) scores were significantly higher in BALB/c mice treated with DNCB than in sham mice (**Figure 1B**). On days 14–21, the decrease in the ADI score was steeper in the AD + SHCGT group than in the AD group [from 8.1 to 6.6 (AD group) and from 5.8 to 3.3 (AD + SHCGT group)]; furthermore, the ADI score was significantly lower in the AD + SHCGT group than in the AD group on day 14 and day 21 (**Figure 1B**). IgE levels were also significantly higher in the AD group than in the sham group (**Figure 1C**). Histological analysis revealed that ear skin tissue was thicker (due to epidermal keratinocyte hyperplasia) in the AD and AD + SHCGT groups than in the sham group, but ear skin in AD + SHCGT mice was thinner than that in AD mice (**Figure 1D**), indicating a favorable inhibitory effect of SHCGT on DNCB-induced thickening of the epidermal tissue.

We also measured the numbers of circulating white blood cells (WBCs), eosinophils, and neutrophils. The AD group had 4.1-fold, 9.0-fold, and 18.0-fold higher WBC, eosinophil, and neutrophil counts, respectively, than the sham group (**Figure 1E**). However, compared with the AD group, treatment with SHCGT reduced the WBC, eosinophil, and neutrophil counts by 35.5, 30.0, and 21.5%, respectively (**Figure 1E**). Furthermore, the ADI index, the percentage of neutrophil, and corticosterone were changed in dose-dependent manners (Supplementary Results and **Supplementary Figure S2**).

A significantly greater number of cells including mast cells infiltrated the skin in the AD group and the AD + SHCGT group than in the sham group (**Figure 3A**). There was a 37.9% decrease in the number of mast cells in the AD + SHCGT group compared to the AD group. Furthermore, immunohistochemistry showed that the expression of TSLP-positive and ICAM-1-positive cells in the epidermis and dermis of the ear skin was significantly higher in the AD group and AD + SHCGT group than in the sham group (**Figure 3B**). Administration of SHCGT decreased the populations of epidermal and dermal TSLP-positive and ICAM-1-positive cells by 54 and 33%, respectively, in the AD group, indicating that SHCGT reduced the inflammatory reaction.

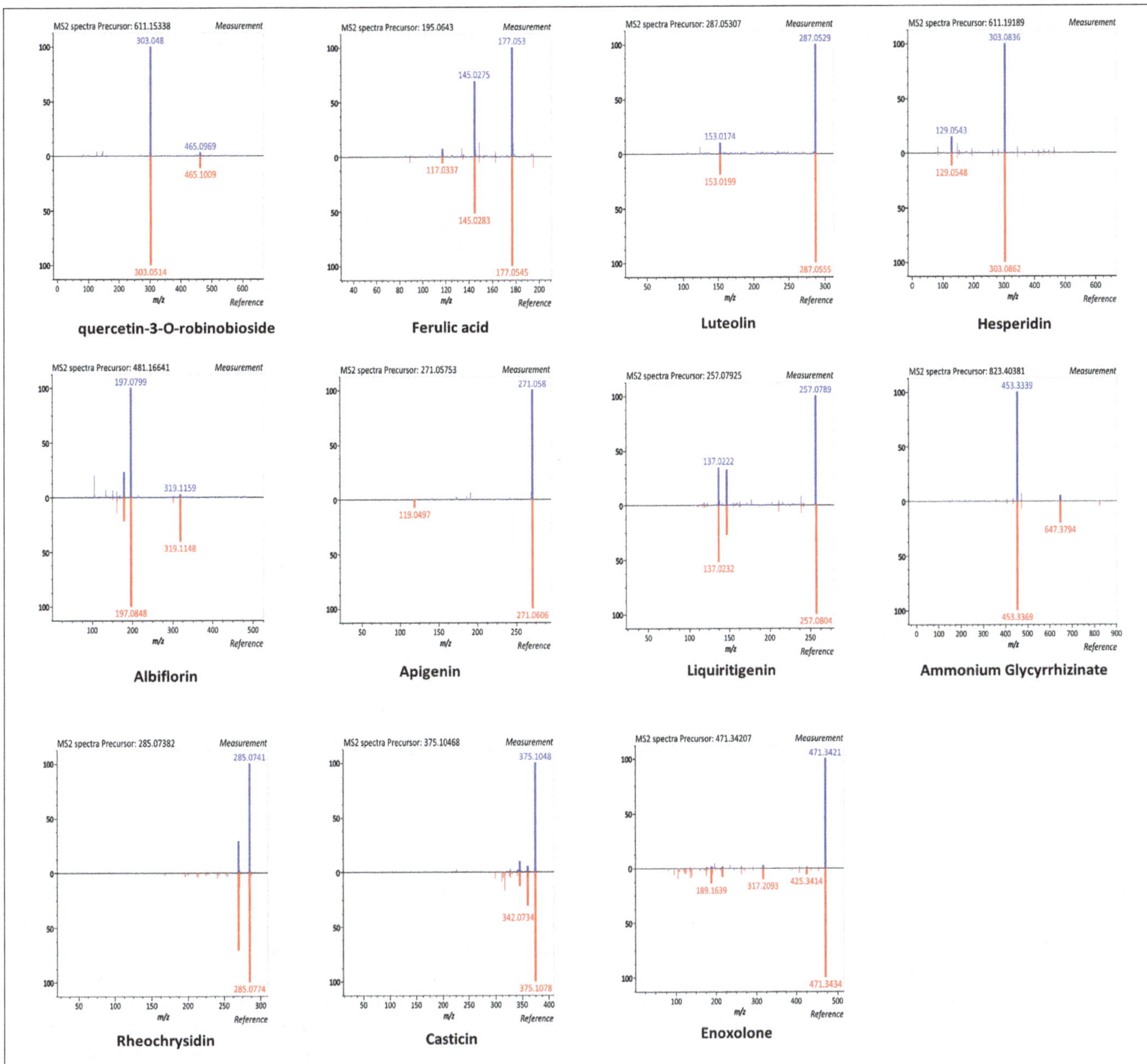

FIGURE 2 | The mirror plots of secondary metabolites in SHCGT. The mirror plots that illustrate MS/MS spectral match of measured peaks of secondary metabolites in SHCGT and reference peaks for authentic standard compounds.

Effect of SHCGT on the Immune Response in Mice With DNCB-Induced AD

We examined the lymph nodes to determine whether topical exposure to DNCB provoked immune activation in mice. DNCB resulted in an increase in lymph node size compared with that of the sham group; this increase was reduced by SHCGT (**Figure 4A**).

The production of IgE is a characteristic of AD. Increased total IgE levels reflect a switch from Th1 to Th2 (Elghazali et al., 1997). In addition, Foxp3+ Treg cells control the recruitment of inflammatory cells and the expression of Th2 cytokines, as well as elevated serum IgE levels (Fyhrquist et al., 2012). In this study, we also observed marked hypertrophic changes with a decrease in Foxp3+ cells in lymph nodes in the AD group compared with those in the sham group (**Figure 4A**). However, compared with that of the AD group, the expression of Foxp3+ cells in lymph node tissues was significantly increased in the AD + SHCGT group, and there were changes in Th2 cytokines, including IL-4 and IL-10, in the spleen. IL-4 and IL-10 levels were significantly increased in the AD group and attenuated by administration of SHCGT (**Figure 4B**).

A surge in Th1 cytokines is characteristic of the chronic and late phases of AD (Chen et al., 2004). In this study, we observed a

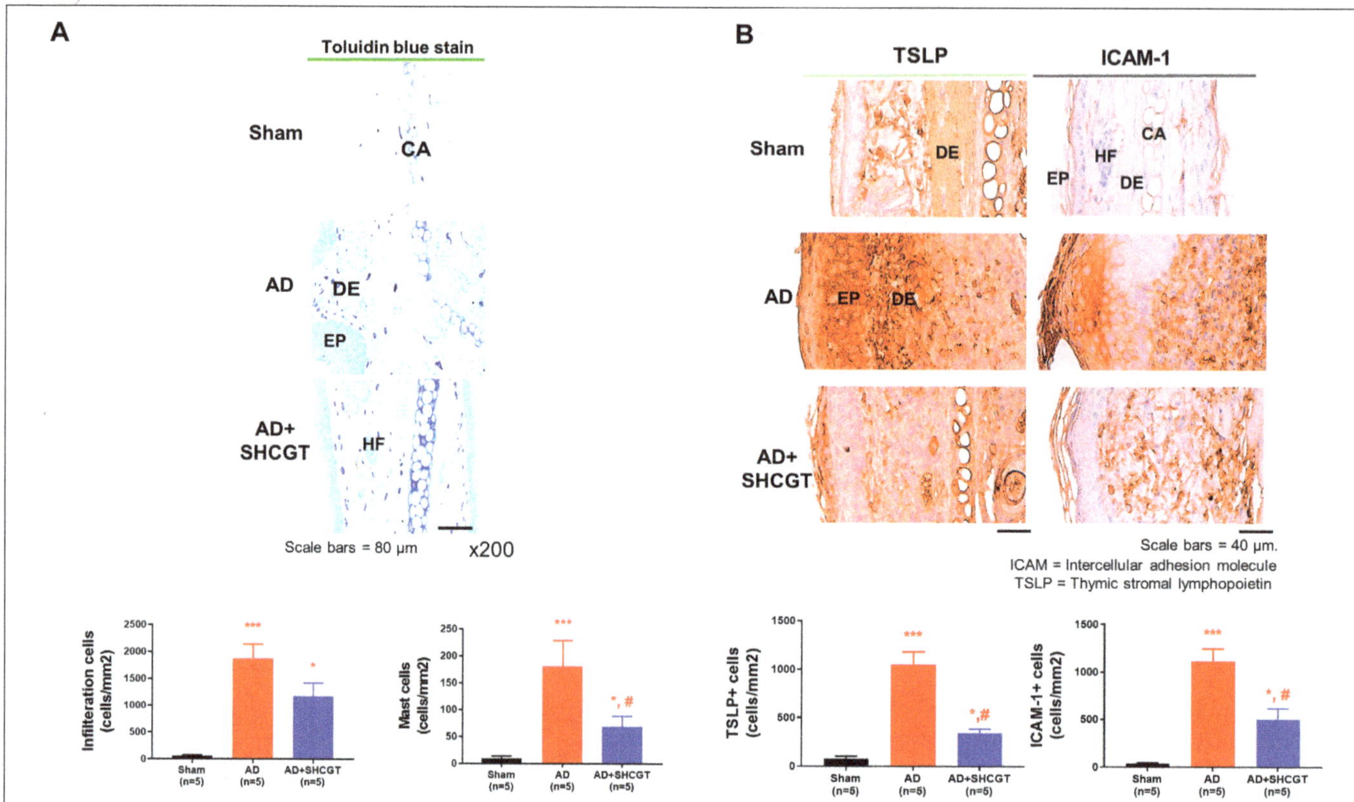

FIGURE 3 | SHCGT inhibited the infiltration of inflammatory cells and the expression of TSLP and ICAM-1 in mice with DNCB-induced AD. **(A)** Toluidine blue-stained mast cells in ear skin tissue. SHCGT reduced the infiltration of inflammatory cells, including mast cells, in the ear skin of mice with DNCB-induced AD. **(B)** Immunohistochemistry staining for TSLP and ICAM-1 in ear skin. SHCGT significantly decreased the expression of TSLP and ICAM-1 in mice with DNCB-induced AD. *p < 0.05, ***p < 0.001 vs. sham; #p < 0.05 vs. AD. AD, atopic dermatitis; DNBC, 2,4-dinitrochlorobenzene; ICAM-1, intercellular adhesion molecule-1; IgE, immunoglobulin E; SHCGT, *Sihocheonggan-Tang*; TSLP, thymic stromal lymphopoietin.

significant increase in TNF-α and IFN-γ levels in the AD group in comparison with those in the sham group; however, compared with those in the AD group, there was a significant decrease in TNF-α and IFN-γ levels in the AD + SHCGT group (**Figure 4B**). Furthermore, the decreasing trend of IL-4, IL-10, TNF-α, and INF-γ in the spleen showed a more clearly SHCGT dose-dependent change (Supplementary Results and **Supplementary Figure S2**).

SHCGT-Induced Changes in the Gut Microbiome in Mice With DNCB-Induced AD

Recent studies have reported that the gut microbiome plays an important role in AD by regulating metabolites and the immune response (Penders et al., 2007; Song et al., 2016). Therefore, we investigated the changes in the microbiome population after treatment with SHCGT. As shown in **Figure 5A**, the microbiome in sham mice was dominated by *Bacteroidetes* and *Firmicutes* at the phylum level in terms of relative abundance. *Verrucomicrobia*, which includes *Akkermansia* at the species level, was present in only the sham mice. The relative abundance of *Deferribacteres* was significantly higher in the AD group and was restored by SHCGT (**Figure 5B**). However, the Shannon index values, which represent community richness and evenness, were not significantly different between the sham, AD, and AD + SHCGT groups (**Figure 5C**).

A three-dimensional score plot obtained by principal coordinates analysis of weighted UniFrac distances showed different microbiome patterns between the sham, AD, and AD + SHCGT groups (**Figure 5D**). LEfSe analysis revealed significant alterations in 50 species based on the p-value (<0.05) and linear discriminant analysis score (>3; **Supplementary Table S2**). Based on the results of a pattern search, 17 of these species (*Mucispirillum schaedleri, Bacteroides faecichinchillae, AB021165, EU509745, EF098405, EU474208, EF098277, HQ786508, FJ880834, EF404944, KI535319, DQ815703, EF603669, DQ905725, AB606259, HM124343*, and *Staphylococcus simiae*) showed significant patterns of recovery in the AD + SHCGT group (**Figure 5E, Supplementary Figure S3**). In particular, the relative abundances of *AB606259* and *M. schaedleri* in the AD group were significantly higher than those in the sham group but improved after treatment with SHCGT (**Figure 5F**).

Change in the Intestinal Barrier System and Microbiome Producing SCFAs in Mice With AD After Treatment With SHCGT

Changes in the gut microbiome impaired the intestinal barrier system, leading to inflammatory events involved in the

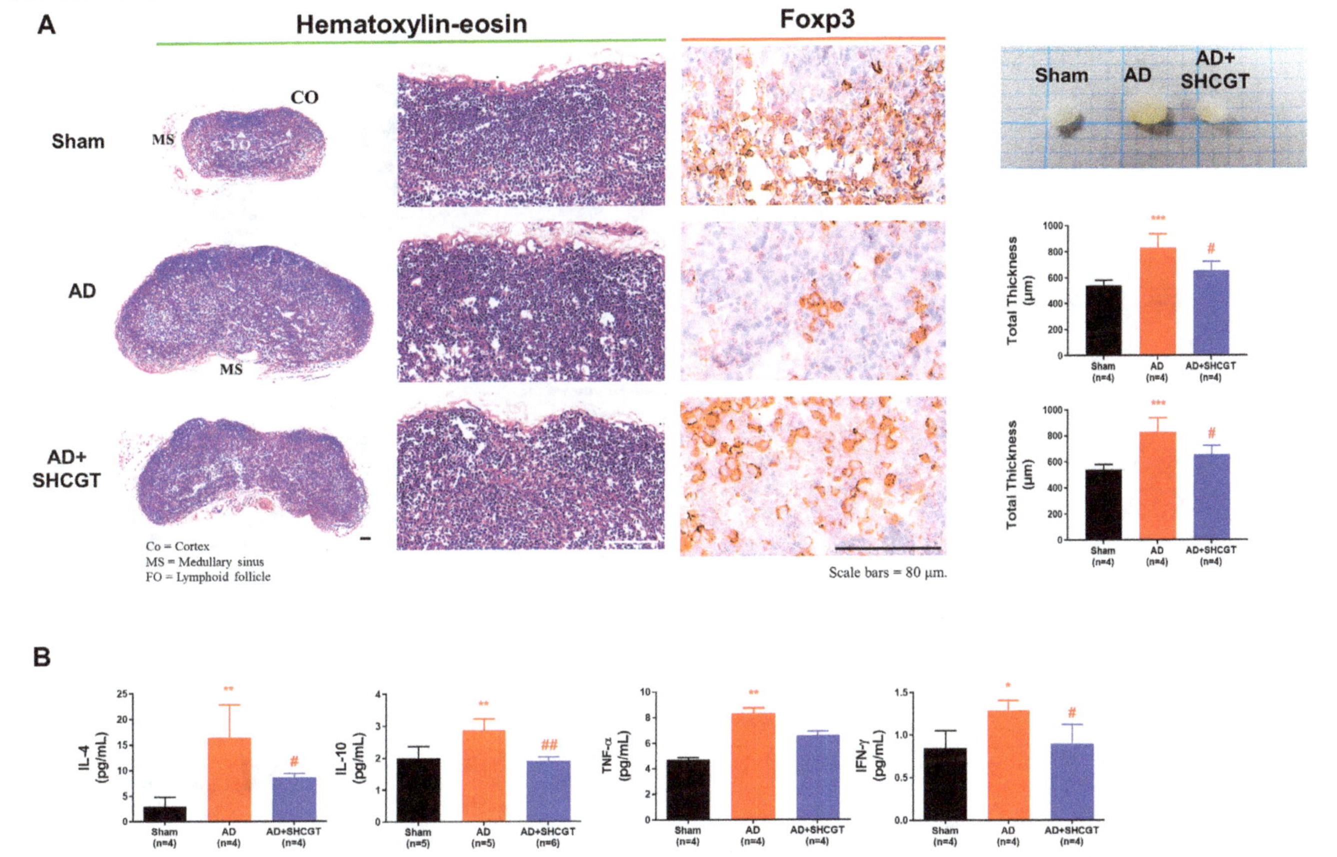

FIGURE 4 | SHCGT suppressed enlargement of peripheral lymph nodes and secretion of cytokines in the spleens of mice with DNCB-induced AD. **(A)** Immunohistochemical lymph node profiles showing that SHCGT reduced the marked hypertrophic changes in the expression of Foxp3, a marker of regulatory T-cell activity, in lymph node tissue from mice with DNCB-induced AD. **(B)** IL-4, IL-10, TNF-α, and IFN-γ levels in the spleen. Increased Th2 (IL-4 and IL-10)-related and Th1 (TNF-α and IFN-γ)-related cytokines were decreased by SHCGT in mice with AD. *$p < 0.05$, **$p < 0.01$, ***$p < 0.001$ vs. sham; #$p < 0.05$, ##$p < 0.01$ vs. AD. AD, atopic dermatitis; CO, cortex; DNCB, 2,4-dinitrochlorobenzene; FO, lymphoid follicle; ICAM-1, intercellular adhesion molecule-1; IFN-γ, interferon-gamma; IL, interleukin; MS, medullary sinus; SHCGT, *Sihocheonggan-Tang*; TNF-α, tumor necrosis factor-alpha.

occurrence and development of human AD via changes in microbiota-derived metabolites, including SCFAs (Craig, 2016; Levy et al., 2016).

We also observed marked intestinal villous atrophy in the group with DNCB-induced AD in comparison with the sham group (**Figure 6A**). However, administration of SHCGT caused a significant decrease in mean villus height and width, reduced numbers of PAS-positive cells, and increased total and cortex thicknesses and numbers of cortical lymphoid follicles (**Figure 6A**). Furthermore, dysfunction of the barrier system, that is, loss of tight junction markers (claudin-5, occludin, and ZO-1), was observed in the group with DNCB-induced AD compared with the sham group (**Figure 6B**). Similarly, there was significant recovery of mean claudin-5, occludin, and ZO-1+ levels in the mucosal tissues of the small intestine after treatment with SHCGT (**Figure 6B**). These results suggest that DNCB-induced AD and related immune responses are mediated by hypersensitivity and small intestinal dysfunction and that administration of SHCGT attenuates the loss of tight junctional proteins and related villus atrophy.

Gut microbiota-derived metabolites, including SCFAs, take part in maintaining the integrity of the epithelial barrier and regulating inflammatory responses. As shown in **Figure 7**, the concentrations of isobutyrate, propionate, and valerate were lower in the mice with DNCB-induced AD than in the sham mice. Administration of SHCGT restored the decreased levels of isobutyrate, propionate, and valerate in the AD group (**Figure 7A**). However, endotoxin levels in the AD group were not significantly different from those in the sham group but were decreased by SHCGT (**Figure 7B**). These findings indicate that the reduction in endotoxin levels by SHCGT may contribute to the mitigation of AD, although endotoxins would not be the main cause of AD (Kim and Kim, 2019).

Effect of SHCGT, Compounds, and SCFAs on TNF-α/IFN-γ-Induced mRNA Expression in HaCaT Cells

Inflammatory keratinocytes are important in the pathogenesis of AD. Exposure of keratinocytes to TNF-α and IFN-γ induces abnormal expression of cytokines and adhesion molecules, such

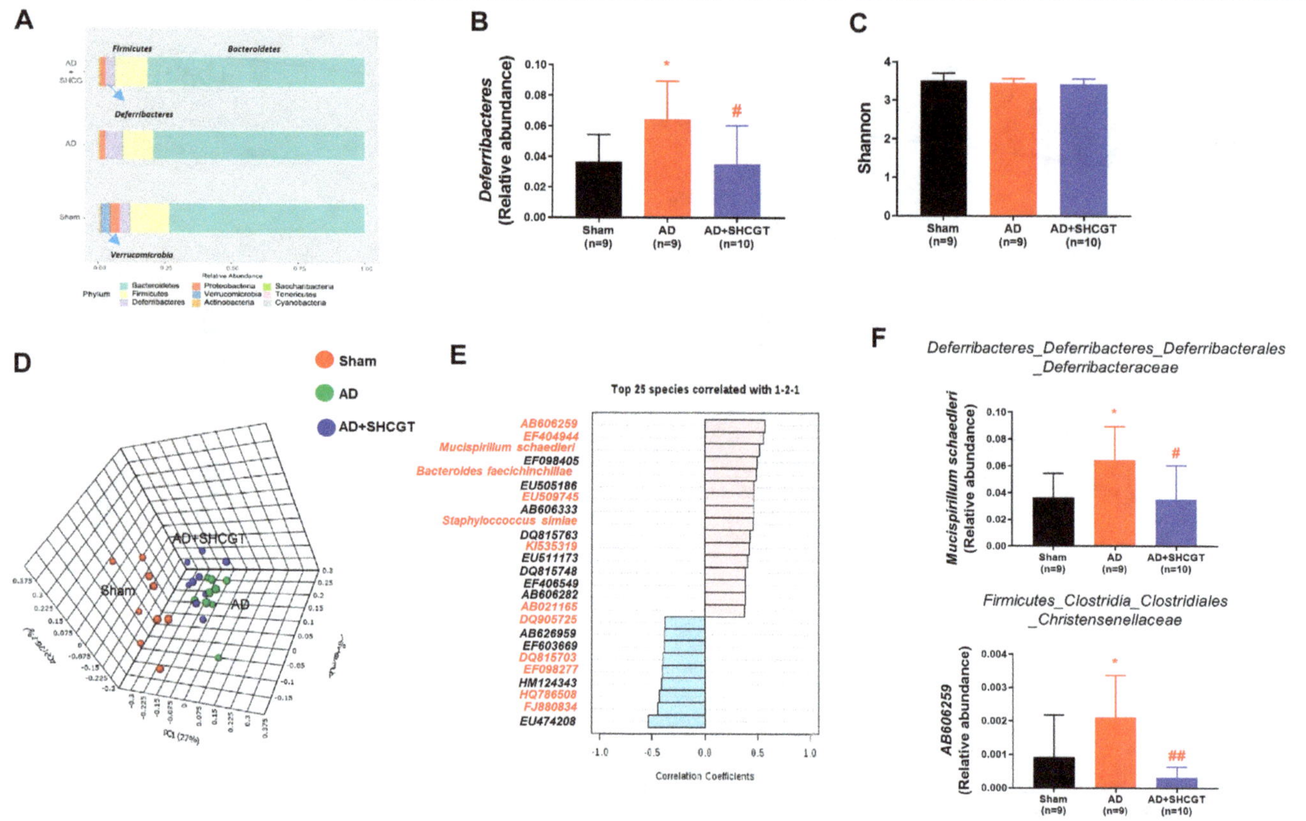

FIGURE 5 | SHCGT changed the gut microbiome in mice with DNCB-induced AD. **(A)** Taxonomic composition of the microbial community in the gut at the phylum level. **(B)** The increased relative abundance of *Deferribacteres* was attenuated by SHCGT in mice with AD. **(C)** Alpha diversity using the Shannon index score at the species level. No significant differences were observed. **(D)** A three-dimensional score plot based on principal coordinates analysis of weighted UniFrac distances showing different microbiome patterns in each group. **(E)** Top 25 species detected in pattern search analysis. The red letters indicate the gut microbiota components also detected by LEfSe analysis. **(F)** A significantly altered gut microbiota profile was identified by a combination of pattern search analysis, LEfSe, and univariate analysis. $^{*}p < 0.05$ vs. sham; $^{\#}p < 0.05$, $^{\#\#}p < 0.01$ vs. AD. AD, atopic dermatitis; DNCB, 2,4-dinitrochlorobenzene; LEfSe, linear discriminant analysis effect size; SHCGT, *Sihocheonggan-Tang*.

as IL-6 and ICAM-1, which are associated with infiltration of monocytes into skin. To identify other possible effects of microbiota-derived SCFAs on AD, we treated HaCaT cells with isobutyrate, propionate, and valerate.

No cytotoxicity was observed in HaCaT cells treated with 1.25–2.5 mM SFCAs (**Supplementary Figure S4**). As shown in **Figure 8**, TNF-α/IFN-γ upregulated IL-6 and ICAM-1 expression in HaCaT cells. However, SHCGT directly downregulated the expression of IL-6 but not that of ICAM-1. Instead, treatment with isobutyrate and propionate significantly downregulated TNF-α/IFN-γ-induced IL-6 and ICAM-1 in these cells, suggesting that the gut microbiome-derived metabolites isobutyrate and propionate are involved in the attenuation of inflammation in AD.

Furthermore, we examined the mRNA expression of IL-6 in TNF-α/IFN-γ-induced HaCaT cells to evaluate whether SHCGT dose-dependently affects the atopic dermatitis. No cytotoxicity was observed with SHCGT up to 1,000 μg/ml in HaCaT cells (**Supplementary Figure S4**). However, SHCGT dose-dependently decreased the TNF-α/IFN-γ-induced mRNA expression of IL-6 in HaCaT cells (**Figure 9A**). In addition, the detailed chemical investigation was done to predict the most active compounds responsible for its anti-atopic dermatitis effect. We determined the concentration of each compound, not having cytotoxicity by CCK-8 assay (**Supplementary Figure S4**). Albiflorin (100 μM), baicalin (50 μM), geniposide (100 μM), glycyrrhizic acid (100 μM), paeoniflorin (100 μM), apigenin (25 μM), luteolin (25 μM), berberine hydrochloride (50 μM), and physcion (100 μM) were used to confirm the inhibitory effect of IL-6 mRNA expression in HaCaT cells. The results showed that apigenin, baicalin, luteolin, and paeoniflorin could be associated with anti-atopic dermatitis effect of SHCGT (**Figure 9B**).

Taken all results together, we suggested that SHCGT relieves the atopic dermatitis in a dose-dependent manner, and SCFAs produced by intestinal microorganisms changed by SHCGT also play a role in improving the atopic dermatitis.

DISCUSSION

Topical steroids and oral antihistamines are the first-line treatment for AS (Eichenfield et al., 2014). However, these

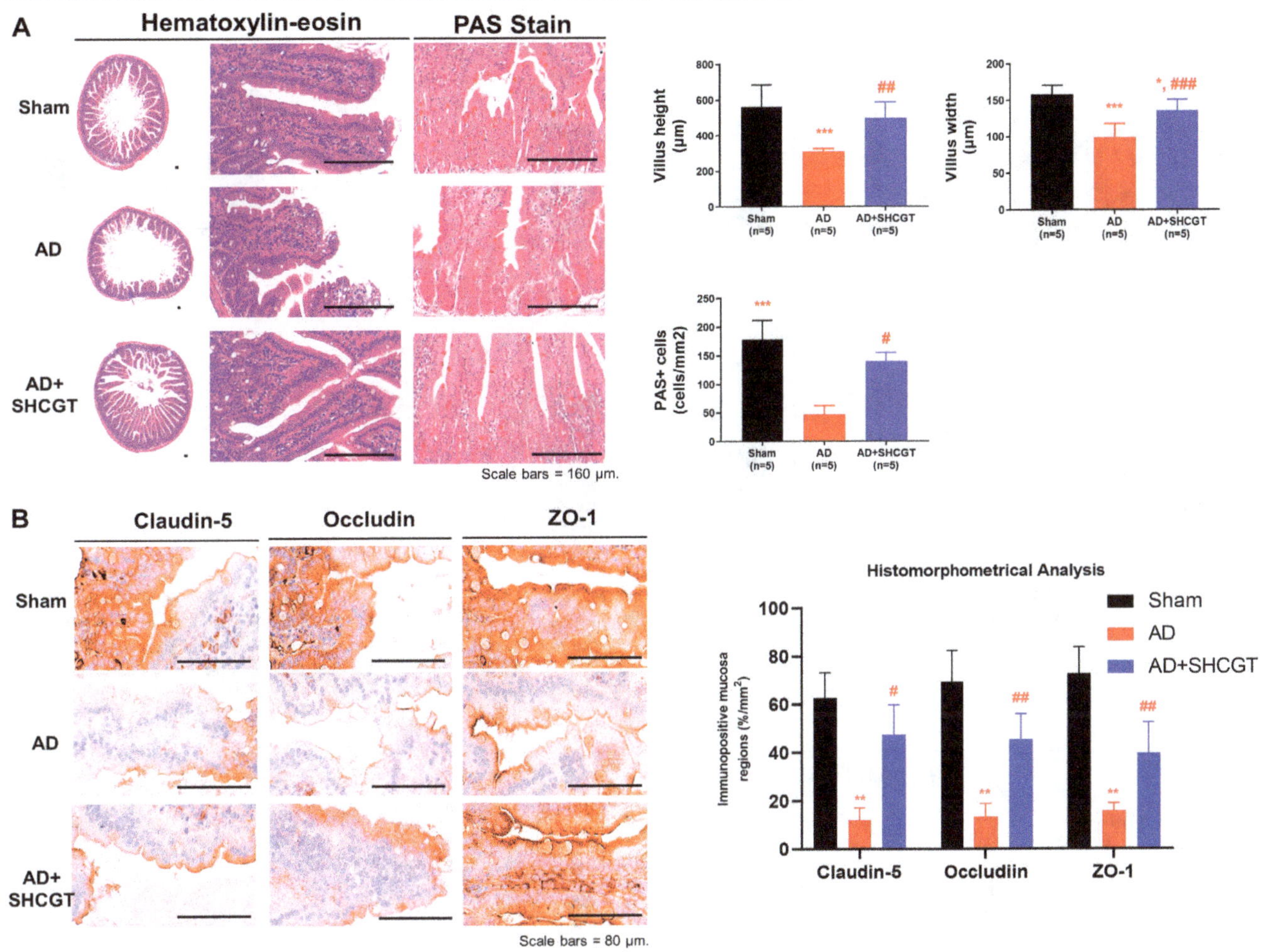

FIGURE 6 | SHCGT improved the damaged intestinal barrier system in mice with DNCB-induced AD. **(A)** Hematoxylin-eosin and PAS staining of intestinal villi. SHCGT significantly reduced the mean villus height and width as well as PAS+ cell numbers in mice with DNCB-induced AD. **(B)** Immunohistochemistry staining for claudin-1, occludin, and ZO-1 in the intestine. Quantitative imaging analysis showed that SHCGT recovered the function of the intestinal barrier system, with losses of tight junctional markers (claudin-5, occludin, and ZO-1). $^{**}p < 0.01$, $^{***}p < 0.001$ vs. sham; $^{\#}p < 0.05$, $^{\#\#}p < 0.01$, $^{\#\#\#}p < 0.001$ vs. AD. AD, atopic dermatitis; DNCB, 2,4-dinitrochlorobenzene; PAS, periodic acid Schiff; SHCGT, *Sihocheonggan-Tang*; ZO-1, zonula occludens-1.

agents have several adverse effects, and many patients with AD are reluctant to use steroids in the long term (Kojima et al., 2013). Therefore, there is increasing interest in herbal medicines as a treatment for AD worldwide, given that many herbs and traditional Chinese medicines are commonly used to treat allergic disorders, including AD, asthma, and arthritis (Ma et al., 2013). Furthermore, several studies have investigated the potential role of herbal medicines as prebiotics for modulation of the growth and activity of microorganisms that play a crucial role in metabolism and the immune response in various diseases (Hutkins et al., 2016; Lee et al., 2020).

SHCGT is an herbal medicine that has been used to treat AD in Korea (An et al., 2017). However, detailed mechanistic studies in animal models have not been reported. In this study, we demonstrated the pharmacological effects of SHCGT in a mouse model of DNBC-induced AD and investigated the ability of SHCGT to regulate the gut microbiome in mice with AD.

Several studies have suggested that abnormalities in the composition and function of the gut microbiome contribute substantially to the onset of AD and atopic march (Kim and Kim, 2019). Watanabe et al. (2003) reported a significantly lower *Bifidobacterium* count and a significantly higher *Staphylococcus* count in patients with AD than in healthy controls and that the levels of these microorganisms differed according to disease state. Interestingly, in our study, we found that mice with AD had increased levels of *S. simiae*, a coagulase-negative bacterium that is closely related to *S. aureus*, which is frequently isolated from the skin in patients with AD during flares (Suzuki et al., 2012; Geoghegan et al., 2018).

Moreover, Song et al. (2016) showed that enrichment of subspecies of *Faecalibacterium prausnitzii* (F06) decreased

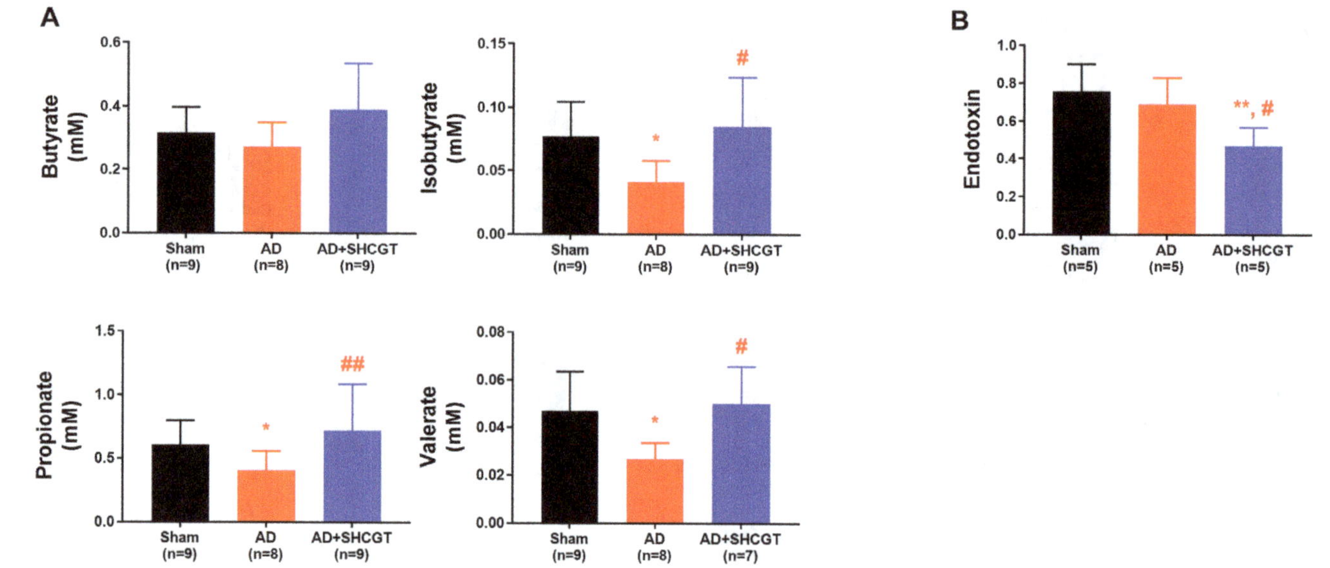

FIGURE 7 | SHCGT regulated gut microbiome-related metabolites and short-chain fatty acids and reduced endotoxin levels. **(A)** Concentrations of short-chain fatty acids, including butyrate, isobutyrate, propionate, and valerate. SHCGT significantly increased the isobutyrate, propionate, and valerate levels in mice with DNCB-induced AD. **(B)** Change in plasma endotoxin levels. The endotoxin level was lower in the group with SHCGT-treated AD than in the sham and AD groups. $^{*}p < 0.05$, $^{**}p < 0.01$ vs. sham; $^{\#}p < 0.05$, $^{\#\#}p < 0.01$ vs. AD. AD, atopic dermatitis; DNCB, 2,4-dinitrochlorobenzene; SHCGT, *Sihocheonggan-Tang*.

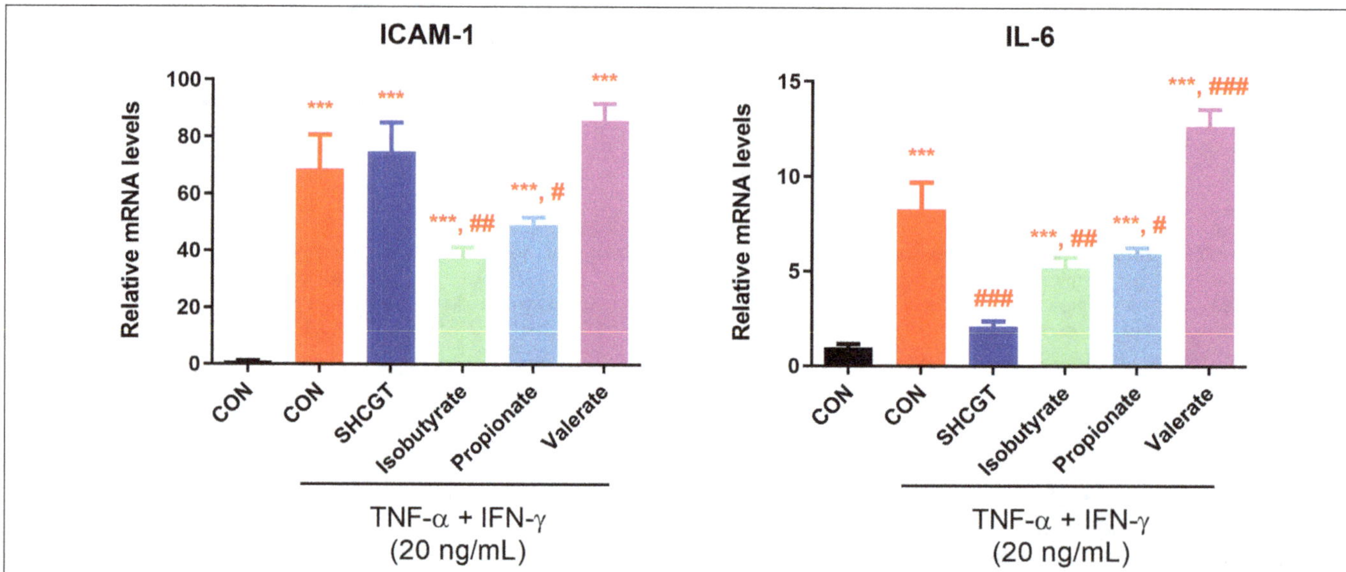

FIGURE 8 | Gut microbiome-related metabolites (short-chain fatty acids) had a beneficial effect on TNF-α/IFN-γ-treated HaCaT cells. Isobutyrate and propionate directly reduced the expression levels of ICAM-1 and IL-6 in TNF-α/IFN-γ-treated HaCaT cells. $^{***}p < 0.001$ vs. CON; $^{\#}p < 0.05$, $^{\#\#}p < 0.01$, $^{\#\#\#}p < 0.001$ vs. TNF-α/IFN-γ-treated CON (CON + TNF-α/IFN-γ). AD, atopic dermatitis; CON, control HaCaT cells; DNCB, 2,4-dinitrochlorobenzene; ICAM-1, intercellular adhesion molecule-1; IFN-γ, interferon-gamma; IL-6, interleukin-6; SHCGT, *Sihocheonggan-Tang*; TNF-α, tumor necrosis factor-alpha.

high butyrate and propionate producers, contributing to impairment of the gut epithelial barrier in patients with AD. In particular, they suggested that damaged epithelium with increased permeability might allow systemic circulation of undigested foods, toxins, and pathogenic microorganisms, ultimately leading to an aberrant Th2-type immune response in the skin of these patients (Pike et al., 1986; Noverr and Huffnagle, 2004). In the present study, treatment with SHCGT significantly decreased the endotoxin level in the AD group, but there was no significant difference in the endotoxin level between the sham and AD groups, indicating that endotoxins may not be the main cause of AD.

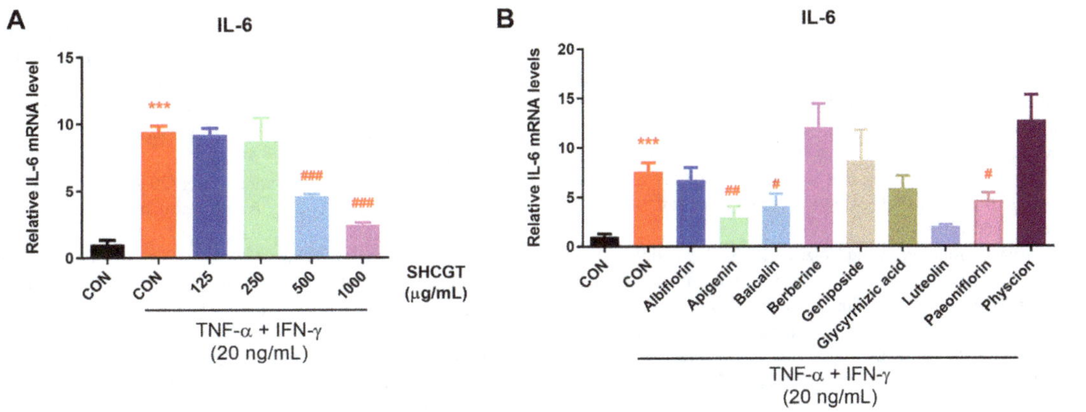

FIGURE 9 | SHCGT dose-dependently affected the atopic dermatitis and bioactive compounds in SHCGT had an inhibitory effect in TNF-α/IFN-γ-treated HaCaT cells. **(A)** SHCGT regulated the expression of IL-6 mRNA expression in TNF-α/IFN-γ-treated HaCaT cells in dose-dependent manners. **(B)** The compounds in SHCGT showed inhibitory effect on IL-6 mRNA expression in TNF-α/IFN-γ-treated HaCaT cells. HaCaT cells were pretreated with SHCGT or compounds at predetermined concentrations (SHCGT, 125–1,000 μg/ml; albiflorin, 100 μM; baicalin, 50 μM; geniposide, 100 μM; glycyrrhizic acid, 100 μM; paeoniflorin, 100 μM; apigenin, 25 μM; luteolin, 25 μM; berberine hydrochloride, 50 μM; and physcion, 100 μM) for 6 h and then stimulated with TNF-α (20 ng/ml) and IFN-γ (20 ng/ml) for an additional 18 h. $^{***}p < 0.001$ vs. CON; $^{\#}p < 0.05$, $^{\#\#}p < 0.01$, $^{\#\#\#}p < 0.001$ vs. TNF-α/IFN-γ-treated CON (CON + TNF-α/IFN-γ). CON, control; TNF-α, tumor necrosis factor-alpha; IFN-γ, interferon-gamma; IL-6, interleukin-6; SHCGT, *Sihocheonggan-Tang*.

SHCGT-induced attenuation of damage to the intestinal barrier system in mice with AD was accompanied by a change in the composition of the gut microbiome, including in *AB606259* and *M. schaedleri*. *M. schaedleri* is found in abundance in the mucosal layer of the intestine. This organism has been suggested to be a pathobiont that modifies gene expression in the host mucosal tissue and has proinflammatory properties that affect inflammation status or susceptibility to disease (Loy et al., 2017). *M. schaedleri* has limited ability to degrade complex polysaccharides and uses monosaccharides, oligopeptides, amino acids, glycerol, and SCFAs, that is, the breakdown products of other members of the microbiota, as substrates for energy metabolism (El Kaoutari et al., 2013; Loy et al., 2017). In accordance with these properties, we found that the levels of SCFAs, including isobutyrate, propionate, and valerate, were significantly lower in mice with AD than in sham mice and returned to the sham levels after treatment with SHCGT.

SCFAs, which are derived from the degradation of polysaccharides by the gut microbiome, participate in the proliferation and differentiation of both B-cells and T-cells and have anti-inflammatory effects (Nguyen et al., 2016; Kim and Kim, 2019). In this study, we found that SHCGT suppressed the increased Th2 and Th1 immune responses in mice with AD and that SCFAs also directly reduced the expression of IL-6 and ICAM-1 in TNF-α/INF-γ-induced keratinocytes. SHCGT contains several compounds that are known to attenuate AD, including berberine and paeoniflorin (Tsang et al., 2016; Jo et al., 2018), and was also found to decrease the expression of IL-6 in an *in vitro* model of AD in our study. However, the actual concentrations of these active compounds in SHCGT may be extremely low in the circulation after oral administration. Therefore, it is possible that SHCGT influences the gut microbiome and that the polysaccharides and indigestible fibers in SHCGT could act as prebiotics by supplying SCFAs to the host circulation (Peterson et al., 2018).

CONCLUSION

In this study, we found that oral administration of SHCGT ameliorated AD-like symptoms and modulated the composition of the gut microbiota, with beneficial effects on AD. However, further studies are necessary to determine the crucial component of SHCGT that controls intestinal bacteria and to identify the underlying mechanism of the effect of the microbiota on AD. The dose of SHCGT was determined by considering the dose used in clinical practice, but it was much higher than the concentration given in a consensus document (Heinrich et al., 2020). Therefore, more experiments with appropriate concentrations are needed to optimize the dosage and explore the effect of SHCGT. Nevertheless, findings in this study advance our knowledge about SHCGT and successfully demonstrate the potential role of herbal medicines as prebiotics for the management of AD.

AUTHOR CONTRIBUTIONS

Conceptualization, HY and JJ; formal analysis, JC and SL; funding acquisition, JJ; investigation, JC, SL, M-GB, and SS; methodology, SL and M-GB; project administration, HY and JJ; visualization, JC and JJ; writing – original draft, JC and JJ; writing – review & editing, JC, YA, and JJ.

ACKNOWLEDGMENTS

We thank Dr. S. K. Gu for providing technical support for the animal experiments.

REFERENCES

Akdis, C. A., Akdis, M., Trautmann, A., and Blaser, K. (2000). Immune Regulation in Atopic Dermatitis. *Curr. Opin. Immunol.* 12, 641–646. doi:10.1016/s0952-7915(00)00156-4

An, J. H., Hwang, M. L., Yoon, H. J., and Jung, H. A. (2017). A Review on the *Sihocheonggan-Tang* & *Sihocheonggan-San* for the Treatablity of Atopic Dermatitis. *J. Korean Med. Ophthalmol. Otolaryngol. Dermatol.* 30, 10–16. doi:10.6114/jkood.2017.30.1.010

Biedermann, T., Skabytska, Y., Kaesler, S., and Volz, T. (2015). Regulation of T Cell Immunity in Atopic Dermatitis by Microbes: the Yin and Yang of Cutaneous Inflammation. *Front. Immunol.* 6, 353. doi:10.3389/fimmu.2015.00353

Caporaso, J. G., Kuczynski, J., Stombaugh, J., Bittinger, K., Bushman, F. D., Costello, E. K., et al. (2010). QIIME Allows Analysis of High-Throughput Community Sequencing Data. *Nat. Methods* 7, 335–336. doi:10.1038/nmeth.f.303

Chen, L., Martinez, O., Overbergh, L., Mathieu, C., Prabhakar, B. S., and Chan, L. S. (2004). Early Up-Regulation of Th2 Cytokines and Late Surge of Th1 Cytokines in an Atopic Dermatitis Model. *Clin. Exp. Immunol.* 138, 375–387. doi:10.1111/j.1365-2249.2004.02649.x

Chong, J., Liu, P., Zhou, G., and Xia, J. (2020). Using Microbiomeanalyst for Comprehensive Statistical, Functional, and Meta-Analysis of Microbiome Data. *Nat. Protoc.* 15, 799–821. doi:10.1038/s41596-019-0264-1

Craig, J. M. (2016). Atopic Dermatitis and the Intestinal Microbiota in Humans and Dogs. *Vet. Med. Sci.* 2, 95–105. doi:10.1002/vms3.24

Eichenfield, L. F., Tom, W. L., Berger, T. G., Krol, A., Paller, A. S., Schwarzenberger, K., et al. (2014). Guidelines of Care for the Management of Atopic Dermatitis: Section 2. Management and Treatment of Atopic Dermatitis with Topical Therapies. *J. Am. Acad. Dermatol.* 71, 116–132. doi:10.1016/j.jaad.2014.03.023

El Kaoutari, A., Armougom, F., Gordon, J. I., Raoult, D., and Henrissat, B. (2013). The Abundance and Variety of Carbohydrate-Active Enzymes in the Human Gut Microbiota. *Nat. Rev. Microbiol.* 11, 497–504. doi:10.1038/nrmicro3050

Elghazali, G., Perlmann, H., Rutta, A. S., Perlmann, P., and Troye-Blomberg, M. (1997). Elevated Plasma Levels of IgE in *Plasmodium Falciparum*-primed Individuals Reflect an Increased Ratio of IL-4 to Interferon-Gamma (IFN-Gamma)-Producing Cells. *Clin. Exp. Immunol.* 109, 84–89. doi:10.1046/j.1365-2249.1997.4401337.x

Foolad, N., Brezinski, E. A., Chase, E. P., and Armstrong, A. W. (2013). Effect of Nutrient Supplementation on Atopic Dermatitis in Children: a Systematic Review of Probiotics, Prebiotics, Formula, and Fatty Acids. *JAMA Dermatol.* 149, 350–355. doi:10.1001/jamadermatol.2013.1495

Fyhrquist, N., Lehtimäki, S., Lahl, K., Savinko, T., Lappeteläinen, A. M., Sparwasser, T., et al. (2012). Foxp3+ Cells Control Th2 Responses in a Murine Model of Atopic Dermatitis. *J. Invest. Dermatol.* 132, 1672–1680. doi:10.1038/jid.2012.40

Geoghegan, J. A., Irvine, A. D., and Foster, T. J. (2018). *Staphylococcus aureus* and Atopic Dermatitis: a Complex and Evolving Relationship. *Trends Microbiol.* 26, 484–497. doi:10.1016/j.tim.2017.11.008

Grüber, C., van Stuijvenberg, M., Mosca, F., Moro, G., Chirico, G., Braegger, C. P., et al. (2010). Reduced Occurrence of Early Atopic Dermatitis Because of Immunoactive Prebiotics Among Low-Atopy-Risk Infants. *J. Allergy Clin. Immunol.* 126, 791–797. doi:10.1016/j.jaci.2010.07.022

Heinrich, M., Appendino, G., Efferth, T., Fürst, R., Izzo, A. A., Kayser, O., et al. (2020). Best Practice in Research - Overcoming Common Challenges in Phytopharmacological Research. *J. Ethnopharmacol.* 246, 112230. doi:10.1016/j.jep.2019.112230

Hutkins, R. W., Krumbeck, J. A., Bindels, L. B., Cani, P. D., Fahey, G., Goh, Y. J., et al. (2016). Prebiotics: Why Definitions Matter. *Curr. Opin. Biotechnol.* 37, 1–7. doi:10.1016/j.copbio.2015.09.001

Isolauri, E., Arvola, T., Sütas, Y., Moilanen, E., and Salminen, S. (2000). Probiotics in the Management of Atopic Eczema. *Clin. Exp. Allergy* 30, 1604–1610. doi:10.1046/j.1365-2222.2000.00943.x

Jo, G. H., Kim, S. N., Kim, M. J., and Heo, Y. (2018). Protective Effect of Paeoniae Radix alba Root Extract on Immune Alterations in Mice with Atopic Dermatitis. *J. Toxicol. Environ. Health A.* 81, 502–511. doi:10.1080/15287394.2018.1460785

Kamada, N., Seo, S. U., Chen, G. Y., and Núñez, G. (2013). Role of the Gut Microbiota in Immunity and Inflammatory Disease. *Nat. Rev. Immunol.* 13, 321–335. doi:10.1038/nri3430

Kim, J. E., and Kim, H. S. (2019). Microbiome of the Skin and Gut in Atopic Dermatitis (AD): Understanding the Pathophysiology and Finding Novel Management Strategies. *J. Clin. Med.* 8, 444. doi:10.3390/jcm8040444

Kojima, R., Fujiwara, T., Matsuda, A., Narita, M., Matsubara, O., Nonoyama, S., et al. (2013). Factors Associated with Steroid Phobia in Caregivers of Children with Atopic Dermatitis. *Pediatr. Dermatol.* 30, 29–35. doi:10.1111/j.1525-1470.2012.01808.x

Korea pharmaceutical information center (2000). Hanpoonng Sihocheongkantang. Available at: http://www.health.kr/searchDrug/result_drug.asp?drug_cd=A11AKP08G2401 (Accessed July 29, 2000).

Lee, J. E., Lee, S. M., and Jung, J. (2020). Integrated Omics Analysis Unraveled the Microbiome-Mediated Effects of Yijin-Tang on Hepatosteatosis and Insulin Resistance in Obese Mouse. *Phytomedicine* 79, 153354. doi:10.1016/j.phymed.2020.153354

Levy, M., Thaiss, C. A., and Elinav, E. (2016). Metabolites: Messengers between the Microbiota and the Immune System. *Genes Dev.* 30, 1589–1597. doi:10.1101/gad.284091.116

Lin, L., Luo, L., Zhong, M., Xie, T., Liu, Y., Li, H., et al. (2019). Gut Microbiota: a New Angle for Traditional Herbal Medicine Research. *RSC Adv.* 9, 17457–17472. doi:10.1039/C9RA01838G

Loy, A., Pfann, C., Steinberger, M., Hanson, B., Herp, S., Brugiroux, S., et al. (2017). Lifestyle and Horizontal Gene Transfer-Mediated Evolution of Mucispirillum Schaedleri, a Core Member of the Murine Gut Microbiota. *mSystems* 2, e00171. doi:10.1128/mSystems.00171-16

Ma, H. D., Deng, Y. R., Tian, Z., and Lian, Z. X. (2013). Traditional Chinese Medicine and Immune Regulation. *Clin. Rev. Allergy Immunol.* 44, 229–241. doi:10.1007/s12016-012-8332-0

Makki, K., Deehan, E. C., Walter, J., and Bäckhed, F. (2018). The Impact of Dietary Fiber on Gut Microbiota in Host Health and Disease. *Cell Host Microbe* 23, 705–715. doi:10.1016/j.chom.2018.05.012

Moreno, A. S., McPhee, R., Arruda, L. K., and Howell, M. D. (2016). Targeting the T Helper 2 Inflammatory axis in Atopic Dermatitis. *Int. Arch. Allergy Immunol.* 171, 71–80. doi:10.1159/000451083

Nair, A. B., and Jacob, S. (2016). A Simple Practice Guide for Dose Conversion between Animals and Human. *J. Basic Clin. Pharm.* 7, 27–31. doi:10.4103/0976-0105.177703

Nguyen, Q. N., Himes, J. E., Martinez, D. R., and Permar, S. R. (2016). The Impact of the Gut Microbiota on Humoral Immunity to Pathogens and Vaccination in Early Infancy. *Plos Pathog.* 12, e1005997. doi:10.1371/journal.ppat.1005997

Noverr, M. C., and Huffnagle, G. B. (2004). Does the Microbiota Regulate Immune Responses outside the Gut? *Trends Microbiol.* 12, 562–568. doi:10.1016/j.tim.2004.10.008

Paller, A. S., Kabashima, K., and Bieber, T. (2017). Therapeutic Pipeline for Atopic Dermatitis: End of the Drought? *J. Allergy Clin. Immunol.* 140, 633–643. doi:10.1016/j.jaci.2017.07.006

Penders, J., Thijs, C., van den Brandt, P. A., Kummeling, I., Snijders, B., Stelma, F., et al. (2007). Gut Microbiota Composition and Development of Atopic Manifestations in Infancy: the KOALA Birth Cohort Study. *Gut* 56, 661–667. doi:10.1136/gut.2006.100164

Peterson, C. T., Sharma, V., Uchitel, S., Denniston, K., Chopra, D., Mills, P. J., et al. (2018). Prebiotic Potential of Herbal Medicines Used in Digestive Health and Disease. *J. Altern. Complement. Med.* 24, 656–665. doi:10.1089/acm.2017.0422

Pike, M. G., Heddle, R. J., Boulton, P., Turner, M. W., and Atherton, D. J. (1986). Increased Intestinal Permeability in Atopic Eczema. *J. Invest. Dermatol.* 86, 101–104. doi:10.1111/1523-1747.ep12284035

Richards, J. L., Yap, Y. A., McLeod, K. H., Mackay, C. R., and Mariño, E. (2016). Dietary Metabolites and the Gut Microbiota: an Alternative Approach to Control Inflammatory and Autoimmune Diseases. *Clin. Transl. Immunol.* 5, e82. doi:10.1038/cti.2016.29

Salem, I., Ramser, A., Isham, N., and Ghannoum, M. A. (2018). The Gut Microbiome as a Major Regulator of the Gut-Skin Axis. *Front. Microbiol.* 9, 1459. doi:10.3389/fmicb.2018.01459

Segata, N., Izard, J., Waldron, L., Gevers, D., Miropolsky, L., Garrett, W. S., et al. (2011). Metagenomic Biomarker Discovery and Explanation. *Genome Biol.* 12, R60. doi:10.1186/gb-2011-12-6-r60

Song, H., Yoo, Y., Hwang, J., Na, Y. C., and Kim, H. S. (2016). *Faecalibacterium Prausnitzii* Subspecies-Level Dysbiosis in the Human Gut Microbiome Underlying Atopic Dermatitis. *J. Allergy Clin. Immunol.* 137, 852–860. doi:10.1016/j.jaci.2015.08.021

Suto, H., Matsuda, H., Mitsuishi, K., Hira, K., Uchida, T., Unno, T., et al. (1999). NC/Nga Mice: a Mouse Model for Atopic Dermatitis. *Int. Arch. Allergy Immunol.* 120 (Suppl. 1), 70–75. doi:10.1159/000053599

Suzuki, H., Lefébure, T., Bitar, P. P., and Stanhope, M. J. (2012). Comparative Genomic Analysis of the Genus *Staphylococcus* Including *Staphylococcus Aureus* and its Newly Described Sister Species *Staphylococcus Simiae. BMC Genomics* 13, 38. doi:10.1186/1471-2164-13-38

Tsang, M. S., Jiao, D., Chan, B. C., Hon, K. L., Leung, P. C., Lau, C. B., et al. (2016). Anti-inflammatory Activities of Pentaherbs Formula, Berberine, Gallic Acid and Chlorogenic Acid in Atopic Dermatitis-like Skin Inflammation. *Molecules* 21, 519. doi:10.3390/molecules21040519

Tsugawa, H., Cajka, T., Kind, T., Ma, Y., Higgins, B., Ikeda, K., et al. (2015). MS-DIAL: Data-independent MS/MS Deconvolution for Comprehensive Metabolome Analysis. *Nat. Methods* 12, 523–526. doi:10.1038/nmeth.3393

Watanabe, S., Narisawa, Y., Arase, S., Okamatsu, H., Ikenaga, T., Tajiri, Y., et al. (2003). Differences in Fecal Microflora between Patients with Atopic Dermatitis and Healthy Control Subjects. *J. Allergy Clin. Immunol.* 111, 587–591. doi:10.1067/mai.2003.105

Yoon, S. H., Ha, S. M., Kwon, S., Lim, J., Kim, Y., Seo, H., et al. (2017). Introducing EzBioCloud: a Taxonomically United Database of 16S rRNA Gene Sequences and Whole-Genome Assemblies. *Int. J. Syst. Evol. Microbiol.* 67, 1613–1617. doi:10.1099/ijsem.0.001755

11

Sulforaphane Ameliorates the Severity of Psoriasis and SLE by Modulating Effector Cells and Reducing Oxidative Stress

Pei Du[1,2,3,4]*, Wenqian Zhang*[1,2,3,4]*, Haobo Cui*[5]*, Wei He*[5]*, Shuang Lu*[1,2,3,4]*, Sujie Jia*[2,5]* and Ming Zhao*[1,2,3,4]*

[1]Department of Dermatology, Second Xiangya Hospital, Central South University, Changsha, China, [2]Hunan Key Laboratory of Medical Epigenomics, Second Xiangya Hospital, Central South University, Changsha, China, [3]Research Unit of Key Technologies of Diagnosis and Treatment for Immune-related Skin Diseases, Chinese Academy of Medical Sciences, Changsha, China, [4]Clinical Medical Research Center of Major Skin Diseases and Skin Health of Hunan Province, Changsha, China, [5]Department of Pharmacy, The Third Xiangya Hospital, Central South University, Changsha, China

Correspondence:
Ming Zhao
zhaoming307@csu.edu.cn
Sujie Jia
sujiejia@csu.edu.cn

Background: Sulforaphane, which is found in cruciferous vegetables, has been reported to have anti-inflammatory, antioxidant, and antitumour activities. However, whether sulforaphane has therapeutic effects on inflammatory or autoimmune skin diseases, including psoriasis and systemic lupus erythematosus (SLE), is unclear.

Methods: The therapeutic effects of sulforaphane were analyzed in Imiquimod (IMQ)-induced psoriasis-like mice and lupus-prone MRL/lpr mice. In IMQ-induced psoriasis-like mice treated with sulforaphane (55.3 and 110.6 μmol/kg) or vehicle control, the pathological phenotypes were assessed by the psoriasis area and severity index (PASI) score, haematoxylin-eosin staining (H&E) and quantifying of acanthosis and dermal inflammatory cell infiltration. The proportions of T cell subsets in draining lymph nodes (dLNs) and spleens were examined by flow cytometry. In MRL/lpr mice treated with sulforaphane (82.9 μmol/kg) or vehicle control, mortality and proteinuria were observed, and the glomerular pathology was examined by H&E staining. C3 and IgG depositions in kidney sections were examined by immunofluorescence staining. The proportions of plasma cells, follicular helper T (Tfh) cells, neutrophils and dendritic cells in the dLNs and spleens were examined by flow cytometry. Finally, we examined the Malondialdehyde (MDA) concentration by thiobarbituric acid reactive substance assay and the expression of *Prdx1*, *Nqo1*, *Hmox1*, and *Gss* by reverse transcription-quantitative polymerase chain reaction (RT-qPCR).

Results: Sulforaphane ameliorated the skin lesions in IMQ-induced psoriasis-like mice and the renal damage in lupus-prone MRL/lpr mice. In IMQ-induced psoriasis-like mice, sulforaphane reduced the proportions of Th1 and Th17 cells and increased the expression of antioxidant gene *Prdx1*. In lupus-prone MRL/lpr mice, sulforaphane increased the lifespan and the expression of *Prdx1*, and decreased the proportions of plasma cells, Tfh cells, neutrophils, and dendritic cells in the dLNs and spleens and the concentration of MDA.

Conclusion: Sulforaphane has significant therapeutic effects on IMQ-induced psoriasis-like mice and lupus-like MRL/Lpr mice by reducing inflammatory and autoimmune-related cells and oxidative stress. These findings provide new evidence for developing natural products to treat inflammatory and autoimmune diseases.

Keywords: antioxidant effect, sulforaphane, natural compounds, psoriasis, SLE

INTRODUCTION

Recently, a growing number of studies have shown that natural compounds extracted from plants have satisfying effects for the treatment of human diseases. For example, artemisinin, which is extracted from *Artemisia annua L.*, is the most widely used natural compound against malaria and plays a vital role in the treatment of malaria worldwide (Ma et al., 2020). Cruciferous vegetables have been considered sanatory, and can reduce the risk of chronic diseases (Raiola et al., 2017). The bioactive compounds that have been reported are ascorbic acid, phenolics, carotenoids, and glucosinolates (Peluso and Palmery, 2014). Sulforaphane, also known as isothiocyanate 1-isothiocyanato-(4R)-(methylsulfinyl) butane (**Figure 1A**), is a kind of isothiocyanate that is a hydrolysate of glucosinolates produced by the enzyme myrosinase in cruciferous vegetables (Raiola et al., 2017). Sulforaphane has been reported to exhibit the anti-inflammatory, antioxidant, and antitumour activities. Sulforaphane exerted an anti-inflammatory effect by regulating MAPK signaling in lipopolysaccharide (LPS)-induced microglia (Subedi et al., 2019). Furthermore, sulforaphane exerts therapeutic effects on diabetic nephropathy by upregulating nuclear factor-like 2 (Nrf2) antioxidant signaling (Li et al., 2020). In addition, the antitumour effects of sulforaphane in clinical therapy range from the attenuation of DNA damage to regulation of the cell cycle by activating the transcription factor Nrf2 (Russo et al., 2018). However, whether sulforaphane has therapeutic effects on inflammatory or autoimmune skin diseases, including psoriasis and systemic lupus erythematosus (SLE), is unclear.

Psoriasis is a chronic inflammatory immune-related skin disease characterized by erythema, scales, epidermal hyperplasia, and infiltration of inflammatory cells (Beek and van Reede, 1977). The release of proinflammatory mediators and cytokines has been identified in the skin and systemically (Nickoloff et al., 2007). Dysfunction of T lymphocytes, especially Th1 and Th17 subtypes, causes the overexpression of interferon-γ, interleukins, and tumor necrosis factor (Wu et al., 2018). Notably, oxidative stress is involved in the pathogenesis of psoriasis. A number of oxidative stress-related markers are increased in the plasma or serum of psoriatic patients, such as ischaemia-modified albumin (Kirmit et al., 2020), catalase (Kirmit et al., 2020), malondialdehyde (Kadam et al., 2010), and nitric oxide (Gabr and Al-Ghadir, 2012). Furthermore, the elevated levels of reactive oxygen species (ROS) are caused by active oxidative stress and initially trigger the abnormal activation of Th1 and Th17 cells (Lai et al., 2018). Moreover, ROS act as secondary messengers that induce activation of the MAPK, NF-κB, and JAK-STAT signaling pathways, amplifying the inflammatory response (Lin and Huang, 2016). Therefore, targeting oxidative stress may be a therapeutic strategy for psoriasis. IMQ-induced psoriasis-like skin inflammation is characterized by acanthosis, parakeratosis, and infiltration of inflammatory cells, which resemble human psoriasis. The mouse model uses the daily topical application of imiquimod (IMQ), a TLR7/8 ligand, to induce the inflammation of skin (Singh et al., 2019). The model is used to investigate the molecular and cellular pathogenesis of psoriasis in preclinical studies, as well as in the evaluation of potential therapies.

SLE is a systemic autoimmune disease that affects multiple organs, including the skin, kidney, and joints. The pathogenesis of SLE has not yet been clarified. The loss of immunologic tolerance causes the aberrant activation of autoreactive T cells and B cells, inducing massive autoantibodies production. Eventually, complement activation and the deposition of immune complexes lead to organ damage. In SLE, neutrophil extracellular traps released by neutrophils enhance the activation of inflammasomes and accumulate due to impaired degradation, causing increased anti-dsDNA production (Yu and Su, 2013). Dysfunction of dendritic cells is associated with the development of SLE. Inappropriate antigen presentation by dendritic cells promotes the loss of immunologic tolerance, accelerating the progression of SLE (Tsokos et al., 2016). Oxidative stress is closely related to the progression of SLE. Excessive production and impaired clearance of ROS induce dysfunction in T cells (Perl, 2013). In addition, oxidative modification of self-antigens triggers autoimmunity, leading to the acceleration of SLE (Perl, 2013). Studies have demonstrated that blocking the antioxidant signaling pathway reduces lifespan and increases autoantibodies, aggravating renal damage (Yoh et al., 2001). The elevated oxidative stress correlates with disease activity and organ damage. Thus, antioxidant therapy might provide an important strategy to ameliorate SLE. MRL/MpJ-$Fas^{lpr/lpr}$ (MRL/lpr) mice are the defect of *Fas* gene on MRL/MpJ background, which fail to eliminate autoreactive lymphocytes, inducing spontaneous autoimmune phenotypes. The clinical manifestations of MRL/lpr mice resemble human SLE, including skin lesion, glomerulonephritis, arthritis, circulating anti-nuclear antibodies (ANA), and depositions of immune complexes and complements (Watanabe-Fukunaga et al., 1992). MRL/lpr mice are used to study molecular and cellular pathogenesis of SLE in preclinical studies and evaluation of potential therapies.

To clarify the effects of sulforaphane on psoriasis, we studied the differences in skin inflammation and changes in Th subtypes

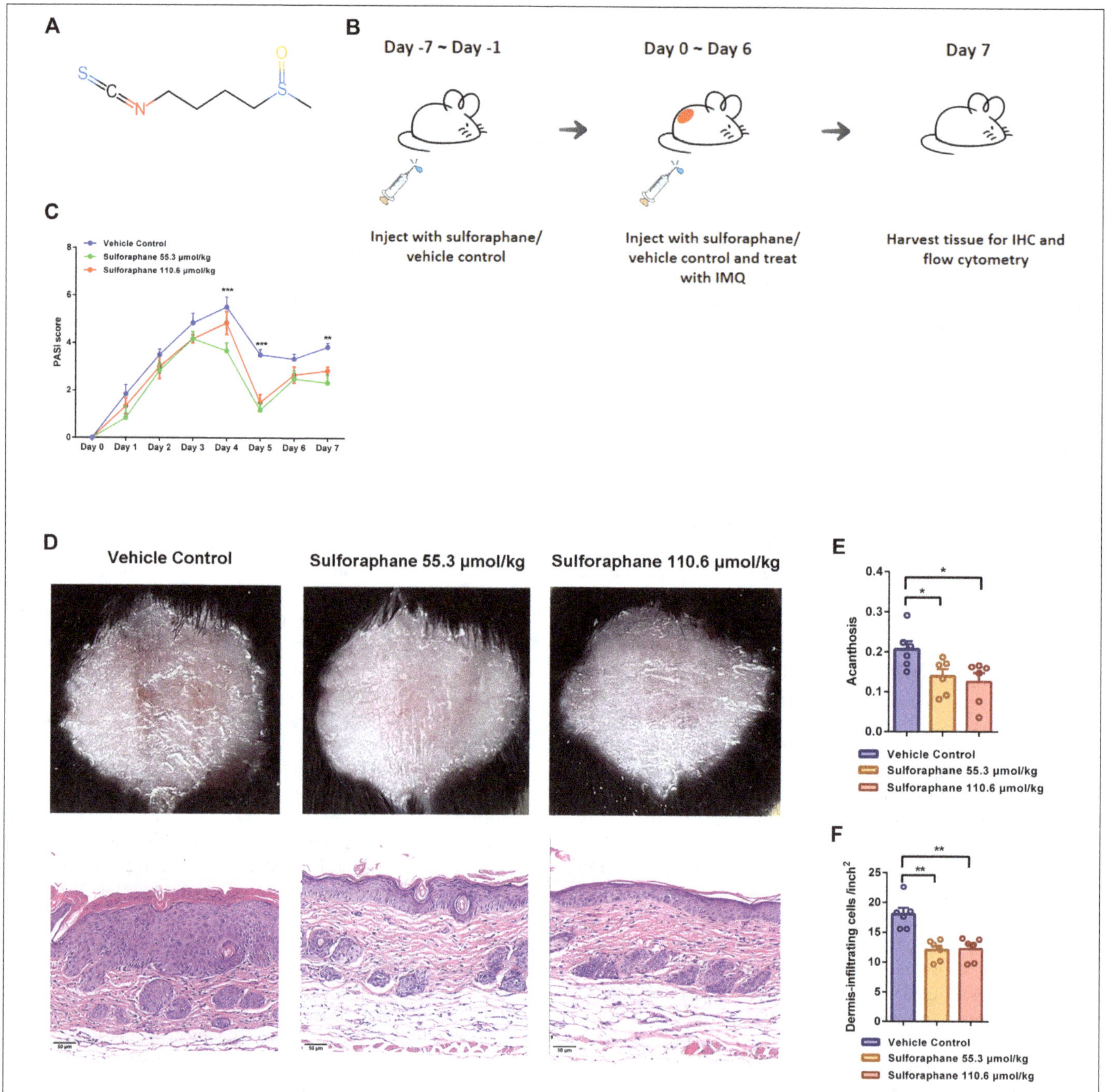

FIGURE 1 | Effects of sulforaphane on IMQ-induced psoriasis-like mouse model. **(A)** The structure of sulforaphane. **(B)** Schematic diagram of sulforaphane administration (55.3 and 110.6 μmol/kg, i.p.) or vehicle control for 7 consecutive days before IMQ treatment, followed by daily treatment with 78 mg of IMQ cream (5%) on the shaved back and injection with sulforaphane or vehicle control for 7 consecutive days. **(C)** PASI scores of mice in each group (n = 6). Compared with vehicle control, PASI scores were significantly decreased in mice treated with sulforaphane (55.3 μmol/kg) on Day 4, 5, and 7 and in mice treated with sulforaphane (110.6 μmol/kg) on Day 5. **(D)** Appearance and H&E staining of lesional skin from mice that were administrated with sulforaphane or vehicle control. Scale bars: 50 μm. **(E, F)** Quantitation of acanthosis and dermal inflammatory cell infiltration was performed in each group. The data represent the mean ± SEM. *$p < 0.05$, **$p < 0.01$, ***$p < 0.001$.

in IMQ-induced psoriasis-like mice treated with sulforaphane or vehicle control Our findings suggested that sulforaphane reduced the percentages of Th1 and Th17 cells to inhibit skin inflammation. Moreover, we investigated the potential therapeutic effect of sulforaphane on SLE. Sulforaphane increased the lifespan and reduced the renal damage in lupus-like mice and decreased the percentages of plasma cells, Tfh cells, neutrophils, and dendritic cells. These results indicated that sulforaphane is a natural compound with therapeutic effects on skin inflammation and autoimmune diseases.

MATERIALS AND METHODS

Mice

Female C57BL/6 mice aged 6–8 weeks were purchased from Slack and were used for the IMQ-induced psoriasis-like model. Female MRL/lpr mice aged 8 weeks were purchased from Sibeifu Experimental Animal Co. Ltd. All mice were housed under specific pathogen-free conditions at a controlled temperature of 20–25°C and 35–75% humidity with a 12-h light/dark cycle and were provided sterile food and water ad libitum. Animal experiments were performed according to the Institutional Animal Care Guidelines and were approved by the Animal Care Committee of Second Xiangya Hospital of Central South University.

Sulforaphane Administration to IMQ-Induced Psoriasis-Like Mice and MRL/Lpr Mice

Sulforaphane is a single compound purchased from APExBIO (Cat. C4733). Female C57BL/6 mice (6–8 weeks of age) were divided into 3 groups. Before being treated with IMQ, all mice were injected daily with sulforaphane (55.3 and 110.6 µmol/kg, intraperitoneal injection) or vehicle control (i.p.) for 1 week. Then, all mice were administered 78 mg of IMQ cream (5%) (Sichuan Med-shine Pharmaceutical) daily on their shaved backs and continually injected with sulforaphane (55.3 and 110.6 µmol/kg, i.p.) or vehicle control (i.p.) daily for 7 consecutive days. The skin, dLNs, and spleens of IMQ-induced psoriasis-like mice were obtained for further detection. After 6 weeks, female MRL/lpr mice (14 weeks of age) were divided into 2 groups. All mice were injected with sulforaphane (82.9 µmol/kg i.p.) or vehicle control (i.p.) daily for 27 consecutive days. The proteinuria was detected once a week to evaluate injury of kidney. The kidneys, dLNs, and spleens of MRL/lpr mice were obtained for further detection. Cell suspensions of spleens and dLNs were obtained by passing the tissues through a 70 µm strainer for flow cytometry analysis.

Evaluation of the Severity of Skin Inflammation in a Psoriasis-Like Mouse Model

The severity of skin inflammation in each mouse was scored once per day according to the criteria. The severity of skin inflammation was assessed according to 3 symptoms: erythema, scaling, and thickening. The score of each symptom ranged from 0 to 4 as follows: 0, none; 1, slight; 2, moderate; 3, marked; and 4, very marked. The total score was the sum of the 3 index scores (score 0–12).

Histological Analysis

Mouse skin and kidney tissues were fixed in 4% paraformaldehyde for 24 h at room temperature and embedded in paraffin. Sections (6 µm) were stained with haematoxylin and eosin (H&E). Acanthosis and the number of dermis-infiltrating cells were assessed as histological features of skin inflammation. The histological analysis of skin was performed as reported (Wu et al., 2018). The relative area of the epidermis was calculated for each mouse. The number of dermis-infiltrating cells in each section was calculated from three random fields of view at ×20 magnification.

Flow Cytometry

The following monoclonal antibodies were used for flow cytometric analysis of immune cells: anti-mouse CD4 (BD Pharmingen, Cat. 553088), anti-mouse IFN-γ (BD Pharmingen, Cat. 560660), anti-mouse IL-4 (BD Pharmingen, Cat. 560699), IL-17a (BD Pharmingen, Cat. 561020), CD8 (Biolegend, Cat. 100744), B220 (BD Pharmingen, Cat. 563894), CD11c (BD Pharmingen, Cat. 746392), CXCR5 (Biolegend, Cat. 560617), CD138 (BD Pharmingen, Cat. 568626), IgD (BD Pharmingen, Cat. 553510), CD19 (Biolegend, Cat. 115530), CD45 (BD Pharmingen, Cat. 560510), CD11b (BD Pharmingen, Cat. 564454), and Gr-1 (Biolegend, Cat. 108410). For cytokine analysis, cells were stimulated in RPMI 1640 medium (Gibco) supplemented with 10% fetal bovine serum (FBS, HyClone), PMA, ionomycin, and GolgiPlug (BD Biosciences, Cat. 550583) at 37°C and 5% CO_2 for 6 h. For intracellular staining, cells were fixed and permeabilized with a Human Foxp3 Buffer Set (BD Biosciences, Cat. 562574) or Cytofix/Cytoperm (BD Biosciences, 554722) according to the manufacturer's instructions.

RNA Isolation, Reverse Transcription and Real-Time PCR

Total RNA was extracted from cells or tissues with TRIzol reagent (Invitrogen) and reverse transcribed with the PrimeScript RT reagent kit with gDNA Eraser (TaKaRa Biotech Co.) according to the manufacturer's instructions. qPCR was performed with SYBR Premix Ex Taq II (Tli RNaseH Plus) (TaKaRa Biotech Co.) in a LightCycler 96 (Roche) thermocycler. Relative mRNA expression was calculated using the $2^{-\Delta Ct}$ ($\Delta Ct = Ct_{target\ gene} - Ct_{housekeeping\ gene}$) method in the experimental group compared with the control group. The primer sequences are shown in **Supplementary Table 1.**

Immunofluorescence Staining

Frozen sections of mouse kidneys were stained with a rat anti-C3 antibodies (11H9, Abcam) and Cy3-conjugated goat anti-rat IgG (GB21302, Servicebio) overnight at 4°C. The same procedure was performed for mouse IgG and direct immunofluorescence analysis with Alexa Fluor 488-conjugated goat anti-mouse IgG (150113, Abcam) overnight at 4°C.

Assay of Malondialdehyde Concentration

The MDA concentrations in skin of IMQ-induced psoriasis-like mice and spleens and dLNs of MRL/lpr mice were detected with the Micro Malondialdehyde Assay Kit (Beijing Solarbio Science and Technology Co.) following the manufacturer's instructions.

Statistics

The data was shown as the mean ± standard error of the mean (SEM). Statistical analysis was performed with GraphPad Prism. A two-tailed t test was used for statistical analysis. When the data were normally distributed, ANOVA and Dunnett's multiple comparisons test were used for grouped data analysis. When the data were not normally distributed or displayed unequal variances between two groups, we used the two-tailed Mann-Whitney U test for statistical analysis. When the data were normally distributed or displayed unequal variances between two groups, we used the unpaired Student's t test. The log-rank (Mantel-Cox) test was used for survival analysis. $p < 0.05$ was considered statistically significant. Sample sizes for all data shown can be found in the figure legends.

RESULTS

Sulforaphane Ameliorates the Skin Lesions in IMQ-Induced Psoriasis-Like Mice

We investigated whether sulforaphane exerted the anti-inflammatory effect on IMQ-induced psoriasis-like mice. Previous study has shown that the pathological phenotypes in 2,4-dinitrochlorobenzene-induced atopic dermatitis-like mice were significantly improved when sulforaphane was used three times a week for 3 weeks with a concentration gradient of 13.8, 27.6, and 55.3 μmol/kg (Wu et al., 2019). As a short course of IMQ-induced psoriasis-like mice model, skin lesions healed themselves after 7 days of induction, we chose two relatively high doses (55.3 and 110.6 μmol/kg) of sulforaphane to treat IMQ-induced mice in this study. Sulforaphane or vehicle control was injected daily (i.p.) in C57BL/6 mice for 7 consecutive days before IMQ stimulation. Then, all mice were treated with 78 mg of IMQ cream (5%) on their shaved backs and injected with sulforaphane or vehicle control (i.p.) daily for 7 consecutive days. The experimental design is shown in **Figure 1B**. As expected, the PASI scores, which indicate the severity of skin lesions in mice, were reduced in the sulforaphane treatment group compared with the vehicle control group (**Figure 1C**). Gross appearance and H&E staining indicated that skin lesions were significantly alleviated in mice treated with sulforaphane (**Figure 1D**). In addition, acanthosis and dermal inflammatory cell infiltration were significantly decreased after sulforaphane treatment (**Figures 1E,F**).

Sulforaphane Reduced the Percentages of Th1 Cells and Th17 Cells in IMQ-Induced Psoriasis-Like Mice

Increasing evidence has demonstrated that inflammatory T cells such as Th1 and Th17 cells in skin lesions play important roles in the pathogenesis of psoriasis (Kagami et al., 2010; Jiang et al., 2020, Diani et al., 2015). Therefore, we sought to evaluate whether the amelioration of skin inflammation was attributed to the decreased differentiation of inflammatory T cells after sulforaphane administration. We examined the percentages of Th1, Th2, and Th17 cells in dLNs and spleens from IMQ-induced psoriasis-like mice. The gating strategy is shown in **Supplementary Figure S1**. Notably, we found that the percentage of Th1 cells in the spleens was significantly reduced in the sulforaphane-treated (110.6 μmol/kg) group (**Figures 2A,B**). The percentage of Th17 cells in the dLN was significantly reduced in the sulforaphane-treated (110.6 μmol/kg) group (**Figures 2C,D**). The percentage of Th17 cells in the spleens was decreased in the sulforaphane-treated groups, but the difference was not significant (**Figures 2C,D**).

Sulforaphane Alleviates Renal Damage in Lupus-Prone MRL/Lpr Mice

Because of the anti-inflammatory effect of sulforaphane on IMQ-induced psoriasis-like mice, we hypothesized that sulforaphane was involved in regulating the autoimmune lymphocytes to alleviate kidney injury in lupus-prone MRL/lpr mice. Since both concentrations (55.3 and 110.6 μmol/kg) significantly improved skin lesions of IMQ-induced psoriasis-like mice, with no side effects, we chose a medium dose of sulforaphane (82.9 μmol/kg i.p.) to treat MRL/lpr mice for 27 consecutive days. The administration of sulforaphane significantly reduced the mortality of MRL/lpr mice (**Figure 3B**). Proteinuria was decreased in the sulforaphane-treated group compared with the vehicle control group (**Figure 3C**). In addition, sulforaphane-treated MRL/lpr mice had reduced glomerular enlargement as shown by H&E staining (**Figure 3D**). Immunofluorescent staining indicated that the deposition of C3 and IgG was dramatically decreased in the sulforaphane-treated group (**Figure 3E**). These results indicate that sulforaphane alleviates the autoimmune responses in the kidneys of lupus-prone MRL/lpr mice.

Sulforaphane Reduces the Proportions of Plasma Cells, Tfh Cells, Neutrophils, and Dendritic Cells in MRL/Lpr Mice

Accumulating evidence has demonstrated that the aberrant responses of the innate and adaptive immune systems are involved in the pathogenesis of lupus. Next, we sought to explore whether sulforaphane influenced the activation and differentiation of B cells, Tfh cells, and innate immune cells in the spleens and dLNs of a lupus-like mouse model. The gating strategy is shown in **Supplementary Figures S2, S3**. We found that the percentages of plasma cells in the dLNs and spleens were significantly reduced in the sulforaphane-treated group (**Figures 4A,E**). And the proportions of Tfh cells, neutrophils, and dendritic cells were significantly decreased in the dLNs of sulforaphane-treated mice compared with vehicle control mice (**Figures 4B–D,F–H**). These results indicate that sulforaphane alleviates autoimmune response by inhibiting the activation or differentiation of plasma cells, Tfh cells, neutrophils, and dendritic cells in MRL/lpr mice.

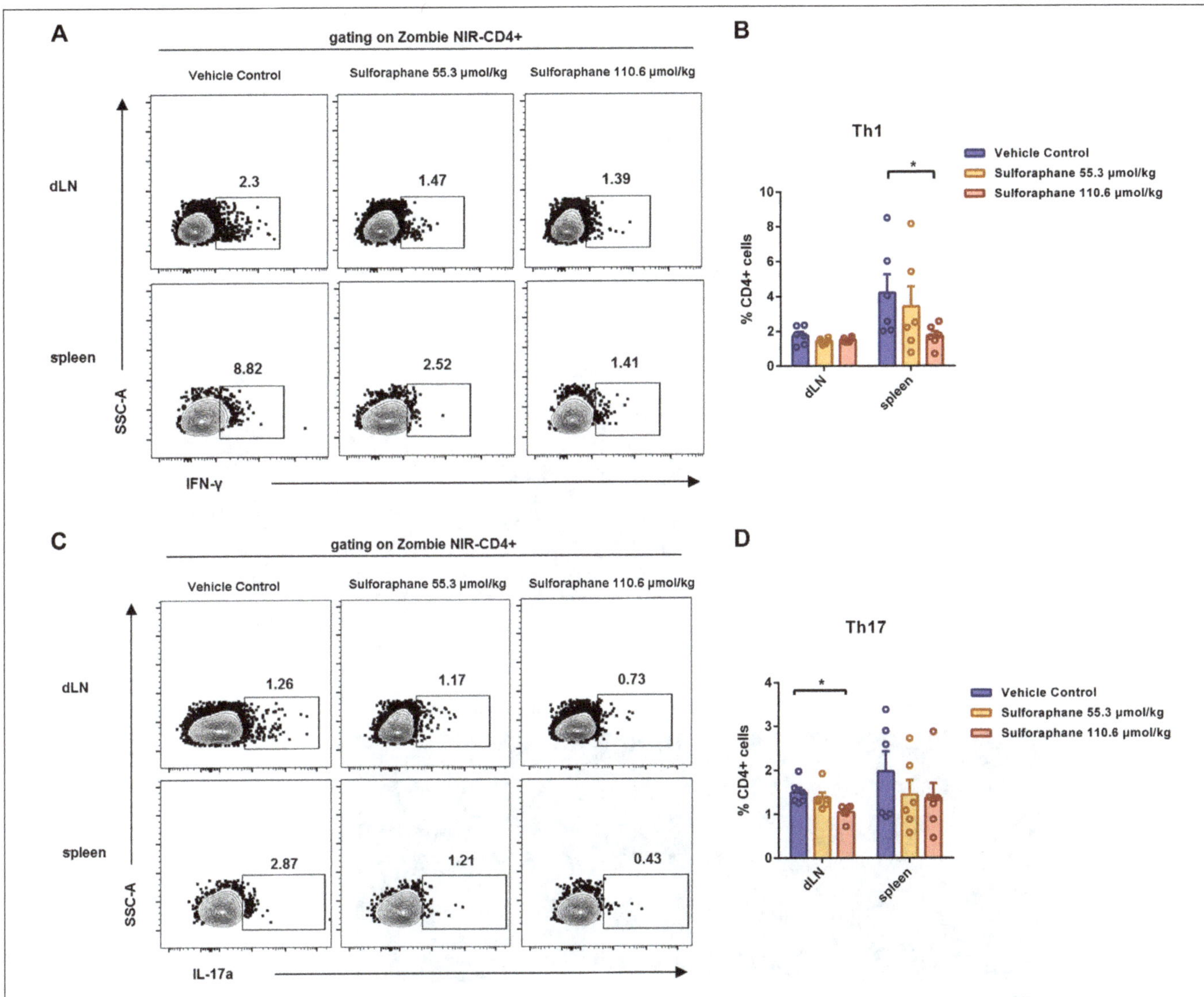

FIGURE 2 | Sulforaphane reduced the proportions of Th1 cells and Th17 cells in IMQ-induced psoriasis-like mice. **(A)** Representative flow cytometric analysis of Th1 cells in the dLNs and spleens from IMQ-induced psoriasis-like mice treated with sulforaphane or vehicle control (n = 6). **(B)** Statistical analysis of **(A)**. **(C)** Representative flow cytometric analysis of Th17 cells in the dLNs and spleens from IMQ-induced psoriasis-like mice treated with sulforaphane or vehicle control. **(D)** Statistical analysis of **(C)**. The data represent the mean ± SEM. $^{*}p < 0.05$.

Sulforaphane Upregulates the Expression of Antioxidant Gene *Prdx1* to Reduce Oxidative Stress

We next investigated the MDA concentrations in skin of IMQ-induced psoriasis-like mice and spleens and dLNs of MRL/lpr mice to indicate the level of oxidative stress between the sulforaphane-treated group and vehicle control-treated group. The treatment of sulforaphane reduced the concentrations of MDA in the skin of IMQ-induced psoriasis-like mice and spleens and dLNs of MRL/lpr mice (**Figures 5A–C**). Then, we explored whether the expression of sulforaphane-induced genes was involved in mediating inflammation and autoimmunity. We examined the expression of *Prdx1*, *Nqo1*, *Hmox1*, and *Gss*. The RT-qPCR results showed that *Prdx1* expression was upregulated in the skin lesions of IMQ-induced psoriasis-like mice and in the spleens and dLNs of MRL/lpr mice with sulforaphane administration (**Figures 5D,E**). These results suggest that sulforaphane may protect against inflammation and autoimmunity in mice *via* upregulating antioxidant gene *Prdx1* expression to reduce the level of oxidative stress.

DISCUSSION

We found that the administration of sulforaphane ameliorated the IMQ-induced psoriasis-like skin inflammation and renal

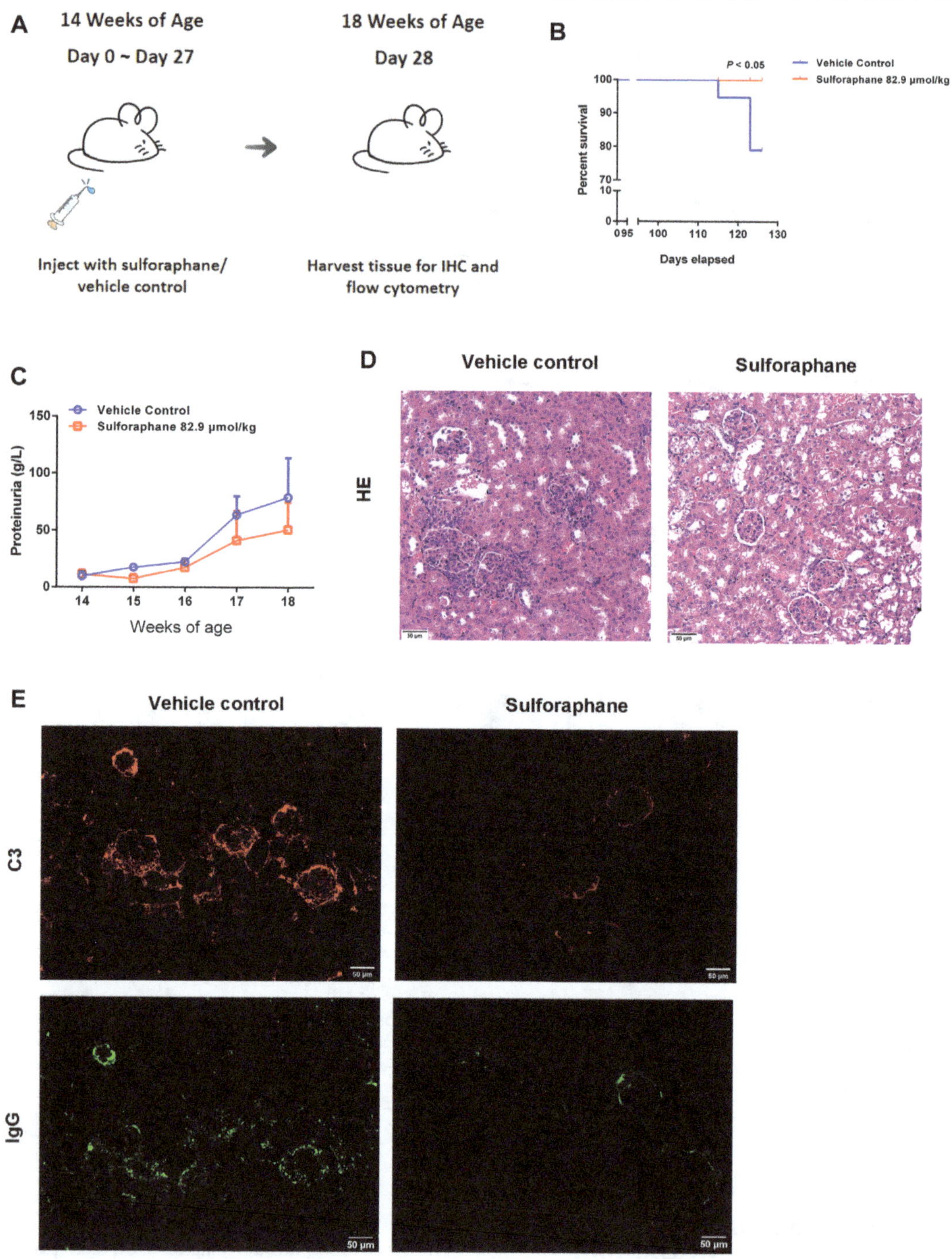

FIGURE 3 | Sulforaphane alleviates renal damage in lupus-prone MRL/lpr mice. **(A)** Schematic diagram of the administration of sulforaphane (82.9 μmol/kg) or vehicle control for 27 consecutive days in MRL/lpr mice at the age of 14 weeks (n = 5–6). **(B)** The lifespan of MRL/lpr mice treated with sulforaphane or vehicle control. **(C)** The changes of urine protein levels in MRL/lpr mice treated with sulforaphane or vehicle control. **(D)** Renal pathology was examined by immunohistochemistry of haematoxylin-eosin staining (H&E) in MRL/lpr mice treated with sulforaphane or vehicle control. Scale bars: 50 μm. **(E)** C3 and IgG deposition in kidney sections was examined by immunofluorescence staining in MRL/lpr mice treated with sulforaphane or vehicle control. Scale bars: 50 μm.

damage in lupus-prone MRL/lpr mice. In IMQ-induced psoriasis-like mice, sulforaphane reduced the proportions of Th1 and Th17 cells and induced the expression of the antioxidant gene *Prdx1*. Furthermore, our results demonstrated that sulforaphane increased the lifespan and reduced renal damage in lupus-prone MRL/lpr mice,

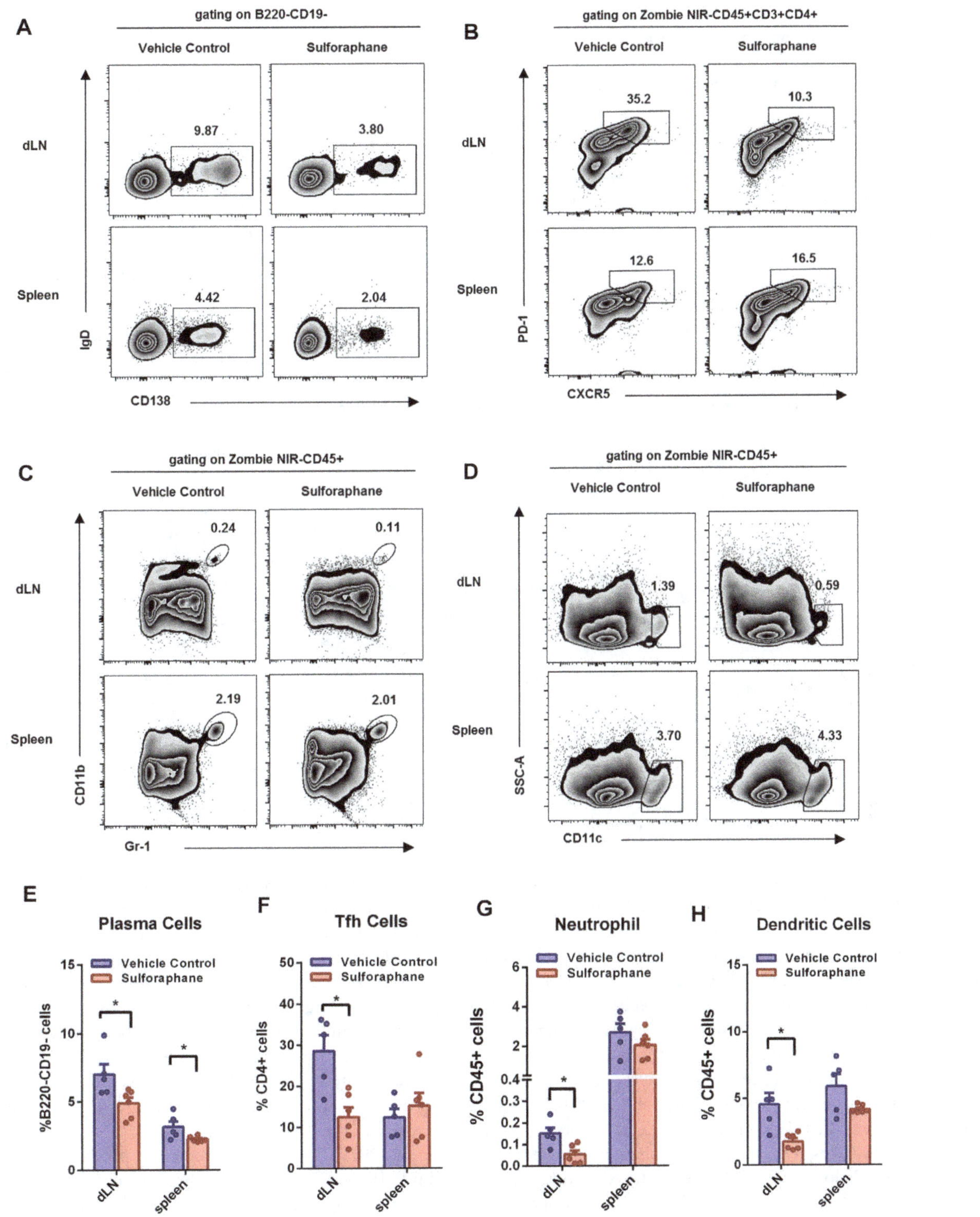

FIGURE 4 | Sulforaphane reduced the percentages of plasma cells, Tfh cells, neutrophils, and dendritic cells in lupus-prone MRL/lpr mice (n = 6). **(A–D)** Representative flow cytometric analysis of plasma cells **(A)**, Tfh cells **(B)**, neutrophils **(C)** and dendritic cells **(D)** in the dLNs and spleens from MRL/lpr mice treated with sulforaphane or vehicle control. **(E–H)** Statistical analysis of **(A–D)**. The data represent the mean ± SEM. $^*p < 0.05$.

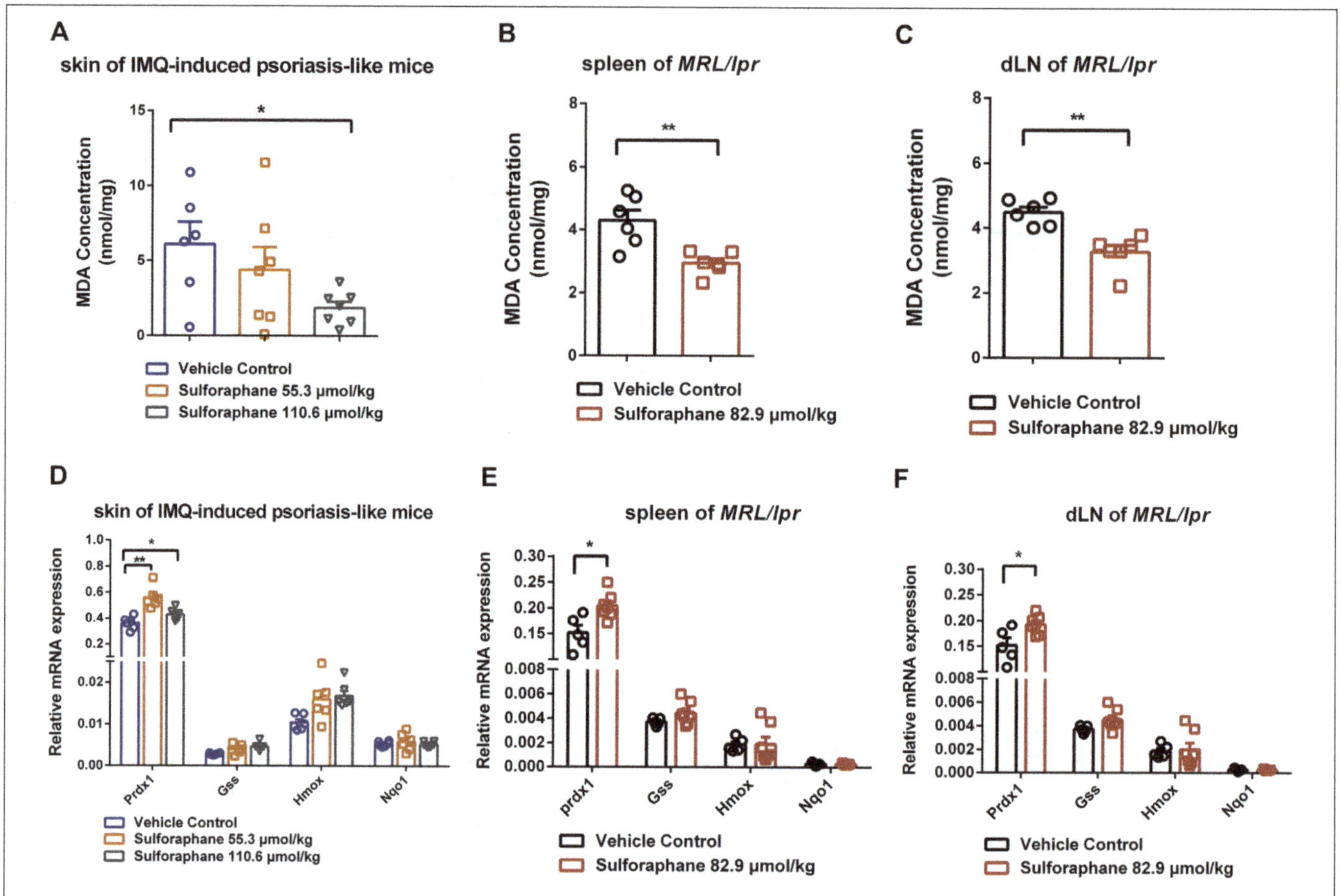

FIGURE 5 | Sulforaphane upregulated the antioxidant gene *Prdx1* expression to reduce the level of oxidative stress. **(A)** The concentrations of MDA in skin of IMQ-induced psoriasis-like mice treated with sulforaphane or vehicle control (n = 5–6). **(B, C)** The concentrations of MDA in the spleens **(B)** and dLNs **(C)** of MRL/lpr mice treated with sulforaphane or vehicle control (n = 5–6). **(D)** The relative mRNA expression of *Prdx1*, *Gss*, *Hmox1*, and *Nqo1* in skin of IMQ-induced psoriasis-like mice treated with sulforaphane or vehicle control (n = 5–6). **(E, F)** The relative mRNA expression of *Prdx1*, *Gss*, *Hmox1*, and *Nqo1* in the spleens **(E)** and dLNs **(F)** of MRL/lpr mice treated with sulforaphane or vehicle control (n = 5–6). The data represent the mean ± SEM. $^{*}p < 0.05$, $^{**}p < 0.01$.

decreased the proportions of plasma cells, Tfh cells, neutrophils, dendritic cells, and the concentration of MDA and induced the expression of antioxidant gene *Prdx1*.

Sulforaphane, which is found in cruciferous vegetables, is an activator of nuclear factor E2-related factor 2 (Nrf2). The antioxidant Nrf2 can suppress lupus nephritis by reducing oxidative stress and the NF-κB signaling pathway (Jiang et al., 2014). Peroxiredoxin 1 (Prdx1) is a member of the peroxiredoxin family that acts as an antioxidant enzyme to catalyze the reduction of hydrogen peroxide (Park et al., 2016). Studies have shown that Prdx1 decreased ROS to protect against oxidative stress (Ding et al., 2017). Quinone oxidoreductase (NQO1), which belongs to the Phase II detoxification enzyme family, catalyzes the two-electron reduction of quinone to the redox-stable hydroquinone (Luo et al., 2019). Nqo1, which exerts antioxidant activity to protect against oxidative stress, is induced by sulforaphane and reduces the neuro-cytotoxicity of DA quinone (Han et al., 2007). Haem oxygenase-1 (Hmox1) and glutathione synthetase (Gss) are also antioxidant enzymes, downstream of the Nrf2 signaling pathway (Lu, 2009; Zhao et al., 2019). We found that Prdx1 expression was upregulated in IMQ-induced psoriasis-like mice and MRL/lpr mice after treatment with sulforaphane, suggesting that sulforaphane exerted the antioxidant effects dependent on the activation of Prdx1.

Psoriasis is a chronic hyperplastic skin disease induced by multiple genetic and environmental factors that affects approximately 0.1–3% of the global population (Boehncke, 2018; Rendon and Schakel, 2019). The abnormally differentiated Th1 and Th17 cells release proinflammatory cytokines, including IFN-γ, IL-17, IL-22, and TNF-α, to increase the cutaneous inflammatory response (Benhadou et al., 2019). Th1 cells increase the production of IL-2, TNF-α, and IFN-γ, participating in the development of psoriasis (Rodriguez-Cerdeira et al., 2019). The enhanced Th1 response increases inflammation by upregulating many cytokines, including IL-1, IL-6, IL-8, IL-12, IL-15, interferon-inducible protein-10, and iNOS, to promote keratinocyte proliferation (Grossman et al., 1989; Xie et al., 1993; Rich and Kupper, 2001; Behnam et al., 2005). IL-17 targets innate immune cells, keratinocytes, and endothelial cells, and is the major effector cytokine that drives the pathogenesis of psoriasis (Blauvelt and

Chiricozzi, 2018). In this study, our results demonstrated that sulforaphane reduced the percentages of Th1 and Th17 cells to ameliorate acanthosis and dermal inflammatory cell infiltration in IMQ-induced psoriasis-like skin inflammation. ROS-mediated oxidative stress is involved in numerous signaling pathways related to the inflammatory response, contributing to the progression of psoriasis (Briganti and Picardo, 2003). As an antioxidant therapy, dimethylfumarate (DMF) has been used for the treatment of psoriasis and has shown a high degree of efficacy (Rostami and Mrowietz, 2008). Sulforaphane, as an antioxidant, induces the expression of antioxidant gene *Prdx1*, contributing to the recovery of psoriasis.

SLE is a complicated multifactorial autoimmune disease. The molecular mechanisms remain voluminously unknown. An imbalance in the production and degradation of ROS causes the oxidative modification of DNA, inducing DNA damage (Shah et al., 2014). Dendritic cells recognize the self-antigens and present them to B cells, triggering the autoimmune response and excessive production of autoantibodies (Herrada et al., 2019). Tfh cells assist B cells in inducing autoimmune response, playing an important role in the pathogenesis of SLE (Blanco et al., 2016). The deposition of immune complexes recruits neutrophils, inducing local inflammation and damage (Kaplan, 2011). In our study, the administration of sulforaphane decreased the percentages of plasma cells, Tfh cells, neutrophils, and dendritic cells. Moreover, sulforaphane induced the expression of Prdx1 to protect against oxidative stress. N-acetyl cysteine has been reported to attenuate oxidative stress in SLE, suggesting that the antioxidant therapy might be a promising strategy for the treatment of SLE.

In this study, we found that sulforaphane reduced the proportions of Th1 and Th17 cells and the concentration of MDA. Similarly, sulforaphane decreased the proportions of plasma cells, Tfh cells, neutrophils, and dendritic cells. We also found that the expression of antioxidative gene *Prdx1* was upregulated in the sulforaphane-treated group. It was reported that CYP11A1-derived vitamin D3- and lumisterol-hydroxy derivatives protected primary human keratinocytes against radiation and UVB-induced damage, which is associated with Nrf2-regulated antioxidants responses (Chaiprasongsuk et al., 2019; Slominski et al., 2020). Previous study showed that the oxidative stress and molecular modifications induced by oxidative stress caused the massive activation of immune cells (Lightfoot et al., 2017). We speculated that the activation of NRF2 signaling and reduced oxidative stress contributed to inhibition of activation of immune cells. Moreover, there are other possible mechanisms that sulforaphane ameliorate skin lesion and renal damage. $20(OH)D_3$ and $20,23(OH)_2D_3$ play as antagonists of RORα and RORγ to inhibit the activity of *IL17* promoter (Slominski et al., 2014). In addition, we suppose that sulforaphane functions as a ligand of transcription factor to inhibit differentiation of immune cells. We conducted the macromolecular docking using the crystal structure of RORγT and sulforaphane. Interestingly, the docking score revealed that sulforaphane might bind to RORγT as a ligand (**Supplementary Figure S4** and **Supplementary Table 2**). We will further study the underlying molecular mechanisms of sulforaphane-induced antioxidation and repression of autoimmune activities in psoriasis and SLE. Moreover, because this condition involves a local inflammatory response, sulforaphane might have a higher degree of efficacy when administered locally in IMQ-induced psoriasis-like skin inflammation.

In conclusion, the results of this study showed that sulforaphane improve the skin lesion of IMQ-induced psoriasis-like mice and the renal damage in lupus-like mice by inhibiting inflammatory and autoimmune responses and oxidative stress. This evidence suggests the potential value of sulforaphane in treating psoriasis and SLE and highlights the use of antioxidant therapy in inflammatory and autoimmune diseases.

AUTHOR CONTRIBUTIONS

SJ and MZ designed the research and revised the manuscript. PD and WZ conducted the research. PD drafted the manuscript. WH and SL analyzed the data. HC performed statistical analysis. All authors read and approved the final version of manuscript.

SUPPLEMENTARY MATERIAL

Supplementary Figure S1 | The gating strategy of Th subtypes.

Supplementary Figure S2 | The gating strategy of plasma cells.

Supplementary Figure S3 | The gating strategy of Tfh cells, neutrophils, and dendritic cells.

Supplementary Figure S4 | The docking result of RORγT and sulforaphane.

REFERENCES

Beek, C. H., and van Reede, E. C. (1977). The Nature and Frequency of the Histological Changes Found in Psoriasis Vulgaris. *Arch. Dermatol. Res.* 257 (3), 255–264. doi:10.1007/BF00741841

Behnam, S. M., Behnam, S. E., and Koo, J. Y. (2005). Smoking and Psoriasis. *Skinmed* 4 (3), 174–176. doi:10.1111/j.1540-9740.2005.03716.x

Benhadou, F., Mintoff, D., and Del Marmol, V. (2019). Psoriasis: Keratinocytes or Immune Cells - Which Is the Trigger? *Dermatology* 235 (2), 91–100. doi:10.1159/000495291

Blanco, P., Ueno, H., and Schmitt, N. (2016). T Follicular Helper (Tfh) Cells in Lupus: Activation and Involvement in SLE Pathogenesis. *Eur. J. Immunol.* 46 (2), 281–290. doi:10.1002/eji.201545760

Blauvelt, A., and Chiricozzi, A. (2018). The Immunologic Role of IL-17 in Psoriasis and Psoriatic Arthritis Pathogenesis. *Clin. Rev. Allergy Immunol.* 55 (3), 379–390. doi:10.1007/s12016-018-8702-3

Boehncke, W. H. (2018). Systemic Inflammation and Cardiovascular Comorbidity in Psoriasis Patients: Causes and Consequences. *Front. Immunol.* 9, 579. doi:10.3389/fimmu.2018.00579

Briganti, S., and Picardo, M. (2003). Antioxidant Activity, Lipid Peroxidation and Skin Diseases. What's New. *J. Eur. Acad. Dermatol. Venereol.* 17 (6), 663–669. doi:10.1046/j.1468-3083.2003.00751.x

Chaiprasongsuk, A., Janjetovic, Z., Kim, T. K., Jarrett, S. G., D'Orazio, J. A., Holick, M. F., et al. (2019). Protective Effects of Novel Derivatives of Vitamin D3 and Lumisterol against UVB-Induced Damage in Human Keratinocytes Involve Activation of Nrf2 and P53 Defense Mechanisms. *Redox Biol.* 24, 101206. doi:10.1016/j.redox.2019.101206

Diani, M., Altomare, G., and Reali, E. (2015). T Cell Responses in Psoriasis and Psoriatic Arthritis. *Autoimmun. Rev.* 14 (4), 286–292. doi:10.1016/j.autrev.2014.11.012

Ding, C., Fan, X., and Wu, G. (2017). Peroxiredoxin 1 - an Antioxidant Enzyme in Cancer. *J. Cel Mol Med* 21 (1), 193–202. doi:10.1111/jcmm.12955

Gabr, S. A., and Al-Ghadir, A. H. (2012). Role of Cellular Oxidative Stress and Cytochrome C in the Pathogenesis of Psoriasis. *Arch. Dermatol. Res.* 304 (6), 451–457. doi:10.1007/s00403-012-1230-8

Grossman, R. M., Krueger, J., Yourish, D., Granelli-Piperno, A., Murphy, D. P., May, L. T., et al. (1989). Interleukin 6 Is Expressed in High Levels in Psoriatic Skin and Stimulates Proliferation of Cultured Human Keratinocytes. *Proc. Natl. Acad. Sci. U S A.* 86 (16), 6367–6371. doi:10.1073/pnas.86.16.6367

Han, J. M., Lee, Y. J., Lee, S. Y., Kim, E. M., Moon, Y., Kim, H. W., et al. (2007). Protective Effect of Sulforaphane against Dopaminergic Cell Death. *J. Pharmacol. Exp. Ther.* 321 (1), 249–256. doi:10.1124/jpet.106.110866

Herrada, A. A., Escobedo, N., Iruretagoyena, M., Valenzuela, R. A., Burgos, P. I., Cuitino, L., et al. (2019). Innate Immune Cells' Contribution to Systemic Lupus Erythematosus. *Front. Immunol.* 10, 772. doi:10.3389/fimmu.2019.00772

Jiang, T., Tian, F., Zheng, H., Whitman, S. A., Lin, Y., Zhang, Z., et al. (2014). Nrf2 Suppresses Lupus Nephritis through Inhibition of Oxidative Injury and the NF-Kb-Mediated Inflammatory Response. *Kidney Int.* 85 (2), 333–343. doi:10.1038/ki.2013.343

Jiang, Y., Wang, W., Zheng, X., and Jin, H. (2020). Immune Regulation of TNFAIP3 in Psoriasis through its Association with Th1 and Th17 Cell Differentiation and P38 Activation. *J. Immunol. Res.* 2020, 5980190. doi:10.1155/2020/5980190

Kadam, D. P., Suryakar, A. N., Ankush, R. D., Kadam, C. Y., and Deshpande, K. H. (2010). Role of Oxidative Stress in Various Stages of Psoriasis. *Indian J. Clin. Biochem.* 25 (4), 388–392. doi:10.1007/s12291-010-0043-9

Kagami, S., Rizzo, H. L., Lee, J. J., Koguchi, Y., and Blauvelt, A. (2010). Circulating Th17, Th22, and Th1 Cells Are Increased in Psoriasis. *J. Invest. Dermatol.* 1305, 1373–1383. doi:10.1038/jid.2009.399

Kaplan, M. J. (2011). Neutrophils in the Pathogenesis and Manifestations of SLE. *Nat. Rev. Rheumatol.* 7 (12), 691–699. doi:10.1038/nrrheum.2011.132

Kirmit, A., Kader, S., Aksoy, M., Bal, C., Nural, C., and Aslan, O. (2020). Trace Elements and Oxidative Stress Status in Patients with Psoriasis. *Postepy Dermatol. Alergol* 37 (3), 333–339. doi:10.5114/ada.2020.94265

Lai, R., Xian, D., Xiong, X., Yang, L., Song, J., and Zhong, J. (2018). Proanthocyanidins: Novel Treatment for Psoriasis that Reduces Oxidative Stress and Modulates Th17 and Treg Cells. *Redox Rep.* 23, 130–135. doi:10.1080/13510002.2018.1462027

Li, Z., Guo, H., Li, J., Ma, T., Zhou, S., Zhang, Z., et al. (2020). Sulforaphane Prevents Type 2 Diabetes-Induced Nephropathy via AMPK-Mediated Activation of Lipid Metabolic Pathways and Nrf2 Antioxidative Function. *Clin. Sci. (Lond)* 134, 2469–2487. doi:10.1042/CS20191088

Lightfoot, Y. L., Blanco, L. P., and Kaplan, M. J. (2017). Metabolic Abnormalities and Oxidative Stress in Lupus. *Curr. Opin. Rheumatol.* 29, 442–449. doi:10.1097/BOR.0000000000000413

Lin, X., and Huang, T. (2016). Oxidative Stress in Psoriasis and Potential Therapeutic Use of Antioxidants. *Free Radic. Res.* 50, 585–595. doi:10.3109/10715762.2016.1162301

Lu, S. C. (2009). Regulation of Glutathione Synthesis. *Mol. Aspects Med.* 30, 42–59. doi:10.1016/j.mam.2008.05.005

Luo, S., Kang, S. S., Wang, Z. H., Liu, X., Day, J. X., Wu, Z., et al. (2019). Akt Phosphorylates NQO1 and Triggers its Degradation, Abolishing its Antioxidative Activities in Parkinson's Disease. *J. Neurosci.* 39, 7291–7305. doi:10.1523/JNEUROSCI.0625-19.2019

Ma, N., Zhang, Z., Liao, F., Jiang, T., and Tu, Y. (2020). The Birth of Artemisinin. *Pharmacol. Ther.* 216, 107658. doi:10.1016/j.pharmthera.2020.107658

Nickoloff, B. J., Xin, H., Nestle, F. O., and Qin, J. Z. (2007). The Cytokine and Chemokine Network in Psoriasis. *Clin. Dermatol.* 25, 568–573. doi:10.1016/j.clindermatol.2007.08.011

Park, M. H., Jo, M., Kim, Y. R., Lee, C. K., and Hong, J. T. (2016). Roles of Peroxiredoxins in Cancer, Neurodegenerative Diseases and Inflammatory Diseases. *Pharmacol. Ther.* 163, 1–23. doi:10.1016/j.pharmthera.2016.03.018

Peluso, I., and Palmery, M. (2014). Is a Flavonoid-Rich Diet with Steamer Cooking Safe during Calcineurin Inhibitors Therapy? *J. Clin. Pharm. Ther.* 39, 471–474. doi:10.1111/jcpt.12186

Perl, A. (2013). Oxidative Stress in the Pathology and Treatment of Systemic Lupus Erythematosus. *Nat. Rev. Rheumatol.* 9, 674–686. doi:10.1038/nrrheum.2013.147

Raiola, A., Errico, A., Petruk, G., Monti, D. M., Barone, A., and Rigano, M. M. (2017). Bioactive Compounds in Brassicaceae Vegetables with a Role in the Prevention of Chronic Diseases. *Molecules* 23, 1. doi:10.3390/molecules23010015

Rendon, A., and Schäkel, K. (2019). Psoriasis Pathogenesis and Treatment. *Int. J. Mol. Sci.* 20, 6. doi:10.3390/ijms20061475

Rich, B. E., and Kupper, T. S. (2001). Cytokines: IL-20 - a New Effector in Skin Inflammation. *Curr. Biol.* 11, R531–R534. doi:10.1016/s0960-9822(01)00312-8

Rodríguez-Cerdeira, C., Cordeiro-Rodríguez, M., Carnero-Gregorio, M., López-Barcenas, A., Martínez-Herrera, E., Fabbrocini, G., et al. (2019). Biomarkers of Inflammation in Obesity-Psoriatic Patients. *Mediators Inflamm.* 2019, 7353420. doi:10.1155/2019/7353420

Rostami Yazdi, M., and Mrowietz, U. (2008). Fumaric Acid Esters. *Clin. Dermatol.* 26, 522–526. doi:10.1016/j.clindermatol.2008.07.001

Russo, M., Spagnuolo, C., Russo, G. L., Skalicka-Woźniak, K., Daglia, M., Sobarzo-Sánchez, E., et al. (2018). Nrf2 Targeting by Sulforaphane: A Potential Therapy for Cancer Treatment. *Crit. Rev. Food Sci. Nutr.* 58, 1391–1405. doi:10.1080/10408398.2016.1259983

Shah, D., Mahajan, N., Sah, S., Nath, S. K., and Paudyal, B. (2014). Oxidative Stress and its Biomarkers in Systemic Lupus Erythematosus. *J. Biomed. Sci.* 21, 23. doi:10.1186/1423-0127-21-23

Singh, T. P., Zhang, H. H., Hwang, S. T., and Farber, J. M. (2019). IL-23- and Imiquimod-Induced Models of Experimental Psoriasis in Mice. *Curr. Protoc. Immunol.* 125 (1), e71. doi:10.1002/cpim.71

Slominski, A. T., Chaiprasongsuk, A., Janjetovic, Z., Kim, T. K., Stefan, J., Slominski, R. M., et al. (2020). Photoprotective Properties of Vitamin D and Lumisterol Hydroxyderivatives. *Cell Biochem Biophys* 78 (2), 165–180. doi:10.1007/s12013-020-00913-6

Slominski, A. T., Kim, T. K., Takeda, Y., Janjetovic, Z., Brozyna, A. A., Skobowiat, C., et al. (2014). RORα and ROR γ Are Expressed in Human Skin and Serve as Receptors for Endogenously Produced Noncalcemic 20-hydroxy- and 20,23-dihydroxyvitamin D. *FASEB J.* 28 (7), 2775–2789. doi:10.1096/fj.13-242040

Subedi, L., Lee, J. H., Yumnam, S., Ji, E., and Kim, S. Y. (2019). Anti-Inflammatory Effect of Sulforaphane on LPS-Activated Microglia Potentially through JNK/AP-1/NF-κB Inhibition and Nrf2/HO-1 Activation. *Cells* 8, 2. doi:10.3390/cells8020194

Tsokos, G. C., Lo, M. S., Costa Reis, P., and Sullivan, K. E. (2016). New Insights into the Immunopathogenesis of Systemic Lupus Erythematosus. *Nat. Rev. Rheumatol.* 12, 716–730. doi:10.1038/nrrheum.2016.186

Watanabe-Fukunaga, R., Brannan, C. I., Copeland, N. G., Jenkins, N. A., and Nagata, S. (1992). Lymphoproliferation Disorder in Mice Explained by Defects in Fas Antigen that Mediates Apoptosis. *Nature* 356, 314–317. doi:10.1038/356314a0

Wu, R., Zeng, J., Yuan, J., Deng, X., Huang, Y., Chen, L., et al. (2018). MicroRNA-210 Overexpression Promotes Psoriasis-like Inflammation by Inducing Th1 and Th17 Cell Differentiation. *J. Clin. Invest.* 128 (6), 2551–2568. doi:10.1172/JCI97426

Xie, Q. W., Whisnant, R., and Nathan, C. (1993). Promoter of the Mouse Gene Encoding Calcium-independent Nitric Oxide Synthase Confers Inducibility by Interferon Gamma and Bacterial Lipopolysaccharide. *J. Exp. Med.* 177, 1779–1784. doi:10.1084/jem.177.6.1779

Yoh, K., Itoh, K., Enomoto, A., Hirayama, A., Yamaguchi, N., Kobayashi, M., et al. (2001). Nrf2-deficient Female Mice Develop Lupus-like Autoimmune Nephritis. *Kidney Int.* 60, 1343–1353. doi:10.1046/j.1523-1755.2001.00939.x

Yu, Y., and Su, K. (2013). Neutrophil Extracellular Traps and Systemic Lupus Erythematosus. *J. Clin. Cel Immunol* 4, 139. doi:10.4172/2155-9899.1000139

Zhao, Y., Sun, Y., Wang, G., Ge, S., and Liu, H. (2019). Dendrobium Officinale Polysaccharides Protect against MNNG-Induced PLGC in Rats via Activating the NRF2 and Antioxidant Enzymes HO-1 and NQO-1. *Oxid Med. Cel Longev* 2019, 9310245. doi:10.1155/2019/9310245

12

Burn Ointment Promotes Cutaneous Wound Healing by Modulating the PI3K/AKT/mTOR Signaling Pathway

Dali Gan[1†], Qiyuan Su[2†], Hanwen Su[3†], Li Wu[1], Jun Chen[4], Bing Han[5] and Meixian Xiang[1*]*

[1]School of Pharmaceutical Sciences, South-Central University for Nationalities, Wuhan, China, [2]Department of Statistics, University of Illinois at Urbana-Champaign, Urbana, IL, United States, [3]Department of Clinical Laboratory, Renmin Hospital of Wuhan University, Wuhan, China, [4]Department of Pharmacy, Wuhan No.1 Hospital (Wuhan Hospital of Traditional Chinese and Western Medicine), Wuhan, China, [5]Department of Pathology, Penn State College of Medicine, Milton S. Hershey Medical Center, Hershey, PA, United States

***Correspondence:**
Bing Han
bhan@pennstatehealth.psu.edu
Meixian Xiang
756626131@qq.com

[†]These authors have contributed equally to this work

Burn ointment (BO) is a clinically useful medicine for the treatment of burns and scalds. However, there is no enough scientific evidence to report the effect of BO on wound healing and its analgesic and anti-inflammatory efficacy. The aim of this work was to evaluate the anti-inflammatory and analgesic efficacy of BO and to reveal the potential wound healing properties and related mechanisms of BO. In this work, the content of active ingredients of BO was determined by high-performance liquid chromatography (HPLC). Two animal models of inflammation were used to study its anti-inflammatory activity, and a hot plate method was used to evaluate its analgesic effect. In addition, mouse incision and rat burn models were used to investigate the effect of BO on the anti-inflammatory and wound healing mechanisms. The results showed that BO was safe for topical application, and BO could significantly inhibit auricular swelling in mice and paw swelling in rats and significantly prolong the latency period of paw licking in the hot plate experiment in mice. It can also accelerate wound healing and repair scars by promoting the formation of new epithelial tissues in rat burn models. In addition, BO significantly downregulated the serum level of TNF-α and significantly increased the serum levels of VEGF and TGF-β1. Also, BO promoted the expression of collagen I and increased the ratio in p-PI3K/PI3K, p-AKT/AKT, and p-mTOR/mTOR pathways. Our results demonstrate the safety and efficacy of BO and suggest that activation of the PI3K/AKT/mTOR signaling pathway may play an important role in the promotion of wound healing by BO.

Keywords: burn ointment, safety evaluation, burn wounds healing, analgesia, anti-inflammatory, PI3K/AKT/mTOR pathway

---

Abbreviations: AKT, protein kinase B; AST, aspartate transaminase; BMS, burn moisturizing scald ointment; BO, burn ointment; Cr, creatinine; DAB, diaminobenzidine; ELISA, enzyme-linked immunosorbent assay; H&E, hematoxylin-eosin; GAPDH, glyceraldehyde phosphate dehydrogenase; mTOR, mammalian target of rapamycin; PAGE, SDS-polyacrylamide gel electrophoresis; PBS, phosphate buffered saline; PDK-1, 3-phosphoinositide-dependent kinases; PI3K, phosphatidylinositol 3-kinase; PIP3: phosphatidylinositol (3,4,5) P3; PVDF, polyvinylidene difluoride; SDS, sodium dodecyl sulfate; TCM, traditional Chinese medicine; TGF-β1, transforming growth factor-beta1; TNF-α, tumor necrosis factor-alpha; VEGF, vascular endothelial growth factor; PIP2, phosphorylates phosphatidylinositol (4, 5) P2.

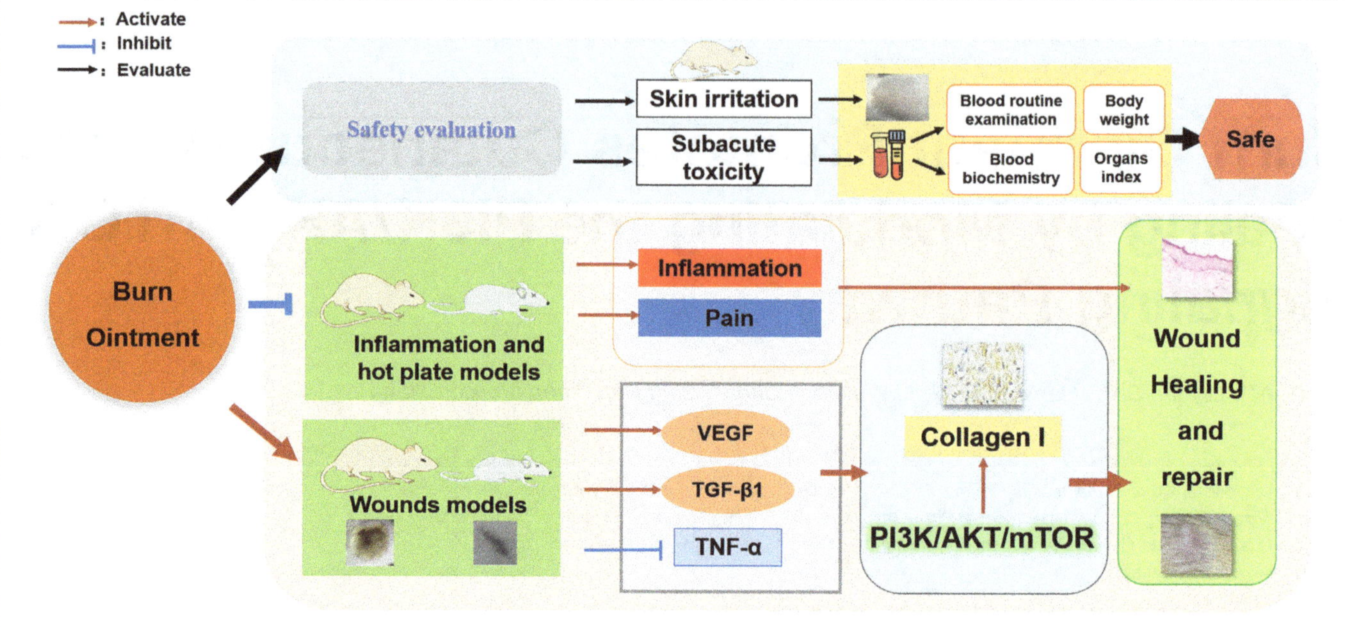

Graphical Abstract |

1 INTRODUCTION

Burns are one of the most serious skin-related injuries, and their incidence is on the rise globally (Shan et al., 2015). In the United States, the number of burn victims is estimated as 1.2 million per year. Of these injuries, an average of 50,000 burn victims are severely burned and require hospital treatment (Kaddoura et al., 2017).

The largest organ of the human body is the skin, and it is able to resist external infections and maintain the stability of the internal environment of our body (Riepl, 2020). Mild scalding will damage the skin tissue, but severe burns will be life-threatening. Additionally, the burns can cause inflammation, pain, and other complications (Wang et al., 2018). There are three phases that can be concluded in the dynamic healing process of wounds, including the inflammatory phase, the proliferation phase, and the maturation phase.

Many researches have indicated that several key cellular factors are involved in the process of burn repair, such as tumor necrosis factor-alpha (TNF-α), vascular endothelial growth factor (VEGF), and transforming growth factor-beta1 (TGF-β1) (Kim et al., 2020; Yaseen et al., 2020). If the body acquires an infection when the skin is damaged, it is stimulated to secrete the proinflammatory cytokines, such as TNF-α. After a while, the cytokine initiates an inflammatory cascade reaction to remove necrotic tissues and cells (Zelova and Hosek, 2013). However, overactive inflammation can cause systemic inflammatory response syndrome and immune dysfunction in patients, which will endanger their lives (Boldeanu et al., 2020). Therefore, anti-inflammatory treatments are essential for burn wound healing processes. Once the inflammation subsides, macrophages and other cells begin to secrete growth factors, such as VEGF. VEGF is an essential cell factor for forming new blood vessels, and it can promote vascular endothelial cell proliferation to produce new blood vessels (Roskoski, 2017). The new blood vessels can provide nutrition to the injured area and accelerate wound healing (Eming et al., 2014). Besides, TGF-β1 is also a necessary cell factor for the healing process, because it promotes fibroblasts to proliferate and differentiate, forms granulation tissues, and synthesizes type I collagen (Kim et al., 2018a). Collagens help with wound contraction and restore skin elasticity to heal the burn wound by filling the space between cells (Gonzalez et al., 2016).

Currently, most of the known medications for burns have the obvious limitation of leaving scars easily. Traditional Chinese medicine compound burn ointment offers a more advanced alternative that avoids such limitations. BO is a traditional Chinese medical formulation, which contains *Rheum palmatum* L., *Angelica sinensis* (Oliv.) Diels, *Codonopsis pilosula* (Franch.) Nannf., *Asarum sieboldii* Miq., *Borneolum syntheticum*, and *Calomelas*. Traditionally, *Rheum palmatum* L. can be used to cure burn wounds *in vitro* (Committee of the Pharmacopoeia of PR China, 2015) due to its antimicrobial and anti-inflammatory qualities (Cao et al., 2017), and it can promote recovery of muscle; *Angelica sinensis* (Oliv.) Diels and *Codonopsis pilosula* (Franch.) Nannf. can remove stasis and analgesia (Wei et al., 2016; Gao et al., 2018), promoting the skin recovery of the wounded area. Modern research has revealed that the extract of *Rheum palmatum* L. could accelerate the progress of wound healing in rats, and its efficacy was better when it combined with the extract of *Angelica dahurica* (Fisch. Ex Hoffm.) Benth. et Hook. f (Yang et al., 2017). Moreover, many studies have shown the enormous potential of BO in treating burns as well, such that many chemicals of *Rheum palmatum* L.

and *Angelica sinensis* (Oliv.) Diels could reduce the liberation of proinflammatory cytokines, including IL-1β, IL-6, TNF-alpha, and IL-33 (Kim et al., 2018b; Shen et al., 2019). They have an anti-inflammatory and analgesic effect (Wei et al., 2016), induce cell proliferation (Gundogdu et al., 2019), and protect cells from injuries (Zhang et al., 2019b). But, the activity of BO in anti-inflammation, analgesia, and promoting skin wound healing, and its specific mechanism are still unclear. Therefore, this study attempted to elucidate the efficacy, the involved molecular mechanisms of BO in the healing process of burn wounds, and their complications. This research would contribute to the development and application of new drugs to treat burns and scalds.

2 MATERIAL AND METHODS

2.1 Materials and Reagents

BO (pharmaceutical batch number: 201671HZ) was supplied by the Department of Pharmacy at the Wuhan Integrated Traditional and Western Medicine Hospital (Wuhan, China). The BO used in this study is a hospital preparation which contains *Rheum palmatum* L., *Angelica sinensis* (Oliv.) Diels, *Codonopsis pilosula* (Franch.) Nannf., *Asarum sieboldii* Miq., *Borneolum syntheticum,* and Calomelas. Burn moisturizing scald ointment (BMS) was purchased from Meibao Pharmaceutical Co., Ltd. (Shantou, China); ELISA kits were obtained from Neobioscience Technology Co., Ltd. (Shenzhen, China); Collagen I primary antibody; phosphorylated PI3K, AKT, and mTOR; unphosphorylated PI3K, AKT, and mTOR polyclonal antibody; and HRP-labeled secondary antibody were purchased from Servicebio (Wuhan, China); Microscope (XSP-C204) was from Motic China group and microscope camera was purchased from Cognex (Massachusetts, United States); Toe volume measuring instrument (PV-200) was from TECHMEN Co., Ltd. (Chengdu, China); full-wavelength microplate reader 1,510 was obtained from Thermo Fisher Scientific (Massachusetts, United States); Ultimate 3000 series HPLC system consisting of the computer-controlled system with the CHROMELEONTM software and a SQL database, equipped with a WPS-3000 autosampler, was from Dionex (California, United States).

2.2 Animals

Kunming (KM) mice (20 ± 2 g), Sprague Dawley (SD) rats (200 ± 20 g), and Sprague Dawley (SD) rats (90 ± 10 g) were purchased from the Experimental Animal Center (certificate of experimental animals: SCXK 2015–0089 for rats and SCXK 2015–0018 for mice), Institute of Health and Epidemic Prevention (Wuhan, China), and housed in the standard specific pathogen-free (SPF) environment for three days. License number of the experimental unit was SYXK (Hubei province) 2016–0089, Experimental Animal Center of Central South University for Nationalities. All animals were allowed free access to food and water. The animal experiments were approved by the Institutional Animal Ethical Committee of Central South University for Nationalities and were performed under the guidelines of the committee; the permit number for the use of animals was no. 2020-scuec-029.

2.3 HPLC Analysis of BO's Chemical Components and Stability

20 mg BO was extracted with 10 ml methanol for 20 min using the ultrasonic method. The obtained extract was separated and transferred to a 10 mL volumetric flask and the volume was adjusted to 10 ml with methanol to obtain a 1 mg/mL sample solution. HPLC was then used to analyze the sample solution to quantify the content of aloe-emodin, emodin, rhein, chrysophanol, ferulic acid, lobetyolin, asarinin, and borneol and evaluate their stability on the 30th day or beyond. The samples were subjected to HPLC analysis on a C_{18} column (Agilent 250 mm × 4.6 mm, 5 μm) by a single injection of 10 μl detected at 254 nm; mobile phase: gradient elution by methyl alcohol (A) and water (B). The gradient program was set as follows: 0–4 min, 5–21% A; 4–8 min, 21–26% A; 8–10 min, 26–32% A; 10–14 min, 32–36% A; 14–18 min, 36–48% A; 18–22 min, 48–55% A; 22–25 min, 55–65% A; 25–30 min, 65% A; column temperature: 25°C; flow rate: 0.8 ml/min.

2.4 Doses and Methods of BO in Animal Models

Mice were randomly divided into several groups: canola oil (Con) group, burn moisturizing scald ointment (BMS) group, and BO group, with 10 mice in each group. The BO dosages of 0.1 g, 0.2 g, and 0.4 g/cm^2 were used to assess the subacute toxicity.

2.5 Skin Irritation Experiment in Rats

One day before the experiment, twenty SD rats were shaved for an area of approximately 4 × 2 cm^2 on the dorsal side. These shaved rats were randomly divided into two groups of ten: the canola oil group (Con) and the BO-treated group (BO). Then 0.2 g/cm^2 BO or Con was applied evenly on the shaved area of animals three times per day for one day. One hour after the last treatment, the treated skin was cleaned with cotton and water. After the application of BO, any signs, symptoms, and other skin changes were observed for 4 h (Ghosh et al., 2019).

2.6 Subacute Toxicity Assessment

Forty SD rats were shaved, weighed, and categorized into four groups of ten: 0.1 g, 0.2 g, and 0.4 g/cm^2 with BO and 0.2 g/cm^2 with Con. All animals received BO or Con 3 times per day for a total of 28 days. The body weight was recorded once per week. At the end of the experiment, all animals were fasted for 12 h and then anesthetized for blood and organ collection (Upadhyay et al., 2009). Hematological and biochemical analyses were run in a clinical laboratory, Wuhan University Renmin Hospital.

2.7 The Hot-Plate Test

The hot-plate test was used to examine the potential analgesic effect of BO. First, 40 KM mice were screened for their pain threshold within 5–30 s. In brief, the temperature of the plate surface was kept at 54 ± 1°C. The interval time that the mice licked its toe or jumped from the plate was detected three times. Twenty-seven mice were selected and randomly divided into the following groups: the Con group, the BO group, and the BMS group. All mice were applied 0.2 g/cm^2 drug each time on the hind paws, 3 times per day for 7 days. The response latency of mice at the first hind paw lick or jump was recorded and analyzed 30 min after the last dose on day 1 and day 7, respectively (Ariyo et al., 2020). The following formula was used to calculate the pain threshold change:

Pain threshold change (s) = Pain threshold after treatment (s) − Pain threshold before treatment (s).

2.8 The Xylene-Induced Mouse Ear Swelling

Thirty KM mice were randomly divided into three groups of ten: the Con, the BO, and the BMS groups. The animals' ears were treated with 0.2 g/cm^2 drug each time, 3 times per day for 5 days. On the sixth day, 100 μl of xylene was dripped on the right ear with a pipette. After the model was established successfully, the animals were immediately sacrificed, and both ears were removed. The samples were immediately weighed after being punched (Xavier-Santos et al., 2018). The following formula was used to calculate the degree of the ear swelling:

The degree of ear swelling: Δm (mg) = The right ear mass (mg) − The left ear mass (mg).

2.9 Carrageenan-Induced Toe Swelling

Thirty SD rats were randomly divided into three groups of ten, the Con group, the BO group, and the BMS group, with 0.2 g/cm^2 drug topically applied evenly on the right hind paw 3 times/day for a total of 5 days. On the sixth day, each rat's right hind paw was injected with 0.1 ml carrageenan (1%). Rats' right hind paw was marked by black marker at its ankle, then, the paw volume before and after injection at 1–5 h was measured by Toes Volume Measuring Instrument, with three measurements each time point (Zahra et al., 2020). The following formula was used to calculate the toe swelling:

The swelling volume (ΔV) (ml) = V_t (ml) − V_0 (ml), where Vt is the right hind paw volume (ml) at test time and V_0 is the right bind paw volume (ml) before carrageenan injection.

2.10 Incision Wound Model

Twenty mice were randomly divided into two groups of ten, the Con group and the BO group. After dorsal fur shaving and anesthesia, a 1.5-cm long, lateral incision near the tail's root was made on the back. Then, 0.2 g/cm^2 of Con or BO was topically applied over the incision three times per day for 16 days (Getachew et al., 2019). The changes in the wound were observed and recorded.

2.11 Thermal Burn Wounds Model

The dorsal hairs of 36 SD rats were shaved 24 h before the induction of burn. After disinfection and anesthesia, the thermal burn injuries were induced on the dorsal of rats by a metal block (1.5 cm^2) heated over the flame for 10 s. After half an hour, all animals were awakened and randomly evenly divided into the Con group, the BO group, and the BMS group, with 0.2 g/cm^2 drug topically applied each time, 3 times per day for 28 days. The wounded skin tissue was collected for H&E staining and Western blot test at the 1st, 7th, 14th, and 28th day after the model was established. Blood samples were collected from the abdominal aorta for TNF-α, VEGF, and TGF-β1 measurements, following the commercial kit instructions (Neobioscience, Shenzhen, China).

The wound contraction was evaluated by tracing the wound, using transparent paper and permanent marker, on the 1st, 7th, 14th, and 28th postwounding day. The wound area was retraced on the paper, and the changes in area were calculated, which indicated the wound contraction (Ghosh et al., 2019). The percentage of wound closure was calculated using this formula:

Wound contraction = [(wound area day1 − wound area day n)/ wound area day1] ×100%, n = 7th, 14th, and 28th after wound.

2.12 Histopathological Evaluation and Type I Collagen Staining on Burn Wound Tissue

The burn wound tissue was collected and H&E stained for histopathological evaluation. The pretreated sample tissues from rats were embedded in paraffin wax. The embedded wax blocks were then cut into 4-μm sections. The sections were routinely deparaffinized with xylene and different concentration alcohol. After the conventional staining, alcohol gradient dehydration, then, the samples were sealed with neutral resin. The observations included the epidermis, dermis, blood vessels, cells, and organelles. Two pathologists blindly read and evaluated histopathological changes with a scoring system. The detail score criteria included the regeneration of epithelial tissues, inflammatory cell infiltration, angiogenesis, and the thickness of the granulation; scores from 0 to 3 indicated from lack of recovery to full recovery. The four variables were summed to represent the histopathological score (total score: 0–12, respectively) (Kazemi et al., 2020).

The immunohistochemistry was applied to determine the type I collagen expression. In brief, after head-based antigen retrieval, each section was incubated with collagen I rabbit poly-Ab (Servicebio, 1:100), 4°C overnight. Then these sections were incubated with HRP-labeled goat anti-rabbit Ab (Servicebio, 1:200) for 2 h at room temperature. Finally, the section was stained with DAB and counterstained with hematoxylin. The sections were observed and photographed. The type I collagen expression was analyzed using ImageJ software (National Institutes of Health, Bethesda, MD, United States). The immunohistochemistry (IHC) Image Analysis Toolbox Plug-tool was first used to identify areas of positive staining. Thirty-six images were then converted to the RGB scale and the threshold tool was used to calculate the percentage area positively stained (SenthilKumar et al., 2020).

2.13 Western Blot Analysis

The protein samples (30 μg) from wound skin tissue lysates of burn rats were concentrated and separated respectively by 5 and 10% SDS-polyacrylamide gel electrophoresis (PAGE). Then, they

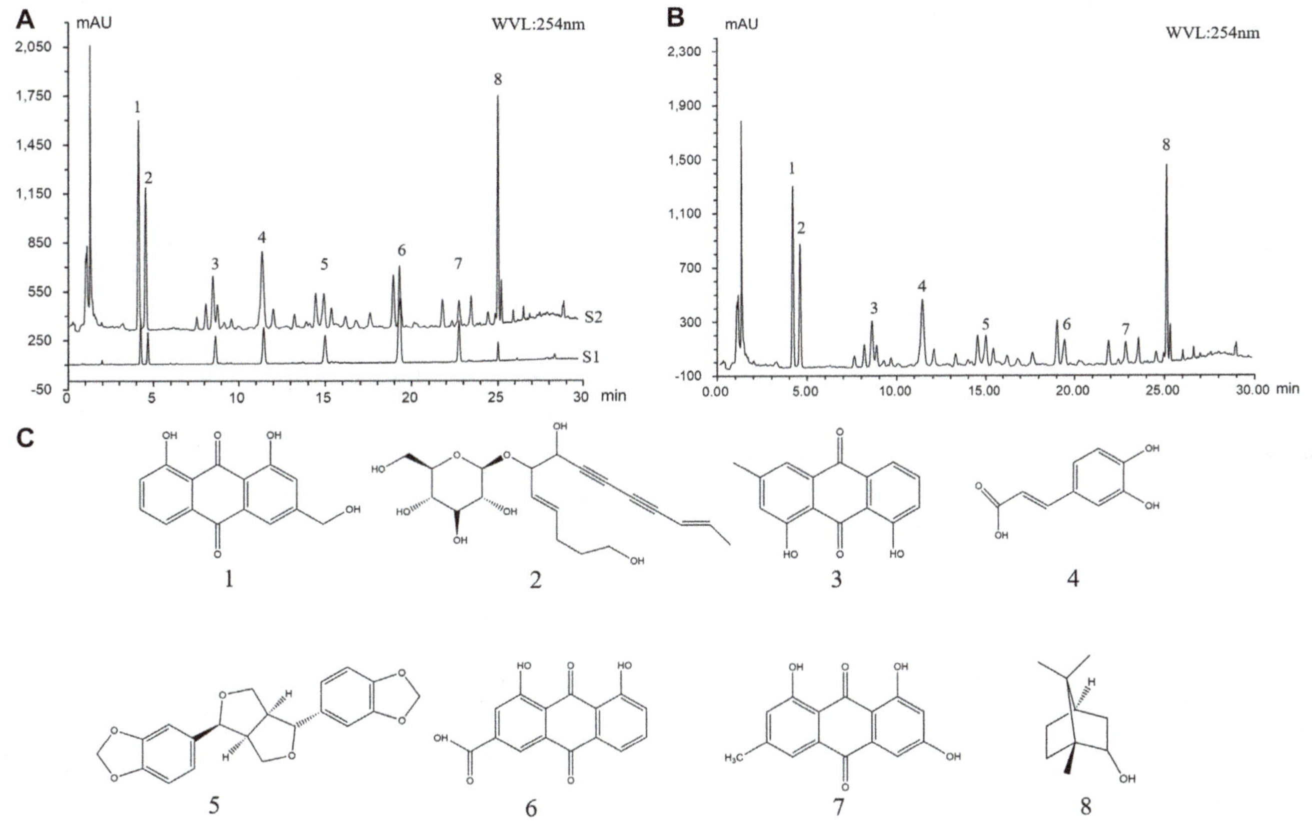

FIGURE 1 | High-performance liquid chromatography (HPLC) analysis of the standard and the BO extract. **(A)** The content determination of standards (S1) and sample (S2). **(B)** The stability of BO after 30 days. **(C)** Compound structure. 1. Aloe-emodin; 2. lobetyolin; 3. rhein; 4. ferulic acid; 5. asarinin; 6. emodin; 7 chrysophanol; 8. borneol.

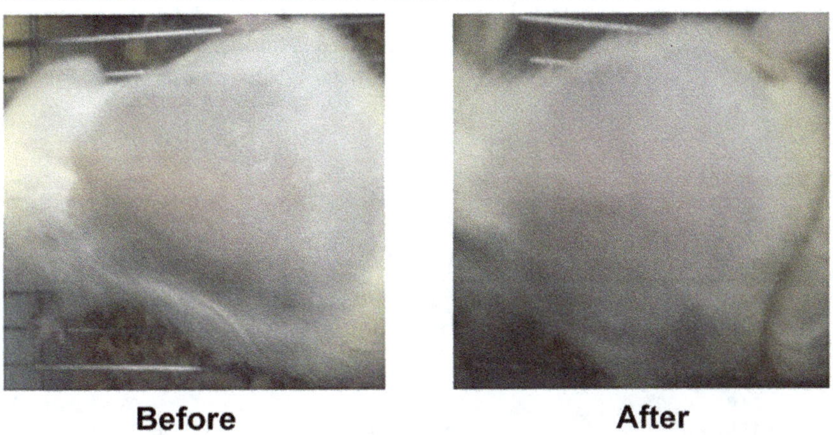

FIGURE 2 | Representative imaging of rat skin before and 24 h after BO administration. 0.2 g/cm^2 BO or Con was applied evenly on the shaved area of animals 8 h per time for 3 times. One hour after the last times, the skin condition was observed (n = 10 each group).

were electrotransferred to PVDF membranes. Then, the membranes were blocked with a Western blocking solution (Tris-buffered saline with 0.05% Tween-20 and 5% nonfat dry milk) for 90 min and incubated at 4°C overnight with primary antibodies, phosphorylated and unphosphorylated PI3K, AKT, and mTOR polyclonal antibody (1:1000, Servicebio, Wuhan,

TABLE 1 | Changes of weight in rats (n = 10, mean ± SEM).

Days	Con	BO		
		0.1 g/cm^2	0.2 g/cm^2	0.4 g/cm^2
1	100.75 ± 0.99	100.63 ± 1.65	102.63 ± 1.09	103.63 ± 1.83
7	127.25 ± 1.56	132.25 ± 2.44	131.13 ± 1.88	135.25 ± 3.50
14	196.50 ± 1.58	200.88 ± 4.10	207.88 ± 3.73	199.88 ± 5.35
21	239.38 ± 2.32	251.13 ± 6.24	261.13 ± 4.78	252.00 ± 4.52
28	288.25 ± 3.10	300.50 ± 8.42	310.38 ± 5.16	302.38 ± 6.00

*Con: canola oil and BO: burn ointment. The data are expressed as the mean ± SEM (n = 10), compared with the Con group; *p < 0.05, **p < 0.01.*

TABLE 2 | Effect of BO on rat organ coefficient (mg/g) (n = 10, mean ± SEM).

Organs	Con	BO		
		0.1 g/cm^2	0.2 g/cm^2	0.4 g/cm^2
Heart	3.38 ± 0.02	3.60 ± 0.09	3.65 ± 0.07	3.66 ± 0.08
Liver	27.22 ± 0.67	28.58 ± 2.29	28.12 ± 0.4	27.89 ± 0.42
Spleen	2.07 ± 0.02	1.94 ± 0.05	2.34 ± 0.09	2.15 ± 0.17
Lungs	4.19 ± 0.20	4.27 ± 0.15	3.93 ± 0.13	4.03 ± 0.01
Kidney L	3.45 ± 0.08	3.60 ± 0.04	3.49 ± 0.01	3.69 ± 0.09
Kidney R	3.51 ± 0.03	3.72 ± 0.08	3.59 ± 0.08	3.79 ± 0.09
Testes L	6.65 ± 0.17	6.54 ± 0.05	6.26 ± 0.18	6.49 ± 0.02
Testes R	6.67 ± 0.19	6.58 ± 0.03	6.86 ± 0.01	6.53 ± 0.08
Thymus	1.64 ± 0.01	1.85 ± 0.09	1.71 ± 0.13	1.73 ± 0.06

*Con: canola oil and BO: burn ointment. The data are expressed as the mean ± SEM (n = 10), compared with the Con group; *p < 0.05, **p < 0.01.*

China), followed by washing 3 times in TBST, 5 min/time and incubation with the HPR-labeled goat anti-rabbit secondary antibodies (1:1000, Servicebio, Wuhan, China) at room temperature for 1 h. The membranes were washed 3 times in TBST, 5 min/time. Finally, the protein levels were detected by gel imaging analyzing system (Bio-Rad, California, United States) and normalized to GAPDH.

TABLE 4 | The effect of BO on blood biochemistry in rats (n = 10, mean ± SEM).

	Con	BO		
		0.1 g/cm^2	0.2 g/cm^2	0.4 g/cm^2
ALT (U/L)	44.33 ± 1.11	45.00 ± 1.38	48.00 ± 1.92	40.67 ± 2.46
AST (U/L)	167.67 ± 4.79	191.33 ± 9.87	156.67 ± 4.13	142.33 ± 9.34
Urea (mmol/L)	7.67 ± 0.15	7.57 ± 0.21	9.23 ± 0.17	8.33 ± 0.05
Cr (μmol/L)	25.33 ± 1.46	24.33 ± 0.36	24.00 ± 0.84	22.33 ± 0.48

*ALT: alanine transaminase; AST: aspartate transaminase; Cr, creatinine; Con: canola oil, BO: burn ointment. The data are expressed as the mean ± SEM (n = 10), compared with the Con group; *p < 0.05, **p < 0.01.*

2.14 Statistical Analysis

The data were expressed as the means ± standard error of mean (SEM). Statistical analysis was performed via Student's *T* test and one-way ANOVA (SPSS Program, version 11.5; SPSS, Inc., Chicago, IL, United States). Significant differences were considered when $p < 0.05$.

3 RESULTS

3.1 Result of HPLC Analysis

HPLC was used to detect the active ingredients in the BO and its stability within 30 days. Eight main peaks were obtained, indicating aloe emodin, emodin, rhein, chrysophanol, ferulic acid, lobetyolin, asarinin, and borneol, respectively. (**Figure 1**). The result was identical with the peaks of a single compound of aloe emodin, emodin, rhein, chrysophanol, ferulic acid, lobetyolin, asarinin, and borneol. And the result suggested that BO was stable within 30 days (**Figure 1B**).

3.2 Safety Assessment of BO

The skin irritation experiment in rats was used to evaluate the safety of BO. We did not observe significant differences in the exposed skin in terms of irritation, swelling, inflammation, redness, or other abnormal changes before and after treatment

TABLE 3 | Effect of BO on blood routine (n = 10, mean ± SEM).

	Con	BO		
		0.1 g/cm^2	0.2 g/cm^2	0.4 g/cm^2
WBC (×109/L)	9.61 ± 1.18	10.45 ± 1.44	9.33 ± 1.37	8.34 ± 0.21
RBC (×1,012/L)	8.37 ± 0.13	7.67 ± 0.27	8.02 ± 0.23	8.35 ± 0.07
HB(g/L)	149.00 ± 2.39	147.67 ± 1.74	155.33 ± 1.59	160.67 ± 1.20
HCT (L/L)	0.46 ± 0.01	0.46 ± 0.00	0.48 ± 0.00	0.50 ± 0.00
MCV (fL)	54.60 ± 0.30	59.93 ± 1.55	60.03 ± 1.24	59.50 ± 0.65
MCH (pg)	17.80 ± 0.14	19.40 ± 0.44	19.43 ± 0.36	19.23 ± 0.15
MCHC (g/L)	326.00 ± 0.84	323.33 ± 1.32	324.00 ± 0.55	323.33 ± 1.80
PLT (×109/L)	1098.67 ± 46.97	896.33 ± 51.98	1184.33 ± 18.58	1140.00 ± 24.26
PCT (%)	1098.67 ± 46.97	896.33 ± 51.98	1184.33 ± 18.58	1140.00 ± 24.26
MPV (fL)	7.73 ± 0.08	7.90 ± 0.09	7.87 ± 0.10	7.80 ± 0.06
PDW (fL)	8.30 ± 0.11	8.47 ± 0.15	8.53 ± 0.08	8.40 ± 0.08
P-LCR (%)	9.53 ± 0.43	10.13 ± 0.69	10.10 ± 0.57	9.70 ± 0.46

*WBC: leukocyte; RBC: erythrocyte; HB: hemoglobin; HCT: hematocrit value; MCV: mean corpuscular volume; MCH: mean corpuscular hemoglobin; MCHC: mean corpuscular hemoglobin concentration; PLT: platelet; PCT: procalcitonin; MPV: mean platelet volume; PDW: platelet distribution width; P-LCR: platelet-larger cell ratio; Con: canola oil, BO: burn ointment. The data are expressed as the mean ± SEM (n = 10), compared with the Con group; *p < 0.05, **p < 0.01.*

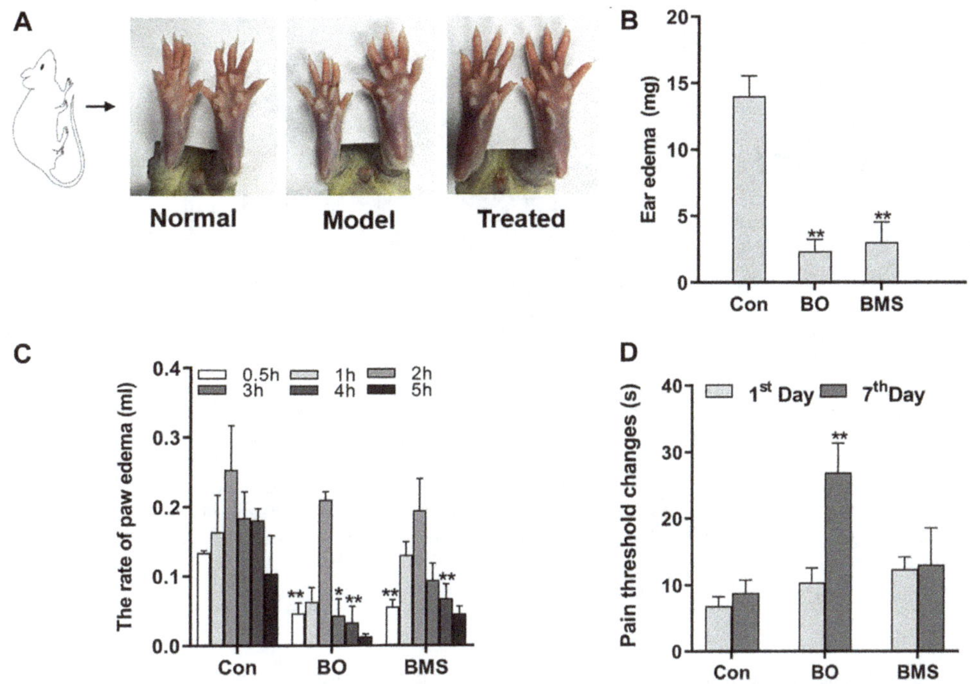

FIGURE 3 | The anti-inflammatory and analgesic effects among Con, BO and BMS. **(A)** Representative imaging of rat toe before and after model induction, before and after treatment. **(B)** On the 6th day, BO pretreatment reduced mouse ear edema; the data were shown as the mean ± SEM (n = 10 each group), compared with the control group; $^*p < 0.05$, $^{**}p < 0.01$. **(C)** On the 6th day, BO pretreatment decreased rats' toe swelling; the data are expressed as the mean ± SEM (n = 10 each group), compared with the control group; $^*p < 0.05$, $^{**}p < 0.01$. **(D)** BO pretreatment enhanced pain threshold; the data were expressed as the mean ± SEM (n = 9 each group), compared with the control group; $^*p < 0.05$, $^{**}p < 0.01$.

(**Figure 2**). Similarly, the preclinical trial for subacute toxicity showed no striking difference among rats treated with BO groups (0.1 g, 0.2 g, and 0.4 g/cm^2) and Con group in rat body weight (**Table 1**), the relative organ weight (**Table 2**), blood routine (**Table 3**), and biochemical analysis (**Table 4**). Thus, our results indicated that BO was safe for rats.

3.3 Effect of BO on Analgesic

As revealed in **Figure 3D**, on the 7th day, the pain threshold of the BO group was significantly increased compared to that of the Con group ($p < 0.01$), while there was no difference in the Con and the BMS group. The results indicated that BO had an analgesic effect.

3.4 Effect of BO on Inhibiting Inflammation

In the model of carrageenan-induced toe swelling, we observed that the rats treated with BO demonstrated a significant reduction in swelling at 3 h after injection ($^*p < 0.05$ or $^{**}p < 0.01$, respectively) (**Figure 3C**). In the second model, auricle swelling was significantly reduced in the BO-treated group ($^{**}p < 0.01$) (**Figure 3B**). These results indicated that BO could inhibit inflammation.

3.5 Effects of BO on Promoting Wounds Healing

The healing process of the incision wound was observed on the 1st, 5th, 10th, and 16th day after wounding, which is demonstrated in **Figure 4A**. The observation revealed that incision wounds treated with BO healed considerably faster in comparison with that of the Con on the 16th day. The wounds treated with BO initiated to form scar and shed the eschar gradually in contrast with the Con group. On the 16th day after the incision wound, the wounds of the BO group almost completely disappeared, whereas the scar in the Con group was still predominant. Consistent with the scar change, hair grew vigorously in the wound area in the BO-treated mice, which were entirely covered by the new epidermis.

The impact of BO on the healing process was also observed using the rat burn wound model, in which the percentage contraction ability on the 1st, 7th, 14th, and 28th day after wounding was recorded, as shown in **Figure 4B,C**. The result showed a significant ($p < 0.01$) increase in wound closure in the BO-treated group compared with the Con group on the 14th dayafter wound. On the last day, compared with the Con group, the scar of the BO group had entirely cured, and new fur had been growing on the scar, with the percentage of wound healing at 90.27 ± 2.06, which was significantly higher than that of the Con group (71.92 ± 5.92, $p < 0.01$). These results suggested that BO could promote wound healing.

3.6 Effects of BO on Skin Tissue Development

The representative H&E images of the burn wound skin (100 × magnificent) are shown in **Figure 5A**, and the histopathological assessment is given in **Figure 5B**. The epidermis was fragmented,

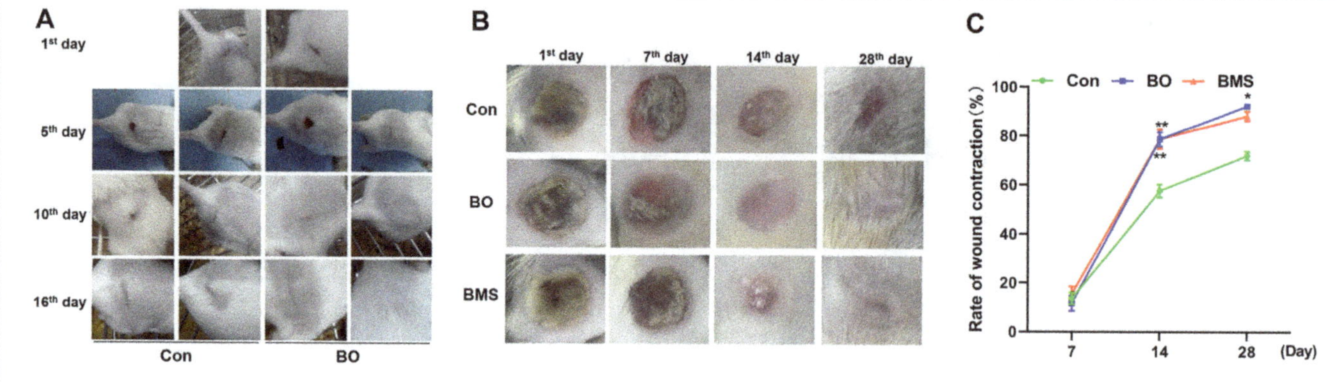

FIGURE 4 | Representative imaging wound healing in mouse incision wound model and rat thermal burn wounds model, and the wound contraction quantification in the thermal burn wounds model. **(A)** Wound healing in mouse incision wound model. The healing process was observed and photographed on the 1st, 5th, 10th, and 16th day. The control group (Con) and the treatment group (BO), which were observed 3 times per day for 16 days (n = 10 each group). Representative pictures revealing that BO pretreatment accelerate the healing process of incision wound. **(B)** Rats thermal burn wounds model. The process of healing was followed and photographed at intervals of the 1st, 7th, 14th, and 28th day for the negative control group (Con), the treatment group (BO), and the positive group burn moisturizing scald (BMS), with 3 times/day for 28 days (n = 12 each group). Representative pictures revealing that BO pretreatment accelerate the healing process of thermal burn wounds. **(C)** The percentage of thermal wound contraction. BO pretreatment enhanced wound contraction observed in the rat thermal burn wounds model. The data were expressed as the mean ± SEM (n = 12 each group), compared with the control group, $^{*}p < 0.05$, $^{**}p < 0.01$.

blood vessels and subcutaneous tissues under the dermis were severely damaged upon the burn wound creation. The BO-treated group healed faster than that of the Con group, with reduced inflammatory cell infiltration, increased fibroblast and blood vessels, and accelerated dermal and epidermal formation, at different time points. On the 28th day, the group treated with BO demonstrated an almost completely healed skin structure with normal epithelization, few inflammatory cell infiltrations, and the junction between the epidermis and dermis layers was tight and seamless when compared with the Con group. Moreover, the epidermis of rats treated with BO was much more uniform in thickness than that of the BMS group. The histopathological evaluation is shown in **Figure 5B**, which supported that the BO group was significantly improved than the Con group on the 7th, 14th, and 28th day ($p < 0.05$, respectively).

3.7 Effects of BO on Increasing Type I Collagen

The microscopic images of IHC stained burn wound skin (100× magnificent) and the percentage of collagen I changes are presented in **Figure 5C,D**, respectively. The results showed a significant increase ($p < 0.05$) in the percentage of collagen I in the BO group when compared with the Con group. In the total study period of 28 days, the irregular collagen I areas of the BO group were increased and arranged tightly and evenly. In contrast, the group treated with canola oil was slowly increased. Similarly, the maximum positive area of collagen I observed was on the 28th day in the BO group ($p < 0.01$). The results indicated that BO played an important role in promoting an increase in cellular type I collagen.

3.8 Effects of BO on Regulating the Cytokine Production

The TNF-α, VEGF, and TGF-β1 levels were detected by using the ELISA method, as shown in **Figure 6**. The levels of TNF-α were significantly lower after BO treatment than in the Con group ($p < 0.001$), indicating a potential anti-inflammatory effect of BO (**Figure 6A**).

The VEGF levels of the BO group were significantly increased on the 14th day compared with the Con group ($p < 0.05$). And the maximum significant differences ($p < 0.01$) of the content of VEGF between the BO-treated group and the Con group were obtained on the 28th day (**Figure 6B**). These results showed that BO could increase the content of VEGF in serum after scalding.

As presented in **Figure 6C**, in the first two weeks after wounding, the content of TGF-β1 of the BO group was significantly increased, compared with the content of the Con group. However, compared with the Con group on the 28th day, the content of the BO-treated group was significantly decreased. These results showed that BO could regulate the content of TGF-β1 in blood with time after burning.

3.9 Effects of BO on Activating the PI3K-AKT-mTOR Pathway

As is evidenced in **Figure 7A**, the application of BO resulted in increased phosphorylation of PI3K, AKT, and mTOR. Densitometry of bands showed that BO did not alter the expression of the unphosphorylated protein of PI3K, AKT, and mTOR. However, it significantly upregulated its phosphorylation compared with the Con group in the last two weeks after wounding ($p < 0.01$) (**Figure 7B–D**). These results suggested that BO could upregulate the expression of the PI3K/AKT/mTOR pathway.

4 DISCUSSION

Burn and scald cause local damage to the body and systemic inflammatory response mediated by neuroendocrine (Gokakin et al., 2013), cytokine, and inflammatory mediators. These biomediators resulted in the delay of the healing of local burn

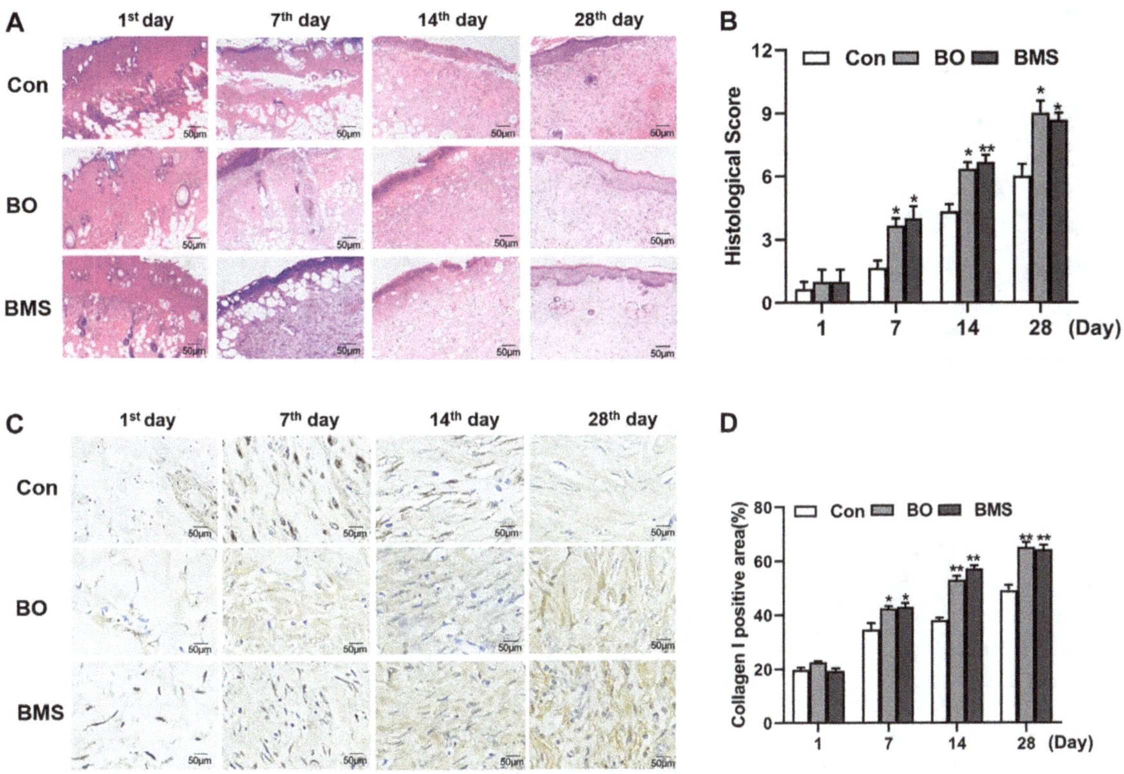

FIGURE 5 | Histopathological evaluation and the type I collagen expression before and after Con, BO, and BMS treatment in the rat thermal burn wounds model. **(A)** Representative H&E imaging of scald wound in rats. Specimens were taken from the 1st, 7th, 14th, and 28th day after modeling. The negative control group (Con), the treatment group (BO), and the positive group burn moisturizing scald (BMS) (n = 12 each group). **(B)** The results of the histological score. Comparing with the Con group, the BO group's wound was significantly healing on the 28th day (*$p < 0.05$), BMS group's wound was prominently healing on the 14th day, and the data were expressed as the mean ± SEM, (*$p < 0.05$, **$p < 0.01$, respectively, n = 12 each group). **(C)** Increased type I collagen expression in the rat scald wound after BO treatment. Specimens were taken from the 1st, 7th, 14th, and 28th day after modeling. The negative control group (Con), the treatment group (BO), and the positive group burn moisturizing scald (BMS) (n = 12 each group). **(D)** The results of collagen ⊠ expression semiquantitation, compared with the control group. BO could upregulate the collagen ⊠ of wound area markedly from the 7th day; the data were expressed as the mean ± SEM (n = 12 each group); *$p < 0.05$, **$p < 0.01$, respectively.

and scald wounds and trigger of various, severe complications, such as pain, making treatment difficult (Naseri et al., 2018). The healing of burn and scald wounds involves three complex processes: inflammation, tissue hyperplasia, and regeneration. These three processes are not independent but overlap and develop in a particular order (Govindaraju et al., 2019). Exogenous damage will stimulate the body to secrete various growth factors, such as VEGF and TGF-β1, which can promote cell migration, proliferation,

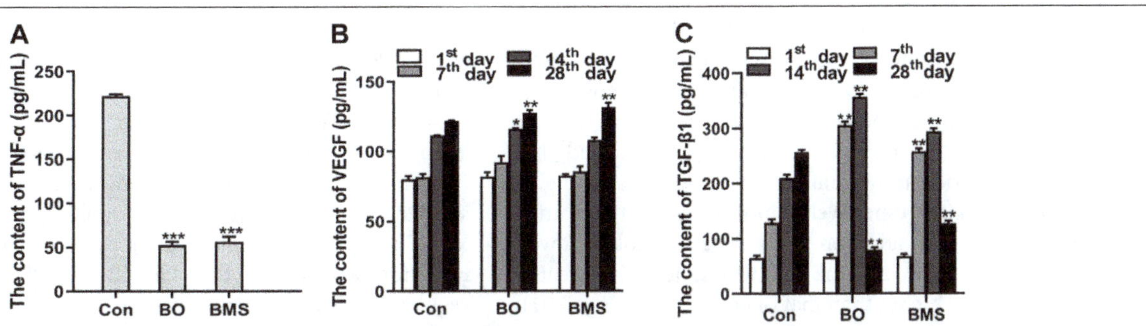

FIGURE 6 | The serum cytokine level before and after Con, BO, and BMS treatment. **(A)** Downregulated TNF-α level after BO treatment. The data are expressed as the mean ± SEM (n = 12 each group), compared with the Con group, ***$p < 0.001$. **(B)** The content of VEGF, which was tested on the 1st, 7th, 14th, and 28th day. The data were expressed as the mean ± SEM (n = 12 each group), compared with the control group; *$p < 0.05$, **$p < 0.01$, respectively. **(C)** The content of TGF-β1, which was tested at the 1st, 7th, 14th, and 28th day. The data were expressed as the mean ± SEM (n = 12 each group), compared with the control group, **$p < 0.01$.

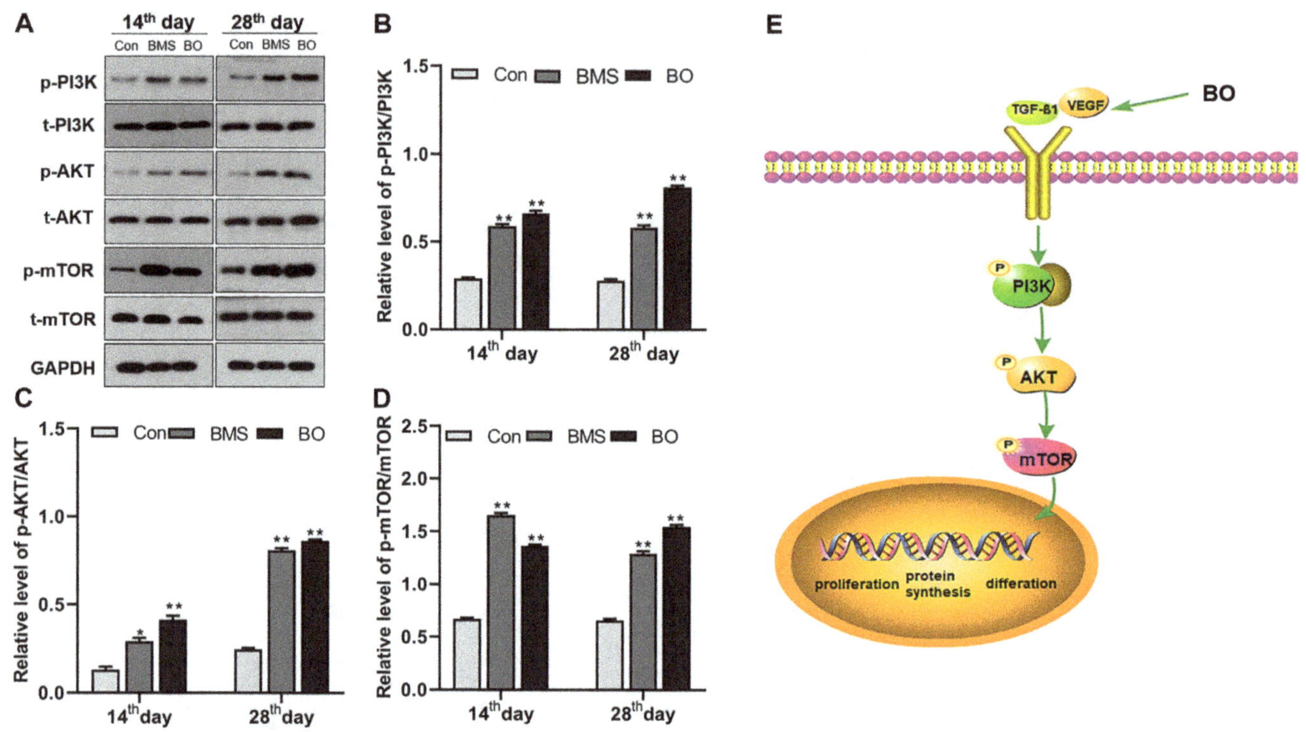

FIGURE 7 | The ;xpression of the PI3K/AKT/mTOR signaling pathway proteins. **(A)** Representative Western blot bands of relevant proteins. Protein levels of **(B)** p-PI3K/t-PI3K, **(C)** p-AKT/t-AKT, and **(D)** p-mTOR/t-mTOR. Data were presented as the mean ± SEM of three independent experiments. Compared with the control group; $^{*}p < 0.05$, $^{**}p < 0.01$, respectively. **(E)** The illustrated picture of the BO-activated signal pathway within this study.

and differentiation, to help wound constriction and recovery. The damaged wound and these biomediators can also activate signaling pathways associated with wound repair, such as the PI3K/AKT/mTOR pathway (Cho et al., 2019; Zhang et al., 2020).

The inflammatory response is the first step after tissue damage and is essential for skin repair (Glim et al., 2015). A prolonged inflammatory response will be harmful to the body and lead to unexpected complications. Therefore, it is crucial to suppress inflammation and pain during tissue recovery. The clinical signs of inflammation are redness, swelling, heat, and pain (Yu et al., 2014). Swelling is a pathological manifestation of inflammation, and it is generally believed that eliminating swelling can achieve anti-inflammatory effects (Srivastava et al., 2018; Chen et al., 2019). To investigate the anti-inflammatory and analgesic effects of BO, we used a variety of classical animal models of inflammation, including mouse auricular swelling, rat toe swelling, and mouse hot plate test. These results showed that BO could inhibit auricular swelling in mice and toe swelling in rats ($p < 0.05$, $p < 0.01$, respectively), indicating its strong anti-inflammatory activity. In addition, the analgesic results showed that BO could relieve pain, and the pain threshold of BO-treated mice was significantly higher than that of control mice ($p < 0.01$), supporting the analgesic effect of BO.

When the wound presents with early inflammation, the body's defense system is activated, with the formation of a protective barrier and several growth factors production (Silvestre et al., 2018). TNF-α and VEGF are two of those cytokines and are critical in the wound healing process. TNF-α, one of the most vital proinflammatory cytokines, can induce vasodilatation, edema, and leukocyte adhesion to the epithelium. It can also regulate blood coagulation and contribute to oxidative stress in inflammation (Zelova and Hosek., 2013). Studies have shown that medications could decrease the release of inflammatory cytokines, such as TNF-α, reduce the inflammatory response, and promote wound healing (Weimann et al., 2018). In the present study, we found that BO could inhibit TNF-α release, which might be one potential anti-inflammatory mechanism of BO.

The secretion of VEGF in the healing process also exerts a significant effect, as VEGF can promote vascular endothelial cell proliferation and survival, accelerating the formation of new blood vessels (Peng et al., 2016; Wagner et al., 2016; Yan et al., 2017; Yen et al., 2018). The blood vessels are the channels of nutrient delivery in the body (Johnson and Wilgus, 2014), and it will ensure that the tissues and organs are provided with sufficient requirements for new skin formation (Sorg et al., 2018). Our results indicated that when the skin was scalded by high temperature, BO could upregulate the release of VEGF to facilitate wound healing. Also, collagen is necessary for repairing wounds. Studies had illustrated that TGF-β1 could regulate type I collagen gene expression and translation (Guo et al., 2018). However, the continuous increase of collagen I in the tissue will cause pathological scars to develop. Our results showed that the TGF-β1 content in the BO-treated group tended to increase early but decreased later. Based on these results, we speculated that with BO treatment, TGF-β1 stimulated the release of type I collagen at the early course to promote skin repair. At the later stage, to avoid collagen over-proliferation and scar formation, TGF-β1 expression is downregulated to inhibit the increase of collagen I.

The PI3K/AKT/mTOR signaling pathway is found in various cells and participates in cell growth, proliferation, apoptosis, and differentiation (Polivka and Janku., 2014; Peng et al., 2016; Dong et al., 2020). PI3K can be activated by growth factors, such as VEGF and TGF-β1 (Cui et al., 2017; Kim et al., 2018a; Zhang et al., 2019c). The activated state of growth factor receptors quickly phosphorylates phosphatidylinositol (4,5) P2 (PIP2) to obtain phosphatidylinositol (3,4,5) P3 (PI3P) (Zhang et al., 2019a). Protein kinase B (AKT) is one of the proteins downstream of PI3K; it is recruited by PI3P and phosphorylated by 3-phosphoinositide-dependent kinases (PDK-1) (Yudushkin, 2019). Then, p-AKT can regulate the protein level of phosphorylated mTOR to promote cellular growth and reproduction (Xu et al., 2018). Fibroblasts are a significant factor involved in wound healing. When tissue injury occurs, this signaling pathway is activated by increased VEGF and TGF-β1 levels, initiating fibroblasts migration to the wound site, proliferation, and differentiation into myofiibroblasts (Eming et al., 2014). These cells can help contract the wound border and contribute to producing collagen-like proteins, which are necessary for healing wounds and forming new skin tissue, accelerating the repair of burn wounds (Ohlund et al., 2014; Brenner et al., 2016; Xiao et al., 2017). Our Western blotting analysis showed that compared with the Con group, the BO-treated group had significantly increased activation of the PI3K/AKT/mTOR signaling pathway, with gradually upregulated phosphorylated proteins of this pathway. This finding suggested that the preliminary mechanism by which BO promoted burn repair might be related to the activation of the PI3K/AKT/mTOR signaling pathway.

In order to evaluate the quality and standard of preparations of BO, we detected and analyzed eight quality marker components in BO by HPLC, which contained aloe emodin, emodin, rhein, chrysophanol, ferulic acid, lobetyolin, asarinin, and borneol. The active compounds aloe emodin, emodin, rhein, and chrysophanol were reported to be quality markers of *Rheum palmatum* L. with anti-inflammatory activity and to promote wound healing, and their pathways of action may be involved in the proliferation and differentiation of skin epithelial cells through the regulation of PI3K/AKT pathway (Dong et al., 2016; Wu et al., 2017; Dong et al., 2019; Su et al., 2020). Ferulic acid is a quality marker of *Angelica sinensis* (Oliv.) Diels, which can promote wound healing (Wei et al., 2016). Lobetyolin is a quality marker of *Codonopsis pilosula* (Franch.) Nannf. Ferulic acid and lobetyolin can increase the content of VEGF in blood vessels and promote angiogenesis (Lin et al., 2010; Wang et al., 2020). Asarinin, a quality marker of *Asarum sieboldii* Miq., increases TGF-β content, reduces toe swelling, and regulates inflammation in arthritis model mice through the NF-κB pathway (Dai et al., 2019). And *Borneolum syntheticum*, whose chemical component is borneol, is a natural transdermal absorption enhancer that promotes BO absorption (Dai et al., 2018).

All of the above compounds have been reported to exhibit anti-inflammatory, analgesic, and skin healing promoting effects individually, but the combined effects of these compounds have not been investigated. In the present report, we investigated the role and mechanism of BO containing a mixture of active ingredients in anti-inflammatory and skin healing promotion. Our study showed that BO had a promising effect, which was most likely achieved by modulating the P13K/AKT transduction pathway.

5 CONCLUSION

In conclusion, this study demonstrated that BO is a pharmacologically active traditional Chinese medical formulation for promoting wound healing. It can accelerate wound healing through PI3K/AKT/mTOR signaling pathway and increase the key cytokines VEGF and TGF-β1 to further help tissue recovery. This study provides an insight into the in vivo effects of this preparation and its mechanism of action of BO in the treatment of burns and scalds, which will provide some guidance for the clinical application and development of BO.

AUTHOR CONTRIBUTIONS

MX and BH designed the research and wrote the paper. DG and LW performed animal experiments. QS carried out data sorting and statistics. HS performed biochemistry and immunology tests. JC supplied BO. All authors reviewed the manuscript.

REFERENCES

Ariyo, O. O., Ajayi, A. M., Ben-Azu, B., and Aderibigbe, A. O. (2020). Anti-nociceptive and anti-inflammatory activities of ethanol extract and fractions of Morus mesozygia Stapf (Moraceae) leaves and its underlying mechanisms in rodents. *J. Ethnopharmacol.* 259, 112934. doi:10.1016/j.jep.2020.11293410.1016/j.jep.2020.112934

Boldeanu, L., Boldeanu, M. V., Bogdan, M., Meca, A. D., Coman, C. G., Buca, B. R., et al. (2020). Immunological approaches and therapy in burns (review). *Exp. Ther. Med.* 20 (3), 2361–2367. doi:10.3892/etm.2020.8932

Brenner, A. K., Andersson, T. T., and Bruserud, O. (2016). The complexity of targeting PI3K-Akt-mTOR signalling in human acute myeloid leukaemia: the importance of leukemic cell heterogeneity, neighbouring mesenchymal stem cells and immunocompetent cells. *Molecules* 21 (11), 1512. doi:10.3390/molecules21111512

Cao, Y. J., Pu, Z. J., Tang, Y. P., Shen, J., Chen, Y. Y., Kang, A., et al. (2017). Advances in bio-active constituents, pharmacology and clinical applications of rhubarb. *Chin. Med.* 12, 36. doi:10.1186/s13020-017-0158-5

Chen, J., Si, M., Wang, Y., Liu, L., Zhang, Y., Zhou, A., et al. (2019). Ginsenoside metabolite compound K exerts anti-inflammatory and analgesic effects via downregulating COX_2. *Inflammopharmacology* 27 (1), 157–166. doi:10.1007/s10787-018-0504-y

Cho, H., Kim, J., Park, J., Hong, S., Kim, D., and Seo, K. (2019). Kochia scoparia seed extract suppresses VEGF-induced angiogenesis via modulating VEGF receptor 2 and PI3K/AKT/mTOR pathways. *Pharm. Biol.* 57 (1), 684–693. doi:10.1080/13880209.2019.1672753

Cui, J., Li, Z., Jin, C., and Jin, Z. (2020). Knockdown of fibronectin extra domain B suppresses TGF-β1-mediated cell proliferation and collagen deposition in keloid fibroblasts via AKT/ERK signaling pathway. *Biochem. Bioph. Res. Co.* 526 (4), 1131–1137. doi:10.1016/j.bbrc.2020.04.021

Cui, M., Pan, Z., and Pan, L. (2017). Danggui Buxue extract-loaded liposomes in thermosensitive gel enhance *in vivo* dermal wound healing via activation of the VEGF/PI3K/Akt and TGF-β/Smads signaling pathway. *Evid. Based Complement. Alternat. Med.* 2017, 8407249. doi:10.1155/2017/8407249

Dai, Q., Wang, M., Li, Y., and Li, J. (2019). Amelioration of CIA by asarinin is associated to a downregulation of TLR9/NF-κB and regulation of Th1/Th2/Treg expression. *Biol. Pharm. Bull.* 42 (7), 1172–1178. doi:10.1248/bpb.b19-00083

Dai, X., Wang, R., Wu, Z., Guo, S., Yang, C., Ma, L., et al. (2018). Permeation-enhancing effects and mechanisms of borneol and menthol on ligustrazine: a multiscale study using *in vitro* and coarse-grained molecular dynamics simulation methods. *Chem. Biol. Drug Des.* 92 (5), 1830–1837. doi:10.1111/cbdd.13350

Dong, X., Fu, J., Yin, X., Cao, S., Li, X., Lin, L., et al. (2016). Emodin: a review of its pharmacology, toxicity and pharmacokinetics. *Phytother Res.* 30 (8), 1207–1218. doi:10.1002/ptr.5631

Dong, X., He, Z., Xiang, G., Cai, L., Xu, Z., Mao, C., et al. (2020). Paeoniflorin promotes angiogenesis and tissue regeneration in a full-thickness cutaneous wound model through the PI3K/AKT pathway. *J. Cel Physiol.* 235 (12), 9933–9945. doi:10.1002/jcp.29808

Dong, X., Zeng, Y., Liu, Y., You, L., Yin, X., Fu, J., et al. (2019). Aloe-emodin: a review of its pharmacology, toxicity, and pharmacokinetics. *Phytother Res.* 34 (2), 270–281. doi:10.1002/ptr.6532

Eming, S. A., Martin, P., and Tomic-Canic, M. (2014). Wound repair and regeneration: mechanisms, signaling, and translation. *Sci. Transl. Med.* 6 (265), 265sr6. doi:10.1126/scitranslmed.3009337

Gao, S. M., Liu, J. S., Wang, M., Cao, T. T., Qi, Y. D., Zhang, B. G., et al. (2018). Traditional uses, phytochemistry, pharmacology and toxicology of Codonopsis: a review. *J. Ethnopharmacol.* 219, 50–70. doi:10.1016/j.jep.2018.02.039

Getachew, A., Assefa, B., and Wubayehu, K. (2019). Evaluation of wound healing and anti-inflammatory activity of the leaves of Calpurnia aurea (Ait.) Benth (fabaceae) in mice. *Wound Med.* 25 (1), 100151. doi:10.1016/j.wndm.2019.100151

Ghosh, D., Mondal, S., and Ramakrishna, K. (2019). A topical ointment formulation containing leaves extract of Aegialitis rotundifolia Roxb., accelerates excision, incision and burn wound healing in rats. *Wound Med.* 26 (1), 100168. doi:10.1016/j.wndm.2019.100168

Glim, J. E., Beelen, R. H., Niessen, F. B., Everts, V., and Ulrich, M. M. (2015). The number of immune cells is lower in healthy oral mucosa compared to skin and does not increase after scarring. *Arch. Oral Biol.* 60 (2), 272–281. doi:10.1016/j.archoralbio.2014.10.008

Gokakin, A. K., Deveci, K., Kurt, A., Karakus, B. C., Duger, C., Tuzcu, M., et al. (2013). The protective effects of sildenafil in acute lung injury in a rat model of severe scald burn: A biochemical and histopathological study. *Burns* 39 (6), 1193–1199. doi:10.1016/j.burns.2012.12.017

Gonzalez, A. C., Costa, T. F., Andrade, Z. A., and Medrado, A. R. (2016). Wound healing - a literature review. *Bras Dermatol.* 91 (5), 614–620. doi:10.1590/abd1806-4841.20164741

Govindaraju, P., Todd, L., Shetye, S., Monslow, J., and Puré, E. (2019). CD44-dependent inflammation, fibrogenesis, and collagenolysis regulates extracellular matrix remodeling and tensile strength during cutaneous wound healing. *Matrix Biol.* 75–76, 314–330. doi:10.1016/j.matbio.2018.06.004

Gundogdu, G., Gundogdu, K., Nalci, K. A., Demirkaya, A. K., Yilmaz, T. S., Demirkaya, M. F., et al. (2019). The effect of parietin isolated from *Rheum ribes* L. on *in vitro* wound model using human dermal fibroblast cells. *Int. J. Low Extrem. Wounds* 18 (1), 56–64. doi:10.1177/1534734618819660

Guo, S., Meng, X. W., Yang, X. S., Liu, X. F., Ou-Yang, C. H., and Liu, C. (2018). Curcumin administration suppresses collagen synthesis in the hearts of rats with experimental diabetes. *Acta Pharmacol. Sin.* 39 (2), 195–204. doi:10.1038/aps.2017.92

Johnson, K. E., and Wilgus, T. A. (2014). Vascular endothelial growth factor and angiogenesis in the regulation of cutaneous wound repair. *Adv. Wound Care* 3 (10), 647–661. doi:10.1089/wound.2013.0517

Kaddoura, I., Abu-Sittah, G., Ibrahim, A., Karamanoukian, R., and Papazian, N. (2017). Burn injury: review of pathophysiology and therapeutic modalities in major burns. *Ann. Burns Fire Disasters* 30 (2), 95–102.

Kazemi, M., Mohammadifar, M., Aghadavoud, E., Vakili, Z., Aarabi, M. H., and Talaei, S. A. (2020). Deep skin wound healing potential of lavender essential oil and licorice extract in a nanoemulsion form: biochemical, histopathological and gene expression evidences. *J. Tissue Viability* 29 (2), 116–124. doi:10.1016/j.jtv.2020.03.004

Kim, D., Jo, Y., Garagiola, U., Choi, J., Kang, Y., Oh, J., et al. (2020). Increased level of vascular endothelial growth factors by 4-hexylresorcinol is mediated by transforming growth factor-β1 and accelerates capillary regeneration in the burns in diabetic animals. *Int. J. Mol. Sci.* 21 (10), 3473. doi:10.3390/ijms21103473

Kim, K. K., Sheppard, D., and Chapman, H. A. (2018a). TGF-β1 signaling and tissue fibrosis. *Cold Spring Harb Perspect. Biol.* 10 (4), a022293. doi:10.1101/cshperspect.a022293

Kim, Y. J., Lee, J. Y., Kim, H. J., Kim, D. H., Lee, T. H., Kang, M. S., et al. (2018b). Anti-inflammatory effects of Angelica sinensis (Oliv.) Diels water extract on RAW 264.7 induced with lipopolysaccharide. *Nutrients* 10 (5), 647. doi:10.3390/nu10050647

Lin, C. M., Chiu, J. H., Wu, I. H., Wang, B. W., Pan, C. M., and Chen, Y. H. (2010). Ferulic acid augments angiogenesis via VEGF, PDGF and HIF-1 alpha. *J. Nutr. Biochem.* 21 (7), 627–633. doi:10.1016/j.jnutbio.2009.04.001

lund, D., Elyada, E., and Tuveson, D. (2014). Fibroblast heterogeneity in the cancer wound. *J. Exp. Med.* 211 (8), 1503–1523. doi:10.1084/jem.20140692

Naseri, N., Kalantar, K., and Amirghofran, Z. (2018). Anti-inflammatory activity of *Echium amoenum* extract on macrophages mediated by inhibition of inflammatory mediators and cytokines expression. *Res. Pharm. Sci.* 13 (1), 73–81. doi:10.4103/1735-5362.220970

Peng, N., Gao, S., Guo, X., Wang, G., Cheng, C., Li, M., et al. (2016). Silencing of VEGF inhibits human osteosarcoma angiogenesis and promotes cell apoptosis via VEGF/PI3K/AKT signaling pathway. *Am. J. Transl. Res.* 8 (2), 1005–1015.

Polivka, J. J., and Janku, F. (2014). Molecular targets for cancer therapy in the PI3K/AKT/mTOR pathway. *Pharmacol. Ther.* 142 (2), 164–175. doi:10.1016/j.pharmthera.2013.12.004

Riepl, M. (2020). Compounding pearls: wound care: burn healing, part 1. *Int. J. Pharm. Compd.* 24 (3), 188–193.

Roskoski, R. J. (2017). Vascular endothelial growth factor (VEGF) and VEGF receptor inhibitors in the treatment of renal cell carcinomas. *Pharmacol. Res.* 120, 116–132. doi:10.1016/j.phrs.2017.03.010

SenthilKumar, G., Fisher, M. M., Skiba, J. H., Miller, M. C., Brennan, S. R., Kaushik, S., et al. (2020). FGFR inhibition enhances sensitivity to radiation in non-small cell lung cancer. *Mol. Cancer Ther.* 19 (6), 1255–1265. doi:10.1158/1535-7163.MCT-19-0931

Shan, Y., Peng, L., Liu, X., Chen, X., Xiong, J., and Gao, J. (2015). Silk fibroin/gelatin electrospun nanofibrous dressing functionalized with astragaloside IV induces healing and anti-scar effects on burn wound. *Int. J. Pharm.* 479 (2), 291–301. doi:10.1016/j.ijpharm.2014.12.067

Shen, C., Zhang, Z., Xie, T., Ji, J., Xu, J., Lin, L., et al. (2019). Rhein suppresses lung inflammatory injury induced by human respiratory syncytial virus through inhibiting NLRP3 inflammasome activation via NF-κB pathway in mice. *Front. Pharmacol.* 10, 1600. doi:10.3389/fphar.2019.01600

Silvestre, M. C., Sato, M. N., and Reis, V. M. S. D. (2018). Innate immunity and effector and regulatory mechanisms involved in allergic contact dermatitis. *Bras Dermatol.* 93 (2), 242–250. doi:10.1590/abd1806-4841.20186340

Sorg, H., Tilkorn, D. J., Mirastschijski, U., Hauser, J., and Kraemer, R. (2018). Panta Rhei: neovascularization, angiogenesis and nutritive perfusion in wound healing. *Eur. Surg. Res.* 59 (3–4), 232–241. doi:10.1159/000492410

Srivastava, R. A. K., Cornicelli, J. A., Markham, B., and Bisgaier, C. L. (2018). Gemcabene, a first-in-class hypolipidemic small molecule in clinical development, attenuates osteoarthritis and pain in animal models of arthritis and pain. *Front. Pharmacol.* 9, 471. doi:10.3389/fphar.2018.00471

Su, S., Wu, J., Gao, Y., Luo, Y., Yang, D., and Wang, P. (2020). The pharmacological properties of chrysophanol, the recent advances. *Biomed. Pharmacother.* 125, 110002. doi:10.1016/j.biopha.2020.110002

Upadhyay, N. K., Kumar, R., Mandotra, S. K., Meena, R. N., Siddiqui, M. S., Sawhney, R. C., et al. (2009). Safety and healing efficacy of Sea buckthorn (*Hippophae rhamnoides* L.) seed oil on burn wounds in rats. *Food Chem. Toxicol.* 47 (6), 1146–1153. doi:10.1016/j.fct.2009.02.002

Wagner, V. P., Curra, M., Webber, L. P., Nor, C., Matte, U., Meurer, L., et al. (2016). Photobiomodulation regulates cytokine release and new blood vessel formation during oral wound healing in rats. *Lasers Med. Sci.* 31 (4), 665–671. doi:10.1007/s10103-016-1904-0

Wang, C., Hui, J., Zhu, X., Cui, S., Cui, Z., and Xu, D. (2020). Lobetyolin efficiently promotes angiogenesis and neuronal development in transgenic zebrafish. *Nat. Product. Commun.* 15 (8), 1–7. doi:10.1177/1934578X20937174

Wang, Y., Beekman, J., Hew, J., Jackson, S., Issler-Fisher, A. C., Parungao, R., et al. (2018). Burn injury: challenges and advances in burn wound healing, infection, pain and scarring. *Adv. Drug Deliv. Rev.* 123, 3–17. doi:10.1016/j.addr.2017.09.018

Wei, W. L., Zeng, R., Gu, C. M., Qu, Y., and Huang, L. F. (2016). Angelica sinensis in China-A review of botanical profile, ethnopharmacology, phytochemistry and chemical analysis. *J. Ethnopharmacol.* 190, 116–141. doi:10.1016/j.jep.2016.05.023

Weimann, E., Silva, M., Murata, G. M., Bortolon, J. R., Dermargos, A., Curi, R., et al. (2018). Topical anti-inflammatory activity of palmitoleic acid improves wound healing. *Plos One* 13 (10), e0205338. doi:10.1371/journal.pone.0205338

Wu, C., Cao, H., Zhou, H., Sun, L., Xue, J., Li, J., et al. (2017). Research progress on the antitumor effects of Rhein: literature review. *Anticancer Agents Med. Chem.* 17 (12), 1624–1632. doi:10.2174/1871520615666150930112631

Xavier-Santos, J. B., Félix-Silva, J., Passos, J. G. R., Gomes, J. A. S., Fernandes, J. M., Garcia, V. B., et al. (2018). Development of an effective and safe topical anti-inflammatory gel containing *Jatropha gossypiifolia* leaf extract: results from a pre-clinical trial in mice. *J. Ethnopharmacol.* 227, 268–278. doi:10.1016/j.jep.2018.09.007

Xiao, W., Tang, H., Wu, M., Liao, Y., Li, K., Li, L., et al. (2017). Ozone oil promotes wound healing by increasing the migration of fibroblasts via PI3K/Akt/mTOR signaling pathway. *Biosci. Rep.* 37 (6), BSR20170658. doi:10.1042/BSR20170658

Xu, J., Wang, S., Feng, T., Chen, Y., and Yang, G. (2018). Hypoglycemic and hypolipidemic effects of total saponins from Stauntonia chinensis in diabetic db/db mice. *J. Cell. Mol. Med.* 22 (12), 6026–6038. doi:10.1111/jcmm.13876

Yan, D., He, Y., Dai, J., Yang, L., Wang, X., and Ruan, Q. (2017). Vascular endothelial growth factor modified macrophages transdifferentiate into endothelial-like cells and decrease foam cell formation. *Biosci. Rep.* 37 (3), BSR20170002. doi:10.1042/BSR20170002

Yang, W. T., Ke, C. Y., Wu, W. T., Harn, H. J., Tseng, Y. H., and Lee, R. P. (2017). Effects of Angelica dahurica and Rheum officinale extracts on excisional wound healing in rats. *Evid. Based Complement. Alternat. Med.* 2017, 1583031. doi:10.1155/2017/1583031

Yaseen, H. S., Asif, M., Saadullah, M., MahrukhAsghar, S., Shams, M. U., et al. (2020). Methanolic extract of Ephedra ciliata promotes wound healing and arrests inflammatory cascade *in vivo* through downregulation of TNF-α. *Inflammopharmacology* 28 (6), 1691–1704. doi:10.1007/s10787-020-00713-7

Yen, Y. H., Pu, C. M., Liu, C. W., Chen, Y. C., Chen, Y. C., Liang, C. J., et al. (2018). Curcumin accelerates cutaneous wound healing via multiple biological actions: the involvement of TNF-α, MMP-9, α-SMA, and collagen. *Int. Wound J.* 15 (4), 605–617. doi:10.1111/iwj.12904

Yu, T., Li, Y. J., Bian, A. H., Zuo, H. B., Zhu, T. W., Ji, S. X., et al. (2014). The regulatory role of activating transcription factor 2 in inflammation. *Mediators Inflamm.* 2014, 950472. doi:10.1155/2014/950472

Yudushkin, I. (2019). Getting the AKT together: guiding intracellular AKT activity by PI3K. *Biomolecules* 9 (2), 67. doi:10.3390/biom9020067

Zahra, Z., Khan, M. R., Shah, S. A., Maryam, S., Majid, M., Younis, T., et al. (2020). Vincetoxicum arnottianum ameliorate inflammation by suppressing oxidative stress and pro-inflammatory mediators in rat. *J. Ethnopharmacol.* 252, 112565. doi:10.1016/j.jep.2020.112565

Zelova, H., and Hosek, J. (2013). TNF-α signaling and inflammation: interactions between old acquaintances. *Inflamm. Res.* 62 (7), 641–651. doi:10.1007/s00011-013-0633-0

Zhang, M., Jang, H., and Nussinov, R. (2019a). The mechanism of PI3Kα activation at the atomic level. *Chem. Sci.* 10 (12), 3671–3680. doi:10.1039/c8sc04498h

Zhang, Q., Hu, F., Guo, F., Zhou, Q., Xiang, H., and Shang, D. (2019b). Emodin attenuates adenosine triphosphate-induced pancreatic ductal cell injury *in vitro* via the inhibition of the P2X7/NLRP3 signaling pathway. *Oncol. Rep.* 42, 1589–1597. doi:10.3892/or.2019.7270

Zhang, Z., Zhang, X., Zhao, D., Liu, B., Wang, B., Yu, W., et al. (2019c). TGF-β1 promotes the osteoinduction of human osteoblasts via the PI3K/AKT/mTOR/S6K1 signaling pathway. *Mol. Med. Rep.* 19 (5), 3505–3518. doi:10.3892/mmr.2019.10051

Zhang, Y., Cai, W., Han, G., Zhou, S., Li, J., Chen, M., et al. (2020). Panax notoginseng saponins prevent senescence and inhibit apoptosis by regulating the PI3K-AKT-mTOR pathway in osteoarthritic chondrocytes. *Int. J. Mol. Med.* 45 (4), 1225–1236. doi:10.3892/ijmm.2020.4491

13

Plant-Derived Compounds as Promising Therapeutics for Vitiligo

Yaobin Pang[1], Shi Wu[1], Yingjie He[1], Qing Nian[1], Jing Lei[1], Yejing Yao[1], Jing Guo[1] and Jinhao Zeng[2,3]**

[1]Dermatological Department, Hospital of Chengdu University of Traditional Chinese Medicine, Chengdu, China, [2]Geriatric Department, Hospital of Chengdu University of Traditional Chinese Medicine, Chengdu, China, [3]TCM Regulating Metabolic Diseases Key Laboratory of Sichuan Province, Hospital of Chengdu University of Traditional Chinese Medicine, Chengdu, China

***Correspondence:**
Jing Guo
guojing66@cdutcm.edu.cn
Jinhao Zeng
zengjinhao@cdutcm.edu.cn

Vitiligo is the most common depigmenting disorder characterized by white patches in the skin. The pathogenetic origin of vitiligo revolves around autoimmune destruction of melanocytes in which, for instance, oxidative stress is responsible for melanocyte molecular, organelle dysfunction and melanocyte specific antigen exposure as well as melanocyte cell death and thus serves as an important contributor for vitiligo progression. In recent years, natural products have shown a wide range of pharmacological bioactivities against many skin diseases, and this review focuses on the effects and mechanisms of natural compounds against vitiligo models. It is showed that some natural compounds such as flavonoids, phenols, glycosides and coumarins have a protective role in melanocytes and thereby arrest the depigmentation, and, additionally, Nrf2/HO-1, MAPK, JAK/STAT, cAMP/PKA, and Wnt/β-catenin signaling pathways were reported to be implicated in these protective effects. This review discusses the great potential of plant derived natural products as anti-vitiligo agents, as well as the future directions to explore.

Keywords: vitiligo, oxidative stress, natural product, melanocytes, flavonoids, phenols, glycosides

INTRODUCTION

Pathogenesis of Vitiligo

Vitiligo is a chronic autoimmune destruction of melanocytes, leading to the pigment loss on the surface of skin and mucosa and then the gradual expansion of decolorized skin plaque (Seneschal et al., 2021). The severity of the disease affects about 1% of humans (Whitton et al., 2015). Clinically, vitiligo is divided into segmental vitiligo (SV), non-segmental vitiligo (NSV) and mixed vitiligo (MV) (Ezzedine et al., 2015). NSV is the most common type of vitiligo. Its clinical features are clear boundary, reticular, different size, different distribution, depigmentation and milky white. SV is a piece or several pieces, along the skin area dominated by a certain cutaneous ganglion segment,

---

Abbreviations: HO-1, heme oxygenase-1; Nrf2, The nuclear factor erythroid 2-like factor 2; NE, Norepinephrine; GCLM, g-glutamylcystine ligase modulatory subunit; GCLC, g-glutamylcystine ligase catalytic subunit; Cyt-4, cytochrome c; ROS, reactive oxygen species; TYR, tyrosinase; TRP-1, tyrosinase-related protein 1; TRP-2, tyrosinase-related protein 2; MITF, microphthalmia-associated transcription factor; MAPK, mitogen-activated protein kinase; ERK, extracellular signal-regulated kinase; JNK, c-Jun N-terminal kinase; cAMP, intracellular cyclic adenosine monophosphate; GSK-3β, glycogen synthase kinase 3β; cRE, cAMP-response element; cREB, cAMP-response element binding protein; PKA, protein kinase A; α-MSH, α melanocyte stimulating hormone; PI3K, phosphoinositide 3-kinase; Akt, protein kinase B; c-Kit, proto-oncogene; TNF-α, tumor necrosis factor alpha; IFN-γ, interferon-γ; ARE, antioxidant response element; SOD, Superoxide dismutase; CAT, catalase; HEMn, normal human epidermal melanocytes; HEKn, normal human epidermal keratinocytes

generally unilateral, accounting for 5–16% of all vitiligo cases (Speeckaert et al., 2020). MV includes the combination of SV and then bilateral NSV plaque after a period of time (Ezzedine et al., 2015). The debilitating nature of vitiligo leads to poor quality of life and mental health (Patel et al., 2017). Dermal exposure to UV light from depigmented skin increases the risk of skin irritation and cancer (Ahluwalia et al., 2017).

The main theories of the pathogenesis of vitiligo are: 1) oxidative stress theory, 2) autoimmune theory, 3) neural theory and 4) biochemical theory. The autoimmune theory is the most accepted one (Rodrigues et al., 2017). More than half of the 40 susceptibility genes revealed by genome-wide analysis are involved in immunoregulatory activities (Jin et al., 2016). Strong evidence shows that oxidative stress is a key factor in the occurrence and development of diseases (Denat et al., 2014). Several endogenous and exogenous stimuli are related to the occurrence of diseases. Endogenous factors include melanin synthesis, proliferation, differentiation, cell metabolism, immune response and apoptosis (Al-Shobaili and Rasheed 2015). Exogenous stimuli include exposure to the environment (e.g., cytotoxic chemicals, trauma, UV exposure, monophenones and other phenolics), other diseases (severe infections, neurological disorders, malignancies, calcium imbalance), and pharmaceutical applications (e.g., certain hormones, vaccination, drugs) (Xie et al., 2016). These all induce oxidative stress in melanocytes, which may be important in activating autoimmune responses associated with vitiligo (Abdel-Malek et al., 2020; Chen X. et al., 2019; Xie et al., 2016). The decrease of the level and activity of antioxidant enzymes (such as catalase and glutathione peroxidase) and the imbalance of Pro oxidation/anti oxidation balance are also the reasons for the production and accumulation of ROS (Wang Y. et al., 2019). Nrf2-ARE regulates cellular protective genes related to oxidative stress (Jian et al., 2011). In vitiligo melanocytes, Nrf2 has nuclear translocation and decreased transcriptional activity, resulting in decreased HO-1 expression and abnormal redox balance (Jian et al., 2014). Due to the deficiency of antioxidant function, melanocytes in vitiligo are particularly sensitive to ROS accumulation, which leads to DNA damage, protein oxidation/breakage, mitochondrial dysfunction, endoplasmic reticulum abnormalities and lipid peroxidation (Bickers and Athar 2006; Chen J. et al., 2021). Increased ROS levels even modified tyrosinase (Tyr) and other melanin proteins into new antigens (Rodrigues et al., 2017). Oxidative stress leads to the accumulation of misfolded proteins in the lumen of the endoplasmic reticulum (ER), which in turn activates the unfolded protein response (UPR) to restore cellular homeostasis and maintain cell survival. The disturbance of endoplasmic reticulum Ca2+ triggered by oxidative stress may also induce UPR and apoptosis (Carreras-Sureda et al., 2018). Under continuous cell pressure, UPR promotes autoimmune response through apoptosis cascade, and then activates $CD8^+$ T cells to produce adaptive immune response, and T cells release interferon-γ (INF-γ), It binds to receptors on keratinocytes, further releases and presents inflammatory cytokines such as CXC-L16 and IL-15, and further recruits T cells to the skin through a positive feedback loop (Bergqvist and Ezzedine 2021). The recruitment of $CD8^+$and T cells induced by cytokines and chemokines ensure the final destruction of epidermal melanocytes (**Figure 1**). After naive T cells are activated by antigen-presenting cells, a small subset of these precursor cells eventually develop into several subsets of memory T cells, including effector memory T (T_{EM}) cells, tissue resident memory T (T_{RM}) cells and central memory T (T_{CM}) cells. T_{RM} play a major role in vitiligo recurrence (Chen and Shen 2020). In the process, melanocytes, fibroblasts, innate lymphoid cells, natural killer cells, and keratinocytes collectively contribute to the pathogenesis of vitiligo (Seneschal et al., 2021).

Vitiligo Therapy

However, there is no clear treatment for local and systemic vitiligo. The most widely used therapy is local steroid and narrowband ultraviolet B monotherapy (Grimes and Nashawati 2017), they are not effective in all patients and are expensive, not easily accepted, and are associated with side effects (Huo et al., 2014). Local corticosteroids, calcineurin inhibitors and phototherapy are still the basis of treatment, and long-term use of steroids can lead to decreased immunity (Whitton et al., 2016). Among the numerous treatments currently available, including medical, physical, or surgical approaches, each modality has its disadvantages and side effects (Yamaguchi et al., 2007).

In vivo and *in vitro* experiments, natural products have been shown to promote melanin production and prevent melanin from being destroyed in a network way. It mainly includes scavenging free radicals (NOS) to alleviate the damage of melanocytes caused by oxidative stress, activating melanogenesis related pathways, increasing the expression of tyrosinase gene, reducing the expression of chemokines and inflammatory cytokines, preventing the migration of CD8 + T cells. This paper reviews several natural drugs for the treatment of vitiligo. Among the natural products that we screened, 16 compounds (such as baicalein, quercetin, paeonol. etc) exert antioxidant effects to protect melanocytes by scavenging free radicals, activating the Nrf2/HO-1 pathway, while maintaining normal cell morphology, slowing down apoptosis and preventing injury. Four compounds (vitexin, baicalin, EGCG and berberine) achieved repigmentation of vitiligo skin lesions via anti-inflammatory effects, the process of which involved the activation of the JAK/STAT pathway as well as the inhibition of autoimmunity caused by the migration of immune cells such as CD8 + T. In mammals, there are three major melanocyte specific enzymes catalyzing melanin biosynthesis: tyrosinase (TYR), tyrosinase associated protein 1 (TRP-1) and TRP-2. TRP-1 and Trp-2 are downstream functional proteins of TYR (Yin et al., 2018). Microphthalmia associated transcription factor (MITF) is a transcription factor important for melanogenesis genes (Hearing 1999). Previous studies summarized three main pathways of melanin biosynthesis regulated by tyrosinase: MAPK, cAMP/PKA, Wnt/β - catenin signaling pathway, and reviewed the effects of several natural products on melanin synthesis and tyrosinase activity (Niu and Aisa 2017; Pillaiyar et al., 2017). Among the compounds we screened, 37 compounds (such as quercetin, afzelin, puerarin, geniposide, etc) promote melanocyte generation through the above pathways (**Figure 2**).

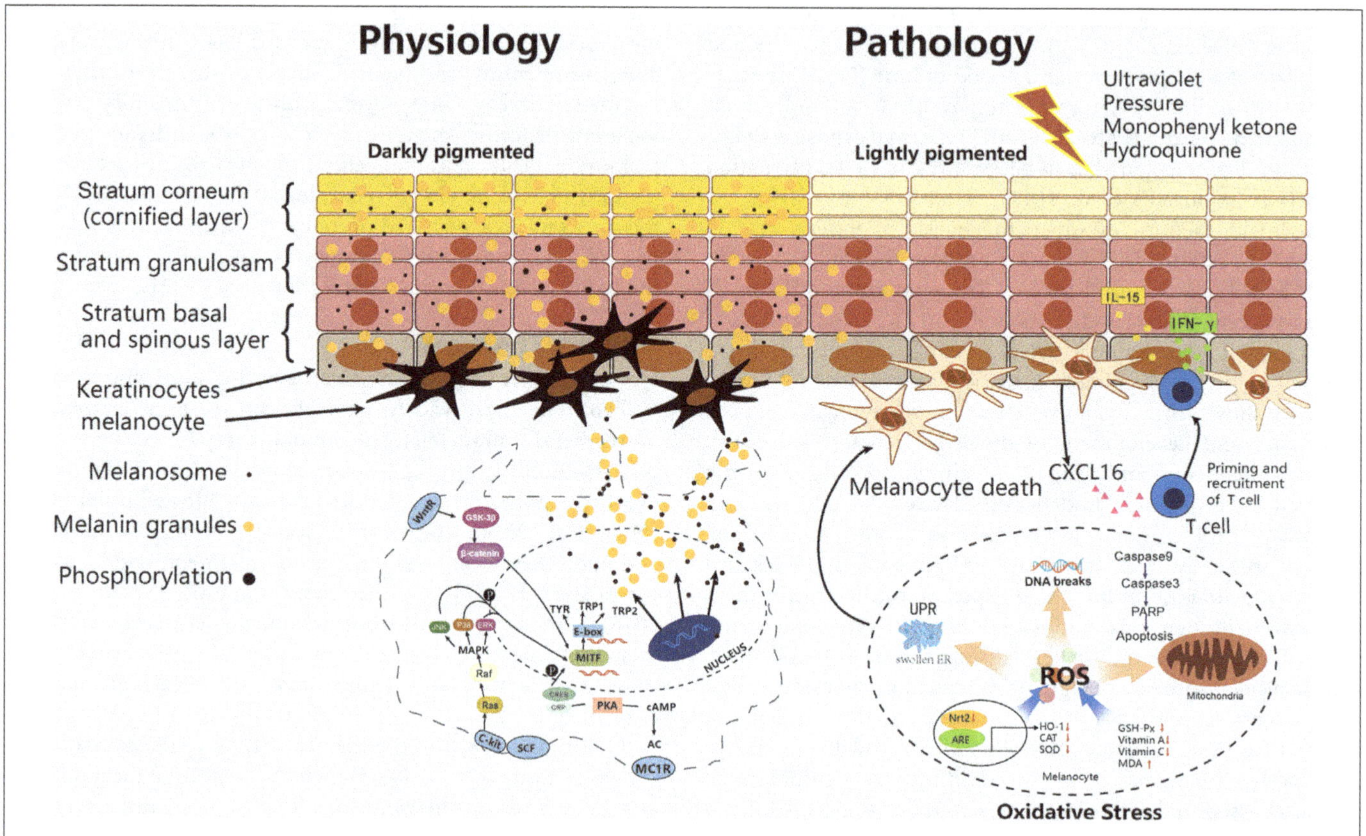

FIGURE 1 | Melanocyte pathophysiology in vitiligo.

Flavonoids

Baicalein

Baicalein is a flavonoid extracted from the roots of Scutellaria baicalensis Georgi that has been extensively applied in Traditional Medicine in Asia (**Figure 3A**) (Kim et al., 2014). It has been reported to have anti-cytotoxic, anti-inflammatory, and anti-tumor effects (Huang et al., 2005; Hwang et al., 2005; Yarla et al., 2016). In addition, the antioxidant effects of baicalein have received special attention during the past decades, including reducing the levels of reactive oxygen species (ROS) generated by chemical agents (Chiu et al., 2010; Choi et al., 2016; Zhao et al., 2018) or ultraviolet radiation (Wang et al., 2018). Baicalein has strong antioxidant properties, partly because compounds scavenge ROS by oxidative consumption of the three 5, 6, 7-position OH–groups in its structure (de Oliveira et al., 2015), and it form stable semiquinone radicals, which also underlie its powerful antioxidant activity (Gao et al., 1999). The apoptosis of PIG1 cells induced by H_2O_2 may be mediated by mitochondrial pathway. In the *in vitro* model of H_2O_2-induced oxidative stress of PIG1, baicalein protected PIG1 cells from H_2O_2-induced oxidative stress and apoptosis, maintained mitochondrial membrane potential, released cytochrome c, and decreased the Bax/Bcl-2 ratio. The mechanism mainly involves the activation of mitochondrial dependent caspase and the regulation of p38MAPK pathway. Baicalein at the concentration of 40 μM had the strongest protective effect on melanocytes (Liu et al., 2012). In human vitiligo melanocytes (PIG3V) induced by hydrogen peroxide, baicalein increased the expression of Nrf2 and its downstream gene HO-1 in PIG3V cells, promoted the translocation of Nrf2 from cytoplasm to nucleus, indicating that the protective effect of baicalein on melanocytes depends on Nrf2 signaling pathway (Ma et al., 2018). Baicalein also has antioxidant effect on keratinocytes (Wang et al., 2018), therefore, the development of baicalein topical preparation for the treatment of vitiligo may be a feasible method.

Quercetin

Quercetin is a kind of polyhydroxy flavonoid, which is chemically named 3,3,4,5,7-pentahydroxyflavone (**Figure 3B**). It has high content in apple, onion and green tea, and also exists in *Asparagus racemosus* Willd., Ficus ingens (Miq.) Miq., Coriandrum sativum L. and Capparis spinosa L. It is one of the most consumed flavonoids in people's daily diet (Alvarez-Arellano et al., 2020). Quercetin has a variety of biological activities, such as antioxidant and scavenging free radicals (Wang et al., 2021e), anti-cancer, anti-aging (Zhu et al., 2015), anti-inflammatory (Rauf et al., 2018; Cui et al., 2019) anti-virus and immune regulation (Zhu et al., 2015; Alvarez-Arellano et al., 2020). It has a very important clinical significance in the treatment of bacterial infection, viral infection, hyperlipidemia and immune system diseases, especially for those caused by increased oxidative stress Cell damage and even mitochondrial dysfunction related diseases have potential

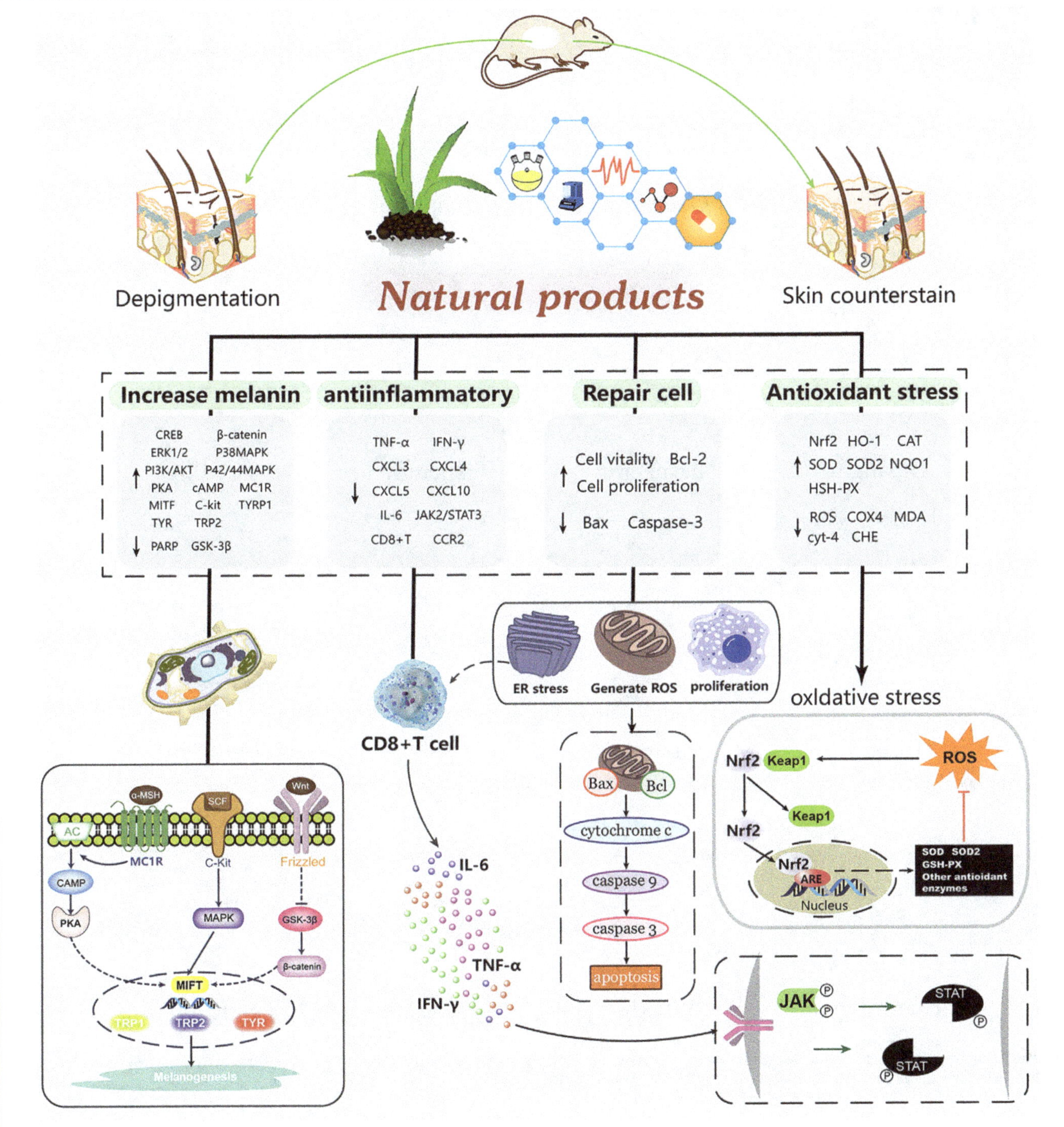

FIGURE 2 | Mechanism of natural products in the treatment of vitiligo.

therapeutic effects. Quercetin treatment of cultured melanoma cells or NHEM promote melanin synthesis and tyrosinase activity. In cell experiment, treatment of HMVII cells with quercetin at different doses (1, 5, 10, 20 μm) and for different times (1, 3, 5, 7 days) resulted in a dose and time-dependent increase in melanin content. The mechanism of action may be reflected by the genomic mechanism of new messenger RNA and protein synthesis (Nagata et al., 2004). Interestingly, the triple combination of GT extract/quercetin/folic acid prevented H_2O_2-induced cell damage in a synergistic manner, suggesting that effective antioxidant combinations should be studied to combat ROS types. Among them, quercetin and GT extract had strong protective effect on H_2O_2 induced cell death, and 100 μm quercetin had the most significant protective effect (Jeong

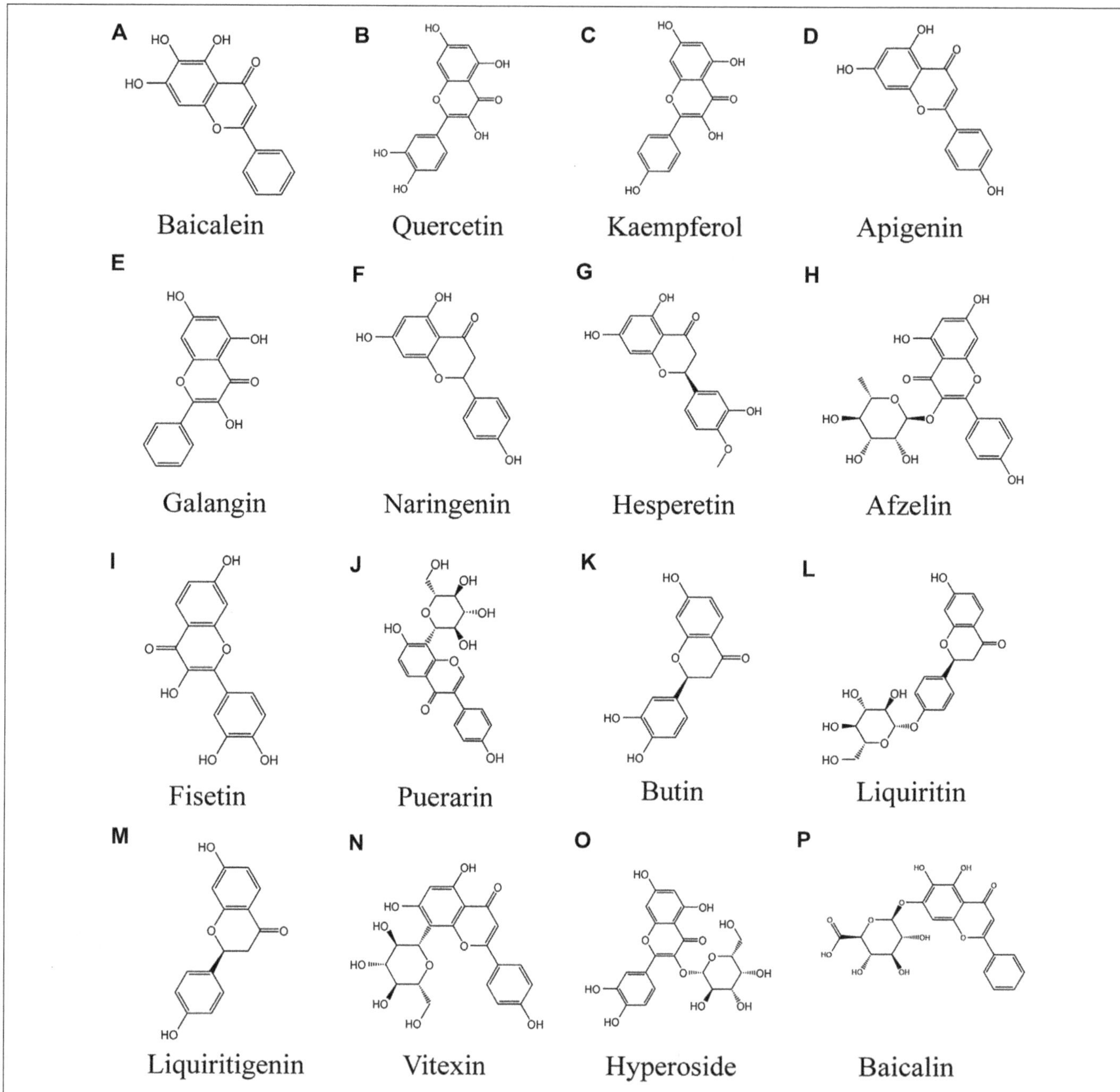

FIGURE 3 | Anti vitiligo flavonoids **(A)** Baicalein, **(B)** Quercetin, **(C)** Kaempferol, **(D)** Apigenin, **(E)** Galangin, **(F)** Naringenin, **(G)** Hesperetin, **(H)** Afzelin, **(I)** Fisetin, **(J)** Puerarin, **(K)** Butin, **(L)** Liquiritin, **(M)** Liquiritigenin, **(N)** Vitexin, **(O)** Hyperoside, **(P)** Baicalin.

et al., 2005). Cuiping Guan et al. observed endoplasmic reticulum expansion and configuration changes in cells treated with H_2O_2 and $NaOH/H_2O_2$. Quercetin alleviated the increase of ROS level induced by H_2O_2, and weakened the inhibition of tyrosinase expression by hydrogen peroxide. The mechanism may be to prevent oxidative stress damage, and tyrosinase is effectively exported from endoplasmic reticulum (Guan et al., 2015). Different nanoparticles, such as transporter, solid lipid nanoparticles, nanostructured lipid carriers, liposomes, nano emulsions and polymer nanoparticles, maximize the ideal properties and/or therapeutic activity of quercetin (Nasr and Al-Karaki 2020), which provides a feasibility for the external treatment of vitiligo with quercetin.

Kaempferol

Kaempferol (**Figure 3C**) is a kind of flavonoids, which mainly comes from the rhizome of Kaempferia galanga L. (Liu Z. Q. et al., 2021). It widely exists in all kinds of fruits, vegetables and beverages, hazelnut, tea, propolis, broccoli and grapefruit (Calderón-Montaño et al., 2011). Kaempferol can be used to combat cardiovascular disease, cancer outbreak, immune dysfunction, diabetes, oxidative stress and other diseases (Imran et al., 2019). Kaempferol has no obvious cytotoxic effect on B16F10 cells at the concentration of 16–32 μm for 24 h (Wang et al., 2017). Kaliziri is an extract from Baccharoides anthelmintica (L.) Moench, which has showed relatively good therapeutic effects for vitiligo (Maimaiti et al., 2017). Kaempferol is one of the main active components of *Baccharoides anthelmintica* (L.) Moench extract (Tuerxuntayi et al., 2014). After treatment with 1, 5, 10 and 20 μm kaempferol for 7 days, melanin content in hmvii cells increased significantly. It enhanced tyrosinase activity in HMVII cells and mouse buccal hair follicles by inducing tyrosinase protein expression (Takekoshi et al., 2014). Based on the SDTNBI method and experimental verification, kaempferol markedly increased tyrosinase activity and melanin biosynthesis gene expression in B16F10 cells, and effectively promoted melanin synthesis (Wang et al., 2017).

Apigenin

Apigenin (4′, 5,7-trihydroxyflavone; (**Figure 3D**) natural plant flavone, widely exists in common fruits and vegetables. It is considered to be a flavonoid with biological activity (Liu et al., 2017). Compared with other flavonoids, apigenin is relatively non-toxic and non-mutagenic, and has significant effects on normal cells and cancer cells (Patel et al., 2007). It has demonstrated a variety of pharmacological effects, including antidepressant (Li et al., 2015; Zhang X. et al., 2019), anti-inflammatory, liver protection, antithrombotic, anticancer, anti-aging (Lim et al., 2015), anti-oxidant (Wang J. et al., 2020). Apigenin significantly increased the activities of glutathione peroxidase (GSH PX), catalase (CAT) and superoxide dismutase (SOD), in a dose-dependent manner, and significantly inhibited the level of malondialdehyde (MDA), a biomarker of oxidative stress, in a H_2O_2 induced cell line PIG3V. Interestingly, apigenin markedly increased protein expression levels of Nrf2 and its downstream NQO1 and HO-1 in a dose-dependent manner, but had no effect on Nrf2 knockout cells. The results showed that apigenin protects melanocytes from oxidative damage dependent Nrf2 pathway (Zhang et al., 2020). In the dopamine (DA)—induced melanocyte model, 10 μm apigenin treatment significantly reduced ROS aggregation, reduced Da induced melanocyte apoptosis, and inhibited caspase-3 and PARP activities, which may be involved in the anti-apoptotic effect of apigenin. The mechanisms include inhibition of JNK, p38MAPK and Akt (Lin M. et al., 2011). *In vitro*, HMVII cells were treated with apigenin at 1, 5, 10 and 20 μm for 7 days, and the melanin content increased significantly (Takekoshi et al., 2014). So far, there is little evidence that apigenin promote adverse metabolic reactions *in vivo* when ingesting nutrition related amounts (Shukla and Gupta 2010; Takekoshi et al., 2014; Weng et al., 2016). Apigenin's local drug delivery system transports apigenin to local skin tissue instead of penetrating into blood circulation (Li et al., 1996). Therefore, apigenin may be a relatively safe method for the treatment of vitiligo.

Galangin

Galangin (GA, 3,5,7-trihydroxyflavone; **Figure 3E**) is an important natural active flavone, which is mainly extracted from the roots of Alpinia officinarum Hance, it has long been used as herbs and spices in South Africa and Asia (Yang et al., 2018). GA has been reported to possess a variety of biological activities, including antibacterial (Skiba et al., 2016), antiviral, anti-inflammatory (Cushnie et al., 2007), anti-obesity (Ma et al., 2019) and antioxidant (Sinha et al., 2014), it is reported that these effects are exerted by regulating NF - κ B, Nrf2 and cAMP/CREB signaling pathways (Yang C.-C. et al., 2020). 4.25 mg/kg GA significantly increased the number of basal melanocytes and melanoepidermal cells in shaving area of mice with hydroquinone induced vitiligo, and promote the melanin hair follicles to increase, the mechanism is to prevent oxidative stress by reducing cholinesterase (CHE) activity and MDA content and increase the expression of TYR protein. Malondialdehyde (MDA) is the final product of lipid peroxidation, which is considered as a specific indicator of oxidative stress (Huo et al., 2014). However, GA metabolism is fast and its bioavailability is low. 90% of GA is metabolized in 1 h and is metabolized in 2 h in hepatocytes. Therefore, it is necessary to modify GA by methylation to slow down its metabolism and improve its bioavailability (Fang et al., 2019).

Naringenin and Hesperetin

Naringenin (**Figure 2F**) and hesperetin (**Figure 3G**) are two main flavonoids identified from Citrus × limon (L.) Osbeck extract (Singh et al., 2020). The flavonoids in sweet orange peel include flavonoid glycosides, flavones and flavonols, among which flavanones exist in the form of glycosides (hesperidin and naringenin) or aglycones (hesperidin and naringenin) (Ramful et al., 2010). Citrus flavonoids have many biological activities, such as anti-tumor, anti-oxidation and anti-inflammatory (Salehi et al., 2019). It was found that flavonoids from navel orange peel extract had antioxidant activity (Long et al., 2021). Citrus products stimulate cell melanin production and tyrosinase expression, thereby preventing skin damage caused by ultraviolet light (Chiang et al., 2011). Huang et al. (2012) used 20 μg/ml citrus extract for melanin synthesis experiment. Citrus are rich in hesperidin, neohesperidin or naringin, and acid hydrolytic extracts of these three species of Citrus promote melanin synthesis. In this experiment, 50 μm hesperetin increased the expression of β-catenin, induced the rapid phosphorylation of p38MAPK, ERK and Akt, and activated the downstream transcription factor CREB phosphorylation in less than 1 h. Hesperidin stimulates melanogenesis by activating CREB and MAPKs in Wnt/β-catenin pathway (Huang et al., 2012). Naringenin enhanced tyrosinase activity of B16 mouse melanocytes in a time-dependent manner and increased melanin content in a concentration dependent manner, reaching the maximum at 100 μM. The mechanism included increasing the expression level of melanin producing enzyme (TYRP1 and DCT) and MITF (Ohguchi et al., 2006). Another study also confirmed that naringenin up-regulated tyrosinase activity of B16-F10 cells in a concentration dependent manner. Naringenin up regulated the expression of MITF by increasing the expression of β-catenin and the phosphorylation of Akt or GSK3, and then increased the activity of tyrosinase, so as to improve the melanin synthesis of B16-F10 cells, rather than through cAMP pathway (Huang et al., 2011). These results suggest that hesperetin induced melanogenesis in cell models may contribute to the development of topical beauty agents.

Afzelin

Afzelin (3-O-α-L-rhamnopyranoside; **Figure 3H**) is a flavonoid isolated from Thesium chinense Turcz. and widely distributed in Korea and China (Li G.-H. et al., 2021). Previous studies have shown that afzelin has antibacterial, anticancer and anti-inflammatory effects (Satthakarn et al., 2015). Afzelin markedly alleviated ultraviolet induced oxidative stress in human skin, damage of mitochondrial membrane potential and mitochondrial permeability (Shin et al., 2013). Afzelin showed strong anti-oxidant activity in DPPH radical scavenging experiment (Kim et al., 2008). Many studies have shown that afzelin could effectively treat skin diseases (Lee et al., 2014). In the experiment of melanogenesis induced by afzelin in human epidermal melanocytes, 100 μm afzelin increased the protein levels of TRP-1 and TYR by up regulating MITF, but did not increase the protein levels of TRP-2. The mechanism is p38MAPK phosphorylation, which up regulates MITF, and is independent of cAMP/PKA pathway (Jung et al., 2016).

Fisetin

Fisetin (3,30,40,7-tetrahydroxyflavone; **Figure 3I**) is a dietary flavone, which exists in a variety of vegetables and fruits, including apples, strawberries, grapes, cucumbers and onions (Khan et al., 2018). Studies have found that fisetin has anti allergic, anti-arthritis and neuroprotective effects (Ahmad et al., 2017; Ahmad et al., 2019). New data also showed that fisetin had anti-cancer activity (Jie et al., 2015; Khan and Mukhtar 2015; Ding et al., 2020). In particular, it has recently been found that it inhibited inflammation and antioxidant stress (Silva et al., 2007; Ahmad et al., 2019). Interestingly, fisetin has a two-way regulatory effect on melanin production. Takekoshi et al. first reported that fisetin could promote Tyr activity and melanin content of human melanoma cells (Takekoshi et al., 2014). However, Shon et al. found that fisetin inhibited the melanin content in and out of mouse B16F10 melanoma cells mediated by α - MSH(Shon et al., 2016). A recent study found that the difference of dual effects of fisetin was related to its concentration, because high concentration of fisetin inhibited the synthesis of melanin in zebrafish larvae (400 μm) and B16F10 melanoma cells (40 μm). When the concentration of fisetin exceeded 25 μm, the inhibitory activity increased slightly, and 200 μ m had the highest inhibitory rate on mushroom tyrosinase activity *in vitro*. Surprisingly, 5 μm fisetin slightly increased the content of spontaneous melanin and extracellular melanin, fisetin (at 20 μm) markedly increased the content and release of melanin in B16F10 cells by up regulating the expression of TYR and MITF, and promoted the melanin synthesis of zebrafish larvae. The mechanism is that fistein inhibits GSK-3 β, which activates β - Catenin, which leads to melanogenesis by activating MITF and tyrosinase (Molagoda et al., 2020). Therefore, low dose of fisetin may be an effective drug in the treatment of vitiligo.

Puerarin

Puerarin (7,40-dihydroxyisoflavone-8b-glucopyranoside; **Figure 3J**) is an isoflavonoid derivative isolated from the root of the traditional Chinese medicine *Pueraria lobata* (Willd.) Ohwi (Zhang 2019). Puerarin exhibits a wide range of antioxidant activities in cardiovascular diseases, diabetes, obesity, osteoporosis, and other diseases (Xu et al., 2021; Chang et al., 2021; Liu Y. et al., 2021; Xiao et al., 2020). In addition, puerarin has anti-inflammatory, anti-viral and other pharmacological activities (Wang Z.-K. et al., 2020; Wang H. X. et al., 2021). Puerarin exhibited obvious pharmacological activities against vitiligo *in vitro* and *in vivo*. Park et al. found that puerarin could increase the melanin content of melanocytes *in vitro*, and topical application could improve the melanin content of mouse skin tissue, the mechanism is via activation of the cAMP pathway, followed by elevation of MITF, tyrosinase, Trp-2, and Bcl-2 to increase melanocyte survival and melanin content (Park et al., 2014). In the 4-benzyloxyphenol-induced vitiligo mouse model, after one week of Puerarin Treatment, HE staining of the skin at the depigmented sites showed increased hair follicles, which were surrounded by a large number of melanocytes. Puerarin at 40 μmol/L significantly increased the melanin content of human melanocytes by decreasing the phosphorylation of ERK in the cells to promote TRP-1 and MITF expression, which led to an increase in melanin content (Ding et al., 2019).

Butin

Butin (7, 30, 40-trihydroxydihydroflavone, BUT; (**Figure 3K**) flavonoid with antioxidant activity, isolated from *Alpinia officinarum* Hance, *Dalbergia odorifera* T.C.Chen (Duan et al., 2017). BUT exhibited a wide range of pharmacological activities for the treatment of aging, diabetes, liver diseases, and cancer (Zhang et al., 2011). In the hydroquinone-induced vitiligo mouse model, (4.25, 42.5 mg/kg) butin increased the melanin content in the skin lesions by increasing the expression of Tyr and TRP-1 protein, reducing the serum cholinesterase activity and malondialdehyde content. Besides, BUT promoted the proliferation of basal melanocytes (Huo et al., 2017). A recent study found that butin induced melanin production both *in vivo* and *in vitro* when the concentration was 40 μmol/L, while tyrosinase activity peaked. Meanwhile, in a H_2O_2-induced zebrafish model, butin reduced the levels of reactive oxygen species *in vivo* (Lai et al., 2021).

Liquiritin and Liquiritigenin

Liquiritigenin (LQ; **Figure 3L**) and liquiritigenin (LQG; **Figure 3M**) are flavonoids extracted from *Glycyrrhiza uralensis* Fisch. ex DC. (Du et al., 2021; Mou et al., 2021). They have many biological activities, such as antiviral, anti-inflammatory, anti-oxidation, anti-tumor and so on (Pastorino et al., 2018). LQ and LQG were used to treat mouse melanoma B16-F1 cells and human melanoma hmvii cells with different doses for 72 h. The results showed that both natural drugs significantly increased the content of melanin in melanocytes in a dose-dependent manner, and had no effect on cell viability. Interestingly, both LQ and LQG could significantly up regulate tyrosinase activity and the expression of MITF and its downstream TRP-1 and Trp-2. Further studies have found that 50 μm LQ and LQG trigger melanin synthesis through p38 phosphorylation and activation of PKA/CREB signaling pathway (Uto et al., 2019).

Vitexin

Vitexin (apigenin-8-C-β-D-glucopyranoside; **Figure 3N**) is a natural flavonoid present in various medicinal plants such as: *Crataegus* L., *Vigna* Savi, *Passiflora cristalina* Vanderpl. & Zappi, *Mimosa* L., bamboo, etc (He et al., 2016). It has many pharmacological activities, anti-inflammatory, antiviral, anticancer, antihypertensive (Ding et al., 2021; Chen Y. et al., 2021). At the same time, Vitexin is an antioxidant (Ożarowski and Karpiński 2020). In H_2O_2-induced human melanocyte PIG1, Vitexin inhibited hydrogen peroxide induced apoptosis and promoted cell proliferation by activating the MAPK-Nrf2/ARE pathway, including decreasing IL-1β. The expression of IL-17A, Bax, caspase-3 and ROS, up-regulated the expression of p53, Bcl-2, Nrf2, HO-1, NQO-1, SOD (Li et al., 2020).

Hyperoside

Hyperoside (quercetin-3-O-galactoside, Hyp; **Figure 3O**) belongs to flavonol glycosides isolated from *Rhododendron brachycarpum* D. Don ex g. don, *Abelmoschus manihot* (L.) Medik. *Rhododendron* L.(Zhou et al., 2021). Studies have shown that Hyp possesses antioxidant, anticancer, antifibrotic, antiallergic, anti-inflammatory and other pharmacological activities (Huang et al., 2020). Hyperoside markly increased the proliferation of melanocytes in a dose - and time-dependent manner *in vitro*. In the H_2O_2-induced melanocyte model, Hyp protected melanocytes from oxidative damage by regulating the PI3K/Akt pathway, inhibiting p38 phosphorylation and suppressing mitochondrial apoptotic signaling, which included upregulation of the Bcl-2/Bax ratio and expression of Akt, and downregulation of caspase 3, p38 (Yang et al., 2016).

Baicalin

Baicalin (7-glucuronic acid-5,6-dihydroxy-flavone, BA; **Figure 3P**) is a kind of small molecular flavonoids extracted from *Scutellaria baicalensis* Georgi (Fan et al., 2021). BA has a variety of pharmacological activities, such as antioxidant stress, regulation of immunity, regulation of lipid metabolism disorders, anti-inflammatory and improve cell apoptosis (Xin et al., 2020). Recent studies have found that baicalin mediates antioxidant stress by activating Nrf2 signaling pathway (Wang X. et al., 2021). In the 40% monobenzone cream-induced vitiligo model, BA intraperitoneal injection inhibited the infiltration of leukocytes and CD8 + T cells in vitiligo lesions, increased the tyrosinase activity in the lesion area, reduced the expression of chemokine CXCL10 and its receptor CXCR3, and reduced the expression of inflammatory factors in serum samples, including IL-6 and TNF-α, IFN- γ And IL-13 (Zhu et al., 2019). The results of this study are obviously exciting. The infiltration of active CD8 + T cells occurs around the lesions of vitiligo, which is an important reason for the immune destruction of melanocytes (Wu et al., 2013). *In vivo* experiments, BA could inhibit the infiltration of immune T cells, remove inflammatory factors to slow down the appearance of leukoplakia, and reduce the area of decolorized spots. So it is a potential drug for the treatment of vitiligo.

Polyphenol

Epigallocatechin-3-Gallate

Epigallocatechin-3-gallate (EGCG, **Figure 4A**) belongs to catechin polyphenols and is one of the main bioactive substances in Camellia sinensis (L.) Kuntze (Huang et al., 2021). It has many pharmacological effects, including anti-inflammatory, anti-atherosclerotic and anti-cancer effects (Mereles and Hunstein 2011), it's also an antioxidant (Kalaiselvi et al., 2013). Katiyar et al. suggested that EGCG could be a topical preparation to resist UVB-induced ROS-related inflammatory skin diseases, photocarcinogenesis and photoaging (Katiyar et al., 1999). In a model of monobenzone-stimulated vitiligo in mice, EGCG delayed the time to depigmentation, the area of depigmentation and reduced the incidence of hyperpigmentation in the dorsal skin of mice. The underlying mechanism was the inhibition of CD8 + T cell migration and inflammatory cytokine expression. Meanwhile, EGCG decreased the expression of IFN-γ, TNF-α, and IL-6 in serum. 5%EGCG cream is the optimal concentration for the treatment of vitiligo (Zhu et al., 2014). IFN - γ, which plays a key role in vitiligo pathogenesis, feedback through crosstalk to promote CD8 + T cell recruitment to the skin (Harris et al., 2012). High levels of CXC chemokines induced by IFN - γ such as CXCL9, CXCL10 and CXCL11 were also found in patient serum, being the most highly expressed genes in the transcriptional profile of skin lesions from vitiligo patients (Rashighi et al., 2014). Excitingly, EGCG inhibited IFN - γ - induced phosphorylation activation of JAK2, STAT1 and STAT3 in human melanocytes and significantly suppressed the levels of ICAM-1, CXCL10 and MCP-1 in a dose-dependent manner. In primary cultured human melanocytes. EGCG reduced the expression of CXCR3, CCR2, and CD11a in purified CD8 + T cells derived from the CD4 + T leukemia cell line Jurkat and peripheral blood monoclonal cells (PBMCs) in a dose-dependent character (Ning et al., 2015).

Cannabidiol

Cannabinediol (CBD; (**Figure 4B**) non-psychoactive compound extracted from Cannabis sativa L., is an open pyran ring analogue. CBD has anti-inflammatory, antioxidant and anti-apoptotic effects (Iuvone et al., 2009). In addition, it has immunomodulatory properties (Mechoulam and Hanus 2002). In recent years, it has attracted great attention due to its potential in the treatment of various pathological diseases, including skin and cosmetic diseases (Baswan et al., 2020). CBD increaseed melanin content by binding to CB1 receptor of human epidermal melanocytes. The mechanism is to up regulate the expression of MITF by activating p42/44MAPK and p38MAPK signaling

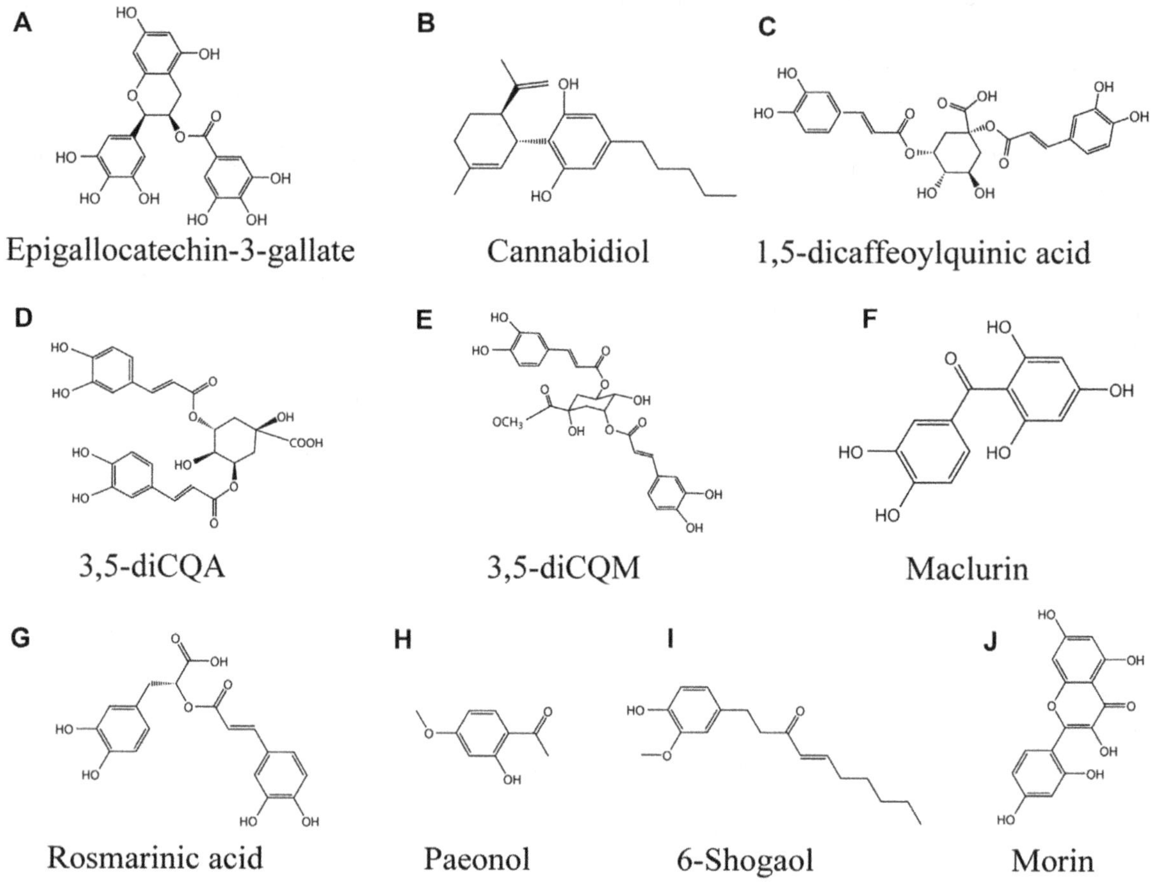

FIGURE 4 | Phenolic compounds against vitiligo **(A)** EGCG, **(B)** Cannabidiol, **(C)** 1,5-dicQA, **(D)** 3,5-diCQA, **(E)** 3,5-diCQM, **(F)** Maclurin, **(G)** Rosmarinic acid, **(H)** Paeonol, **(I)** 6-Shogaol, **(J)** Morin.

pathways, and then promote melanogenesis (Hwang et al., 2017). The safety of CBD transdermal drug delivery system is also under development (Paudel et al., 2010).

1,5-Dicaffeoylquinic Acid

1,5-dicaffeoylquinic acid (1,5-dicQA; **Figure 4C**) is a natural polyphenol widely found in Baccharoides anthelmintica (L.) Moench and Helianthus annuus L. (Cheevarungnapakul et al., 2019; Dogra et al., 2020). 1, 5-diCQA has a wide range of pharmacological effects, such as antioxidant, neuroprotective, antifibrotic and other biological activities (Cao et al., 2010). Plant seeds containing 1, 5-diCQA are used in traditional medicine to treat vitiligo (Tuerxuntayi et al., 2014). A previous study found that 1,5-dicqa exerts antioxidant activity through reducing intracellular ROS level and Nrf2 dependent pathway (Cao et al., 2010). 1, 5-diCQA inhibited Aβ42-induced neurotoxicity by activating PI3K/Akt, decreasing GSK3 β level and regulating Bcl-2/Bax ratio (Xiao et al., 2011). B16 cells treated with 0, 5, 50 or 100 μM 1, 5-dicQA significantly up-regulated the transcription levels of MITF, TYR, TRP1 and TRP2 in a dose-dependent manner without cytotoxicity. The mechanism is to activate p38 MAPK, ERK MAPK and PKA signaling pathway to promote the melanin synthesis of B16 cells. In conclusion, these studies suggest that 1,5-dicQA may be an effective drug for the treatment of hypopigmented skin diseases (Mamat et al., 2018).

3,5-diCQA

3,5-caffeoylquinic acid (3,5-diCQA; **Figure 4D**) is a polyphenolic compound extracted from the root of Cichorium intybus L. (Legrand et al., 2016), it also accumulated in *Achillea millefolium* L. and *Artemisia dracunculus* L. 3,5-diCQA has high free radical scavenging activity (Bernard et al., 2020). Phenolic compounds are beneficial to human health, especially their anti-inflammatory and antioxidant properties (Miguel et al., 2020). Plant polyphenols help the skin resist the damage caused by sunlight (Perez-Sanchez et al., 2016). 3,5-diCQA increased the content of melanin in melanocytes in a dose-dependent manner, the possible mechanism is that 3,5-diCQA promoted the phosphorylation of Akt and GSK-3 β, leading to the accumulation of β - Catenin in the cytoplasm. Subsequently, β - Catenin transferred to the nucleus and bound to LEF, which increased the protein expression of downstream MITF, TYR, TRP1 and TRP2. Therefore, 3,5-diCQA may restore skin pigmentation under the loss of antioxidant enzymes or melanocyte dysfunction (Mamat et al., 2017).

3,5-diCQM

3,5-dicaffeoylquinic acids (3,5-diCQM; **Figure 4E**) is a sort of natural phenolic acids condensed from quinic acid and caffeic acid by esterification. It is widely found in plants such as Gloriosa superba L., Inula helenium L., *Xanthium strumarium* subsp. strumarium, Crataegus azarolus L. and other fruit trees (Bernard et al., 2020). Caffeoylquinic acid derivatives have been used in traditional medicine in the east to treat a variety of diseases and show a diversity of pharmacological effects, such as liver protection (Basnet et al., 1996), anti-microbial (Zhu et al., 2004), anti-inflammatory (Góngora et al., 2002). In addition, the antioxidant activity of caffeoylquinic acid derivatives has been reported (Lin Y.-L. et al., 2011; Jang and Koh 2019). In the experiment of B16F10 melanoma cells treated with 0–50 μm 3, 5-dicCQM, the results showed that 3,5-diCQM could induce pigmentation. 3,5-diCQM drives melanogenesis in a dose-dependent manner, and the molecular mechanism underlying its ability to induce pigmentation is through activation of the p38 signaling pathway, phosphorylation and activation of CREB, and a cAMP/PKA dependent signaling pathway, which in turn upregulates the transcription factor MITF, thereby activating tyrosinase activity (Kim et al., 2015).

Maclurin

Maclurin [(3,4-dihydroxyphenyl) -(2,4,6-trihydroxyphenyl; **Figure 4F**) methanone] is a natural phenolic compound that belongs to the benzophenone family and is found in *Morus alba* L., *Garcinia mangostana* L. Previous studies have found that maclurin has pharmacological activities such as anticancer, antioxidant and anti-skin aging (Lee 2018; Lee et al., 2018; Mi Moon et al., 2019). The content of melanin in melanocytes was increased by maclurin in a dose-dependent manner, by a mechanism involving the activation of the cAMP/PKA/CREB signaling pathway, which in turn increased tyrosinase, MITF and their downstream TRP-1 and Trp-2 protein content, while also involving the activation of p38 MAPK and p44/42 MAPK pathways. *In vitro*, maclurin significantly attenuated UVB induced ROS production, inhibited hydrogen peroxide induced reduction of melanin and decreased cell survival (Hwang et al., 2019).

Rosmarinic Acid

Rosmarinic acid (a-o-caffeoyl-3,4-dihydroxyphenyl lacticacid; **Figure 4G**) is a natural phenolic compound, which exists in many Labiatae plants, such as *Perilla L.*, *Rosmarinus officinalis* L., *Prunella vulgaris* L. (Zhang et al., 2021). Rosmarinic acid has anti-inflammatory, anti-oxidation, anti-cancer and other pharmacological activities (Wang L. et al., 2019; Zhang et al., 2021). Incubation of 50 μm rosmarinic acid with B16 melanoma cells for 48 h resulted in a significant increase in melanin content and tyrosinase protein expression, the mechanism being that rosmarinic acid induces melanin synthesis by activating the PKA/CREB signaling pathway via phosphorylation (Shomirzoeva et al., 2019). Recently, ultradeformable liposomes (UL) have been developed by scientific researchers, which greatly increased the skin permeation ability of rosmarinic acid by UL containing oleic acid, exhibiting potential as a formulation for development for external use (Subongkot et al., 2021).

Paeonol

Paeonol (Pae; 2′-hydroxy-4-methoxyacetophenone; **Figure 4H**) is a natural phenolic compound extracted from the *Paeonia × suffruticosa* Andrews (Miao et al., 2021). Paeonol has been used in traditional Chinese medicine as an anti-inflammatory and antipyretic drug with cardiovascular, anti-inflammatory, neuroprotective, antitumour and other pharmacological activities (Zhang L. et al., 2019; Tsai et al., 2020). Paeonol alleviated UVB-induced skin photoaging by activating Nrf2 and the antioxidant response element (Sun et al., 2018). Paeonol exhibits anti-inflammatory, anti-allergic activity in animal models of atopic dermatitis and psoriasis (Meng et al., 2017; Meng et al., 2019). In H_2O_2-induced PIG1 oxidative stress model of normal human epidermal melanocytes, paeonol inhibited hydrogen peroxide induced decrease in cell viability in a dose-dependent manner. 20 μM paeonol increased the enzymatic activities of SOD, CAT, GSH-Px and the expression of HO-1, NQO1, and SOD2 by activating the Nrf2 signaling pathway, but paeonol was unable to affect melanogenesis in PIG1 cells and acted only as a protective agent (Guo and Zhang 2021).

6-Shogaol

6-shogaol (**Figure 4I**), a natural phenolic compound, is the major active ingredient in *Zingiber officinale* Roscoe. Studies have found that 6-shogao possesses antiemetic, anti-inflammatory, antioxidant, and anticancer activities, as well as cardiovascular and neuroprotective effects (Kou et al., 2018; Chen et al., 2020; Yadav and Jang 2020). Jin et al. found that 6-shogaol exerts cellular antioxidant activity by mediating Nrf2 signaling through activation of the JNK pathway (Kim and Jang 2016). Feng et al. found that 6-shogaol inhibited UVB induced inflammation and oxidative stress in keratinocytes (Chen F. et al., 2019). Pretreatment of HEMn-MPs with 5 μM 6-shogaol for 6 h protected melanocytes from rhododendrol-induced cytotoxicity and maintained their original cell viability. In the oxidative stress-induced HEMn-MPs model, cells pretreated with 6-shogao maintained the initial cellular morphology, and 6-shogao significantly attenuated H_2O_2 induced oxidative stress and death and melanogenesis inhibition in melanocytes (Yang L. et al., 2020).

Morin

Morin (2′,3,4′,5,7-pentahydroxyflavone; **Figure 4J**) is a natural polyphenol found in onion, fig, guava leaves, apple and other Moraceae families such as *Psidium guajava* L., *Maclura pomifera* (Raf.) C.K.Schneid., as well as the medicinal plant *Alpinia officinarum* Hance (Lotito and Frei 2006). Studies have found that Morin has antitumor, antihypertensive, antioxidant, anti-inflammatory, antidiabetic, neuroprotective, antibacterial and other pharmacological effects (Caselli et al., 2016; Heeba et al., 2021). 50 μM Morin significantly upregulated the expression of MITF, as well as its downstream TRP-1 and Trp-2 to increase melanin production in B16F10 mouse melanoma cells, and the mechanisms include the activation of ERK and p38 signaling pathways via the phosphorylated MAPK pathway (Shin et al.,

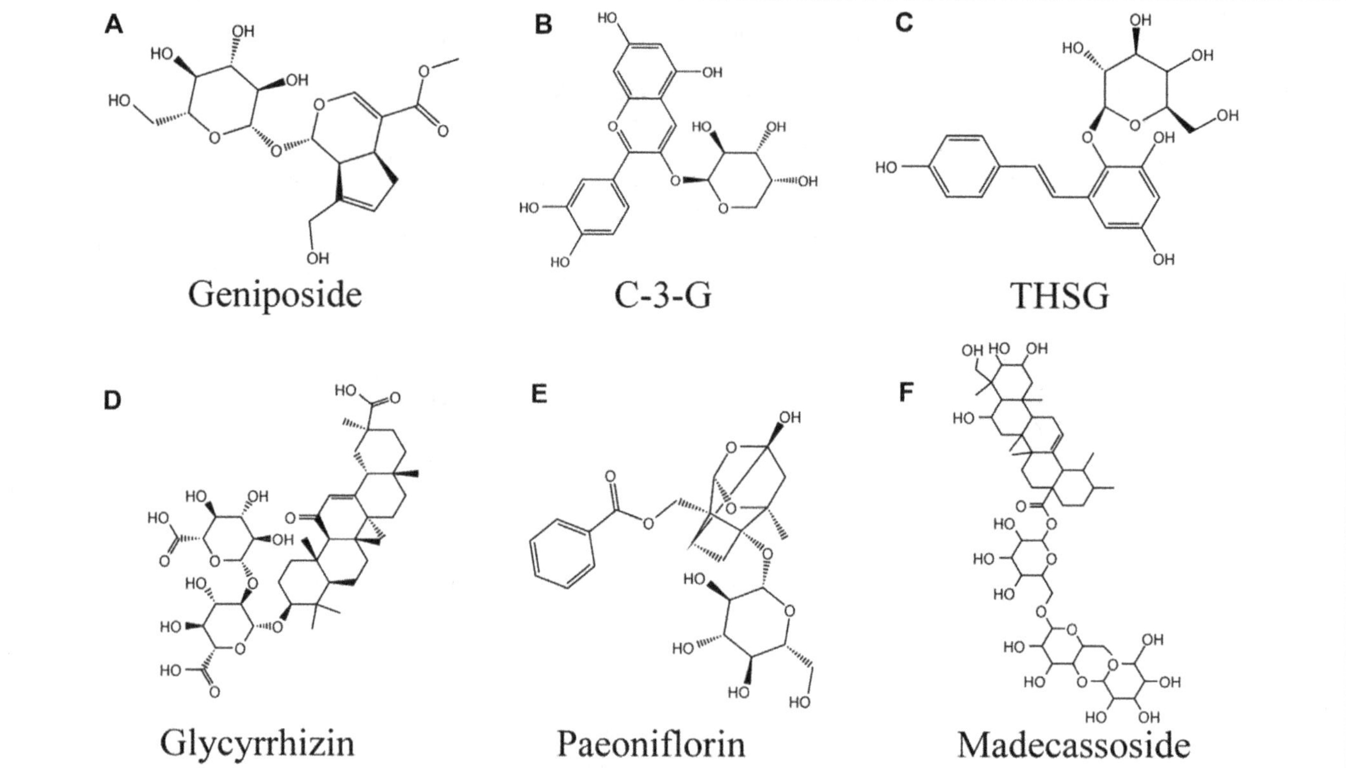

FIGURE 5 | Glycosides against vitiligo **(A)** Geniposide, **(B)** C-3-G, **(C)** THSG, **(D)** Glycyrrhizin, **(E)** Paeoniflorin, **(F)** Madecassoside.

2021). Excitingly, long-term doses of oral Morin did not exhibit any toxicity (Cho et al., 2006).

GLYCOSIDES

Geniposide

Geniposide (GP; **Figure 5A**) (C17H24O10) is a sort of iridoid glycoside extracted from Gardenia jasminoides J. Ellis fruits, which widely exists in nearly 40 species of plants in various families, especially Rubiaceae (Shan et al., 2017). In terms of biological activity, GP has been found to have a variety of pharmacological effects, such as anti-diabetes (Zhang et al., 2016), neuroprotective (Zhao et al., 2017), anti-inflammatory, antioxidant, etc (Zhou et al., 2019). GP is also an important component in many traditional Chinese herbal medicines for the treatment of vitiligo, such as Eucommia ulmoides Oliv. and Rehmannia glutinosa (Gaertn.) DC. (Zhou et al., 2019). In HEMn or HEKn models induced by norepinephrine (NE), GP significantly abolished the inhibitory effect of NE on HEMn melanogenesis in the presence of recombinant SCF. The binding of NE to α 1-adrenoceptor in melanocytes decreased cAMP level, resulting in decreased intracellular calcium uptake associated with c-kit production. The mechanism of GP promoting melanogenesis was through activating GLP-1R/c-kit receptor signal to enhance the expression of c-kit receptor, so as to eliminate the depigmentation caused by norepinephrine (Wen-Jun et al., 2008). In the melanocytes induced by H_2O_2, GP increased the activities of SOD and CAT, reduced the accumulation of ROS, thus increased the antioxidant capacity of melanocytes and inhibited melanocyte apoptosis by upregulating the Bcl-2/Bax ratio, while increasing cell viability. This process involves activation of PI3K/Akt signaling pathway (Zhou et al., 2019).

Cyanidin-3-o-β-Glucopyranoside

Cyanidin-3-o-β-glucopyranoside (C-3-G; **Figure 5B**) is a kind of anthocyanin flavonoids widely found in vegetables and fruits. Chinese *Myrica cerifera* L. is a rich source of C-3-G, which is one of the most common anthocyanins (Sun et al., 2013). Anthocyanins are beneficial to human body. Known pharmacological actions include anti-inflammatory, anti-fatigue, anti-oxidation, anti-tumor and so on (Cui et al., 2018). In addition to the ability to significantly reduce ROS mediated oxidative damage, C-3-G inhibited UVA induced damage to primary human dermal fibroblasts (HDFS) by inducing autophagy (Wu et al., 2019). In one study, TVM-A12 human melanoma cells were incubated with 5 μm C-3-G, and the cells return to the differentiation state from the proliferation state. In addition, two human melanoma cell lines A-375 and M14 also obtained dendritic phenotypes after C-3-G treatment. At the concentration used, the cells treated with C-3-G showed no apoptosis or necrosis. At the same time, C-3-G significantly up-regulated the expression of tyrosinase, thereby inducing the content of melanin in TVM-A12 cells, which was mediated by up regulating cAMP pathway. It is particularly encouraging that the

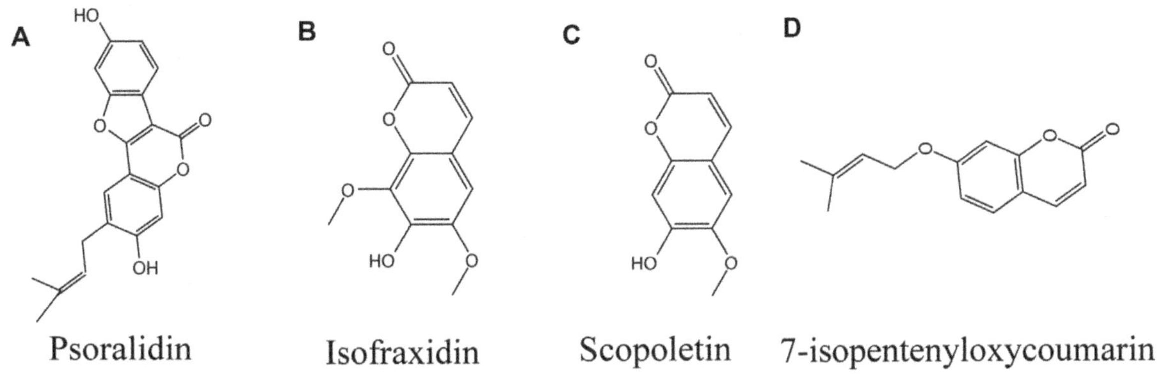

FIGURE 6 | Coumarins against vitiligo **(A)** Psoralidin, **(B)** Isofraxidin, **(C)** Scopoletin, **(D)** 7-isopentenyloxycoumarin.

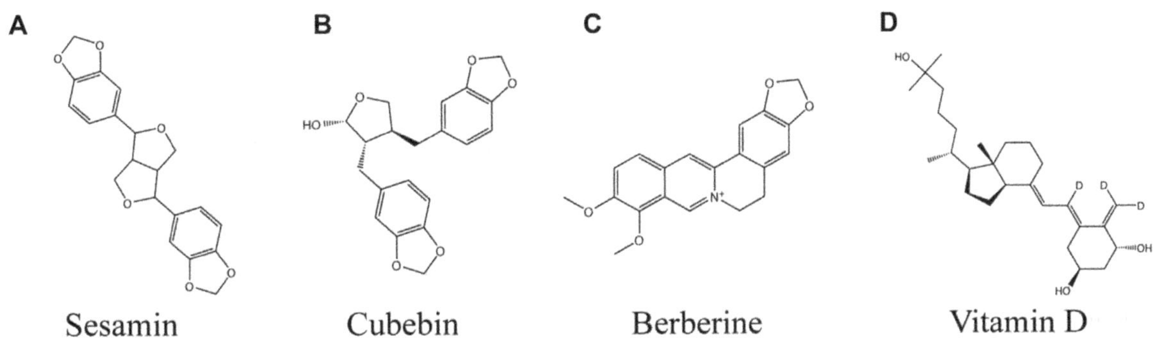

FIGURE 7 | Coumarins against vitiligo **(A)** Sesamin, **(B)** Cubebin, **(C)** Berberine, **(D)** Vitamin D.

active concentration of C-3-G is comparable to food intake (range of μm) and has no toxicity. (Serafino et al., 2004).

2, 3, 5, 4′-Tetrahydroxystilbene-2-O-β-D-Glucoside

2, 3, 5, 4′-tetrahydroxystilbene-2-O-β-D-glucoside (THSG; **Figure 5C**) is a water-soluble active ingredient in Reynoutria multiflora (Thunb.) Moldenke (He et al., 2015). Numerous studies have found that THSG exerts antioxidant effects by protecting cells from oxidative damage caused by H_2O_2 through increasing SOD activity, reducing MDA content, and inhibiting ROS production (Yang et al., 2014; Wu et al., 2020). In hairless skin model, the extract of *Reynoutria multiflora* could up regulate SOD in a dose-dependent manner, thereby reducing UVB-induced oxidative damage, suggesting that the extract of *Reynoutria multiflora* contains anti skin photoaging agent (Hwang et al., 2006). At the first time, it was proved to be an effective tyramine Acid enzyme activators and melanogenesis stimulants (Guan et al., 2008). THSG increased tyrosinase activity in a dose-dependent manner at concentrations ranging from 1 to 10 μg/ml (Jiang et al., 2009). Guan et al. (2008) reached a similar conclusion. The mechanism was that THSG directly activated AC or inhibited PDE, increased cAMP level in cytoplasm, and mediated the activation of MITF/CREB. P38MAPK had a regulatory effect on melanin formation and the induced expression of tyrosinase and MITF in B16 cells induced by THSG (Jiang et al., 2009).

Glycyrrhizin

Glycyrrhizin (GLC; (**Figure 5D**) natural triterpene saponin, is one of the major chemical components extracted from *Glycyrrhiza* Tourn. ex L. and has been widely used in Asia, Europe, the Middle East (Cai et al., 2017). Studies have shown that GLC has antiallergic, immunomodulatory, antiulcer, anticancer, antioxidant, and antiviral effects (Wang G. et al., 2021). Jung et al. were the first to find that GLC induced melanin production in B16 melanoma cells in a dose-dependent manner by upregulating the tyrosinase and Trp-2 genes (Jung et al., 2001). Li et al. also verified this conclusion. Further studies revealed that GLC increases melanin production in melanocytes by three pathways, 1) activating activator protein-1 (AP-1) and CRE promoter to activate p42/44 MAPK signaling, 2) activating cAMP signaling, and 3) decreasing GSK3β phosphorylation while inducing CREB phosphorylation (Lee et al., 2005). Pretreatment with 1 mM GLC significantly inhibited H_2O_2-induced melanocyte apoptosis, and GR protected melanocytes from oxidative stress by reducing ROS production in cells via activation of the Nrf2/HO-1 pathway (Mou et al., 2019). Clinical study

TABLE 1 | Summary of natural products for the treatment of vitiligo in models.

	Natural compounds name	Models	Range of dosage	Targets/pathway/process/ mechanism	References
Flavonoids	Baicalein	H_2O_2-induced PIG3V (human cell)	50 μM	Cell vitality and proliferation, Nrf2, HO-1, SOD2, NQO1, ERK1/2, PI3K/AKT	Ma et al. (2018)
		H_2O_2-induced PIG1 (human cell)	10, 20, and 40 μM	Cell viability, ROS, Bax, Bcl-2, caspase-3, β-actin, COX4, Cyt-4, p38 MAPK, ERK	Liu et al. (2012)
	Quercetin	H_2O_2-induced epidermal melanocytes (human cell)	25 μM	TYRe, Cell viability, ROS production, β-actin	Guan et al. (2015)
	Kaempferol	HMVII (human cell)	1, 5, 10 and 20 μM	TYR activity, melanin content	Takekoshi et al. (2014)
		B16F10	8, 16, 32 μM	Viability, melanin melanin contents, Synthesis, TYR activity, MC1R, MITF, TYRP1, DCT	Wang et al. (2017)
	Apigenin	H_2O_2-induced PIG3V (human cell)	1, 5, 10 and 20 μM	Cell viability, SOD, CAT, GSH-PX, MDA, Nrf2, HO-1, NQO1, β-actin	Zhang et al. (2020)
		Dopamine-induced melanocytes (human cell)	0.3–10 μM	Cell viability, ROS, JNK, p38MAPK, Akt, caspase-3, PARP	Lin et al. (2011a)
	Galangin	Male C57BL/6 (mice)	0.425 mg/kg, 4.25 m g/kg	Melanocytes, TYR activity, CHE activity, MDA	Huo et al. (2014)
	Naringenin	B16 melanocytes 4A5 (mice cell)	0, 10, 25, 50, 100, 200 μM	Tyrp1, Dct, MITF, ERK, PI3K, GSK-3β, β-actin	Ohguchi et al. (2006)
		B16-F10 (mice cell)	3–50 μM	Cell viability, melanin content, TYR, MITF, β-catenin, GSK-3β, Akt	Huang et al. (2011)
	Hesperetin	B16-F10 (mice cell)	3, 10, 30, 50 μM	Cell viability, melanin content, TYR, MITF, β-catenin, p38 MAPK, GSK-3β, p38MAPK, ERK, Akt, CREB	Huang et al. (2012)
	Afzelin	Epidermal melanocytes (human cell)	0, 10, 50, 100 μM	TYR activity, Cell viability, MITF, TRP-1, TRP-2, p42/44MAPK, p38MAPK, JNK, CREB	Jung et al. (2016)
	Fisetin	B16F10 (mice cell), zebrafish model	5, 20 μM	MITF, TYR, cell viability, melanin Content	Molagoda et al. (2020)
	Puerarin	Melan-a cell, zebrafish model, MITFvit/vit mice	50 μM	MITF-M, Bcl-2, TRP-2, TYR, cAMP, melanin content cell	Park et al. (2014)
		40% monobenzone cream-induced emale C57BL/6 (mice), melanocytes from foreskins (human cell)	1, 5, 10, 20, 40 μmol/L	viability, melanin content, TYR, TRP-1, MITF, GAPDH, ERK1/2, p38, JNK	Ding et al. (2019)
	Butin	Hydroquinone-induced mice	0.425, 4.25, 42.5 mg/kg	TYR, Trp-1, CHE, MDA	Huo et al. (2017)
		B16 cell, H_2O_2-induced zebrafish	1, 10, 100 μM	ROS, melanin Content, TYR	Lai et al. (2021)
	Liquiritin	B16-F1 (mice cell), HMVII (human cell)	12.5, 25, 50 μM	Cell viability, melanin Content, TYR, TRP-1, TRP-2, p38, CREB, MITF, GAPDH	Uto et al. (2019)
	Liquiritigenin	B16-F1 (mice cell), HMVII (human cell)	12.5, 25, 50 μM	Cell viability, melanin Content, TYR, TRP-1, TRP-2, p38, CREB, MITF, GAPDH	Uto et al. (2019)
	Vitexin	H_2O_2-induced PIG1	10, 20, 30, 40 μM	Cells viability, IL-1β, IL-17A, Nrf2, HO-1, NQO-1, SOD, cyt-C, ERK, ROS, p53, Bax, Bcl-2, β-actin, caspase-3	Li et al. (2020)
	Hyperoside	H_2O_2-induced epidermal melanocytes (human cell)	2, 10, 50 μg/ml	Cell viability, melanin amount, Bcl-2, Bax, caspase 3, GAPDH, AKT, p38	Yang et al. (2016)
	Baicalin	40% monobenzone-induced C57BL/6 (mice)	20 mg/ml	CD8+T, CXCL10, CXCR3, IL-6, TNF-α, IFN-γ, IL-13	Zhu et al. (2019)
Polyphenol	EGCG	IFN-γ-induced (human cell), CD8+T	0, 10, 20, 40 μM	ICAM-1, CXCL10, and MCP-1, JAK2/STATs, CD11a, CXCR3, CCR2	Ning et al. (2015)
		Female C57BL/6 (mice)	2%, 5% and 10% EGCG cream	$CD8^+$ T cells, TNF-α, IFN-γ, and IL-6, CXCl3, CXCL5, CXCR4, S100B, TGFBR2, c-fos, Rab27A, EGFR, PI3K	Zhu et al. (2014)

(Continued on following page)

TABLE 1 | *(Continued)* Summary of natural products for the treatment of vitiligo in models.

	Natural compounds name	Models	Range of dosage	Targets/pathway/process/ mechanism	References
	Cannabidiol	Epidermal melanocytes (human cell)	1, 3, 6 μM	MITF, TYR, TRP-1, TRP-2, p38MAPK, p42/44 MAPK, TYR activity, cell viability	Hwang et al. (2017)
	1,5-dicQA	B16 (mice cell)	0–400 μM	Tyr activity, MITF, TYR, TRP-1, TRP-2, ERK, JNK, p38, PKA	Mamat et al. (2018)
	3,5-diCQA	B16 (mice cell)	0–200 μM	TYR activity, TYR, TRP1, TRP2, MITF, β-catenin	Mamat et al. (2017)
	3,5-diCQM	B16F10 (mice cell)	0–50 μM	TYR activity, melanin content, TRP-1, TRP-2, MITF, cAMP, ERK, p38MAPK, JNK, AKT	Kim et al. (2015)
	Maclurin	H_2O_2-induced epidermal melanocytes (human cell)	1, 10, 50 μM	TRP-1, TRP-2, MITF, tyrosinase, cAMP, PKA, CREB, p38 MAPK, p44/42 MAPK, PKA	Hwang et al. (2019)
	Rosmarinic acid	B16 (mice cell)	1, 10, 50, 100 μM	Melanin content, CREB, p38mapk, Akt, tyrosinase	Lee et al. (2007)
	Paeonol	H_2O_2-induced PIG1 (human cell)	5, 10, 20, 40 μM	Cell viability, TYR, TRP-1, MITF, CAT, HO-1, NQO1, SOD2, Nrf2, GAPDH, SOD, GSH-Px	Guo and Zhang (2021)
	6-Shogaol	H_2O_2-induced HEMn-MPs (human cell)	5 μM	Cell viability, MITF, HO-1, NQO1, Nrf2, GAPDH	Yang et al. (2020b)
	Morin	B16F10 (mice cell)	25, 50, 100, 250, 500 μM	MITF, TRP-1, TRP-2, GAPDH, ERK, p38	Shin et al. (2021)
Glycosides	Geniposide	NE-induced HEMn (human cell)	0–100 μM	TYR activity, melanin, c-kit receptor, SCF ligand	Wen-Jun et al. (2008)
		H_2O_2-induced primary melanocytes (human cell)		ROS, SOD, CAT, Akt, Bcl-2, Bax, caspase 3, caspase 9, β-actin	Lu et al. (2018)
	C-3-G	TVM-A12,M14,A-375 (human cell)	5, 10 μM	Cell viability, proliferation, NF-68 kDa, NF-160 kDa, NF-200 kDa, Melan-A/MART-1	Serafino et al. (2004)
	THSG	B16F1 (mice cell)	1–10 μg/ml	Melanin amount, TYR activity, MITF, ERK, p38 MAPK, JNK, cAMP	Jiang et al. (2009)
		B16 (mice cell)	0.1–25 μg/ml	TYR activity, melanin content	Guan et al. (2008)
	Glycyrrhizin	B16 (mice cell)	0.2, 0.5, 1.0, 1.5 mM	Cell viability, melanin amount, AP-1, CREB, p42/44 MAPK, cAMP, GSK-3β, MITF	Lee et al. (2005)
		H_2O_2-induced NHEM (human cell)	1 mM	Cell viability, ROS, β-actin, Nrf2, HO-1, GAPDH, NQO-1, GCLC, GCLM	Mou et al. (2019)
	Paeoniflorin	Epidermal melanocytes (human cell), 40% monobenzone-inducedC57BL/6 (mice)	0, 5, 10 μg/ml, 60 mg/kg in 20% propanediol	Cell vitality and proliferation, melanin amount, TRP-1, MITF, TYR, ERK, CREB, GAPDH cell	Hu et al. (2020a)
		H_2O_2-induced PIG1, PIG3V (human cell)	50–400 μM	viability, ROS, SOD, CAT, Nrf2, NQO1, HO-1	Yuan et al. (2020)
	Cistanche deserticola polysaccharide	H_2O_2-induced B16F10 (mice cell) and epidermal melanocytes (human cell), zebrafish	20,40,80 μg/ml	Cell viability, melanin amount, TYR, ROS, MITF, TRP1, TRP2, RAB2 7A, FSCN1, GAPDH, ERK, JNK, p38, ROS, Nrf2, HO-1	Hu et al. (2020b)
	Madecassoside	H_2O_2-induced B16F10 (mice cell), HEM (human cell), zebrafish	20, 40, 80 μg/ml	Cell viability, melanin amount, TYR, MITF, TRP1, TRP2, RAB2 7A, FSCN1, GAPDH, ERK, JNK, p38, ROS, Nrf2, HO-1, MAPK	Ling et al. (2017)
Coumarin	Psoralidin	In silico (no cell)	0.125, 0.25, 0.5, 1 g/ml	TYR, a rate-limiting enzyme of melanogenesis	Shi et al. (2018)
	isofraxidin	B16F10 (mice cell), zebrafish	12.5, 25 μM	Melanocytes, TYR activity, melanin, MIFT, TRP-1	Yim et al. (2017a)
	Scopoletin	B16F10 (mice cell) B16F10 (mice cell), zebrafish	0–50 μM 10–25 μmol/L	TYR activity, melanin content, TYR, MITF, CREB, β-actin, melanin content, TYR activity, melanin content, Cell viability, ROS	Ahn et al. (2014), Heriniaina et al. (2018)
	7-Isopentenyloxycoumarin	Melan-a (mice cell)	1, 10, 20, 40 μM	Cells viability, melanin content, tyrosinase, TRP-1, TRP-2, and MITF	Fiorito et al. (2018)

(Continued on following page)

Vitamin D

Vitamin D (1,25-dihy-droxyvitamin D3, **Figure 7D**) is a cyclopentane phenanthrene compound, which is an essential vitamin for human body, it mainly comes from daily meat (Dominguez et al., 2021). Vitamin D has been used in autoimmune diseases, cancer and osteoporosis (Sintov et al., 2014). Vitamin D deficiency leads to the excessive production of ROS in mitochondria and damages the antioxidant system (Latham et al., 2021). Previous studies have confirmed that vitamin D compounds regulate the proliferation, differentiation, migration and apoptosis of melanocytes and affect T-cell mediated peripheral immune response (Birlea et al., 2008; Kawakami et al., 2014). In H_2O_2-induced oxidative stress models in PIG1 and PIG3V cells, vitamin D activated WNT/β-Catenin signaling pathway exerted antioxidant activity, the mechanism included the promotion of GSK3β inactivation, increased β-catenin nuclear translocation and activation of the downstream Nrf2/ARE pathway. In addition, vitamin D passed through up regulation of MITF in a β-catenin pathway dependent manner promoted melanocyte proliferation and protected melanocytes from H_2O_2-induced apoptosis by suppressing caspase3 expression (Tang et al., 2018).

CONCLUSION AND PROSPECTIVE

In traditional medicine, there are many traditional herbal medicines (Kwon et al., 2018; Xu et al., 2017; Moreira et al., 2012) for the treatment of pigment deficiency. Their extracts significantly improved the activity of tyrosinase (Xu et al., 2017). However, their specific components and mechanism of action are still unclear. Vitiligo is an autoimmune skin disease in which melanocytes are destroyed by autoreactive $CD8^+$ T cells, resulting in cutaneous leukoplakia. Depigmented mouse skin lesions with autoimmune features were fitted to a monobenzone-induced vitiligo model (Zhu et al., 2013). Unfortunately, among all natural drugs mentioned in this review, only four natural products (such as Vitexin, baicalin, EGCG and berberine) currently exhibit anti depigmenting pharmacological activity in this model. We mentioned earlier that oxidative stress may be a driver of autoimmune destruction and that intense and persistent oxidative stress leads to apoptosis, damage, and antigen exposure of melanocytes, which in turn trigger autoimmune destruction. Therefore, recently, researchers have paid more attention to the mechanism of action of natural products against oxidative stress in melanocytes. Some natural drugs (such as baicalein, Vitexin, maclurin, etc.) inhibited the damaging effects of H_2O_2-induced oxidative stress on melanocytes, even counterstaining depigmented mouse skin lesions. Therefore, it is reasonable to speculate that some of these members contribute to protection against autoimmune destruction. 37 natural products can elevate melanin expression by elevating tyrosinase activity in an *in vitro* melanocyte model *in vivo*, but their contribution to intervening in autoimmune destruction is similarly unknown. The above mentioned vitiligo models are all inducible and cannot fully replicate the disease characteristics of human vitiligo, thus increasing the difficulty of developing new drugs. Genetically edited mice have not been widely promoted (Riding et al., 2019). Several natural drugs have been reported for their use in the clinic. For example: observations from clinical studies have shown that oral Glycyrrhizin Combined with UVB therapy improves active systemic vitiligo, but also exposes minor side effects (Mou et al., 2016). In clinical studies, the overall recolor rate of PUVA (psoralen plus UVA) was only 44% (Bishnoi and Parsad 2018). However, due to the lack of large clinical research, they still have a long way to go before they can be promoted as anti-vitiligo agents (Maleš et al., 2019). A systematic review study showed that vitiligo does not generally produce benefi cial outcomes with the use of topical antioxidants, but the added effect of oral intake cannot be ignored (Speeckaert et al., 2018). Developing new natural products against autoimmune destruction will be a hotspot in the future and also provide a new direction to elucidate the pathogenesis of vitiligo. Vitiligo treatment serves two purposes: 1) Controlling vitiligo disease progression during the active phase and 2) increasing melanocyte production during the stationary phase. We propose the hypothesis that in the future natural drugs with anti-oxidant and anti-autoimmune properties are used in vitiligo progression phase and natural drugs with improved tyrosinase activity are used in stability phase.

In conclusion, strong evidence that natural products can prevent or treat vitiligo is still lacking. Appropriately designed clinical trials are needed to further understand the efficacy of natural products against vitiligo. As an auxiliary means of phototherapy, plant derived compounds with antioxidant properties are becoming an attractive choice for the treatment of vitiligo (Dell'Anna et al., 2007). Natural products (NPs) extracted from plants show the effect of increasing the expression of melanin, and have less side effects on human body, which is of great significance for us to continue to develop natural drugs (Yin et al., 2017).

AUTHOR CONTRIBUTIONS

Concepts: YP. Wrote the paper: YP, SW, YH, and JL. Designed the figures: JZ, YP, and YY. Reviewed manuscript: JG and QN. All authors commented on the manuscript. All authors contributed to the article and approved the submitted version.

FUNDING

This work was supported by the National Natural Science Foundation of China (Grant nos. 81804066, 82074443, 81873310), and by Xinglin Scholar Research Promotion Project of Chengdu University of TCM (Grant nos. QNXZ2019017, and QNXZ2020003) and "Hundred Talents Program" of the Hospital of Chengdu University of Traditional Chinese Medicine (Grant nos. 20-B01, 20-Q03, and 20-Q05).

REFERENCES

Abdel-Malek, Z. A., Jordan, C., Ho, T., Upadhyay, P. R., Fleischer, A., and Hamzavi, I. (2020). The enigma and Challenges of Vitiligo Pathophysiology and Treatment. *Pigment Cel Melanoma Res* 33 (6), 778–787. doi:10.1111/pcmr.12878

Ahluwalia, J., Correa-Selm, L. M., and Rao, B. K. (2017). Vitiligo: Not Simply a Skin Disease. *Skinmed* 15 (2), 125–127. doi:10.1080/14725843.2017.1282416

Ahmad, A., Ali, T., Park, H. Y., Badshah, H., Rehman, S. U., and Kim, M. O. (2017). Neuroprotective Effect of Fisetin against Amyloid-Beta-Induced Cognitive/Synaptic Dysfunction, Neuroinflammation, and Neurodegeneration in Adult Mice. *Mol. Neurobiol.* 54 (3), 2269–2285. doi:10.1007/s12035-016-9795-4

Ahmad, A., Ali, T., Rehman, S. U., and Kim, M. O. (2019). Phytomedicine-Based Potent Antioxidant, Fisetin Protects CNS-Insult LPS-Induced Oxidative Stress-Mediated Neurodegeneration and Memory Impairment. *J. Clin. Med.* 8 (6). doi:10.3390/jcm8060850

Ahn, M.-J., Hur, S.-J., Kim, E.-H., Lee, S. H., Shin, J. S., Kim, M.-K., et al. (2014). Scopoletin fromCirsium setidensIncreases Melanin Synthesis via CREB Phosphorylation in B16F10 Cells. *Korean J. Physiol. Pharmacol.* 18 (4), 307–311. doi:10.4196/kjpp.2014.18.4.307

Al-Shobaili, H. A., and Rasheed, Z. (2015). Oxidized Tyrosinase: A Possible Antigenic Stimulus for Non-segmental Vitiligo Autoantibodies. *J. Dermatol. Sci.* 79 (3), 203–213. doi:10.1016/j.jdermsci.2015.06.009

Alvarez-Arellano, L., Salazar-García, M., and Corona, J. C. (2020). Neuroprotective Effects of Quercetin in Pediatric Neurological Diseases. *Molecules* 25 (23). doi:10.3390/molecules25235597

Basnet, P., Matsushige, K., Hase, K., Kadota, S., and Namba, T. (1996). Four Di-O-caffeoyl Quinic Acid Derivatives from Propolis. Potent Hepatoprotective Activity in Experimental Liver Injury Models. *Biol. Pharm. Bull.* 19 (11), 1479–1484. doi:10.1248/bpb.19.1479

Baswan, S. M., Klosner, A. E., Glynn, K., Rajgopal, A., Malik, K., Yim, S., et al. (2020). Therapeutic Potential of Cannabidiol (CBD) for Skin Health and Disorders. *Ccid* 13, 927–942. doi:10.2147/ccid.s286411

Bergqvist, C., and Ezzedine, K. (2021). Vitiligo: A Focus on Pathogenesis and its Therapeutic Implications. *J. Dermatol.* 48 (3), 252–270. doi:10.1111/1346-8138.15743

Bernard, G., Alves Dos Santos, H., Etienne, A., Samaillie, J., Neut, C., Sahpaz, S., et al. (2020). MeJA Elicitation of Chicory Hairy Roots Promotes Efficient Increase of 3,5-diCQA Accumulation, a Potent Antioxidant and Antibacterial Molecule. *Antibiotics (Basel)* 9 (10). doi:10.3390/antibiotics9100659

Bickers, D. R., and Athar, M. (2006). Oxidative Stress in the Pathogenesis of Skin Disease. *J. Invest. Dermatol.* 126 (12), 2565–2575. doi:10.1038/sj.jid.5700340

Birlea, S., Costin, G.-E., and Norris, D. (2008). Cellular and Molecular Mechanisms Involved in the Action of Vitamin D Analogs Targeting Vitiligo Depigmentation. *Cdt* 9 (4), 345–359. doi:10.2174/138945008783954970

Bishnoi, A., and Parsad, D. (2018). Clinical and Molecular Aspects of Vitiligo Treatments. *Int. J. Mol. Sci.* 19 (5). doi:10.3390/ijms19051509

Cai, X., Wang, X., Li, J., and Chen, S. (2017). Protective Effect of Glycyrrhizin on Myocardial Ischemia/reperfusion Injury-Induced Oxidative Stress, Inducible Nitric Oxide Synthase and Inflammatory Reactions through High-Mobility Group Box 1 and Mitogen-Activated Protein Kinase Expression. *Exp. Ther. Med.* 14 (2), 1219–1226. doi:10.3892/etm.2017.4617

Calderón-Montaño, J. M., Burgos-Morón, E., Pérez-Guerrero, C., and López-Lázaro, M. (2011). A Review on the Dietary Flavonoid Kaempferol. *Mini Rev. Med. Chem.* 11 (4), 298–344.

Cao, H.-j., Li, C.-r., Wang, L.-y., Ziadlou, R., Grad, S., Zhang, Y., et al. (2019). Effect and Mechanism of Psoralidin on Promoting Osteogenesis and Inhibiting Adipogenesis. *Phytomedicine* 61, 152860. doi:10.1016/j.phymed.2019.152860

Cao, X., Xiao, H., Zhang, Y., Zou, L., Chu, Y., and Chu, X. (2010). 1, 5-Dicaffeoylquinic Acid-Mediated Glutathione Synthesis through Activation of Nrf2 Protects against OGD/reperfusion-induced Oxidative Stress in Astrocytes. *Brain Res.* 1347, 142–148. doi:10.1016/j.brainres.2010.05.072

Carreras-Sureda, A., Pihán, P., and Hetz, C. (2018). Calcium Signaling at the Endoplasmic Reticulum: fine-tuning Stress Responses. *Cell Calcium* 70, 24–31. doi:10.1016/j.ceca.2017.08.004

Caselli, A., Cirri, P., Santi, A., and Paoli, P. (2016). Morin: A Promising Natural Drug. *Cmc* 23 (8), 774–791. doi:10.2174/0929867323666160106150821

Chaingam, J., Juengwatanatrakul, T., Yusakul, G., Kanchanapoom, T., and Putalun, W. (2020). HPLC-UV-based Simultaneous Determination of Canthin-6-One Alkaloids, Quassinoids,and Scopoletin: the Active Ingredients in Eurycoma Longifolia Jack and Eurycoma Harmandiana Pierre, and Their Anti-inflammatory Activities. *J. AOAC Int.* 104, 802–810. doi:10.1093/jaoacint/qsaa141

Chang, X., Zhang, T., Liu, D., Meng, Q., Yan, P., Luo, D., et al. (2021). Puerarin Attenuates LPS-Induced Inflammatory Responses and Oxidative Stress Injury in Human Umbilical Vein Endothelial Cells through Mitochondrial Quality Control. *Oxid Med. Cel Longev* 2021, 6659240. doi:10.1155/2021/6659240

Cheevarungnapakul, K., Khaksar, G., Panpetch, P., Boonjing, P., and Sirikantaramas, S. (2019). Identification and Functional Characterization of Genes Involved in the Biosynthesis of Caffeoylquinic Acids in Sunflower (Helianthus Annuus L.). *Front. Plant Sci.* 10, 968. doi:10.3389/fpls.2019.00968

Chen, F., Tang, Y., Sun, Y., Veeraraghavan, V. P., Mohan, S. K., and Cui, C. (2019a). 6-shogaol, a Active Constiuents of Ginger Prevents UVB Radiation Mediated Inflammation and Oxidative Stress through Modulating NrF2 Signaling in Human Epidermal Keratinocytes (HaCaT Cells). *J. Photochem. Photobiol. B: Biol.* 197, 111518. doi:10.1016/j.jphotobiol.2019.111518

Chen, J., Li, S., and Li, C. (2021a). Mechanisms of Melanocyte Death in Vitiligo. *Med. Res. Rev.* 41 (2), 1138–1166. doi:10.1002/med.21754

Chen, L., and Shen, Z. (2020). Tissue-resident Memory T Cells and Their Biological Characteristics in the Recurrence of Inflammatory Skin Disorders. *Cell Mol Immunol* 17 (1), 64–75. doi:10.1038/s41423-019-0291-4

Chen, T. C., Yen, C. K., Lu, Y. C., Shi, C. S., Hsieh, R. Z., Chang, S. F., et al. (2020). The Antagonism of 6-shogaol in High-Glucose-Activated NLRP3 Inflammasome and Consequent Calcification of Human Artery Smooth Muscle Cells. *Cell Biosci* 10, 5. doi:10.1186/s13578-019-0372-1

Chen, X., Guo, W., Chang, Y., Chen, J., Kang, P., Yi, X., et al. (2019b). Oxidative Stress-Induced IL-15 Trans-presentation in Keratinocytes Contributes to CD8+ T Cells Activation via JAK-STAT Pathway in Vitiligo. *Free Radic. Biol. Med.* 139, 80–91. doi:10.1016/j.freeradbiomed.2019.05.011

Chen, Y., Wang, B., Yuan, X., Lu, Y., Hu, J., Gao, J., et al. (2021b). Vitexin Prevents Colitis-Associated Carcinogenesis in Mice through Regulating Macrophage Polarization. *Phytomedicine* 83, 153489. doi:10.1016/j.phymed.2021.153489

Chiang, H.-M., Lin, J.-W., Hsiao, P.-L., Tsai, S.-Y., and Wen, K.-C. (2011). Hydrolysates of Citrus Plants Stimulate Melanogenesis Protecting against UV-Induced Dermal Damage. *Phytother. Res.* 25 (4), 569–576. doi:10.1002/ptr.3302

Chiu, W.-T., Shen, S.-C., Chow, J.-M., Lin, C.-W., Shia, L.-T., and Chen, Y.-C. (2010). Contribution of Reactive Oxygen Species to Migration/invasion of Human Glioblastoma Cells U87 via ERK-dependent COX-2/PGE2 Activation. *Neurobiol. Dis.* 37 (1), 118–129. doi:10.1016/j.nbd.2009.09.015

Cho, Y.-M., Onodera, H., Ueda, M., Imai, T., and Hirose, M. (2006). A 13-week Subchronic Toxicity Study of Dietary Administered Morin in F344 Rats. *Food Chem. Toxicol.* 44 (6), 891–897. doi:10.1016/j.fct.2005.12.002

Choi, E.-O., Jeong, J.-W., Park, C., Hong, S. H., Kim, G.-Y., Hwang, H.-J., et al. (2016). Baicalein Protects C6 Glial Cells against Hydrogen Peroxide-Induced Oxidative Stress and Apoptosis through Regulation of the Nrf2 Signaling Pathway. *Int. J. Mol. Med.* 37 (3), 798–806. doi:10.3892/ijmm.2016.2460

Cui, H. X., Chen, J. H., Li, J. W., Cheng, F. R., and Yuan, K. (2018). Protection of Anthocyanin from Myrica Rubra against Cerebral Ischemia-Reperfusion Injury via Modulation of the TLR4/NF-Kb and NLRP3 Pathways. *Molecules* 23 (7). doi:10.3390/molecules23071788

Cui, S., Wu, Q., Wang, J., Li, M., Qian, J., and Li, S. (2019). Quercetin Inhibits LPS-Induced Macrophage Migration by Suppressing the iNOS/FAK/paxillin Pathway and Modulating the Cytoskeleton. *Cell Adhes. Migration* 13 (1), 1–12. doi:10.1080/19336918.2018.1486142

Cushnie, T. P. T., Hamilton, V. E. S., Chapman, D. G., Taylor, P. W., and Lamb, A. J. (2007). Aggregation of *Staphylococcus aureus* Following Treatment with the Antibacterial Flavonol Galangin. *J. Appl. Microbiol.* 103 (5), 1562–1567. doi:10.1111/j.1365-2672.2007.03393.x

de Oliveira, M. R., Nabavi, S. F., Habtemariam, S., Erdogan Orhan, I., Daglia, M., and Nabavi, S. M. (2015). The Effects of Baicalein and Baicalin on Mitochondrial Function and Dynamics: A Review. *Pharmacol. Res.* 100, 296–308. doi:10.1016/j.phrs.2015.08.021

Dell'Anna, M. L., Mastrofrancesco, A., Sala, R., Venturini, M., Ottaviani, M., Vidolin, A. P., et al. (2007). Antioxidants and Narrow Band-UVB in the Treatment of Vitiligo: a Double-Blind Placebo Controlled Trial. *Clin. Exp. Dermatol.* 32 (6), 631–636. doi:10.1111/j.1365-2230.2007.02514.x

Denat, L., Kadekaro, A. L., Marrot, L., Leachman, S. A., and Abdel-Malek, Z. A. (2014). Melanocytes as Instigators and Victims of Oxidative Stress. *J. Invest. Dermatol.* 134 (6), 1512–1518. doi:10.1038/jid.2014.65

Dincer Rota, D., Aksoy Sarac, G., Arca, E., and Onder, M. (2021). Comparison of the Efficacy of Broad-Band Targeted UVB Phototherapy and Topical Psoralen with Targeted UVA Phototherapy in Localized Vitiligo. *Dermatol. Ther.* 34 (1), e14562. doi:10.1111/dth.14562

Ding, G., Xu, X., Li, D., Chen, Y., Wang, W., Ping, D., et al. (2020). Fisetin Inhibits Proliferation of Pancreatic Adenocarcinoma by Inducing DNA Damage via RFXAP/KDM4A-dependent Histone H3K36 Demethylation. *Cell Death Dis* 11 (10), 893. doi:10.1038/s41419-020-03019-2

Ding, T., Zhao, T., Li, Y., Liu, Z., Ding, J., Ji, B., et al. (2021). Vitexin Exerts Protective Effects against Calcium Oxalate crystal-induced Kidney Pyroptosis *In Vivo* and *In Vitro*. *Phytomedicine* 86, 153562. doi:10.1016/j.phymed.2021.153562

Ding, X., Mei, E., Hu, M., Zhou, C., Li, X., Cai, L., et al. (2019). Effect of Puerarin on Melanogenesis in Human Melanocytes and Vitiligo Mouse Models and the Underlying Mechanism. *Phytotherapy Res.* 33 (1), 205–213. doi:10.1002/ptr.6218

Dogra, N. K., Kumar, S., and Kumar, D. (2020). Vernonia Anthelmintica (L.) Willd.: An Ethnomedicinal, Phytochemical, Pharmacological and Toxicological Review. *J. Ethnopharmacology* 256, 112777. doi:10.1016/j.jep.2020.112777

Dominguez, L. J., Farruggia, M., Veronese, N., and Barbagallo, M. (2021). Vitamin D Sources, Metabolism, and Deficiency: Available Compounds and Guidelines for its Treatment. *Metabolites* 11 (4), 255. doi:10.3390/metabo11040255

Du, Y., Luo, M., Du, Y., Xu, M., Yao, Q., Wang, K., et al. (2021). Liquiritigenin Decreases Aβ Levels and Ameliorates Cognitive Decline by Regulating Microglia M1/M2 Transformation in AD Mice. *Neurotox Res.* 39 (2), 349–358. doi:10.1007/s12640-020-00284-z

Duan, J., Guan, Y., Mu, F., Guo, C., Zhang, E., Yin, Y., et al. (2017). Protective Effect of Butin against Ischemia/reperfusion-Induced Myocardial Injury in Diabetic Mice: Involvement of the AMPK/GSK-3β/Nrf2 Signaling Pathway. *Sci. Rep.* 7, 41491. doi:10.1038/srep41491

Ezzedine, K., Eleftheriadou, V., Whitton, M., and van Geel, N. (2015). Vitiligo. *The Lancet* 386 (9988), 74–84. doi:10.1016/s0140-6736(14)60763-7

Fan, Z., Cai, L., Wang, S., Wang, J., and Chen, B. (2021). Baicalin Prevents Myocardial Ischemia/Reperfusion Injury through Inhibiting ACSL4 Mediated Ferroptosis. *Front. Pharmacol.* 12, 628988. doi:10.3389/fphar.2021.628988

Fang, D., Xiong, Z., Xu, J., Yin, J., and Luo, R. (2019). Chemopreventive Mechanisms of Galangin against Hepatocellular Carcinoma: A Review. *Biomed. Pharmacother.* 109, 2054–2061. doi:10.1016/j.biopha.2018.09.154

Fiorito, S., Epifano, F., Palmisano, R., Genovese, S., and Taddeo, V. A. (2017). A Re-investigation of the Phytochemical Composition of the Edible Herb Amaranthus Retroflexus L. *J. Pharm. Biomed. Anal.* 143, 183–187. doi:10.1016/j.jpba.2017.05.051

Fiorito, S., Epifano, F., Preziuso, F., Cacciatore, I., di Stefano, A., Taddeo, V. A., et al. (2018). Natural Oxyprenylated Coumarins Are Modulators of Melanogenesis. *Eur. J. Med. Chem.* 152, 274–282. doi:10.1016/j.ejmech.2018.04.051

Gao, Z., Huang, K., Yang, X., and Xu, H. (1999). Free Radical Scavenging and Antioxidant Activities of Flavonoids Extracted from the Radix of Scutellaria Baicalensis Georgi. *Biochim. Biophys. Acta (Bba) - Gen. Subjects* 1472 (3), 643–650. doi:10.1016/s0304-4165(99)00152-x

Gnonlonfin, B. G., Gbaguidi, F., Gbenou, J. D., Sanni, A., and Brimer, L. (2011). Changes in Scopoletin Concentration in Cassava Chips from Four Varieties during Storage. *J. Sci. Food Agric.* 91 (13), 2344–2347. doi:10.1002/jsfa.4465

Godoy de Lima, R., Barros, M. T., and da Silva Laurentiz, R. (2018). Medicinal Attributes of Lignans Extracted from Piper Cubeba: Current Developments. *ChemistryOpen* 7 (2), 180–191.

Góngora, L., Giner, R. M., Máñez, S., del Carmen Recio, M., Schinella, G., and Rios, J. L. (2002). Effects of Caffeoyl Conjugates of Isoprenyl-Hydroquinone Glucoside and Quinic Acid on Leukocyte Function. *Life Sci.* 71 (25), 2995–3004. doi:10.1016/s0024-3205(02)02167-7

Grimes, P. E., and Nashawati, R. (2017). Depigmentation Therapies for Vitiligo. *Dermatol. Clin.* 35 (2), 219–227. doi:10.1016/j.det.2016.11.010

Gu, C., Yang, X., and Huang, L. (2016). Cistanches Herba: A Neuropharmacology Review. *Front. Pharmacol.* 7, 289. doi:10.3389/fphar.2016.00289

Guan, C., Xu, W., Hong, W., Zhou, M., Lin, F., Fu, L., et al. (2015). Quercetin Attenuates the Effects of H2O2 on Endoplasmic Reticulum Morphology and Tyrosinase export from the Endoplasmic Reticulum in Melanocytes. *Mol. Med. Rep.* 11 (6), 4285–4290. doi:10.3892/mmr.2015.3242

Guan, S., Su, W., Wang, N., Li, P., and Wang, Y. (2008). A Potent Tyrosinase Activator from Radix Polygoni Multiflori and its Melanogenesis Stimulatory Effect in B16 Melanoma Cells. *Phytother. Res.* 22 (5), 660–663. doi:10.1002/ptr.2358

Guo, S., and Zhang, Q. (2021). Paeonol Protects Melanocytes against Hydrogen Peroxide-Induced Oxidative Stress through Activation of Nrf2 Signaling Pathway. *Drug Dev. Res.* doi:10.1002/ddr.21793

Harris, J. E., Harris, T. H., Weninger, W., John Wherry, E., Hunter, C. A., and Turka, L. A. (2012). A Mouse Model of Vitiligo with Focused Epidermal Depigmentation Requires IFN-γ for Autoreactive CD8+ T-Cell Accumulation in the Skin. *J. Invest. Dermatol.* 132 (7), 1869–1876. doi:10.1038/jid.2011.463

He, H., Wang, S., Tian, J., Chen, L., Zhang, W., Zhao, J., et al. (2015). Protective Effects of 2,3,5,4′-Tetrahydroxystilbene-2-O-β-D-Glucoside in the MPTP-Induced Mouse Model of Parkinson's Disease: Involvement of Reactive Oxygen Species-Mediated JNK, P38 and Mitochondrial Pathways. *Eur. J. Pharmacol.* 767, 175–182. doi:10.1016/j.ejphar.2015.10.023

He, M., Min, J.-W., Kong, W.-L., He, X.-H., Li, J.-X., and Peng, B.-W. (2016). A Review on the Pharmacological Effects of Vitexin and Isovitexin. *Fitoterapia* 115, 74–85. doi:10.1016/j.fitote.2016.09.011

Hearing, V. J. (1999). Biochemical Control of Melanogenesis and Melanosomal Organization. *J. Invest. Dermatol. Symp. Proc.* 4 (1), 24–28. doi:10.1038/sj.jidsp.5640176

Heeba, G. H., Rabie, E. M., Abuzeid, M. M., Bekhit, A. A., and Khalifa, M. M. (2021). Morin Alleviates Fructose-Induced Metabolic Syndrome in Rats via Ameliorating Oxidative Stress, Inflammatory and Fibrotic Markers. *Korean J. Physiol. Pharmacol.* 25 (3), 177–187. doi:10.4196/kjpp.2021.25.3.177

Heriniaina, R. M., Dong, J., Kalavagunta, P. K., Wu, H.-L., Yan, D.-S., and Shang, J. (2018). Effects of Six Compounds with Different Chemical Structures on Melanogenesis. *Chin. J. Nat. Medicines* 16 (10), 766–773. doi:10.1016/s1875-5364(18)30116-x

Hirata, N., Naruto, S., Ohguchi, K., Akao, Y., Nozawa, Y., Iinuma, M., et al. (2007). Mechanism of the Melanogenesis Stimulation Activity of (−)-cubebin in Murine B16 Melanoma Cells. *Bioorg. Med. Chem.* 15 (14), 4897–4902. doi:10.1016/j.bmc.2007.04.046

Hu, M., Chen, C., Liu, J., Cai, L., Shao, J., Chen, Z., et al. (2020a). The Melanogenic Effects and Underlying Mechanism of Paeoniflorin in Human Melanocytes and Vitiligo Mice. *Fitoterapia* 140, 104416. doi:10.1016/j.fitote.2019.104416

Hu, Y., Huang, J., Li, Y., Jiang, L., Ouyang, Y., Li, Y., et al. (2020b). Cistanche Deserticola Polysaccharide Induces Melanogenesis in Melanocytes and Reduces Oxidative Stress via Activating NRF2/HO-1 Pathway. *J. Cel Mol Med* 24 (7), 4023–4035. doi:10.1111/jcmm.15038

Huang, J., Tong, X., Zhang, L., Zhang, Y., Wang, L., Wang, D., et al. (2020). Hyperoside Attenuates Bleomycin-Induced Pulmonary Fibrosis Development in Mice. *Front. Pharmacol.* 11, 550955. doi:10.3389/fphar.2020.550955

Huang, K., Li, C., Gao, F., Fan, Y., Zeng, F., Meng, L., et al. (2021). Epigallocatechin-3-Gallate Promotes the *In Vitro* Maturation and Embryo Development Following IVF of Porcine Oocytes. *Dddt* 15, 1013–1020. doi:10.2147/dddt.s295936

Huang, W. H., Lee, A. R., Chien, P. Y., and Chou, T. C. (2005). Synthesis of Baicalein Derivatives as Potential Anti-aggregatory and Anti-inflammatory Agents. *J. Pharm. Pharmacol.* 57 (2), 219–225. doi:10.1211/0022357055371

Huang, Y.-C., Yang, C.-H., and Chiou, Y.-L. (2011). Citrus Flavanone Naringenin Enhances Melanogenesis through the Activation of Wnt/β-Catenin Signalling in Mouse Melanoma Cells. *Phytomedicine* 18 (14), 1244–1249. doi:10.1016/j.phymed.2011.06.028

Huang, Y. C., Liu, K. C., and Chiou, Y. L. (2012). Melanogenesis of Murine Melanoma Cells Induced by Hesperetin, a Citrus Hydrolysate-Derived Flavonoid. *Food Chem. Toxicol.* 50 (3-4), 653–659. doi:10.1016/j.fct.2012.01.012

Huo, S.-X., Liu, X.-M., Ge, C.-H., Gao, L., Peng, X.-M., Zhao, P.-P., et al. (2014). The Effects of Galangin on a Mouse Model of Vitiligo Induced by Hydroquinone. *Phytother. Res.* 28 (10), 1533–1538. doi:10.1002/ptr.5161

Huo, S.-X., Wang, Q., Liu, X.-M., Ge, C.-H., Gao, L., Peng, X.-M., et al. (2017). The Effect of Butin on the Vitiligo Mouse Model Induced by Hydroquinone. *Phytother. Res.* 31 (5), 740–746. doi:10.1002/ptr.5794

Hwang, I. K., Yoo, K.-Y., Kim, D. W., Jeong, S. J., Won, C.-K., Moon, W.-K., et al. (2006). An Extract of Polygonum Multiflorum Protects against Free Radical Damage Induced by Ultraviolet B Irradiation of the Skin. *Braz. J. Med. Biol. Res.* 39 (9), 1181–1188. doi:10.1590/s0100-879x2006000900005

Hwang, J.-M., Tseng, T.-H., Tsai, Y.-Y., Lee, H.-J., Chou, F.-P., Wang, C.-J., et al. (2005). Protective Effects of Baicalein on Tert-Butyl Hydroperoxide-Induced Hepatic Toxicity in Rat Hepatocytes. *J. Biomed. Sci.* 12 (2), 389–397. doi:10.1007/s11373-005-1572-8

Hwang, Y. S., Oh, S. W., Park, S. H., Lee, J., Yoo, J. A., Kwon, K., et al. (2019). Melanogenic Effects of Maclurin Are Mediated through the Activation of cAMP/PKA/CREB and P38 MAPK/CREB Signaling Pathways. *Oxid Med. Cel Longev* 2019, 9827519. doi:10.1155/2019/9827519

Hwang, Y. S., Kim, Y.-J., Kim, M. O., Kang, M., Oh, S. W., Nho, Y. H., et al. (2017). Cannabidiol Upregulates Melanogenesis through CB1 Dependent Pathway by Activating P38 MAPK and P42/44 MAPK. *Chemico-Biological Interactions* 273, 107–114. doi:10.1016/j.cbi.2017.06.005

Imran, M., Rauf, A., Shah, Z. A., Saeed, F., Imran, A., Arshad, M. U., et al. (2019). Chemo-preventive and Therapeutic Effect of the Dietary Flavonoid Kaempferol: A Comprehensive Review. *Phytotherapy Res.* 33 (2), 263–275. doi:10.1002/ptr.6227

Iuvone, T., Esposito, G., De Filippis, D., Scuderi, C., and Steardo, L. (2009). Cannabidiol: a Promising Drug for Neurodegenerative Disorders?. *CNS Neurosci. Ther.* 15 (1), 65–75. doi:10.1111/j.1755-5949.2008.00065.x

Jang, Y., and Koh, E. (2019). Antioxidant Content and Activity in Leaves and Petioles of Six Sweet Potato (Ipomoea Batatas L.) and Antioxidant Properties of Blanched Leaves. *Food Sci. Biotechnol.* 28 (2), 337–345. doi:10.1007/s10068-018-0481-3

Jeng, K.-C. G., Hou, R. C. W., Wang, J.-C., and Ping, L.-I. (2005). Sesamin Inhibits Lipopolysaccharide-Induced Cytokine Production by Suppression of P38 Mitogen-Activated Protein Kinase and Nuclear Factor-Kb. *Immunol. Lett.* 97 (1), 101–106. doi:10.1016/j.imlet.2004.10.004

Jeong, Y.-M., Choi, Y.-G., Kim, D.-S., Park, S.-H., Yoon, J.-A., Kwon, S.-B., et al. (2005). Cytoprotective Effect of green tea Extract and Quercetin against Hydrogen Peroxide-Induced Oxidative Stress. *Arch. Pharm. Res.* 28 (11), 1251–1256. doi:10.1007/bf02978208

Jian, Z., Li, K., Liu, L., Zhang, Y., Zhou, Z., Li, C., et al. (2011). Heme Oxygenase-1 Protects Human Melanocytes from H2O2-Induced Oxidative Stress via the Nrf2-ARE Pathway. *J. Invest. Dermatol.* 131 (7), 1420–1427. doi:10.1038/jid.2011.56

Jian, Z., Li, K., Song, P., Zhu, G., Zhu, L., Cui, T., et al. (2014). Impaired Activation of the Nrf2-ARE Signaling Pathway Undermines H2O2-Induced Oxidative Stress Response: a Possible Mechanism for Melanocyte Degeneration in Vitiligo. *J. Invest. Dermatol.* 134 (8), 2221–2230. doi:10.1038/jid.2014.152

Jiang, W., Li, S., Chen, X., Zhang, W., Chang, Y., He, Y., et al. (2019). Berberine Protects Immortalized Line of Human Melanocytes from H2O2-Induced Oxidative Stress via Activation of Nrf2 and Mitf Signaling Pathway. *J. Dermatol. Sci.* 94 (1), 236–243. doi:10.1016/j.jdermsci.2019.03.007

Jiang, Z., Li, S., Liu, Y., Deng, P., Huang, J., and He, G. (2011). Sesamin Induces Melanogenesis by Microphthalmia-Associated Transcription Factor and Tyrosinase Up-Regulation via cAMP Signaling Pathway. *Acta Biochim. Biophys. Sinica* 43 (10), 763–770. doi:10.1093/abbs/gmr078

Jiang, Z., Xu, J., Long, M., Tu, Z., Yang, G., and He, G. (2009). 2, 3, 5, 4'-Tetrahydroxystilbene-2-O-Beta-D-Glucoside (THSG) Induces Melanogenesis in B16 Cells by MAP Kinase Activation and Tyrosinase Upregulation. *Life Sci.* 85 (9-10), 345–350. doi:10.1016/j.lfs.2009.05.022

Jie, Q., Kodithuwakku, N. D., Yuan, X., He, G., Chen, M., Xu, S., et al. (2015). Anti-allergic and Anti-inflammatory Properties of a Potent Histamine H1 Receptor Antagonist, Desloratadine Citrate Disodium Injection, and its Anti-inflammatory Mechanism on EA.Hy926 Endothelial Cells. *Eur. J. Pharmacol.* 754, 1–10. doi:10.1016/j.ejphar.2015.02.016

Jin, Y., Andersen, G., Yorgov, D., Ferrara, T. M., Ben, S., Brownson, K. M., et al. (2016). Genome-wide Association Studies of Autoimmune Vitiligo Identify 23 New Risk Loci and Highlight Key Pathways and Regulatory Variants. *Nat. Genet.* 48 (11), 1418–1424. doi:10.1038/ng.3680

Jung, E., Kim, J. H., Kim, M. O., Jang, S., Kang, M., Oh, S. W., et al. (2016). Afzelin Positively Regulates Melanogenesis through the P38 MAPK Pathway. *Chemico-Biological Interactions* 254, 167–172. doi:10.1016/j.cbi.2016.06.010

Jung, G.-D., Yang, J.-Y., Song, E.-S., and Park, J.-W. (2001). Stimulation of Melanogenesis by Glycyrrhizin in B16 Melanoma Cells. *Exp. Mol. Med.* 33 (3), 131–135. doi:10.1038/emm.2001.23

Kalaiselvi, P., Rajashree, K., Bharathi Priya, L., and Padma, V. V. (2013). Cytoprotective Effect of Epigallocatechin-3-Gallate against Deoxynivalenol-Induced Toxicity through Anti-oxidative and Anti-inflammatory Mechanisms in HT-29 Cells. *Food Chem. Toxicol.* 56, 110–118. doi:10.1016/j.fct.2013.01.042

Katiyar, S. K., Matsui, M. S., Elmets, C. A., and Mukhtar, H. (1999). Polyphenolic Antioxidant (-)-Epigallocatechin-3-Gallate from Green Tea Reduces UVB-Lnduced Inflammatory Responses and Infiltration of Leukocytes in Human Skin. *Photochem. Photobiol.* 69 (2), 148–153. doi:10.1111/j.1751-1097.1999.tb03267.x

Kawakami, T., Ohgushi, A., Hirobe, T., and Soma, Y. (2014). Effects of 1,25-dihydroxyvitamin D3 on Human Epidermal Melanocytes and Melanoblasts. *J. Dermatol. Sci.* 76 (1), 72–74. doi:10.1016/j.jdermsci.2014.07.005

Khan, H., Marya, S., Amin, S., Kamal, M. A., and Patel, S. (2018). Flavonoids as Acetylcholinesterase Inhibitors: Current Therapeutic Standing and Future Prospects. *Biomed. Pharmacother.* 101, 860–870. doi:10.1016/j.biopha.2018.03.007

Khan, N., and Mukhtar, H. (2015). Dietary Agents for Prevention and Treatment of Lung Cancer. *Cancer Lett.* 359 (2), 155–164. doi:10.1016/j.canlet.2015.01.038

Kim, H. J., Kim, J. S., Woo, J.-T., Lee, I.-S., and Cha, B.-Y. (2015). Hyperpigmentation Mechanism of Methyl 3,5-Di-Caffeoylquinate through Activation of P38 and MITF Induction of Tyrosinase. *Acta Biochim. Biophys. Sin* 47 (7), 548–556. doi:10.1093/abbs/gmv040

Kim, J.-K., and Jang, H.-D. (2016). 6-shogaol Attenuates H2O2-Induced Oxidative Stress via Upregulation of Nrf2-Mediated γ-glutamylcysteine Synthetase and Heme Oxygenase Expression in HepG2 Cells. *Food Sci. Biotechnol.* 25 (1), 319–327. doi:10.1007/s10068-016-0045-3

Kim, J. K., Kim, Y. S., Kim, Y., Uddin, M. R., Kim, Y. B., Kim, H. H., et al. (2014). Comparative Analysis of Flavonoids and Polar Metabolites from Hairy Roots of Scutellaria Baicalensis and Scutellaria Lateriflora. *World J. Microbiol. Biotechnol.* 30 (3), 887–892. doi:10.1007/s11274-013-1498-7

Kim, S. K., Kim, H. J., Choi, S. E., Park, K. H., Choi, H. K., and Lee, M. W. (2008). Anti-oxidative and Inhibitory Activities on Nitric Oxide (NO) and Prostaglandin E2 (COX-2) Production of Flavonoids from Seeds of Prunus Tomentosa Thunberg. *Arch. Pharm. Res.* 31 (4), 424–428. doi:10.1007/s12272-001-1174-9

Kou, X., Wang, X., Ji, R., Liu, L., Qiao, Y., Lou, Z., et al. (2018). Occurrence, Biological Activity and Metabolism of 6-shogaol. *Food Funct.* 9 (3), 1310–1327. doi:10.1039/c7fo01354j

Kwon, S.-J., Kim, Y.-M., Jang, H.-J., and Seo, Y.-K. (2018). Synergistic Effect of rice Bran Extract and Extremely Low-Frequency Electromagnetic fields on Dermal Papilla/melanocytes in Melanogenesis. *Bioelectromagnetics* 39 (8), 595–603. doi:10.1002/bem.22151

Lai, Y., Feng, Q., Zhang, R., Shang, J., and Zhong, H. (2021). The Great Capacity on Promoting Melanogenesis of Three Compatible Components in Vernonia Anthelmintica (L.) Willd. *Int. J. Mol. Sci.* 22 (8). doi:10.3390/ijms22084073

Latham, C. M., Brightwell, C. R., Keeble, A. R., Munson, B. D., Thomas, N. T., Zagzoog, A. M., et al. (2021). Vitamin D Promotes Skeletal Muscle Regeneration and Mitochondrial Health. *Front. Physiol.* 12, 660498. doi:10.3389/fphys.2021.660498

Lau, K. M., Yue, G. G., Chan, Y. Y., Kwok, H. F., Gao, S., Wong, C. W., et al. (2019). A Review on the Immunomodulatory Activity of Acanthopanax Senticosus and its Active Components. *Chin. Med.* 14, 25. doi:10.1186/s13020-019-0250-0

Lee, J., Jung, E., Park, J., Jung, K., Park, E., Kim, J., et al. (2005). Glycyrrhizin Induces Melanogenesis by Elevating a cAMP Level in B16 Melanoma Cells. *J. Invest. Dermatol.* 124 (2), 405–411. doi:10.1111/j.0022-202x.2004.23606.x

Lee, J., Kim, Y. S., and Park, D. (2007). Rosmarinic Acid Induces Melanogenesis through Protein Kinase A Activation Signaling. *Biochem. Pharmacol.* 74 (7), 960–968. doi:10.1016/j.bcp.2007.06.007

Lee, S., So, Y.-J., Shin, M., Cho, J., and Lee, J. (2014). Antibacterial Effects of Afzelin Isolated from Cornus Macrophylla on *Pseudomonas aeruginosa*, a Leading Cause of Illness in Immunocompromised Individuals. *Molecules* 19 (3), 3173–3180. doi:10.3390/molecules19033173

Lee, S. Y. (2018). Synergistic Effect of Maclurin on Ginsenoside Compound K Induced Inhibition of the Transcriptional Expression of Matrix Metalloproteinase-1 in HaCaT Human Keratinocyte Cells. *J. Ginseng Res.* 42 (2), 229–232. doi:10.1016/j.jgr.2017.11.003

Lee, Y. J., Jung, O., Lee, J., Son, J., Cho, J. Y., Ryou, C., et al. (2018). Maclurin Exerts Anti-cancer Effects on PC3 Human Prostate Cancer Cells via Activation of P38 and Inhibitions of JNK, FAK, AKT, and C-Myc Signaling Pathways. *Nutr. Res.* 58, 62–71. doi:10.1016/j.nutres.2018.07.003

Legrand, G., Delporte, M., Khelifi, C., Harant, A., Vuylsteker, C., Mörchen, M., et al. (2016). Identification and Characterization of Five BAHD Acyltransferases Involved in Hydroxycinnamoyl Ester Metabolism in Chicory. *Front. Plant Sci.* 7, 741. doi:10.3389/fpls.2016.00741

Li, B., Pinch, H., and Birt, D. R. (1996). Influence of Vehicle, Distant Topical Delivery, and Biotransformation on the Chemopreventive Activity of Apigenin, a Plant Flavonoid, in Mouse Skin. *Pharm. Res.* 13 (10), 1530–1534. doi:10.1023/a:1016083613916

Li, G.-H., Fang, K.-L., Yang, K., Cheng, X.-P., Wang, X.-N., Shen, T., et al. (2021a). Thesium Chinense Turcz.: An Ethnomedical, Phytochemical and Pharmacological Review. *J. Ethnopharmacology* 273, 113950. doi:10.1016/j.jep.2021.113950

Li, J., Ren, S., Li, M., Bi, J., Yang, G., and Li, E. (2021b). Paeoniflorin Protects against Dextran Sulfate Sodium (DSS)-induced Colitis in Mice through Inhibition of Inflammation and Eosinophil Infiltration. *Int. Immunopharmacology* 97, 107667. doi:10.1016/j.intimp.2021.107667

Li, R., Zhao, D., Qu, R., Fu, Q., and Ma, S. (2015). The Effects of Apigenin on Lipopolysaccharide-Induced Depressive-like Behavior in Mice. *Neurosci. Lett.* 594, 17–22. doi:10.1016/j.neulet.2015.03.040

Li, X.-S., Tang, X.-Y., Su, W., and Li, X. (2020). Vitexin Protects Melanocytes from Oxidative Stress via Activating MAPK-Nrf2/ARE Pathway. *Immunopharmacology and Immunotoxicology* 42 (6), 594–603. doi:10.1080/08923973.2020.1835952

Lim, H., Park, H., and Kim, H. P. (2015). Effects of Flavonoids on Senescence-Associated Secretory Phenotype Formation from Bleomycin-Induced Senescence in BJ Fibroblasts. *Biochem. Pharmacol.* 96 (4), 337–348. doi:10.1016/j.bcp.2015.06.013

Lin, M., Lu, S.-s., Wang, A.-x., Qi, X.-y., Zhao, D., Wang, Z.-h., et al. (2011a). Apigenin Attenuates Dopamine-Induced Apoptosis in Melanocytes via Oxidative Stress-Related P38, C-Jun NH2-terminal Kinase and Akt Signaling. *J. Dermatol. Sci.* 63 (1), 10–16. doi:10.1016/j.jdermsci.2011.03.007

Lin, T. Y., Wu, P. Y., Hou, C. W., Chien, T. Y., Chang, Q. X., Wen, K. C., et al. (2019). Protective Effects of Sesamin against UVB-Induced Skin Inflammation and Photodamage *In Vitro* and *In Vivo*. *Biomolecules* 9 (9). doi:10.3390/biom9090479

Lin, Y.-L., Lu, C.-K., Huang, Y.-J., and Chen, H.-J. (2011b). Antioxidative Caffeoylquinic Acids and Flavonoids from Hemerocallis Fulva Flowers. *J. Agric. Food Chem.* 59 (16), 8789–8795. doi:10.1021/jf201166b

Ling, Y., Gong, Q., Xiong, X., Sun, L., Zhao, W., Zhu, W., et al. (2017). Protective Effect of Madecassoside on H2O2-Induced Oxidative Stress and Autophagy Activation in Human Melanocytes. *Oncotarget* 8 (31), 51066–51075. doi:10.18632/oncotarget.17654

Liu, B., Jian, Z., Li, Q., Li, K., Wang, Z., Liu, L., et al. (2012). Baicalein Protects Human Melanocytes from H2O2-Induced Apoptosis via Inhibiting Mitochondria-dependent Caspase Activation and the P38 MAPK Pathway. *Free Radic. Biol. Med.* 53 (2), 183–193. doi:10.1016/j.freeradbiomed.2012.04.015

Liu, R., Ji, P., Liu, B., Qiao, H., Wang, X., Zhou, L., et al. (2017). Apigenin Enhances the Cisplatin Cytotoxic Effect through P53-Modulated Apoptosis. *Oncol. Lett.* 13 (2), 1024–1030. doi:10.3892/ol.2016.5495

Liu, Y., Qiu, Y., Chen, Q., Han, X., Cai, M., and Hao, L. (2021a). Puerarin Suppresses the Hepatic Gluconeogenesis via Activation of PI3K/Akt Signaling Pathway in Diabetic Rats and HepG2 Cells. *Biomed. Pharmacother.* 137, 111325. doi:10.1016/j.biopha.2021.111325

Liu, Y., Wang, H., Yang, M., Liu, N., Zhao, Y., Qi, X., et al. (2018). Cistanche Deserticola Polysaccharides Protects PC12 Cells against OGD/RP-induced Injury. *Biomed. Pharmacother.* 99, 671–680. doi:10.1016/j.biopha.2018.01.114

Liu, Z. Q., Yao, G. L., Zhai, J. M., Hu, D. W., and Fan, Y. G. (2021b). Kaempferol Suppresses Proliferation and Induces Apoptosis and DNA Damage in Human Gallbladder Cancer Cells through the CDK4/CDK6/cyclin D1 Pathway. *Eur. Rev. Med. Pharmacol. Sci.* 25 (3), 1311–1321.

Long, X., Zeng, X., Yan, H., Xu, M., Zeng, Q., Xu, C., et al. (2021). Flavonoids Composition and Antioxidant Potential Assessment of Extracts from Gannanzao Navel Orange (Citrus Sinensis Osbeck Cv. Gannanzao) Peel. *Nat. Product. Res.* 35 (4), 702–706. doi:10.1080/14786419.2019.1593162

Lotito, S., and Frei, B. (2006). Consumption of Flavonoid-Rich Foods and Increased Plasma Antioxidant Capacity in Humans: Cause, Consequence, or Epiphenomenon?. *Free Radic. Biol. Med.* 41 (12), 1727–1746. doi:10.1016/j.freeradbiomed.2006.04.033

Lu, W., Zhao, Y., Kong, Y., Zhang, W., Ma, W., Li, W., et al. (2018). Geniposide Prevents H2 O2 -induced Oxidative Damage in Melanocytes by Activating the PI3K-Akt Signalling Pathway. *Clin. Exp. Dermatol.* 43 (6), 667–674. doi:10.1111/ced.13409

Ma, J., Li, S., Zhu, L., Guo, S., Yi, X., Cui, T., et al. (2018). Baicalein Protects Human Vitiligo Melanocytes from Oxidative Stress through Activation of NF-E2-Related Factor2 (Nrf2) Signaling Pathway. *Free Radic. Biol. Med.* 129, 492–503. doi:10.1016/j.freeradbiomed.2018.10.421

Ma, Y. L., Zhao, F., Yin, J. T., Liang, C. J., Niu, X. L., Qiu, Z. H., et al. (2019). Two Approaches for Evaluating the Effects of Galangin on the Activities and mRNA Expression of Seven CYP450. *Molecules* 24 (6), 1171. doi:10.3390/molecules24061171

Maimaiti, Z., Turak, A., and Aisa, H. A. (2017). Two New Compounds from the Seeds of Vernonia Anthelmintica. *J. Asian Nat. Prod. Res.* 19 (9), 862–868. doi:10.1080/10286020.2016.1269760

Majnooni, M. B., Fakhri, S., Shokoohinia, Y., Mojarrab, M., Kazemi-Afrakoti, S., and Farzaei, M. H. (2020). Isofraxidin: Synthesis, Biosynthesis, Isolation, Pharmacokinetic and Pharmacological Properties. *Molecules* 25 (9), 2040. doi:10.3390/molecules25092040

Maleš, Ž., Drvar, D. L., Duka, I., and Žužul, K. (2019). Application of Medicinal Plants in Several Dermatovenerological Entities. *Acta Pharm.* 69 (4), 525–531.

Mamat, N., Lu, X. Y., Kabas, M., and Aisa, H. A. (2018). Potential Anti-vitiligo Properties of Cynarine Extracted from Vernonia Anthelmintica (L.) Willd. *Int. J. Mol. Med.* 42 (5), 2665–2675. doi:10.3892/ijmm.2018.3861

Mamat, N., Dou, J., Lu, X., Eblimit, A., and Haji Akber, A. (2017). Isochlorogenic Acid A Promotes Melanin Synthesis in B16 Cell through the β-catenin Signal Pathway. *Acta Biochim. Biophys. Sin (Shanghai)* 49 (9), 800–807. doi:10.1093/abbs/gmx072

Mechoulam, R., and Hanus, L. (2002). Cannabidiol: an Overview of Some Chemical and Pharmacological Aspects. Part I: Chemical Aspects. *Chem. Phys. Lipids* 121 (1-2), 35–43. doi:10.1016/s0009-3084(02)00144-5

Meng, Y., Liu, Z., Zhai, C., Di, T., Zhang, L., Zhang, L., et al. (2019). Paeonol Inhibits the Development of 1-chloro-2,4-dinitrobenzene-induced A-topic D-ermatitis via M-ast and T C-ells in BALB/c M-ice. *Mol. Med. Rep.* 19 (4), 3217–3229. doi:10.3892/mmr.2019.9985

Meng, Y., Wang, M., Xie, X., Di, T., Zhao, J., Lin, Y., et al. (2017). Paeonol Ameliorates Imiquimod-Induced Psoriasis-like Skin Lesions in BALB/c Mice by Inhibiting the Maturation and Activation of Dendritic Cells. *Int. J. Mol. Med.* 39 (5), 1101–1110. doi:10.3892/ijmm.2017.2930

Mereles, D., and Hunstein, W. (2011). Epigallocatechin-3-gallate (EGCG) for Clinical Trials: More Pitfalls Than Promises?. *Ijms* 12 (9), 5592–5603. doi:10.3390/ijms12095592

Mi Moon, K., Young Kim, C., Yeul Ma, J., and Lee, B. (2019). Xanthone-related Compounds as an Anti-browning and Antioxidant Food Additive. *Food Chem.* 274, 345–350. doi:10.1016/j.foodchem.2018.08.144

Miao, J., Zhong, J., Lan, J., Ye, S., Ye, P., Li, S., et al. (2021). Paeonol Attenuates Inflammation by Confining HMGB1 to the Nucleus. *J. Cel Mol Med* 25 (6), 2885–2899. doi:10.1111/jcmm.16319

Miguel, S., Legrand, G., Duriot, L., Delporte, M., Menin, B., Michel, C., et al. (2020). A GDSL Lipase-like from Ipomoea Batatas Catalyzes Efficient Production of 3,5-diCQA when Expressed in Pichia pastoris. *Commun. Biol.* 3 (1), 673. doi:10.1038/s42003-020-01488-x

Molagoda, I. M. N., Karunarathne, W., Park, S. R., Choi, Y. H., Park, E. K., Jin, C. Y., et al. (2020). GSK-3beta-Targeting Fisetin Promotes Melanogenesis in

B16F10 Melanoma Cells and Zebrafish Larvae through Beta-Catenin Activation. *Int. J. Mol. Sci.* 21 (1). doi:10.3390/ijms21010312

Monteiro, É., Chibli, L., Yamamoto, C., Pereira, M., Vilela, F., Rodarte, M., et al. (2014). Antinociceptive and Anti-inflammatory Activities of the Sesame Oil and Sesamin. *Nutrients* 6 (5), 1931–1944. doi:10.3390/nu6051931

Moreira, C. G., Horinouchi, C. D. S., Souza-Filho, C. S., Campos, F. R., Barison, A., Cabrini, D. A., et al. (2012). Hyperpigmentant Activity of Leaves and Flowers Extracts of *Pyrostegia venusta* on Murine B16F10 Melanoma. *J. Ethnopharmacology* 141 (3), 1005–1011. doi:10.1016/j.jep.2012.03.047

Mou, K., Pan, W., Han, D., Wen, X., Cao, F., Miao, Y., et al. (2019). Glycyrrhizin Protects Human Melanocytes from H2O2-induced O-xidative D-amage via the Nrf2-dependent I-nduction of HO-1. *Int. J. Mol. Med.* 44 (1), 253–261. doi:10.3892/ijmm.2019.4200

Mou, K. H., Han, D., Liu, W. L., and Li, P. (2016). Combination Therapy of Orally Administered Glycyrrhizin and UVB Improved Active-Stage Generalized Vitiligo. *Braz. J. Med. Biol. Res.* 49 (8). doi:10.1590/1414-431x20165354

Mou, S. Q., Zhou, Z. Y., Feng, H., Zhang, N., Lin, Z., Aiyasiding, X., et al. (2021). Liquiritin Attenuates Lipopolysaccharides-Induced Cardiomyocyte Injury via an AMP-Activated Protein Kinase-dependent Signaling Pathway. *Front. Pharmacol.* 12, 648688. doi:10.3389/fphar.2021.648688

Nagata, H., Takekoshi, S., Takeyama, R., Homma, T., and Yoshiyuki Osamura, R. (2004). Quercetin Enhances Melanogenesis by Increasing the Activity and Synthesis of Tyrosinase in Human Melanoma Cells and in normal Human Melanocytes. *Pigment Cel Res* 17 (1), 66–73. doi:10.1046/j.1600-0749.2003.00113.x

Nasr, M., and Al-Karaki, R. (2020). Nanotechnological Innovations Enhancing the Topical Therapeutic Efficacy of Quercetin: A Succinct Review. *Cdd* 17 (4), 270–278. doi:10.2174/1567201817666200317123224

Nguyen, D.-V., Li, F., Li, H., Wong, B. S., Low, C. Y., Liu, X.-Y., et al. (2015). Drug Permeation through Skin Is Inversely Correlated with Carrier Gel Rigidity. *Mol. Pharmaceutics* 12 (2), 444–452. doi:10.1021/mp500542a

Ning, W., Wang, S., Dong, X., Liu, D., Fu, L., Jin, R., et al. (2015). Epigallocatechin-3-gallate (EGCG) Suppresses the Trafficking of Lymphocytes to Epidermal Melanocytes via Inhibition of JAK2: Its Implication for Vitiligo Treatment. *Biol. Pharm. Bull.* 38 (11), 1700–1706. doi:10.1248/bpb.b15-00331

Niu, C., and Aisa, H. A. (2017). Upregulation of Melanogenesis and Tyrosinase Activity: Potential Agents for Vitiligo. *Molecules* 22 (8), 1303. doi:10.3390/molecules22081303

Niu, C., Pang, G. X., Li, G., Dou, J., Nie, L. F., Himit, H., et al. (2016). Synthesis and Biological Evaluation of Furocoumarin Derivatives on Melanin Synthesis in Murine B16 Cells for the Treatment of Vitiligo. *Bioorg. Med. Chem.* 24 (22), 5960–5968. doi:10.1016/j.bmc.2016.09.056

Ohguchi, K., Akao, Y., and Nozawa, Y. (2006). Stimulation of Melanogenesis by the Citrus Flavonoid Naringenin in Mouse B16 Melanoma Cells. *Biosci. Biotechnol. Biochem.* 70 (6), 1499–1501. doi:10.1271/bbb.50635

Ożarowski, M., and Karpiński, T. M. (2020). Extracts and Flavonoids of Passiflora Species as Promising Anti-inflammatory and Antioxidant Substances. *Curr. Pharm. Des.* doi:10.2174/1381612826666200526150113

Park, W.-s., Kwon, O., Yoon, T.-J., and Chung, J. H. (2014). Anti-graying Effect of the Extract of Pueraria Thunbergiana via Upregulation of cAMP/MITF-M Signaling Pathway. *J. Dermatol. Sci.* 75 (2), 153–155. doi:10.1016/j.jdermsci.2014.05.003

Pastorino, G., Cornara, L., Soares, S., Rodrigues, F., and Oliveira, M. B. P. P. (2018). Liquorice (Glycyrrhiza Glabra): A Phytochemical and Pharmacological Review. *Phytotherapy Res.* 32 (12), 2323–2339. doi:10.1002/ptr.6178

Patel, D., Shukla, S., and Gupta, S. (2007). Apigenin and Cancer Chemoprevention: Progress, Potential and Promise (Review). *Int. J. Oncol.* 30 (1), 233–245. doi:10.3892/ijo.30.1.233

Patel, S., Rauf, A., Khan, H., Meher, B. R., and Hassan, S. S. U. (2017). A Holistic Review on the Autoimmune Disease Vitiligo with Emphasis on the Causal Factors. *Biomed. Pharmacother.* 92, 501–508. doi:10.1016/j.biopha.2017.05.095

Pathak, N., Rai, A. K., Kumari, R., and Bhat, K. V. (2014). Value Addition in Sesame: A Perspective on Bioactive Components for Enhancing Utility and Profitability. *Pharmacogn Rev.* 8 (16), 147–155. doi:10.4103/0973-7847.134249

Paudel, K. S., Hammell, D. C., Agu, R. U., Valiveti, S., and Stinchcomb, A. L. (2010). Cannabidiol Bioavailability after Nasal and Transdermal Application: Effect of Permeation Enhancers. *Drug Develop. Ind. Pharm.* 36 (9), 1088–1097. doi:10.3109/03639041003657295

Pei, T., Zheng, C., Huang, C., Chen, X., Guo, Z., Fu, Y., et al. (2016). Systematic Understanding the Mechanisms of Vitiligo Pathogenesis and its Treatment by Qubaibabuqi Formula. *J. Ethnopharmacology* 190, 272–287. doi:10.1016/j.jep.2016.06.001

Peng, L. Y., Shi, H. T., Yuan, M., Li, J. H., Song, K., Huang, J. N., et al. (2020). Madecassoside Protects against LPS-Induced Acute Lung Injury via Inhibiting TLR4/NF-Kb Activation and Blood-Air Barrier Permeability. *Front. Pharmacol.* 11, 807. doi:10.3389/fphar.2020.00807

Pérez-Sánchez, A., Barrajón-Catalán, E., Herranz-López, M., Castillo, J., and Micol, V. (2016). Lemon Balm Extract (Melissa Officinalis , L.) Promotes Melanogenesis and Prevents UVB-Induced Oxidative Stress and DNA Damage in a Skin Cell Model. *J. Dermatol. Sci.* 84 (2), 169–177. doi:10.1016/j.jdermsci.2016.08.004

Pillaiyar, T., Manickam, M., and Jung, S.-H. (2017). Recent Development of Signaling Pathways Inhibitors of Melanogenesis. *Cell Signal.* 40, 99–115. doi:10.1016/j.cellsig.2017.09.004

Preziuso, F., Genovese, S., Marchetti, L., Sharifi-Rad, M., Palumbo, L., Epifano, F., et al. (2020). 7-Isopentenyloxycoumarin: What Is New across the Last Decade. *Molecules* 25 (24), 5923. doi:10.3390/molecules25245923

Ramful, D., Bahorun, T., Bourdon, E., Tarnus, E., and Aruoma, O. I. (2010). Bioactive Phenolics and Antioxidant Propensity of Flavedo Extracts of Mauritian Citrus Fruits: Potential Prophylactic Ingredients for Functional Foods Application. *Toxicology* 278 (1), 75–87. doi:10.1016/j.tox.2010.01.012

Rashighi, M., Agarwal, P., Richmond, J. M., Harris, T. H., Dresser, K., Su, M.-W., et al. (2014). CXCL10 Is Critical for the Progression and Maintenance of Depigmentation in a Mouse Model of Vitiligo. *Sci. Translational Med.* 6 (223), 223ra23. doi:10.1126/scitranslmed.3007811

Rauf, A., Imran, M., Khan, I. A., Ur-Rehman, M., Gilani, S. A., Mehmood, Z., et al. (2018). Anticancer Potential of Quercetin: A Comprehensive Review. *Phytotherapy Res.* 32 (11), 2109–2130. doi:10.1002/ptr.6155

Riding, R. L., Richmond, J. M., and Harris, J. E. (2019). Mouse Model for Human Vitiligo. *Curr. Protoc. Immunol.* 124 (1), e63. doi:10.1002/cpim.63

Rodrigues, M., Ezzedine, K., Hamzavi, I., Pandya, A. G., and Harris, J. E. (2017). New Discoveries in the Pathogenesis and Classification of Vitiligo. *J. Am. Acad. Dermatol.* 77 (1), 1–13. doi:10.1016/j.jaad.2016.10.048

Salehi, B., Fokou, P. V. T., Sharifi-Rad, M., Zucca, P., Pezzani, R., Martins, N., et al. (2019). The Therapeutic Potential of Naringenin: A Review of Clinical Trials. *Pharmaceuticals (Basel)* 12 (1), 11. doi:10.3390/ph12010011

Satthakarn, S., Hladik, F., Promsong, A., and Nittayananta, W. (2015). Vaginal Innate Immune Mediators Are Modulated by a Water Extract of Houttuynia Cordata Thunb. *BMC Complement. Altern. Med.* 15, 183. doi:10.1186/s12906-015-0701-9

Seneschal, J., Boniface, K., D'Arino, A., and Picardo, M. (2021). An Update on Vitiligo Pathogenesis. *Pigment Cel Melanoma Res.* 34 (2), 236–243. doi:10.1111/pcmr.12949

Serafino, A., Sinibaldi Vallebona, P., Lazzarino, G., Tavazzi, B., Rasi, G., Pierimarchi, P., et al. (2004). Differentiation of Human Melanoma Cells Induced by Cyanidin-3- O -β-glucopyranoside. *FASEB j.* 18 (15), 1940–1942. doi:10.1096/fj.04-1925fje

Shan, M., Yu, S., Yan, H., Guo, S., Xiao, W., Wang, Z., et al. (2017). A Review on the Phytochemistry, Pharmacology, Pharmacokinetics and Toxicology of Geniposide, a Natural Product. *Molecules* 22 (10), 1689. doi:10.3390/molecules22101689

Sharifi-Rad, J., Kamiloglu, S., Yeskaliyeva, B., Beyatli, A., Alfred, M. A., Salehi, B., et al. (2020). Pharmacological Activities of Psoralidin: A Comprehensive Review of the Molecular Mechanisms of Action. *Front. Pharmacol.* 11, 571459. doi:10.3389/fphar.2020.571459

Shi, M., Zhang, Y., Song, M., Sun, Y., Li, C., and Kang, W. (2018). Screening the Marker Components in Psoralea Corylifolia L. With the Aids of Spectrum-Effect Relationship and Component Knock-Out by UPLC-MS(2). *Int. J. Mol. Sci.* 19 (11), 3439. doi:10.3390/ijms19113439

Shin, S., Ko, J., Kim, M., Song, N., and Park, K. (2021). Morin Induces Melanogenesis via Activation of MAPK Signaling Pathways in B16F10 Mouse Melanoma Cells. *Molecules* 26 (8), 2150. doi:10.3390/molecules26082150

Shin, S. W., Jung, E., Kim, S., Kim, J. H., Kim, E. G., Lee, J., et al. (2013). Antagonizing Effects and Mechanisms of Afzelin against UVB-Induced Cell Damage. *PLoS One* 8 (4), e61971. doi:10.1371/journal.pone.0061971

Shomirzoeva, O., Li, J., Numonov, S., Mamat, N., Shataer, D., Lu, X., et al. (2019). Chemical Components of Hyssopus Seravshanicus: Antioxidant Activity, Activations of Melanogenesis and Tyrosinase, and Quantitative Determination by UPLC-DAD. *Nat. Product. Res.* 33 (6), 866–870. doi:10.1080/14786419.2017.1408105

Shon, M.-S., Kim, R.-H., Kwon, O. J., Roh, S.-S., and Kim, G.-N. (2016). Beneficial Role and Function of Fisetin in Skin Health via Regulation of the CCN2/TGF-β Signaling Pathway. *Food Sci. Biotechnol.* 25 (S1), 133–141. doi:10.1007/s10068-016-0110-y

Shukla, S., and Gupta, S. (2010). Apigenin: a Promising Molecule for Cancer Prevention. *Pharm. Res.* 27 (6), 962–978. doi:10.1007/s11095-010-0089-7

Silva, M. L. A., Coímbra, H. S., Pereira, A. C., Almeida, V. A., Lima, T. C., Costa, E. S., et al. (2007). Evaluation of Piper Cubeba Extract, (-)-cubebin and its Semi-synthetic Derivatives against Oral Pathogens. *Phytother. Res.* 21 (5), 420–422. doi:10.1002/ptr.2088

Singh, B., Singh, J. P., Kaur, A., and Singh, N. (2020). Phenolic Composition, Antioxidant Potential and Health Benefits of Citrus Peel. *Food Res. Int.* 132, 109114. doi:10.1016/j.foodres.2020.109114

Sinha, R., Srivastava, S., Joshi, A., Joshi, U. J., and Govil, G. (2014). In-vitro Anti-proliferative and Anti-oxidant Activity of Galangin, Fisetin and Quercetin: Role of Localization and Intermolecular Interaction in Model Membrane. *Eur. J. Med. Chem.* 79, 102–109. doi:10.1016/j.ejmech.2014.04.002

Sintov, A. C., Yarmolinsky, L., Dahan, A., and Ben-Shabat, S. (2014). Pharmacological Effects of Vitamin D and its Analogs: Recent Developments. *Drug Discov. Today* 19 (11), 1769–1774. doi:10.1016/j.drudis.2014.06.008

Skiba, M. A., Szendzielorz, K., Mazur, B., and Król, W. (2016). The Inhibitory Effect of Flavonoids on Interleukin-8 Release by Human Gastric Adenocarcinoma (AGS) Cells Infected with Cag PAI (+) *Helicobacter pylori. cejoi* 3 (3), 229–235. doi:10.5114/ceji.2016.63119

Somani, G. S., Nahire, M. S., Parikh, A. D., Mulik, M. B., Ghumatkar, P. J., Laddha, K. S., et al. (2017). Neuroprotective Effect of Cubebin: A Dibenzylbutyrolactone Lignan on Scopolamine-Induced Amnesia in Mice. *Indian J. Med. Res.* 146 (2), 255–259. doi:10.4103/ijmr.IJMR_156_14

Souza, G. H. B., da Silva Filho, A. A., de Souza, V. A., Pereira, A. C., de A. Royo, V., e Silva, M. L. A., et al. (2004). Analgesic and Anti-inflammatory Activities Evaluation of (-)-O-Acetyl, (-)-O-Methyl, (-)-O-Dimethylethylamine Cubebin and Their Preparation from (-)-cubebin. *Il Farmaco* 59 (1), 55–61. doi:10.1016/j.farmac.2003.07.012

Speeckaert, R., Dugardin, J., Lambert, J., Lapeere, H., Verhaeghe, E., Speeckaert, M. M., et al. (2018). Critical Appraisal of the Oxidative Stress Pathway in Vitiligo: a Systematic Review and Meta-Analysis. *J. Eur. Acad. Dermatol. Venereol.* 32 (7), 1089–1098. doi:10.1111/jdv.14792

Speeckaert, R., Lambert, J., Bulat, V., Belpaire, A., Speeckaert, M., and van Geel, N. (2020). Autoimmunity in Segmental Vitiligo. *Front. Immunol.* 11, 568447. doi:10.3389/fimmu.2020.568447

Subongkot, T., Ngawhirunpat, T., and Opanasopit, P. (2021). Development of Ultradeformable Liposomes with Fatty Acids for Enhanced Dermal Rosmarinic Acid Delivery. *Pharmaceutics* 13 (3), 404. doi:10.3390/pharmaceutics13030404

Sun, C., Huang, H., Xu, C., Li, X., and Chen, K. (2013). Biological activities of extracts from Chinese bayberry (Myrica rubra Sieb. et Zucc.): a review. *Plant Foods Hum. Nutr.* 68 (2), 97–106. doi:10.1007/s11130-013-0349-x

Sun, Z., Du, J., Hwang, E., and Yi, T.-H. (2018). Paeonol Extracted from Paeonia Suffruticosa Andr. Ameliorated UVB-Induced Skin Photoaging via DLD/Nrf2/ARE and MAPK/AP-1 Pathway. *Phytotherapy Res.* 32 (9), 1741–1749. doi:10.1002/ptr.6100

Takekoshi, S., Nagata, H., and Kitatani, K. (2014). Flavonoids Enhance Melanogenesis in Human Melanoma Cells. *Tokai J. Exp. Clin. Med.* 39 (3), 116–121.

Tal, B., and Robeson, D. J. (1986). The Metabolism of Sunflower Phytoalexins Ayapin and Scopoletin. *Plant Physiol.* 82 (1), 167–172. doi:10.1104/pp.82.1.167

Tang, L., Fang, W., Lin, J., Li, J., Wu, W., and Xu, J. (2018). Vitamin D Protects Human Melanocytes against Oxidative Damage by Activation of Wnt/β-Catenin Signaling. *Lab. Invest.* 98 (12), 1527–1537. doi:10.1038/s41374-018-0126-4

Tsai, C. F., Su, H. H., Chen, K. M., Liao, J. M., Yao, Y. T., Chen, Y. H., et al. (2020). Paeonol Protects against Myocardial Ischemia/Reperfusion-Induced Injury by Mediating Apoptosis and Autophagy Crosstalk. *Front. Pharmacol.* 11, 586498. doi:10.3389/fphar.2020.586498

Tuerxuntayi, A., Liu, Y. Q., Tulake, A., Kabas, M., Eblimit, A., and Aisa, H. A. (2014). Kaliziri Extract Upregulates Tyrosinase, TRP-1, TRP-2 and MITF Expression in Murine B16 Melanoma Cells. *BMC Complement. Altern. Med.* 14, 166. doi:10.1186/1472-6882-14-166

Udomruk, S., Kaewmool, C., Phitak, T., Pothacharoen, P., and Kongtawelert, P. (2020). Sesamin Promotes Neurite Outgrowth under Insufficient Nerve Growth Factor Condition in PC12 Cells through ERK1/2 Pathway and SIRT1 Modulation. *Evid. Based Complement. Alternat Med.* 2020, 9145458. doi:10.1155/2020/9145458

Usman, H., Ullah, M. A., Jan, H., Siddiquah, A., Drouet, S., Anjum, S., et al. (2020). Interactive Effects of Wide-Spectrum Monochromatic Lights on Phytochemical Production, Antioxidant and Biological Activities of Solanum Xanthocarpum Callus Cultures. *Molecules* 25 (9), 2201. doi:10.3390/molecules25092201

Uto, T., Ohta, T., Yamashita, A., Fujii, S., and Shoyama, Y. (2019). Liquiritin and Liquiritigenin Induce Melanogenesis via Enhancement of P38 and PKA Signaling Pathways. *Medicines* 6 (2), 68. doi:10.3390/medicines6020068

Wang, G., Hiramoto, K., Ma, N., Yoshikawa, N., Ohnishi, S., Murata, M., et al. (2021a). Glycyrrhizin Attenuates Carcinogenesis by Inhibiting the Inflammatory Response in a Murine Model of Colorectal Cancer. *Int. J. Mol. Sci.* 22 (5), 2609. doi:10.3390/ijms22052609

Wang, H. X., Zeng, M. S., Ye, Y., Liu, J. Y., and Xu, P. P. (2021b). Antiviral Activity of Puerarin as Potent Inhibitor of Influenza Virus Neuraminidase. *Phytotherapy Res.* 35 (1), 324–336. doi:10.1002/ptr.6803

Wang, J., Wang, S., Sun, S., Lu, Y., Gao, K., Guo, C., et al. (2020a). Apigenin-7-O-β-D-(-6"-p-coumaroyl)-glucopyranoside Treatment Elicits a Neuroprotective Effect through GSK-3β Phosphorylation-Mediated Nrf2 Activation. *Aging* 12 (23), 23872–23888. doi:10.18632/aging.104050

Wang, J. Y., Chen, H., Wang, Y. Y., Wang, X. Q., Chen, H. Y., Zhang, M., et al. (2017). Network Pharmacological Mechanisms of Vernonia Anthelmintica (L.) in the Treatment of Vitiligo: Isorhamnetin Induction of Melanogenesis via Up-Regulation of Melanin-Biosynthetic Genes. *BMC Syst. Biol.* 11 (1), 103. doi:10.1186/s12918-017-0486-1

Wang, L., Yang, H., Wang, C., Shi, X., and Li, K. (2019a). Rosmarinic Acid Inhibits Proliferation and Invasion of Hepatocellular Carcinoma Cells SMMC 7721 via PI3K/AKT/mTOR Signal Pathway. *Biomed. Pharmacother.* 120, 109443. doi:10.1016/j.biopha.2019.109443

Wang, X., Yu, J.-y., Sun, Y., Wang, H., Shan, H., and Wang, S. (2021c). Baicalin Protects LPS-Induced Blood-Brain Barrier Damage and Activates Nrf2-Mediated Antioxidant Stress Pathway. *Int. Immunopharmacology* 96, 107725. doi:10.1016/j.intimp.2021.107725

Wang, Y.-F., Liu, Y.-N., Xiong, W., Yan, D.-M., Zhu, Y., Gao, X.-M., et al. (2014). A UPLC-MS/MS Method for *In Vivo* and *In Vitro* Pharmacokinetic Studies of Psoralenoside, Isopsoralenoside, Psoralen and Isopsoralen from Psoralea Corylifolia Extract. *J. Ethnopharmacology* 151 (1), 609–617. doi:10.1016/j.jep.2013.11.013

Wang, Y.-s., Cho, J.-G., Hwang, E.-S., Yang, J.-E., Gao, W., Fang, M.-z., et al. (2018). Enhancement of Protective Effects of Radix Scutellariae on UVB-Induced Photo Damage in Human HaCaT Keratinocytes. *Appl. Biochem. Biotechnol.* 184 (4), 1073–1093. doi:10.1007/s12010-017-2611-4

Wang, Y., Li, S., and Li, C. (2019b). Perspectives of New Advances in the Pathogenesis of Vitiligo: From Oxidative Stress to Autoimmunity. *Med. Sci. Monit.* 25, 1017–1023. doi:10.12659/msm.914898

Wang, Y., Liu, H., Zheng, M., Yang, Y., Ren, H., Kong, Y., et al. (2021d). Berberine Slows the Progression of Prediabetes to Diabetes in Zucker Diabetic Fatty Rats by Enhancing Intestinal Secretion of Glucagon-like Peptide-2 and Improving the Gut Microbiota. *Front. Endocrinol. (Lausanne)* 12, 609134. doi:10.3389/fendo.2021.609134

Wang, Y., Quan, F., Cao, Q., Lin, Y., Yue, C., Bi, R., et al. (2021e). Quercetin Alleviates Acute Kidney Injury by Inhibiting Ferroptosis. *J. Adv. Res.* 28, 231–243. doi:10.1016/j.jare.2020.07.007

Wang, Z.-K., Chen, R.-R., Li, J.-H., Chen, J.-Y., Li, W., Niu, X.-L., et al. (2020b). Puerarin Protects against Myocardial Ischemia/reperfusion Injury by Inhibiting Inflammation and the NLRP3 Inflammasome: The Role of the SIRT1/NF-Kb Pathway. *Int. Immunopharmacology* 89 (Pt B), 107086. doi:10.1016/j.intimp.2020.107086

Wen-Jun, L., Hai-Yan, W., Wei, L., Ke-Yu, W., and Rui-Ming, W. (2008). Evidence that Geniposide Abrogates Norepinephrine-Induced Hypopigmentation by the Activation of GLP-1r-dependent C-Kit Receptor Signaling in Melanocyte. *J. Ethnopharmacology* 118 (1), 154–158. doi:10.1016/j.jep.2008.03.021

Weng, L., Guo, X., Li, Y., Yang, X., and Han, Y. (2016). Apigenin Reverses Depression-like Behavior Induced by Chronic Corticosterone Treatment in Mice. *Eur. J. Pharmacol.* 774, 50–54. doi:10.1016/j.ejphar.2016.01.015

Whitton, M. E., Pinart, M., Batchelor, J., Leonardi-Bee, J., González, U., Jiyad, Z., et al. (2015). Interventions for Vitiligo. *Cochrane Database Syst. Rev.*, CD003263. doi:10.1002/14651858.cd003263.pub5

Whitton, M., Pinart, M., Batchelor, J. M., Leonardi-Bee, J., Gonzalez, U., Jiyad, Z., et al. (2016). Evidence-based Management of Vitiligo: Summary of a Cochrane Systematic Review. *Br. J. Dermatol.* 174 (5), 962–969. doi:10.1111/bjd.14356

Wu, J., Zhou, M., Wan, Y., and Xu, A. (2013). CD8+ T Cells from Vitiligo Perilesional Margins Induce Autologous Melanocyte Apoptosis. *Mol. Med. Rep.* 7 (1), 237–241. doi:10.3892/mmr.2012.1117

Wu, S., Hu, Y., Bai, W., Zhao, J., Huang, C., Wen, C., et al. (2019). Cyanidin-3-o-glucoside Inhibits UVA-induced Human Dermal Fibroblast Injury by Upregulating Autophagy. *Photodermatol. Photoimmunol Photomed.* 35 (5), 360–368. doi:10.1111/phpp.12493

Wu, T. Y., Lin, J. N., Luo, Z. Y., Hsu, C. J., Wang, J. S., and Wu, H. P. (2020). 2,3,4',5-Tetrahydroxystilbene-2-O-beta-D-Glucoside (THSG) Activates the Nrf2 Antioxidant Pathway and Attenuates Oxidative Stress-Induced Cell Death in Mouse Cochlear UB/OC-2 Cells. *Biomolecules* 10 (3), 465. doi:10.3390/biom10030465

Xiao, H. B., Cao, X., Wang, L., Run, X. Q., Su, Y., Tian, C., et al. (2011). 1,5-dicaffeoylquinic Acid Protects Primary Neurons from Amyloid β 1-42-induced Apoptosis via PI3K/Akt Signaling Pathway. *Chin. Med. J. (Engl)* 124 (17), 2628–2635. doi:10.3760/cma.j.issn.0366-6999.2011.17.012

Xiao, L., Zhong, M., Huang, Y., Zhu, J., Tang, W., Li, D., et al. (2020). Puerarin Alleviates Osteoporosis in the Ovariectomy-Induced Mice by Suppressing Osteoclastogenesis via Inhibition of TRAF6/ROS-dependent MAPK/NF-κB Signaling Pathways. *Aging* 12 (21), 21706–21729. doi:10.18632/aging.103976

Xie, H., Zhou, F., Liu, L., Zhu, G., Li, Q., Li, C., et al. (2016). Vitiligo: How Do Oxidative Stress-Induced Autoantigens Trigger Autoimmunity?. *J. Dermatol. Sci.* 81 (1), 3–9. doi:10.1016/j.jdermsci.2015.09.003

Xin, L., Gao, J., Lin, H., Qu, Y., Shang, C., Wang, Y., et al. (2020). Regulatory Mechanisms of Baicalin in Cardiovascular Diseases: A Review. *Front. Pharmacol.* 11, 583200. doi:10.3389/fphar.2020.583200

Xu, D.-X., Guo, X.-X., Zeng, Z., Wang, Y., and Qiu, J. (2021). Puerarin Improves Hepatic Glucose and Lipid Homeostasis *In Vitro* and *In Vivo* by Regulating the AMPK Pathway. *Food Funct.* 12 (6), 2726–2740. doi:10.1039/d0fo02761h

Xu, P., Su, S., Tan, C., Lai, R.-S., and Min, Z.-S. (2017). Effects of Aqueous Extracts of Ecliptae Herba, Polygoni Multiflori Radix Praeparata and Rehmanniae Radix Praeparata on Melanogenesis and the Migration of Human Melanocytes. *J. Ethnopharmacology* 195, 89–95. doi:10.1016/j.jep.2016.11.045

Yadav, A. K., and Jang, B. C. (2020). Anti-Survival and Pro-apoptotic Effects of 6-Shogaol on SW872 Human Liposarcoma Cells via Control of the Intrinsic Caspase Pathway, STAT-3, AMPK, and ER Stress. *Biomolecules* 10 (10). doi:10.3390/biom10101380

Yamada, Y., Obayashi, M., Ishikawa, T., Kiso, Y., Ono, Y., and Yamashita, K. (2008). Dietary Tocotrienol Reduces UVB-Induced Skin Damage and Sesamin Enhances Tocotrienol Effects in Hairless Mice. *J. Nutr. Sci. Vitaminol* 54 (2), 117–123. doi:10.3177/jnsv.54.117

Yamaguchi, Y., Brenner, M., and Hearing, V. J. (2007). The Regulation of Skin Pigmentation. *J. Biol. Chem.* 282 (38), 27557–27561. doi:10.1074/jbc.r700026200

Yang, B., Yang, Q., Yang, X., Yan, H.-B., and Lu, Q.-P. (2016). Hyperoside Protects Human Primary Melanocytes against H2O2-Induced Oxidative Damage. *Mol. Med. Rep.* 13 (6), 4613–4619. doi:10.3892/mmr.2016.5107

Yang, C.-C., Hsiao, L.-D., and Yang, C.-M. (2020a). Galangin Inhibits LPS-Induced MMP-9 Expression via Suppressing Protein Kinase-dependent AP-1 and FoxO1 Activation in Rat Brain Astrocytes. *Jir* 13, 945–960. doi:10.2147/jir.s276925

Yang, C. C., Lin, C. C., Hsiao, L. D., and Yang, C. M. (2018). Galangin Inhibits Thrombin-Induced MMP-9 Expression in SK-N-SH Cells via Protein Kinase-dependent NF-Kb Phosphorylation. *Int. J. Mol. Sci.* 19 (12), 4084. doi:10.3390/ijms19124084

Yang, L., Yang, F., Teng, L., and Katayama, I. (2020b). 6-Shogaol Protects Human Melanocytes against Oxidative Stress through Activation of the Nrf2-Antioxidant Response Element Signaling Pathway. *Int. J. Mol. Sci.* 21 (10), 3537. doi:10.3390/ijms21103537

Yang, X.-P., Liu, T.-Y., Qin, X.-Y., and Yu, L.-C. (2014). Potential protection of 2,3,5,4′-Tetrahydroxystilbene-2-O-β-D-Glucoside against Staurosporine-Induced Toxicity on Cultured Rat hippocampus Neurons. *Neurosci. Lett.* 576, 79–83. doi:10.1016/j.neulet.2014.05.045

Yarla, N. S., Bishayee, A., Sethi, G., Reddanna, P., Kalle, A. M., Dhananjaya, B. L., et al. (2016). Targeting Arachidonic Acid Pathway by Natural Products for Cancer Prevention and Therapy. *Semin. Cancer Biol.* 40-41, 48–81. doi:10.1016/j.semcancer.2016.02.001

Yim, S. H., Tabassum, N., Kim, W. H., Cho, H., Lee, J. H., and Batkhuu, G. J. (2017b). Isolation and Characterization of Isofraxidin 7-O-(6'-O-P-Coumaroyl)-β-Glucopyranoside from Artemisia Capillaris Thunberg: A Novel, Nontoxic Hyperpigmentation Agent that Is Effective *In Vivo*. *Evid. Based Complement. Alternat Med.* 2017, 1401279. doi:10.1155/2017/1401279

Yim, S. H., Tabassum, N., Kim, W. H., Cho, H., Lee, J. H., Batkhuu, G. J., et al. (2017a). Isolation and Characterization of Isofraxidin 7-O-(6'-O-P-Coumaroyl)-β-Glucopyranoside from Artemisia Capillaris Thunberg: A Novel, Nontoxic Hyperpigmentation Agent that Is Effective *In Vivo*. *Evid. Based Complement. Alternat Med.* 2017, 1401279. doi:10.1155/2017/1401279

Yin, L., Pang, G., Niu, C., Habasi, M., Dou, J., and Aisa, H. A. (2018). A Novel Psoralen Derivative-MPFC Enhances Melanogenesis via Activation of P38 MAPK and PKA Signaling Pathways in B16 Cells. *Int. J. Mol. Med.* 41 (6), 3727–3735. doi:10.3892/ijmm.2018.3529

Yin, L., Niu, C., Liao, L. X., Dou, J., Habasi, M., and Aisa, H. A. (2017). An Isoxazole Chalcone Derivative Enhances Melanogenesis in B16 Melanoma Cells via the Akt/GSK3β/β-Catenin Signaling Pathways. *Molecules* 22 (12), 2077. doi:10.3390/molecules22122077

Yuan, J., Lu, Y., Wang, H., Feng, Y., Jiang, S., Gao, X. H., et al. (2020). Paeoniflorin Resists H(2)O(2)-Induced Oxidative Stress in Melanocytes by JNK/Nrf2/HO-1 Pathway. *Front. Pharmacol.* 11, 536. doi:10.3389/fphar.2020.00536

Zabolinejad, N., Maleki, M., Salehi, M., Ashrafi, Z., Molkara, S., and Layegh, P. (2020). Psoralen and Narrowband UVB Combination Provides Higher Efficacy in Treating Vitiligo Compared with Narrowband UVB Alone: A Randomised Clinical Trial. *Australas. J. Dermatol.* 61 (1), e65–e69. doi:10.1111/ajd.13184

Zang, D., Niu, C., and Aisa, H. A. (2019). Amine Derivatives of Furocoumarin Induce Melanogenesis by Activating Akt/GSK-3β/β-Catenin Signal Pathway. *Drug Des. Develop. Ther.* 13, 623–632. doi:10.2147/DDDT.S180960

Zhai, Y., Wang, Q., Li, Y., Cui, J., Feng, K., Kong, X., et al. (2018). The Higher Osteoprotective Activity of Psoralidin *In Vivo* Than Coumestrol Is Attributed by its Presence of an Isopentenyl Group and through Activated PI3K/Akt axis. *Biomed. Pharmacother.* 102, 1015–1024. doi:10.1016/j.biopha.2018.03.166

Zhang, B., Wang, J., Zhao, G., Lin, M., Lang, Y., Zhang, D., et al. (2020). Apigenin Protects Human Melanocytes against Oxidative Damage by Activation of the Nrf2 Pathway. *Cell Stress and Chaperones* 25 (2), 277–285. doi:10.1007/s12192-020-01071-7

Zhang, F., Zhang, Y., Yang, T., Ye, Z. Q., Tian, J., Fang, H. R., et al. (2019a). Scopoletin Suppresses Activation of Dendritic Cells and Pathogenesis of Experimental Autoimmune Encephalomyelitis by Inhibiting NF-Kb Signaling. *Front. Pharmacol.* 10, 863. doi:10.3389/fphar.2019.01037

Zhang, L., Li, D.-c., and Liu, L.-f. (2019b). Paeonol: Pharmacological Effects and Mechanisms of Action. *Int. Immunopharmacology* 72, 413–421. doi:10.1016/j.intimp.2019.04.033

Zhang, L. (2019). Pharmacokinetics and Drug Delivery Systems for Puerarin, a Bioactive Flavone from Traditional Chinese Medicine. *Drug Deliv.* 26 (1), 860–869. doi:10.1080/10717544.2019.1660732

Zhang, R., Lee, I. K., Piao, M. J., Kim, K. C., Kim, A. D., Kim, H. S., et al. (2011). Butin (7,3′,4′-Trihydroxydihydroflavone) Reduces Oxidative Stress-Induced Cell Death via Inhibition of the Mitochondria-dependent Apoptotic Pathway. *Ijms* 12 (6), 3871–3887. doi:10.3390/ijms12063871

Zhang, W., Cheng, C., Sha, Z., Chen, C., Yu, C., Lv, N., et al. (2021). Rosmarinic Acid Prevents Refractory Bacterial Pneumonia through Regulating Keap1/

Nrf2-Mediated Autophagic Pathway and Mitochondrial Oxidative Stress. *Free Radic. Biol. Med.* 168, 247–257. doi:10.1016/j.freeradbiomed.2021.03.038

Zhang, X., Bu, H., Jiang, Y., Sun, G., Jiang, R., Huang, X., et al. (2019c). The Antidepressant Effects of Apigenin Are Associated with the Promotion of Autophagy via the mTOR/AMPK/ULK1 Pathway. *Mol. Med. Rep.* 20 (3), 2867–2874. doi:10.3892/mmr.2019.10491

Zhang, Y., Ding, Y., Zhong, X., Guo, Q., Wang, H., Gao, J., et al. (2016). Geniposide Acutely Stimulates Insulin Secretion in Pancreatic β-cells by Regulating GLP-1 receptor/cAMP Signaling and Ion Channels. *Mol. Cell Endocrinol.* 430, 89–96. doi:10.1016/j.mce.2016.04.020

Zhao, C., Zhang, H., Li, H., Lv, C., Liu, X., Li, Z., et al. (2017). Geniposide Ameliorates Cognitive Deficits by Attenuating the Cholinergic Defect and Amyloidosis in Middle-Aged Alzheimer Model Mice. *Neuropharmacology* 116, 18–29. doi:10.1016/j.neuropharm.2016.12.002

Zhao, L., Li, H., Gao, Q., Xu, J., Zhu, Y., Zhai, M., et al. (2021). Berberine Attenuates Cerebral Ischemia-Reperfusion Injury Induced Neuronal Apoptosis by Down-Regulating the CNPY2 Signaling Pathway. *Front. Pharmacol.* 12, 609693. doi:10.3389/fphar.2021.609693

Zhao, W.-Z., Wang, H.-T., Huang, H.-J., Lo, Y.-L., and Lin, A. M.-Y. (2018). Neuroprotective Effects of Baicalein on Acrolein-Induced Neurotoxicity in the Nigrostriatal Dopaminergic System of Rat Brain. *Mol. Neurobiol.* 55 (1), 130–137. doi:10.1007/s12035-017-0725-x

Zhou, J., Chen, F., Yan, A., and Xia, X. (2020a). Madecassoside Protects Retinal Pigment Epithelial Cells against Hydrogen Peroxide-Induced Oxidative Stress and Apoptosis through the Activation of Nrf2/HO-1 Pathway. *Biosci. Rep.* 40 (10), 4347. doi:10.1042/bsr20194347

Zhou, J., Zhang, S., Sun, X., Lou, Y., Bao, J., and Yu, J. (2021). Hyperoside Ameliorates Diabetic Nephropathy Induced by STZ via Targeting the miR-499-5p/APC axis. *J. Pharmacol. Sci.* 146 (1), 10–20. doi:10.1016/j.jphs.2021.02.005

Zhou, Y.-X., Gong, X.-H., Zhang, H., and Peng, C. (2020b). A Review on the Pharmacokinetics of Paeoniflorin and its Anti-inflammatory and Immunomodulatory Effects. *Biomed. Pharmacother.* 130, 110505. doi:10.1016/j.biopha.2020.110505

Zhou, Y. X., Zhang, R. Q., Rahman, K., Cao, Z. X., Zhang, H., and Peng, C. (2019). Diverse Pharmacological Activities and Potential Medicinal Benefits of Geniposide. *Evid. Based Complement. Alternat Med.* 2019, 4925682. doi:10.1155/2019/4925682

Zhu, X., Zhang, H., and Lo, R. (2004). Phenolic Compounds from the Leaf Extract of Artichoke (Cynara scolymusL.) and Their Antimicrobial Activities. *J. Agric. Food Chem.* 52 (24), 7272–7278. doi:10.1021/jf0490192

Zhu, Y., Tchkonia, T., Pirtskhalava, T., Gower, A. C., Ding, H., Giorgadze, N., et al. (2015). The Achilles' Heel of Senescent Cells: from Transcriptome to Senolytic Drugs. *Aging Cell* 14 (4), 644–658. doi:10.1111/acel.12344

Zhu, Y., Wang, S., Lin, F., Li, Q., and Xu, A. (2014). The Therapeutic Effects of EGCG on Vitiligo. *Fitoterapia* 99, 243–251. doi:10.1016/j.fitote.2014.08.007

Zhu, Y., Wang, S., and Xu, A. (2013). A Mouse Model of Vitiligo Induced by Monobenzone. *Exp. Dermatol.* 22 (7), 499–501. doi:10.1111/exd.12184

Zhu, Y., Zhong, L., Peng, J., Yuan, Q., and Xu, A. (2019). The Therapeutic Effects of Baicalin on Vitiligo Mice. *Biol. Pharm. Bull.* 42 (9), 1450–1455. doi:10.1248/bpb.b19-00319

14

Management of Atopic Dermatitis via Oral and Topical Administration of Herbs in Murine Model

Vivi Nur Khalieda Mohd Kasim[1†], *Siti Mahirah Noble*[2†], *Kong Yen Liew*[1], *Ji Wei Tan*[2], *Daud Ahmad Israf*[1] *and Chau Ling Tham*[1*]

[1]*Department of Biomedical Science, Faculty of Medicine and Health Sciences, Universiti Putra Malaysia, Serdang, Malaysia,*
[2]*School of Science, Monash University Malaysia, Subang Jaya, Malaysia*

Correspondence:
Chau Ling Tham
chauling@upm.edu.my

†These authors have contributed equally to this work and share first authorship

Over the past few decades, complementary and alternative medicine (CAM) using herbs, or their active constituents have garnered substantial attention in the management of a chronic and relapsing inflammatory skin disorder called atopic dermatitis (AD), particularly in attenuating disease recurrence and maintaining long-term remission. In Eastern Asian countries including China, Korea and Taiwan, herbal medicine available in both topical and oral preparation plays a significant role in treating skin diseases like AD as they possibly confer high anti-inflammatory properties and immunomodulatory functions. Conventional murine models of AD have been employed in drug discovery to provide scientific evidence for conclusive and specific pharmacological effects elicited by the use of traditional herbs and their active constituents. Coupled with the goal to develop safe and effective novel therapeutic agents for AD, this systematic review consists of a summary of 103 articles on both orally and topically administered herbs and their active constituents in the murine model, whereby articles were screened and selected *via* a specialized framework known as PICO (Population, Intervention, Comparator and Outcome). The objectives of this review paper were to identify the efficacy of oral and topical administered herbs along with their active constituents in alleviating AD and the underlying mechanism of actions, as well as the animal models and choice of inducer agents used in these studies. The main outcome on the efficacy of the majority of the herbs and their active constituents illustrated suppression of Th2 response as well as improvements in the severity of AD lesions, suppression of Immunoglobulin E (IgE) concentration and mast cell infiltration. The majority of these studies used BALB/c mice followed by NC/Nga mice (commonly used gender–male; commonly used age group – 6–8 weeks). The most used agent in inducing AD was 2, 4-Dinitrochlorobenzene (DNCB), and the average induction period for both oral and topical administered herbs and their active constituents in AD experiments lasted between 3 and 4 weeks. In light of these findings, this review paper could potentially assist researchers in exploring the potential candidate herbs and their active constituents using murine model for the amelioration of AD.

Keywords: herbs, atopic dermatitis, topical, oral, murine model, IgE, Th2 cytokines, systematic review

INTRODUCTION

Atopic Dermatitis (AD) is a chronic skin inflammatory disorder affecting 20% of children and up to 10% of adults worldwide (Laughter et al., 2021). Clinical manifestations of AD include dryness, erythema, itchy skin, and histological findings illustrate spongiosis and infiltration of inflammatory cells around the upper dermal layer (Han et al., 2016). Immune dysregulation as well as a plethora of genetic and environmental factors significantly contribute to the multifactorial etiology and complexed pathophysiology of a debilitating skin disorder like AD. With regards to immune dysregulation, AD has long been understood to predominantly express skewness towards a systemic T-helper type 2 (Th2)-dominant immune response (Renert-Yuval et al., 2021). With the expression of a Th2-skewed immunity, AD patients tend to exhibit an increase in cytokine expression, with interleukins 4 and 13 (IL-4 and IL-13) being the two pivotal cytokines that orchestrate the pathogenesis of this disease as well as elevated levels of high-affinity IgE receptor known as Fc epsilon receptor I (FcεRI). Studies have reported that the initiation of AD is closely associated with Th2 cytokines whereas the disease progression and chronicity are correlated with a delayed surge of Th1 cytokines mainly interferon- γ (IFN- γ) in the chronic phase, thus presenting itself as a biphasic inflammation (Grewe et al., 1998). Amongst the many prevalent hallmarks of AD, it is often correlated with a high level of circulating IgE and an elevated mast cells (MC) count in AD skin lesions (An et al., 2020).

Originally deriving from the bone marrow, MCs are the only terminally differentiated hematopoietic cells that express the c-Kit tyrosine kinase receptor and its ligand stem cell factor (SCF), to synergistically aid in mast cell proliferation and maturation in peripheral tissues (Mekori et al., 1995). Extensive studies in the literature have established the role of MCs as key contributors in the development and propagation of IgE-mediated hypersensitivity reactions as well as in innate and adaptive immune responses. Additionally, MCs are eminently located around the blood and lymphatic vessels, hair follicles and glandular structures of the skin. Mast cells found in the skin could be easily distinguished from mucosal MCs by their protease content as the former contains both chymase and tryptase in their granules whereas only tryptase is present in the latter (Stone et al., 2010). Upon exposure and sensitization to an allergen, activated B cells undergo differentiation into plasma cells to produce IgE, which readily cross-links with an antigen *via* high-affinity IgE receptors (FcεRI) on the MCs surface. This in turn stimulates IgE-mediated activation of MCs whereby subsequent degranulation induces the release of cytokines (i.e., IL-4, IL-5 and IL-13), preformed lipid mediators namely leukotrienes and platelet activating factor (PAF) which could further intensify the progression of AD (Kulka and Befus, 2003).

To date, the management of AD mainly focuses on the restoration of a normal functional skin barrier as well as to elicit anti-inflammatory and immunosuppressing effects, in a stepwise manner according to disease severity and symptoms (Lebwohl et al., 2013). Currently, standard treatment regimens for AD involve the use of moisturizing emollients, topical corticosteroids (TCs) and topical calcineurin inhibitors (TCIs) for mild-to-moderate AD; and the reliance on systemic immunosuppressant drugs such as azathioprine and mycophenolate mofetil or phototherapy, especially for more severe AD cases (Akhavan and Rudikoff, 2008; Lee HJ et al., 2016). However, studies have emphasized an increased risk of unwanted side effects such as skin atrophy, telangiectasia, acneiform eruptions and many more due to long-term usage of TCs and TCIs. Consequently, to address an unmet need in establishing a "gold standard" treatment for AD, profound interest lies in unravelling the development of a safe, efficacious as well as cost-effective anti-atopic agents derived from traditional herbs or natural sources (Choi JH et al., 2017; Nygaard et al., 2017).

Recent studies are actively demonstrating the potential pharmacological actions of traditional herbs and their active constituents as they might possess anti-inflammatory, antibacterial, antifungal, immunosuppressive activities and many more. *Aloe vera* (L.) Burm.f. is a plant widely prized in the medicinal, skincare and beauty industry owing to its wound healing and immunomodulatory properties. Based on a review carried out by Sánchez et al. (2020), the Chinese, Ayurvedic and Arabian medicine highly utilize *Aloe vera* (L.) Burm.f. as a treatment for constipation, helminth infections, and eczema respectively. In studies performed by Kim et al. (2010) and Finberg et al. (2015), the efficacy of a medicinal plant like *Aloe vera* (L.) Burm.f. in treating AD could be proven by its ability to modulate immunological responses in AD when administered *via* oral and topical routes. Once known as folk medicine, this stemless plant has gained a well-deserved reputation in ameliorating AD due to its profound anti-inflammatory properties and effectiveness in wound healing (Zari and Zari, 2015). Moreover, local inhabitants have been using herbs as one of the methods in managing diseases including skin related problems. As evidently seen in Nigeria, residents in Keffi are known to utilize the leaves of *Senna alata* (L.) Roxb. as a treatment for eczema by applying the herb extract to the affected areas (Mowobi et al., 2016) and this herb was proven to elicit dermatophytic activities due to its bioactive compounds (Oladeji et al., 2020). As reported by Hennebelle et al. (2009), *Senna alata* (L.) Roxb. was used not only as a topical treatment but also as an oral medicament against skin diseases including eczema. In consolidation, *Senna alata* (L.) Roxb. and *Aloe vera* (L.) Burm.f. were administered *via* the two most common routes of drugs administration, which further elucidates the primary focus of this review on highlighting both oral and topical routes of administration. A systematic review can therefore assist in analyzing the recent and relevant data from studies investigating the potential therapeutic effects of herbs and their active constituents on AD *via* two common routes of drug administration namely oral and topical. On top of that, an astonishing array of animal models have been developed in the field of skin diseases for drug discovery particularly in mice whereby they develop spontaneous skin lesions after prolonged exposure to various allergens and closely mimic the features of human AD. Therefore, this systematic review consists of a total of 103 *in vivo* studies of AD models that were being divided into two categories with the first section studying the oral administration of herbs and their active constituents ($n = 48$) followed by the topical route ($n = 55$). This review paper was commissioned:

TABLE 1 | Respective search strategies applied for PubMed and Science Direct.

	PubMed	Science direct
Intervention	(Herb* OR "herbal medicine" OR "medicinal plant" OR "Traditional Chinese Medicine" OR "Korean medicine" OR kampo OR Ayurveda OR ethnobotany)	(Herb* OR "herbal medicine" OR "medicinal plant" OR "Traditional Chinese Medicine" OR "Korean medicine" OR kampo OR Ayurveda OR ethnobotany)
Disease of interest	Atopic dermatitis OR eczema	Atopic dermatitis OR eczema
Outcome measures	Not included in the search term	Not included in the search term
Filter	2014–2020 Full-text available Other animals	2014–2020 Research articles

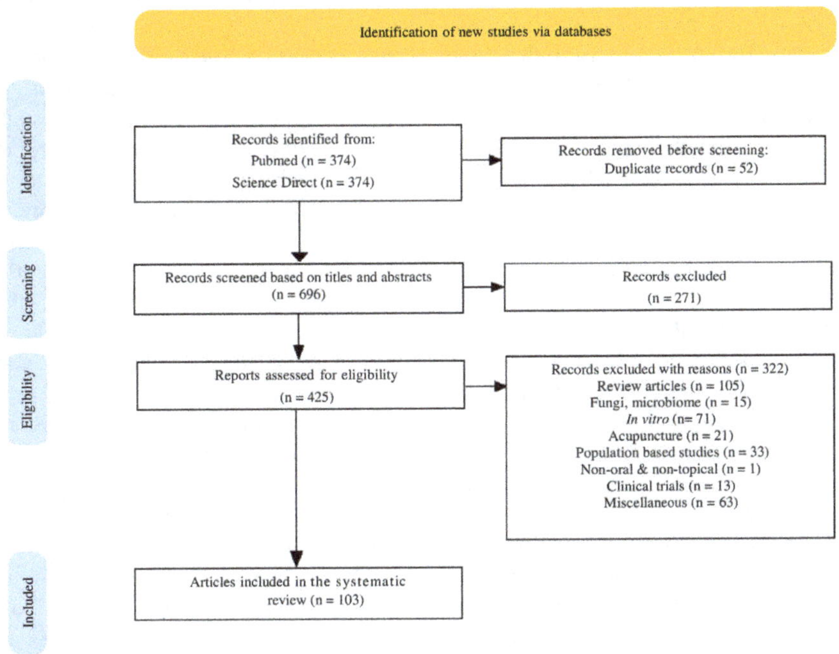

FIGURE 1 | Flow chart illustrating the search strategy and study selection process from Pubmed and Science Direct according to the PRISMA statement.

i. to screen recent 6 years of publications (2014–2020) on oral and topical administration of herbs and their active constituents in murine models of AD
ii. to refine the suitable conditions for animal experimentation on AD by identifying the choice of animal models and inducer agents used
iii. to elucidate the presumed underlying mechanism of actions of oral and topical administered herbs and their active constituents as well as their efficacies

METHODS

Search Strategy

Relevant articles in the literature were identified through systematic searches in two electronic databases, namely PubMed and ScienceDirect. The search terms comprised of two components: *1*) intervention or exposure to herb and *2*) disease of interest, "atopic dermatitis" or "eczema." The Preferred Reporting Items for Systematic Reviews and Meta-analysis (PRISMA) criteria were followed in this study (Shamseer et al., 2015). PubMed thesaurus and MeSH term were used and filter was activated to select full text and publication year from 2014 to 2020. An additional filter on species "Other Animal" was also selected to focus on animal studies. ScienceDirect search was generated by truncating a term with an asterisk (*) as well as with the use of Boolean operators such as "AND" and "OR" to narrow the search to more manageable and relevant articles. After the initial search, refine filter was used to narrow down the articles to those published between 2014 and 2020. Owing to the absence of an animal exclusion search filter on ScienceDirect, manual searching was done to identify all relevant animal studies. The detailed search strategies for the two databases are presented in **Table 1**, where as the process and result of the systematic search are displayed in **Figure 1**. The flow diagram was created using an online tool that conforms to the PRISMA2020 Statement (Haddaway et al., 2021).

Eligibility Criteria

The inclusion criteria are *1)* herbs (extract, mixture and active constituents from the herbs), *2)* AD or eczema in murine model. In contrast, the exclusion criteria are *1)* review articles, *2)* fungi, microbiome, *3) in vitro* studies, *4)* acupuncture, *5)* population-based studies, *6)* non-oral and non-topical route of herb administrations, *7)* clinical trials, *8)* miscellaneous articles (food chemistry, non-english, *etc.*) The eligibility criteria according to the PICO approach (population, intervention, comparator and, outcome) are as follows:

- Population: murine model with no restriction on gender, age and weight.
- Interventions: herbal extracts, complex mixtures of herbs or isolated active constituents from distinct parts of herbs.
- Comparator: a group that received control drugs (corticosteroids, calcineurin inhibitors or others).
- Outcomes: severity of AD lesions, serum IgE levels, infiltration of mast cells, Th1 and Th2 cytokine concentrations and other relevant parameters associated with AD.
- Study design: murine experimental research.

Study Appraisal and Selection

Study selection was conducted independently by two reviewers (VK and SN) who searched the articles in PubMed and ScienceDirect databases. Irrelevant duplicate articles were crosschecked and removed by both authors and the remaining articles were screened based on the titles and abstracts. The relevant articles were further assessed to ensure that they comply with the eligibility criteria. Any contradictions between the authors were settled by consensus. Excluded articles were recorded with reasons. Subsequently, eligible literature was analyzed by the authors to extract the relevant information.

Data Extraction

Data from all articles that met the criteria were extracted. Basic characteristics of the animals (age, gender and species) and experimental procedures including the inducers, the usage of barrier disruption tools, investigation sites and the control drugs were tabulated. Experimental outcomes and proposed mechanisms were listed systematically. This was followed by the preparations and chemical analysis of the herbs and their constituents.

Risk of Bias

Risk of Bias (RoB) assessment was performed using the SYstematic Review Centre for Laboratory Animal Experimentation (SYRCLE). The types of biases under RoB assessment include selection bias (sequence generation, baseline characteristics, allocation concealment), performance bias (random housing, blinding), detection bias (random outcome assessment, blinding), attrition bias (incomplete outcome data), reporting bias (selective outcome reporting) and other sources of bias. For each bias, there are different domains which constitute the ten entries for RoB tool for animal research. Each study was screened for all the entries and jotted with "yes" for a low risk of bias, "no" for a high risk of bias and "unclear" for an unclear risk of bias as presented in **Figure 2**.

RESULTS

Risk of Bias

Risk of Bias (RoB) tool for animal intervention research in this sysmatic review is presented by SYRCLE (Hooijmans et al., 2014). SYRCLE is a tool for assessing the risk of bias in animal studies which consists of six types of bias. Under the selection bias, there are three domains. First is sequence generation. Almost half of the studies (45.54%) reported on the sequence generation that refers to the random sequence of the animal especially on the grouping. Second is baseline characteristics. Most studies (93.07%) mentioned the age, gender and weight of the animal in the methodology which proved that the experiments were started with animals having similar characteristics before the induction of AD. Third is allocation concealment. However, none of the studies mentioned that the information on the allocation of the animals were concealed from the investigators. Next, performance bias that consists of random housing and blinding were not reported in any studies. Under detection bias there are random outcome assessment and blinding. Only one study by Sur et al. (2017) reported random outcome assessment where the investigators randomly picked the animals before proceeding with the assessment. In only 15.84% of the studies, the outcome assessors were reported to be blinded. Incomplete outcome data under attrition bias revealed that 43.56% of the studies included all animals in the analysis. Reporting bias refers to whether or not the published report included all expected outcomes. All 103 studies reported expected oucomes when comparing methods and results section which defined as low risk of reporting bias. Other sources of bias such as the inappropriate influence of funders and the addition of new animals to replace dropout data were not reported in any of the studies. Nevertheless, these findings were expected as a survey disclosed that methodology and materials are poorly reported for experiments using animals, and the users of SYRCLE also mentioned that they had to judge a large number of entries as "unclear" (Kilkenny et al., 2009; Hooijmans et al., 2014).

Oral Administration of Herbs and Their Active Constituents

Basic Characteristics of the Included Studies

In this review, 48 studies on orally administered herbs and their active constituents were analyzed with majority (n = 32) of them being based in Korea, 13 in China and the remaining three articles were from Japan, Taiwan and Pakistan, respectively. All the articles included in this review were rigorously assessed and screened according to a specialized search strategy known as PICO. The choice of intervention used during the screening process was "herb" which was being divided into three categories based on their formulation namely, extract, mixture, and compound. Most of the studies worked on the extracts (n =

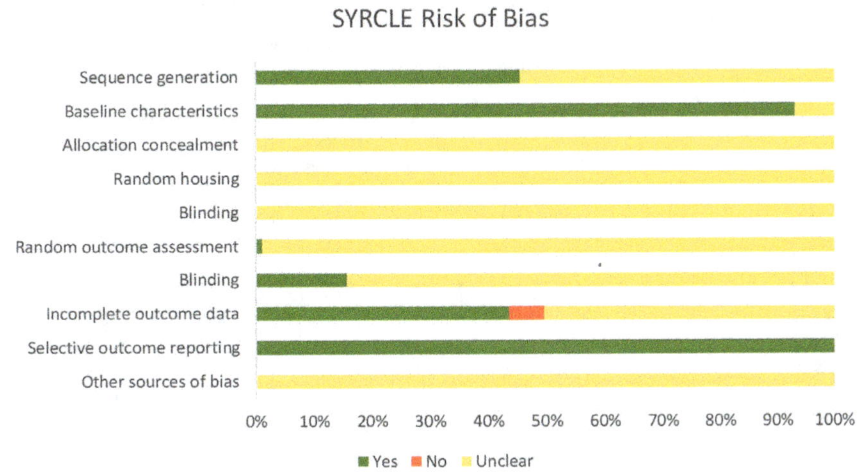

FIGURE 2 | Assessment of the risk of bias (SYRCLE) for selected studies, presented as the percentages of the total.

20), followed by herb mixtures (n = 19) and compounds isolated from herbs (n = 8) as shown in **Supplementary Table S1**. The preparation steps of the herbs and their active constituents were shown in **Supplementary Table S2**. In addition, only one study focused on oil extracted from herb. None of the studies in this review was reported to work on the same herb using same route of administration. Two studies conducted by Tsang et al. (2016) and Aslam et al. (2018) were identified to work on a mixture of herbs named Pentaherbs and compound named Thymoquinone, respectively, *via* both oral and topical routes of administration.

Drug Control

The efficacy and safety of these novel oral herbal agents in the treatment of AD was corroborated with the use of well-established treatment modalities against AD. The choice of positive controls or comparison drugs in these studies varied from dexamethasone (n = 18), prednisolone (n = 5) and four individual studies by Ok et al. (2018) used terfenadine, Wu et al. (2014) used quercetin, Chen et al. (2017) used cetirizine and Aslam et al. (2018) used tacrolimus. However, 20 studies did not include a positive control drug. Lastly, a study by Zheng et al. (2019) was identified to use a total of three positive control drugs namely dexamethasone, loratadine and montelukast.

Animal Models Used

Murine models were the choice of population (P) for all the studies included in this review, to investigate the anti-AD effects of both oral and topical herbal administrations in an *in vivo* setting. Out of the 48 studies involving the oral route of herbal administration, male murine models (n = 28) and female murine models (n = 14) were used, however sex of the mice was not mentioned in six of the remaining studies. Moreover, the animal species also differed as 47 studies were identified to use mice of various strains; with BALB/C mice (n = 31) being the most popular strain, followed by NC/Nga mice (n = 14), C57BL/6J mice (n = 1), IL-4/Luc/CNS-1 transgenic mice (n = 1) and Sprague Dawley rats (n = 1). With reference to **Table 2**, induction of AD-like skin lesions was mostly achieved by the chemical exposure to 2, 4-Dinitrochlorobenzene (DNCB) as stated in 20 studies followed by 2, 4-Dinitrofluorobenzene (DNFB) as mentioned in eight studies. Six studies used *Dermatophagoides farinae* (DfE) and less than five studies used each of these inducers; fluorescein isothiocyanate (FITC), ovalbumin, oxazolone, phthalic anhydride (PA) and trimellitic anhydride (TMA). Interestingly, five studies were investigated to use a combination of inducers namely acetone with DNFB, 2, 4, 6-trinitro-1-chrolobenzene (TNCB) with ovalbumin and lastly, DfE with DNCB. In addition, mice in six studies received treatment with sodium dodecyl sulfate (SDS) to facilitate skin barrier perturbation and surgical tape stripping was performed in seven studies. Most of the studies administered the inducer on areas which include dorsal skin, ear or a combination of both as indicated in **Table 2**.

Topical Administration of Herbs

Basic Characteristics of the Included Studies

In this review, fifty-five studies were conducted across several East and South Asian countries with majority (n = 43) of them being based in Korea, seven in China, two in Japan, two in Taiwan and one study was performed in Pakistan. With cross-reference to **Supplementary Table S3**, the action of three different herbs namely, *Pyrus ussuriensis* Maxim., *Gardenia jasminoides* J.Ellis and *Stellera chamaejasme* L. were investigated repetitively in a few studies, whereas the subsequent 53 studies worked on diverse herbs of interest, in its extract (n = 32), mixture (n = 10) and compound (n = 11) forms. Interestingly, two studies in this review focused on studying the essential oil extracted from herbs. The preparation steps of the herbs and their active constituents were shown in **Supplementary Table S4**.

Drug Control

With close reference to **Table 3**, majority of the studies in this review used the two primary classes of drugs commonly used to treat AD as positive control drugs, which includes topical

TABLE 2 | Basic characteristics of the murine models and experimental procedures from studies involving oral treatments of herbs and their active constituents.

Age/Sex/Model species	Induction of AD-like skin lesions	Barrier disruption	Positive control drug	Investigation site	References
4w/M/BALB/c mouse	DNCB	N/A	1 mg/kg Dexamethasone	Dorsal skin	Lee JH et al. (2019)
5w/M/BALB/c mouse	DNCB	N/A	10 mg/kg Terfenadine	Dorsal skin	Ok et al. (2018)
5w/M/BALB/c mouse	DNCB	N/A	1 mg/kg Dexamethasone	Dorsal skin and ear	Yang et al. (2018)
5w/M/BALB/c mouse	DNCB	N/A	1 mg/kg Dexamethasone	Dorsal skin and ear	Zari and Zari, (2015)
5w/M/BALB/c mouse	DNCB	N/A	N/A	Dorsal skin	Jung et al. (2014)
5w/M/BALB/c mouse	DNCB	N/A	N/A	Dorsal skin	Park JH et al. (2019)
5w/M/BALB/c mouse	DNFB	N/A	N/A	Dorsal skin	Kee et al. (2017)
5w/M/BALB/c mouse	DNFB	N/A	N/A	Dorsal skin	Jeon et al. (2015)
6w/M/BALB/c mouse	DNCB	N/A	N/A	Dorsal skin	Ku et al. (2017)
6w/M/BALB/c mouse	DNCB	N/A	N/A	Dorsal skin	Kim SR et al. (2014)
6–7w/M/BALB/c mouse	DfE	N/A	N/A	Ear	Makino et al. (2014)
12w/M/BALB/c mouse	TMA	N/A	N/A	Ear	Sur et al. (2017)
M/BALB/c mouse	DNCB	N/A	30 mg/kg Prednisolone	Dorsal skin and ear	Song-lin et al. (2014)
4w/F/BALB/c mouse	DNCB and HDM (house dust mite)	Tape	Dexamethasone (dose not indicated)	Ear	Bae et al. (2016)
5w/F/BALB/c mouse	Ovalbumin	Tape	1 mg/kg Dexamethasone	Dorsal skin	Kong et al. (2015)
6w/F/BALB/c mouse	DNCB and DfE	Tape	N/A	Ear	Choi et al. (2014b)
6w/F/BALB/c mouse	DNCB and DfE	Tape	1 mg/kg Dexamethasone	Ear	Jeong et al. (2018)
6w/F/BALB/c mouse	Ovalbumin	Tape	1.3 mg/kg Cetirizine	Dorsal skin	Chen et al. (2017)
6–8w/F/BALB/c mouse	DNCB	N/A	10 mg/kg Prednisolone	Dorsal skin	Meng et al. (2019)
6–8w/F/BALB/c mouse	DNCB	N/A	2.5 mg/kg Dexamethasone	Dorsal skin and ear	Chen et al. (2020)
6–10w/BALB/c mouse	FITC	N/A	N/A	Ear	Tao et al. (2017)
6–10w/BALB/c mouse	FITC	N/A	0.67 mg/kg Dexamethasone	Ear	Wang et al. (2017)
8w/F/BALB/c mouse	DNCB	N/A	N/A	Dorsal skin and ear	Han et al. (2016)
8w/F/BALB/c mouse	Acetone and DNFB	N/A	0.039 mg/kg Dexamethasone	Abdominal and dorsal skin	Han et al. (2018)
8w/F/BALB/c mouse	TNCB and ovalbumin	N/A	1.6 mg/kg Quercetin	Dorsal skin	Wu et al. (2014)
8w/F/BALB/c mouse	DNFB	N/A	10 nM Dexamethasone	Dorsal skin	Moon et al. (2019)
8w/F/BALB/c mouse	Oxazolone	N/A	2.5 mg/ml Dexamethasone	Dorsal skin and ear	Tsang et al. (2016)
F/BALB/c mouse	DNCB	N/A	30 mg/kg Tacrolimus	Ear	Aslam et al. (2018)
5w/BALB/c mouse	DNCB	N/A	N/A	Abdominal and dorsal skin	Zhanxue et al. (2018)
6–8w/BALB/c mouse	FITC	N/A	0.67 mg/kg Dexamethasone	Abdominal skin and ear	Xiao-Tong et al. (2019)
BALB/c mouse	FITC	N/A	0.67 mg/kg Dexamethasone 1.3 mg/kg Loratadine 1.3 mg/kg Montelukast	Abdominal skin and ear	Zheng et al. (2019)
3w/M/NC/Nga mouse	DfE	5% SDS	N/A	Dorsal skin	Kim et al. (2020)
3w/M/NC/Nga mouse	DNFB	Tape and 5% SDS	N/A	Dorsal skin	Cha et al. (2016)
3w/M/NC/Nga mouse	DfE	Tape and 5% SDS	N/A	Dorsal skin	Cha HY et al. (2017)
5w/M/NC/Nga mouse	DNCB	N/A	3 mg/kg Prednisolone	Dorsal skin	Park et al. (2018)
6w/M/NC/Nga mouse	DNCB	N/A	3 mg/kg Dexamethasone	Dorsal skin	Park BK et al. (2014)
6w/M/NC/Nga mouse	DNCB	N/A	3 mg/kg Dexamethasone	Dorsal skin	Park et al. (2015)
6w/M/NC/Nga mouse	DNFB	N/A	N/A	Dorsal skin	Lee et al. (2017)
6w/M/NC/Nga mouse	DfE	4% SDS	5 mg/kg Dexamethasone	Dorsal skin	Kang et al. (2018)
6–8w/M/NC/Nga mouse	DNCB	N/A	3 mg/kg Dexamethasone	Dorsal skin, face and ear	Yan et al. (2019)
8w/M/NC/Nga mouse	DfE	4% SDS	3 mg/kg Prednisolone	Dorsal skin and ear	Lim et al. (2014b)
8w/M/NC/Nga mouse	DfE	4% SDS	3 mg/kg Prednisolone	Dorsal skin and ear	Lim et al. (2015)
M/NC/Nga mouse	DNFB	N/A	N/A	Abdominal and dorsal skin	Han et al. (2014a)
M/NC/Nga mouse	DNFB	N/A	0.039 mg/kg Dexamethasone	Abdominal and dorsal skin	Han et al. (2014b)
5w/F/NC/Nga mouse	DNCB	N/A	5 mg/kg Dexamethasone	Dorsal skin	Cha KJ et al. (2017)
4w/M/C57BL/6J mouse	DNFB	N/A	N/A	Dorsal skin	Park J et al. (2019)
8w/IL-4/Luc/CNS-1 transgenic mouse	PA	N/A	N/A	Ear	Kwak et al. (2017)
4w/M&F Lee/SD rat	DNCB	N/A	N/A	Dorsal skin and ear	Wan et al. (2016)

N/A, Not applicable.

TABLE 3 | Basic characteristics of the murine models and experimental procedures from studies involving topical treatments of herbs and their active constituents.

Age/Sex/ Model species	Induction of AD-like skin lesions	Barrier disruption	Positive control drug	Investigation site	References
5w/M/BALB/c mouse	DNCB	N/A	Betamethasone (% not indicated)	Dorsal skin (thoracic area)	Mechesso et al. (2019)
6w/M/BALB/c mouse	DNCB	N/A	N/A	Dorsal skin	Jung et al. (2015)
6w/M/BALB/c mouse	DNCB	N/A	Tacrolimus (% not indicated)	Dorsal skin	Hong et al. (2019)
6w/M/BALB/c mouse	DNCB	4% SDS	10 μM Dexamethasone	Dorsal skin	Choi et al. (2018)
6w/M/BALB/c mouse	DNCB	N/A	0.1% Tacrolimus	Dorsal skin	Ku et al. (2018)
8–10w/M/BALB/c mouse	DNFB	N/A	N/A	Both ears	Osada-Oka et al. (2018)
5w/F/BALB/c mouse	DNCB	N/A	10 μM Dexamethasone	Dorsal skin	Lee J et al. (2016)
6w/F/BALB/c mouse	DNCB and Oxazolone	N/A	N/A	Dorsal skin, ears	Lee et al. (2018)
6w/F/BALB/c mouse	DNCB	4% SDS	10 μM Dexamethasone	Dorsal skin	Choi et al. (2016)
6w/F/BALB/c mouse	DNCB	4% SDS	10 μM Dexamethasone	Dorsal skin	Choi YY et al. (2017b)
6w/F/BALB/c mouse	DNCB and DfE	Tape	N/A	Both ears	Choi and Kim, (2014a)
6w/F/BALB/c mouse	Oxazolone	N/A	N/A	Both ears	Jo et al. (2018)
6w/SKH-1 hairless mouse	DNCB	N/A	Pimecrolimus (1% Elidel)	Dorsal skin	
6w/F/BALB/c mouse	Oxazolone	N/A	N/A	Both ears	Jung et al. (2018)
6w/F/BALB/c mouse	Oxazolone	N/A	N/A	Both ears	Lee S et al. (2019)
6w/SKH-1 hairless mouse	DNCB	N/A	N/A	Dorsal skin	
6w/F/BALB/c mouse	DNCB	4% SDS	N/A	Dorsal skin	An et al. (2020)
6w/F/BALB/c mouse	DNCB	N/A	10 μM Dexamethasone	Dorsal skin	Choi YY et al. (2017a)
6w/F/BALB/c mouse	Oxazolone	N/A	N/A	Dorsal skin, ears	Jegal et al. (2017)
6w/F/SKH-1 hairless mouse	DNCB	N/A	N/A	Dorsal skin, ears	
7w/F/BALB/c mouse	DNCB	N/A	Wu Dai ointment	Dorsal skin	Wu et al. (2020)
7w/F/BALB/c mouse	DNCB	N/A	N/A	Dorsal skin	Lim et al. (2018)
7w/F/BALB/c mouse	DNCB	4% SDS	0.1 and 0.5% Dexamethasone	Dorsal skin	Lee HJ et al. (2016)
8w/F/BALB/c mouse	DNFB	N/A	5 mg/kg Dexamethasone	Dorsal skin	Ryu et al. (2018)
8w/F/BALB/c mouse	DNCB	N/A	N/A	Dorsal skin, both ears	Fang et al. (2015)
8w/F/BALB/c mouse	DNCB	N/A	N/A	Dorsal skin, ears	Huang et al. (2019)
8w/F/BALB/c mouse	Oxazolone	N/A	2.5 mg/ml Dexamethasone	Both ears	Tsang et al. (2016)
F/BALB/c mouse	DNCB	N/A	1% Tacrolimus	Both ears	Aslam et al. (2018)
4w/M/NC/Nga mouse	DfE	N/A	N/A	Dorsal skin, ears	Yang G et al. (2016)
6w/M/NC/Nga mouse	DNCB	N/A	N/A	Dorsal skin	Yang HJ et al. (2017)
6w/M/NC/Nga mouse	DNFB	N/A	N/A	Dorsal and abdominal skin	Han et al. (2014c)
	Biostir-AD	4% SDS	0.1% Tacrolimus	Dorsal skin	Ngo et al. (2020)

(Continued on following page)

TABLE 3 | *(Continued)* Basic characteristics of the murine models and experimental procedures from studies involving topical treatments of herbs and their active constituents.

Age/Sex/ Model species	Induction of AD-like skin lesions	Barrier disruption	Positive control drug	Investigation site	References
6w/M/NC/Nga mouse					
6w/M/NC/Nga mouse	DNCB	N/A	0.1% Dexamethasone	Dorsal skin	Yang IJ et al. (2016)
6w/M/NC/Nga mouse	DfE	4% SDS	0.1% Tacrolimus	Dorsal skin, ears	Sung and Kim, (2018)
7w/M/NC/Nga mouse	DNCB	N/A	3 mg/kg Dexamethasone	Dorsal skin	Kim et al. (2015)
8w/M/NC/Nga mouse	DfE	4% SDS	0.1% Tacrolimus	Dorsal neck, ears	Park et al. (2020)
8w/M/NC/Nga mouse	DfE	4% SDS	0.1% Tacrolimus	Dorsal skin, ears	Park SH et al. (2019)
8w/M/NC/Nga mouse	DfE	4% SDS	0.1% Tacrolimus	Dorsal skin, both ears	Sung et al. (2016)
8w/M/NC/Nga mouse	DfE	4% SDS	0.1% Tacrolimus	Dorsal skin, both ears	Sung et al. (2014)
8w/M/NC/Nga mouse	DfE	10% (w/v) SDS	0.1% Tacrolimus	Dorsal skin, both ears	Lee et al. (2014)
8w/M/NC/Nga mouse	DfE	4% SDS	0.1% Tacrolimus	Dorsal skin, both ears	Lim et al. (2014a)
8w/M/NC/Nga mouse	DfE	N/A	0.1% Tacrolimus	Upper dorsal skin, both ears	Ha et al. (2014)
8w/M/NC/Nga mouse	DfE	N/A	0.1% Tacrolimus	Upper dorsal skin, both ears	Ha et al. (2015)
4w/F/NC/Nga mouse	DNCB	N/A	0.1% Dexamethasone	Dorsal skin, ears	Cho et al. (2019)
4w/F/NC/Nga mouse	DNCB	N/A	0.1% Dexamethasone	Dorsal skin, ears	Cho et al. (2018)
4w/F/NC/Nga mouse	DNCB	N/A	0.1% Tacrolimus	Dorsal skin, face and both ears	Kim H et al. (2014)
4w/F/NC/Nga mouse	DNCB	N/A	N/A	Dorsal skin	Ham et al. (2019)
5w/F/NC/Nga mouse	DfE	N/A	0.1% Hydrocortisone	Dorsal skin	Park KH et al. (2014)
5w/F/SKH-1 hairless mouse	Oxazolone	N/A	0.1% Hydrocortisone	Dorsal skin	Kang et al. (2017)
6w/F/SKH-1 hairless mouse	DNCB	N/A	Pimecrolimus (1% Elidel)	Dorsal skin	Lee et al. (2020)
6w/F/SKH-1 hairless mouse	DNCB	N/A	N/A	Dorsal skin	Jo et al. (2018)
4w/M/Kunming mouse	DNCB	N/A	Dexamethasone and Paeonol cream (% not indicated)	Dorsal skin, right ear	Yang J et al. (2017)
8w/M/Kunming mouse	DNCB	N/A	Dexamethasone acetate (contain 0.075% dexamethasone)	Dorsal skin, right ear	Fan et al. (2019)
8w/M/Kunming mouse	DNCB	N/A	0.025% Dexamethasone	Dorsal skin, right ear	Fan et al. (2018)
5–8w/F/ICR mouse	DNCB	N/A	0.1% Mometasone furoate cream	Dorsal skin, right ear	Wang et al. (2018)
8w/HR-1 mouse	Phthalic anhydride	N/A	N/A	Dorsal skin, ears	Ho et al. (2018)
6–8w/F/C57BL/6 mouse	MC903 (vitamin D3 analogue)	N/A	N/A	Dorsal side of left ear	Hou et al. (2019)
8–10w/M/NC/Tnd mouse	N/A	N/A	N/A	Dorsal skin	Amagai et al. (2017)

N/A, Not applicable.

corticosteroids (n = 19) i.e., dexamethasone (n = 15), hydrocortisone (n = 2), mometasone (n = 1), betamethasone (n = 1) and topical calcineurin inhibitors (n = 16) i.e., tacrolimus (n = 14) and pimecrolimus (n = 2). However, 19 studies did not include a positive control drug and a study by Wu et al. (2020) confirmed the therapeutic actions of the herbal medicinal treatment against a pre-existing traditional Chinese medicine known as "Wu Dai ointment."

Animal Models Used

Murine models had been used in all the studies to investigate the anti-AD effects of novel topical herbal administration in an *in vivo* setting. Female mice were identified in 30 studies while male mice were used in 25 studies, however, a few studies did not disclose the gender of the mice. Categorically, the BALB/c mice model (n = 25) was most extensively used among the included studies, superseded by NC/Nga (n = 20), hairless mice (n = 6), Kunming mice (n = 3), ICR mice (n = 1), HR-1 mice (n = 1), C57BL/6 (n = 1) and NC/Tnd mice (n = 1). It is also noteworthy that three individual studies conducted by Jegal et al. (2017), Jo et al. (2018) and Lee JH et al. (2019), utilized two different mice species namely BALB/c and SKH-1 hairless mice. According to Erkes and Selvan (2014), variation in the type of mouse strains could lead to a substantial difference in the immune stimulatory ability of haptens used to induce AD, which in these three studies, were DNCB and oxazolone. In order to evoke AD-like skin lesions, repetitive cutaneous sensitization with house dust mite allergen namely *Dermatophagoides farinae* (DfE) and chemical induced irritation *i.e.*, DNCB, DNFB, oxazolone, MC903 (a synthetic derivative of vitamin D) and phthalic anhydride were used in 12 and 42 studies, respectively. However, a study by Amagai et al. (2017) on *Alpinia intermedia* Gagnep., differed substantively from the rest as they used NC/Tnd mice, a sub-strain of Nc/Nga developed from inbreeding to give spontaneous itch and eczematous skin which resembles AD. Hence, no induction agent was needed to elicit AD-like skin lesions in this particular mouse strain. Besides, sodium dodecyl sulfate (SDS) was applied to the AD lesions in 13 of the studies for barrier disruption purposes, in which 12 received treatment with 4% (w/v) SDS, whereas only one study by Lee et al. (2014) applied 10% (w/v) SDS to mice skin. Mechanical skin injury by surgical tape stripping was only performed in a single study by Choi and Kim (2014a). On top of that, the majority of the studies in this review focused on investigating the dorsal skin, ears, or a combination of both as they were representative sites depicting the histological features of AD-like skin lesions.

DISCUSSION

Over the past few decades, there has been a tremendous surge in the public's shifting interest towards the reliance on natural herbal remedies as alternative therapeutic options to conventional Western allopathic medicine to treat AD. Essentially, plant-based or herbal medicine are natural products consisting portions of plants or unpurified plant extracts that possess potential bioactive compounds offering a myriad of medicinal and nutritive values possibly working synergistically, to affect multiple targets that contribute to the pathogenesis of AD. To date, the cornerstone of AD management commonly involves therapeutic intervention with emollients, TCs, TCIs and systemic immunosuppressants, especially for more severe AD cases (Carr, 2013; Nygaard et al., 2017). Nonetheless, inter-individual drug response variability and the potential risk of adverse effects from long-term use such as skin atrophy, tachyphylaxis and telangiectasia, are the key rationale behind a shifting interest towards herbal drug development with lesser side effects (Thomsen 2014; Montes-Torres et al., 2015). With that goal in mind, this systematic review was drawn from 103 studies evaluating the efficacy of novel herbs and their active constituents, synthesized from various preparations including crude extracts, compounds isolated from the herbs or mixtures of different herbs applied *via* oral and topical administration in *in vivo* murine AD models.

The use of murine models is needed to aid in drug discovery and testing of novel treatments as they are capable of mimicking different aspects of the pathophysiology of human AD. Mice models of AD are generally classified into three categories: *1*) mice induced by epicutaneous sensitization with allergens, *2*) spontaneous mice models and *3*) genetically modified mice that either over-express a transgene or lack of selective endogenous genes. In this review paper, the majority of the studies used allergen-induced AD models, which are relatively more convenient as the usage of exogenous allergens permits dose- and time-controlled induction (Kim et al., 2019). Also, out of 48 oral and 55 topical herbs administration studies involving AD in murine models, the majority used BALB/c mice strain (oral: n = 31, topical: n = 25), followed by NC/Nga (oral: n = 14, topical: n = 20). BALB/c mice have been widely known to trigger a Th2-dominant immune response, therefore, propagating the development of AD (Lee et al., 2010). On the other hand, NC/Nga mice were investigated to develop approximately 50% of spontaneous AD-like skin lesions when they are kept in conventional housing with uncontrolled air but remain normal and healthy under specific pathogen-free (SPF) conditions. However, this particular mouse model requires repeated applications of a hapten to fully develop AD (Shiohara et al., 2004).

Gender considerations remain an important facet in *in vivo* pharmacology studies as a substantial body of literature supports the notion that male mice are highly preferred in comparison to female due to the ease of handling, less variation in results and cost-effectiveness. Studies on orally administered herbs in this review correspond to this notion as male mice (n = 28) and female mice (n = 14) were used. Contrastingly, this was not constant with studies involving topical herb administration as female mice were found to lead the number with n = 30 and male (n = 25). However, this gap was not of significant difference and male mice are indeed more favourable in AD research. According to Wald and Wu (2010), female murine models confer a 4-day oestrous cycle which therefore accounts for the use of a larger number of animals as compared to males in order to keep their cycle in synchrony, and this in turn makes it less economical. Additionally, the fluctuation of hormones across their oestrus cycle results in behavioural variability in female mice as seen in the production of a female sex hormone called oestrogen which was reported to negatively regulate the wound healing process of AD-like skin lesions (Mukai et al., 2016). Taken together, researchers more typically eliminate the use of female murine models on the presupposition that they elicit intrinsic variation as compared to males, which could possibly interfere with the efficacy of herbs of interest in ameliorating AD. It was also brought to attention that a range between 6 and 8 weeks were the most commonly used murine age groups across the studies in this review, involving oral (n = 24) and topical (n = 43) herb administration. In murine, the maturation of T cells was at 8 weeks of age, which is crucial for the production of T-cell-dependent antibodies (Holladay and Smialowicz, 2000; Jackson et al., 2017).

A vast array of inducer agents was utilized across the studies on orally and topically administered herbs with the majority of them involving the use of DNCB (n = 52) either individually or in combination with DfE or Biostir-AD ointment (Choi and Kim, 2014a; Choi et al., 2014b; Bae et al., 2016; Jeong et al., 2018) and oxazolone (Jegal et al., 2017; Lee et al., 2018; Jo et al., 2019). DNCB exposure can create covalent conjugates with skin proteins to undergo further processing and presented to T cells for activation. Besides, repeated exposure to DNCB permits the accumulation of macrophages at the sensitization site, hence exemplifying an allergic inflammatory response as seen in AD (Yan et al., 2019). In fact, Ku et al. (2018) mentioned that morphological changes in the skin lesions of DNCB-sensitized mice revealed some of the major histopathological findings associated with human AD such as thickened epidermis, massive infiltration of $CD4^+$ T-cells producing pro-inflammatory cytokines as well as increased infiltration of inflammatory cells i.e., mast cells and eosinophils. Apart from DNCB, several other chemical compounds were also used to induce AD-like lesions in topical application of herb section of this review, including DNFB (n = 3), oxazolone (n = 6), repetitive cutaneous sensitization with DfE ointment (n = 12), MC903 (n = 1), and phthalic anhydride (n = 1). As we dived into the induction period, it was noticeable that the average duration of exposure to an inducer lasted between 3 and 4 weeks, with the shortest being a week. However, in a study conducted by Jung et al. (2015), DNCB exposure lasted for approximately 8 weeks (~55 days). DNFB (n = 8), DfE (n = 6) and FITC (n = 4) are among other inducers that were mentioned in this orally administered herb section of this review. In terms of duration, FITC marked the shortest period of AD induction with only 3 days then the mice were sacrificed. This is because the induction was only for the initial stage of AD and the articles from Tao et al. (2017) and Wang et al. (2017) did not mention any data on dermatitis score, serum IgE level and mast cell count which are the hallmarks of AD hence it was difficult to assess the AD severity. On the other hand, DfE recorded the longest period of AD induction which is 8 weeks.

Interestingly, nine out of 14 studies on topically administered herbs and their active constituents and five out of six studies on orally administered herbs and their active constituents were subjected to repeated application of DfE, subsequently after barrier disruption with a chemical substance mainly known as sodium dodecyl sulfate (SDS). SDS functions to facilitate the development of AD-like skin lesions by eliminating the lipid lamella of the stratum corneum. With reference to **Supplementary Tables S1, S3**, the oral and topical application of herbs and their active constituents was found to ameliorate AD symptoms *via* restoration of the skin barrier function (Cha et al., 2016; Yang JH et al., 2016; Cha HY et al., 2017; Cha KJ et al., 2017; Kang et al., 2018; Lee et al., 2018; Zhanxue et al., 2018; Cho et al., 2019; Jo et al., 2019; Park J et al., 2019; Park JH et al., 2019). Breakdown in the architecture of the stratum corneum in response to barrier disruption methods with either SDS or tape stripping, further permits the entry of allergens across the skin to interact with local antigen-presenting cells and immune effector cells. Previous research in the literature illustrated that repetitive application of DfE is capable of contributing to the onset and development of AD *via* the activation of inflammasomes in the epidermal keratinocytes (Jin et al., 2016). Restoration of an intact skin barrier in AD serves as a valuable therapeutic target since it acts as the first line of defence from various microbes and environmental allergens, as well as decreases in trans-epidermal water loss (TEWL). Subsequently, we found out that two studies of oral herbs and their active constituents' administration and 13 studies using topical herbs and their active constituents' administration were shown to decrease TEWL, whereas five studies on orally treated herbs and their active constituents and seven studies on topically treated herbs and their active constituents showed increased levels of epidermal barrier proteins such as filaggrin, involucrin and loricrin.

Until recently, the etiology of AD could possibly be accounted by two opposing hypotheses brought up by Silverberg and Silverberg (2015). The "outside-in" hypothesis supports the notion impairments in the epidermal barrier are solely responsible for the onset of inflammatory lesions in AD and an essential structural protein filaggrin, possesses a fundamental role in maintaining skin barrier integrity, skin hydration and pH by minimizing water loss (Li, 2014; Malik et al., 2017). In contrast, there are some who propose the "inside-out" hypothesis in which a dysregulated immune response is the key event that propagates the inflammatory cascade in AD and skin barrier disruption is an epiphenomenon (Boguniewicz and Leung, 2011; Silverberg and Silverberg, 2015). In this review, 102 studies could be accounted by the outside-in theory as murine models were introduced to the experimental allergens repeatedly in order to disrupt epidermal barrier integrity. Additionally, 12 studies in this review reported that oral and topical herbs and their active constituents' administration elicited an increase in levels of epidermal barrier proteins such as filaggrin, involucrin and loricrin. Hence, it allows us to justify that orally and topically administered herbs and their active constituents confers the potential to accelerate barrier recovery by up-regulating the expression of such vital structural proteins of the skin.

To fully comprehend the origins of AD, a molecular link has been well-documented between the elevated serum IgE levels and marked infiltration of mast cells. During AD inflammation, an allergen penetrates through the skin and gets readily bound to MCs by cross-linking to the high-affinity IgE receptor, FcεRI, expressed on their cell surface (Brown et al., 2008; Amin, 2012). Upon the activation of MCs, degranulation occurs within seconds, leading to the subsequent release of preformed secretory granules containing biologically active inflammatory mediators and proteins including histamine (cutaneous inductor of itch), PGs and leukotrienes, as well as serine proteases i.e. mast-cell chymase and tryptase (Kawakami et al., 2009; Siebenhaar et al., 2018). Among the 48 studies on orally administered herbs and their active constituents, 37 of them were reported to measure serum IgE levels and 22 studies measured the number of MCs and reported congruent decrease. Decreased levels in both of these crucial parameters suggest that the oral route of herbs and their active constituents' administration is capable of alleviating the allergic responses. On the other hand, across the 45 studies investigating IgE levels as an outcome parameter for topically administered herbs and their active constituents, it was found that 39 of these studies measured serum IgE and six studies investigated plasma IgE levels. Fortunately, serum or blood IgE levels successfully decreased after treatment with topical herbs and their active constituents in all 45 studies. However, it is important to note that total serum IgE may not reflect accurate levels of systemic IgE since raised concentrations are present in many patients who have no evidence of allergy. As a result, accurate measures of allergen-specific IgE could assist in defining the bona fide mechanism of novel topically applied herbal drugs in immunity (Qiu et al., 2020). In addition, from the studies involving topical route of administration, 39 herbs and their active constituents were found to significantly decrease the extent of mast cell infiltration into the skin. Moreover, it seems that the reduction of MCs infiltration can be associated with a decrease in MCs degranulation as well as down-regulation of IL-4 and IL-13 cytokines secretion. Therefore, this implies that MCs may serve as a key contributing factor to the suppression of Th2 cytokines in AD-like skin lesions *via* topical herbs and their active constituents' administration.

The extensive array of mediators secreted from FcεRI-mediated mast cell degranulation can ultimately promote inflammation, resulting in the appearance of macroscopic and microscopic skin lesions which are associated with AD. The severity of AD-like skin lesions could be investigated macroscopically according to the acronym widely known as SCORAD (SCORing Atopic Dermatitis) index. This scoring system serves as a clinical tool to assess the extent and severity of eczema by evaluating the common characteristic skin symptoms of AD including *1*) erythema, *2*), erosion, *3*) dryness and *4*) lichenification. In our review, dermatitis severity was measured in 26 studies using oral administration of herbs in which all 26 herbs and their active constituents were able to reduce the dermatitis severity score. The same results were obtained for treatment with topical herbs and their active constituents as the dermatitis severity score was found to decrease in 19 studies. On top of that, there was a study performed by Aslam et al. (2018), investigating on a single compound named thymoquinone, which used both routes of drug administration. Results from this study illustrated that both routes were able to alleviate the dermatitis severity score in murine models of AD. However, more in-depth studies need to be performed to thoroughly compare the efficacy of thymoquinone *via* different routes of administration before definitive conclusions can be drawn.

The immunological hallmark of AD is characterized by a predominant expression of Th2-inflammatory cytokines (i.e., IL-4, IL-5 and IL-13) in the acute phase followed by a prolonged activation of Th1-type cytokines (i.e., IFN-γ and TNF-α) in the chronic phase of AD (Brunner et al., 2017; Choi et al., 2014b). As demonstrated in **Supplementary Table S1**, 19 studies showed a simultaneous decrease in both Th1 and Th2 cytokines after treatment with orally administered herbs and their active constituents. Apart from that, 11 articles were found to study the Th2 cytokines independently and results showed a reduction in the level of cytokines. Without much anticipation, four studies measured the cytokines released from both types of helper T cells reported an unpredictable finding as orally administered herbs and their active constituents decreased the level of Th2 cytokines but contrastingly, induced an increase in the level of Th1 cytokines (Wu et al., 2014; Kong et al., 2015; Wan et al., 2016; Han et al., 2018). A substantial body of literature have suggested that an aberrant Th2-immune response plays a key proximal role in the pathogenesis of AD, hence the two vital Th2 cytokines, IL-4 and IL-13 were investigated in 38 and 32 studies of topical administration of herb and their active constituents, respectively. Besides, another Th2-mediated cytokine, IL-5 was measured in 11 studies. In all the studies mentioned above, topical application of herbs and their active constituents resulted in a marked reduction of IL-4, IL-5 and IL-13 expression. To address the classical Th1/Th2 paradigm in AD, TNF-α and IFN-γ levels were investigated as representative Th1 cytokines in 24 and 16 studies, respectively. Across all these studies, topical herbal application induced a decrease in TNF-α and IFN-γ levels, however, this was not achieved in a study by Yang HJ et al. (2017) whereby an unexpected asynchronism in both Th1 cytokines was reported after treatment. This finding could be accounted by the "Th1/Th2 imbalance" in the immunological hallmark of AD, in which Th1 responses are capable of antagonizing the development of Th2 cells, hence producing a contrasting effect in the levels of both types of cytokines (Herberth et al., 2010). On the other hand, extremely low and undetected levels of IFN-γ were reported by Yang J et al. (2017), possibly due to a Th2-driven inflammation whereby IL-4 was able to truncate the key Th1 cytokines namely IFN-γ (Brunner et al., 2017).

Recent progress in molecular biology has provided insights into the potential role of nuclear factor kappa B (NF-κB) transcription factor family in the progression and maintenance of AD (Tanaka et al., 2007). Studies have illustrated that activation of the NF-κB pathway is accountable for the regulation and chronicity of inflammatory skin diseases like AD. NF-κB participates in the differentiation of T cells into various subsets comprising of Th1, Th2 and Th17. Moreover, NF-κB functions to increase the expression and transcription of numerous cytokines, growth factors and chemokines such as IL-1β, IL-6 and IL-8, which are highly linked to the inflammatory cascade in AD (Tak and Firestein, 2001; Liu et al., 2017). In this review, 10 articles on orally administered herbs and their active constituents managed to inhibit the NF-κB pathway and similar results were recorded from 10 articles on topically administered herbs and their active constituents. Apart from NF-κB pathway, the phosphorylation of mitogen-activated protein kinases (MAPKs) signalling pathway is closely associated with the production of pro-inflammatory mediators which could trigger and exacerbate AD. Owing to the importance of MAPK signalling molecules i.e. ERK, JNK and p38, in the activation, proliferation, migration and degranulation of immune cells involved in AD,

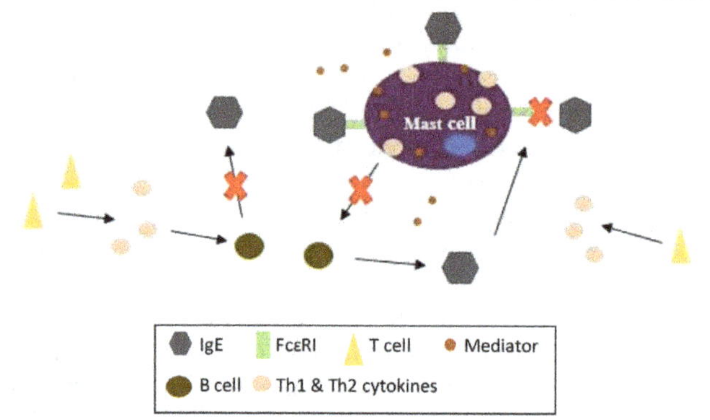

FIGURE 3 | The mechanism of actions of orally and topically administered herbs and their active constituents in murine model of AD.

therefore pharmacological inhibition of this pathway may serve as an attractive strategy for the treatment of allergic disorders (Huang et al., 2019). Inhibition of MAPK activation were seen in eight articles after administration of herbs and their active constituents *via* oral route whereas 11 studies illustrated an inhibition of MAPK phosphorylation after administration of herbs and their active constituents topically, as illustrated by a decrease in ERK, JNK and p38 protein kinases. As such, these findings propose that both NF-κB and MAPK signalling pathway serve as the potential avenues of investigative research in the development of a new therapeutic agent to treat AD.

Throughout this systematic review, we found that serum IgE, infiltration of mast cells and the levels of Th1 and Th2 cytokines were evaluated the most in 82, 62 and 53 studies respectively. These three biomarkers are interrelated in the pathogenesis of AD as depicted in **Figure 3**. In brief, allergen penetration stimulates T cells to secrete cytokines (IL-4, IL-5, IL-13, IFN-γ, *etc*.). The released cytokines in turn trigger nearby B cells to produce IgE which then bind to the high affinity receptor IgE, FcεRI on MCs. The synthesis and release of inflammatory mediators and cytokines can be induced by IgE-dependent mechanism (Williams and Galli, 2000: Kulka and Befus, 2003). The mechanism of action of these herbs and their active constituents may involve the inhibition of *1*) binding of IgE to the FcεRI, *2*) the release of mediators and cytokines from MCs, or *3*) synthesis of IgE from B cells. Although the exact mechanism was not mentioned in each of these studies, the biomarkers of AD related to these three parameters were found to be alleviated. However, it may be difficult to compare the data from different studies as various investigators used different experimental approaches to assess the outcome of AD such as ELISA, histological analysis and dermatitis severity. Reports may also vary considerably depending on the methodological details provided that could potentially lead to risk of bias. Generally, most studies included in this systematic review did not describe their methodologies precisely which could lead to an underestimation or overestimation of the findings. Thus, it is suggested that animal experiments should be properly designed and carried out well with transparency in every step especially blinding in performance and assessment to avoid any bias. Data should be reported entirely and reasons for any dropout data should also be provided. With all the data gathered from 103 studies evaluating the efficacies of oral and topical administered herbs along with their active constituents in alleviating AD and the underlying mechanism of actions using various animal models and inducers, it is hoped that this systematic review will aid in the evidence-based selection of animal models for AD in the future.

CONCLUSION

This systematic review has summarized 103 articles into several aspects based on PICO; in which the most common population (P) or choice of animal model used was BALB/C mice (n = 56), due to the fact that they lean towards a Th2-dominated immune response which, therefore, suit the disease of interest, AD. As for the intervention (I), this review consisted of both oral and topical administration routes of herbs and their active constituents in AD-like murine models and the most common positive control (C) drug chosen among these studies was the topical corticosteroid known as dexamethasone (n = 34). A substantially large number of these studies (n = 75) were conducted in Korea and none of the studies analysed the same herb and only two articles by Aslam et al. (2018) and Tsang et al. (2016) were understood to compare the different routes of administrations of the same herb mixture and compound. Findings from these two studies showed that both oral and topical routes of herb and their active constituents' administration were able to alleviate AD, however, the authors did not make a distinct comparison as to which route was more effective than the other. The common outcome (O) parameters of AD assessed amongst these studies include the histological findings of AD-like skin lesions, serum IgE levels, mast cell count and Th1/Th2 cytokines. Generally, both oral and topical administration of herbs and their active constituents elicited the potential to decrease the AD parameters mentioned above. Besides, large attention was also drawn towards the production and expression of Th2 cytokines in these studies. Upon tabulation of the vast array of findings, a myriad of results obtained from majority of the oral and topical studies demonstrated that herb extracts, mixtures and compounds isolated from herbs could markedly suppress IgE levels and MCs infiltration or degranulation. Theoretically, upon successful inhibition of IgE-mediated activation of MCs, they therefore hinder the subsequent degranulation and secretion of pro-inflammatory cytokines and preformed mediators. Taken together, these findings allow us to propose that the anti-AD effects could be attained by down-regulation of IgE-mediated MCs activation in *in vivo* models. Therewithal, MAPK and NF-κB pathways are worth to dive into for future research endeavours as the inhibition of these signalling pathways have been recognized as a potential therapeutic candidate against AD. It is also important to note that majority of the studies included in this systematic review mentioned about compliance with animal welfare as well as conflict of interest statement among the authors. However, most studies did not distinctly elaborate on examiner blinding, sample size calculation and animal allocation. As a result, there is ample room for methodological improvement in these studies as the authors could declare these aspects in order to circumvent an unclear risk of bias. Therefore, future research should implement these crucial details to enhance the quality of studies.

AUTHOR CONTRIBUTIONS

VM and SN contributed to the conceptualization, investigation, analysis and writing of the manuscript; KL, DI, and JT provided important information and reviewed the manuscript; CT conceived the idea, reviewed the manuscript and significantly refined the manuscript; all authors contributed to the final version of the manuscript.

ACKNOWLEDGMENTS

The authors would like to thank the members of Cell Signaling Lab, Faculty of Medicine and Health Sciences, Universiti Putra Malaysia for providing technical support for this study. The authors wish to express sincere gratitude to Chan Yee Han for her guidance, advice and support through all the stages of writing this systematic review.

REFERENCES

Akhavan, A., and Rudikoff, D. (2008). Atopic Dermatitis: Systemic Immunosuppressive Therapy. *Semin. Cutan. Med. Surg.* 27 (2), 151–155. doi:10.1016/j.sder.2008.04.004

Amagai, Y., Katsuta, C., Nomura, Y., Oida, K., Matsuda, K., Jang, H., et al. (2017). Amelioration of Atopic-like Skin Conditions in NC/Tnd Mice by Topical Application with Distilled *Alpinia Intermedia Gagnep* Extracts. *J. Dermatol* 44 (11), 1238–1247. doi:10.1111/1346-8138.13995

Amin, K. (2012). The Role of Mast Cells in Allergic Inflammation. *Respir. Med.* 106 (1), 9–14. doi:10.1016/j.rmed.2011.09.007

An, E. J., Kim, Y., Lee, S. H., Choi, S. H., Chung, W. S., and Jang, H. J. (2020). Ophiopogonin D Ameliorates DNCB-Induced Atopic Dermatitis-like Lesions in BALB/c Mice and TNF-α- Inflamed HaCaT Cell. *Biochem. Biophys. Res. Commun.* 522 (1), 40–46. doi:10.1016/j.bbrc.2019.10.190

Aslam, H., Shahzad, M., Shabbir, A., and Irshad, S. (2018). Immunomodulatory Effect of Thymoquinone on Atopic Dermatitis. *Mol. Immunol.* 101, 276–283. doi:10.1016/j.molimm.2018.07.013

Bae, M. J., See, H. J., Choi, G., Kang, C. Y., Shon, D. H., and Shin, H. S. (2016). Regulatory T Cell Induced by *Poria Cocos* Bark Exert Therapeutic Effects in Murine Models of Atopic Dermatitis and Food Allergy. *Mediat. Inflamm.* 2016, 3472608. doi:10.1155/2016/3472608

Boguniewicz, M., and Leung, D. Y. (2011). Atopic Dermatitis: a Disease of Altered Skin Barrier and Immune Dysregulation. *Immunol. Rev.* 242 (1), 233–246. doi:10.1111/j.1600-065X.2011.01027.x

Brown, J. M., Wilson, T. M., and Metcalfe, D. D. (2008). The Mast Cell and Allergic Diseases: Role in Pathogenesis and Implications for Therapy. *Clin. Exp. Allergy* 38 (1), 4–18. doi:10.1111/j.1365-2222.2007.02886.x

Brunner, P. M., Guttman-Yassky, E., and Leung, D. Y. (2017). The Immunology of Atopic Dermatitis and its Reversibility with Broad-Spectrum and Targeted Therapies. *J. Allergy Clin. Immunol.* 139 (4S), S65–S76. doi:10.1016/j.jaci.2017.01.011

Carr, W. W. (2013). Topical Calcineurin Inhibitors for Atopic Dermatitis: Review and Treatment Recommendations. *Paediatr. Drugs* 15 (4), 303–310. doi:10.1007/s40272-013-0013-9

Cha, H. Y., Ahn, S. H., Cheon, J. H., Park, I. S., Kim, J. T., and Kim, K. (2016). Hataedock Treatment Has Preventive Therapeutic Effects in Atopic Dermatitis-Induced NC/Nga Mice under High-Fat Diet Conditions. *Evid. Based Complement. Altern. Med.* 2016, 1739760. doi:10.1155/2016/1739760

Cha, H. Y., Ahn, S. H., Cheon, J. H., Park, S. Y., and Kim, K. (2017). Hataedock Treatment Has Preventive Therapeutic Effects for Atopic Dermatitis through Skin Barrier Protection in Dermatophagoides Farinae-Induced NC/Nga Mice. *J. Ethnopharmacol.* 206, 327–336. doi:10.1016/j.jep.2017.06.001

Cha, K. J., Im, M. A., Gu, A., Kim, D. H., Lee, D., Lee, J. S., et al. (2017). Inhibitory Effect of *Patrinia Scabiosifolia* Link on the Development of Atopic Dermatitis-like Lesions in Human Keratinocytes and NC/Nga Mice. *J. Ethnopharmacol.* 206, 135–143. doi:10.1016/j.jep.2017.03.045

Chen, M., Ding, P., Yang, L., He, X., Gao, C., Yang, G., et al. (2017). Evaluation of Anti-inflammatory Activities of Qingre-Qushi Recipe (QRQS) against Atopic Dermatitis: Potential Mechanism of Inhibition of IL-33/ST2 Signal Transduction. *Evid. Based Complement. Altern. Med.* 2017, 2489842. doi:10.1155/2017/2489842

Chen, Y., Xian, Y. F., Loo, S., Lai, Z., Chan, W. Y., Liu, L., et al. (2020). Huang-Lian-Jie-Du Extract Ameliorates Atopic Dermatitis-like Skin Lesions Induced by 2,4-dinitrobenzene in Mice via Suppression of MAPKs and NF-Kb Pathways. *J. Ethnopharmacol.* 249 (112367), 112367. doi:10.1016/j.jep.2019.112367

Cho, K., Kang, M. C., Parveen, A., Yumnam, S., and Kim, S. Y. (2019). Anti-inflammatory Effect of Chloroform Fraction of *Pyrus Ussuriensis Maxim.* Leaf Extract on 2, 4-Dinitrochlorobenzene-Induced Atopic Dermatitis in Nc/nga Mice. *Nutrients* 11 (2), 276. doi:10.3390/nu11020276

Cho, K., Parveen, A., Kang, M. C., Subedi, L., Lee, J. H., Park, S. Y., et al. (2018). *Pyrus Ussuriensis Maxim.* Leaves Extract Ameliorates DNCB-Induced Atopic Dermatitis-like Symptoms in NC/Nga Mice. *Phytomedicine* 48, 76–83. doi:10.1016/j.phymed.2018.05.006

Choi, J. H., Song, Y. S., Lee, H. J., Kim, G. C., and Hong, J. W. (2017). The Topical Application of Low-Temperature Argon Plasma Enhances the Anti-inflammatory Effect of Jaun-Ointment on DNCB-Induced NC/Nga Mice. *BMC Complement. Altern. Med.* 17 (1), 340. doi:10.1186/s12906-017-1850-9

Choi, J. K., and Kim, S. H. (2014a). Inhibitory Effect of Galangin on Atopic Dermatitis-like Skin Lesions. *Food Chem. Toxicol.* 68, 135–141. doi:10.1016/j.fct.2014.03.021

Choi, J. K., Oh, H. M., Lee, S., Kwon, T. K., Shin, T. Y., Rho, M. C., et al. (2014b). *Salvia Plebeia* Suppresses Atopic Dermatitis-like Skin Lesions. *Am J Chin MedAsian Sci. Med.* 42 (4), 967–985. doi:10.1142/S0192415X1450061X

Choi, Y. Y., Kim, M. H., Ahn, K. S., Um, J. Y., Lee, S. G., and Yang, W. M. (2017a). Immunomodulatory Effects of *Pseudostellaria Heterophylla* (Miquel) Pax on Regulation of Th1/Th2 Levels in Mice with Atopic Dermatitis. *Mol. Med. Rep.* 15 (2), 649–656. doi:10.3892/mmr.2016.6093

Choi, Y. Y., Kim, M. H., Hong, J., Kim, K., and Yang, W. M. (2016). Effect of Dangguibohyul-Tang, a Mixed Extract of *Astragalus Membranaceus* and *Angelica Sinensis*, on Allergic and Inflammatory Skin Reaction Compared with Single Extracts of *Astragalus Membranaceus* or *Angelica Sinensis*. *Evid. Based Complement. Altern. Med.* 2016, 5936354. doi:10.1155/2016/5936354

Choi, Y. Y., Kim, M. H., Lee, H., Ahn, K. S., Um, J. Y., Lee, S. G., et al. (2017b). *Cynanchum Atratum* Inhibits the Development of Atopic Dermatitis in 2,4-Dinitrochlorobenzene-Induced Mice. *Biomed. Pharmacother.* 90, 321–327. doi:10.1016/j.biopha.2017.03.065

Choi, Y. Y., Kim, M. H., Lee, H., Jo, S. Y., and Yang, W. M. (2018). (R)-(+)-pulegone Suppresses Allergic and Inflammation Responses on 2,4-Dinitrochlorobenzene-Induced Atopic Dermatitis in Mice Model. *J. Dermatol Sci.* 91 (3), 292–300. doi:10.1016/j.jdermsci.2018.06.002

Erkes, D. A., and Selvan, S. R. (2014). Hapten-induced Contact Hypersensitivity, Autoimmune Reactions, and Tumor Regression: Plausibility of Mediating Antitumor Immunity. *J. Immunol. Res.* 2014, 175265. doi:10.1155/2014/175265

Fan, H. J., Xie, Z. P., Lu, Z. W., Tan, Z. B., Bi, Y. M., Xie, L. P., et al. (2018). Anti-inflammatory and Immune Response Regulation of Si-Ni-San in 2,4-

Dinitrochlorobenzene-Induced Atopic Dermatitis-like Skin Dysfunction. *J. Ethnopharmacol.* 222, 1–10. doi:10.1016/j.jep.2018.04.032

Fan, H. J., Zhao, X. S., Tan, Z. B., Liu, B., Xu, H. L., Wu, Y. T., et al. (2019). Effects and Mechanism of Action of Huang-Lian-Jie-Du-Tang in Atopic Dermatitis-like Skin Dysfunction In Vivo and In Vitro. *J. Ethnopharmacol.* 240 (111937), 111937. doi:10.1016/j.jep.2019.111937

Fang, L. W., Cheng, C. C., Hwang, T. S., Huang, W. C., Liou, C. J., Chen, W. C., et al. (2015). Danggui Buxue Tang Inhibits 2,4-dinitrochlorobenzene: Induced Atopic Dermatitis in Mice. *Evid. Based Complement. Altern. Med.* 2015, 672891. doi:10.1155/2015/672891

Finberg, M. J., Muntingh, G. L., and van Rensburg, C. E. (2015). A Comparison of the Leaf Gel Extracts of *Aloe Ferox* and *Aloe Vera* in the Topical Treatment of Atopic Dermatitis in Balb/c Mice. *Inflammopharmacology* 23 (6), 337–341. doi:10.1007/s10787-015-0251-2

Grewe, M., Bruijnzeel-Koomen, C. A., Schöpf, E., Thepen, T., Langeveld-Wildschut, A. G., Ruzicka, T., et al. (1998). A Role for Th1 and Th2 Cells in the Immunopathogenesis of Atopic Dermatitis. *Immunol. Today* 19 (8), 359–361. doi:10.1016/S0167-5699(98)01285-7

Ha, H., Lee, H., Seo, C. S., Lim, H. S., Lee, J. K., Lee, M. Y., et al. (2014). *Artemisia Capillaris* Inhibits Atopic Dermatitis-like Skin Lesions in Dermatophagoides Farinae-Sensitized Nc/Nga Mice. *BMC Complement. Altern. Med.* 14 (1), 100. doi:10.1186/1472-6882-14-100

Ha, H., Lim, H. S., Lee, M. Y., Shin, I. S., Jeon, W. Y., Kim, J. H., et al. (2015). *Luffa Cylindrica* Suppresses Development of Dermatophagoides Farinae-Induced Atopic Dermatitis-like Skin Lesions in Nc/Nga Mice. *Pharm. Biol.* 53 (4), 555–562. doi:10.3109/13880209.2014.932392

Haddaway, N. R., Pritchard, C. C., and McGuinness, L. A. (2021). *PRISMA2020: R Package and ShinyApp for Producing PRISMA 2020 Compliant Flow Diagrams.* Zenodo. doi:10.5281/zenodo.4287834

Ham, B., Kim, M., Son, Y. J., Chang, S., Jung, S. H., Nho, C. W., et al. (2019). Inhibitory Effects of *Pterocarpus Santalinus* Extract against IgE/antigen-Sensitized Mast Cells and Atopic Dermatitis-like Skin Lesions. *Planta Med.* 85 (7), 599–607. doi:10.1055/a-0824-1282

Han, H. M., Kim, S. J., Kim, J. S., Kim, B. H., Lee, H. W., Lee, Y. T., et al. (2016). Ameliorative Effects of Artemisia Argyi Folium Extract on 2,4-dinitrochlorobenzene-induced A-topic D-ermatitis-like L-esions in BALB/c M-ice. *Mol. Med. Rep.* 14 (4), 3206–3214. doi:10.3892/mmr.2016.5657

Han, N. R., Kang, S. W., Moon, P. D., Jang, J. B., Kim, H. M., and Jeong, H. J. (2014a). Genuine Traditional Korean Medicine, Naju Jjok (Chung-Dae, *Polygonum Tinctorium*) Improves 2,4-Dinitrofluorobenzene-Induced Atopic Dermatitis-like Lesional Skin. *Phytomedicine* 21 (4), 453–460. doi:10.1016/j.phymed.2013.09.021

Han, N. R., Moon, P. D., Kim, H. M., and Jeong, H. J. (2014b). Tryptanthrin Ameliorates Atopic Dermatitis through Down-Regulation of TSLP. *Arch. Biochem. Biophys.* 542, 14–20. doi:10.1016/j.abb.2013.11.010

Han, N. R., Moon, P. D., Yoo, M. S., Ryu, K. J., Kim, H. M., and Jeong, H. J. (2018). Regulatory Effects of Chrysophanol, a Bioactive Compound of AST2017-01 in a Mouse Model of 2,4-Dinitrofluorobenzene-Induced Atopic Dermatitis. *Int. Immunopharmacol.* 62, 220–226. doi:10.1016/j.intimp.2018.06.046

Han, N. R., Park, J. Y., Jang, J. B., Jeong, H. J., and Kim, H. M. (2014c). A Natural Dye, Niram Improves Atopic Dermatitis through Down-Regulation of TSLP. *Environ. Toxicol. Pharmacol.* 38 (3), 982–990. doi:10.1016/j.etap.2014.10.011

Hennebelle, T., Weniger, B., Joseph, H., Sahpaz, S., and Bailleul, F. (2009). *Senna alata. Fitoterapia* 80 (7), 385–393. doi:10.1016/j.fitote.2009.05.008

Herberth, G., Heinrich, J., Röder, S., Figl, A., Weiss, M., Diez, U., et al. (2010). Reduced IFN-Gamma- and Enhanced IL-4-producing CD4+ Cord Blood T Cells Are Associated with a Higher Risk for Atopic Dermatitis during the First 2 Yr of Life. *Pediatr. Allergy Immunol.* 21 (1 Pt 1), 5–13. doi:10.1111/j.1399-3038.2009.00890.x

Holladay, S. D., and Smialowicz, R. J. (2000). Development of the Murine and Human Immune System: Differential Effects of Immunotoxicants Depend on Time of Exposure. *Environ. Health Perspect.* 108 (Suppl. 3), 463–473. doi:10.1289/ehp.00108s3463

Hong, S. H., Ku, J. M., Kim, H. I., Kim, T. Y., Seo, H. S., Shin, Y. C., et al. (2019). Topical Application of KAJD Attenuates 2,4-Dinitrochlorobenzene-Induced Atopic Dermatitis Symptoms through Regulation of IgE and MAPK Pathways in BALB/C Mice and Several Immune Cell Types. *Front. Pharmacol.* 10, 1097. doi:10.3389/fphar.2019.01097

Hooijmans, C. R., Rovers, M. M., de Vries, R. B., Leenaars, M., Ritskes-Hoitinga, M., and Langendam, M. W. (2014). SYRCLE's Risk of Bias Tool for Animal Studies. *BMC Med. Res. Methodol.* 14 (1), 43–49. doi:10.1186/1471-2288-14-43

Hou, D. D., Zhang, W., Gao, Y. L., Sun, Y. Z., Wang, H. X., Qi, R. Q., et al. (2019). Anti-inflammatory Effects of Quercetin in a Mouse Model of MC903-Induced Atopic Dermatitis. *Int. Immunopharmacol.* 74 (105676), 105676. doi:10.1016/j.intimp.2019.105676

Huang, W. C., Huang, C. H., Hu, S., Peng, H. L., and Wu, S. J. (2019). Topical Spilanthol Inhibits MAPK Signaling and Ameliorates Allergic Inflammation in DNCB-Induced Atopic Dermatitis in Mice. *Int. J. Mol. Sci.* 20 (10), 2490. doi:10.3390/ijms20102490

Jackson, S. J., Andrews, N., Ball, D., Bellantuono, I., Gray, J., Hachoumi, L., et al. (2017). Does Age Matter? the Impact of Rodent Age on Study Outcomes. *Lab. Anim.* 51 (2), 160–169. doi:10.1177/0023677216653984

Jegal, J., Park, N. J., Bong, S. K., Jegal, H., Kim, S. N., and Yang, M. (2017). *Dioscorea Quinqueloba* Ameliorates Oxazolone- and 2,4-Dinitrochlorobenzene-Induced Atopic Dermatitis Symptoms in Murine Models. *Nutrients* 9 (12), 1324. doi:10.3390/nu9121324

Jeon, Y. D., Kee, J. Y., Kim, D. S., Han, Y. H., Kim, S. H., Kim, S. J., et al. (2015). Effects of *Ixeris Dentata* Water Extract and Caffeic Acid on Allergic Inflammation In Vivo and In Vitro. *BMC Complement. Altern. Med.* 15 (1), 196. doi:10.1186/s12906-015-0700-x

Jeong, N. H., Yang, E. J., Jin, M., Lee, J. Y., Choi, Y. A., Park, P. H., et al. (2018). Esculetin from *Fraxinus Rhynchophylla* Attenuates Atopic Skin Inflammation by Inhibiting the Expression of Inflammatory Cytokines. *Int. Immunopharmacol.* 59, 209–216. doi:10.1016/j.intimp.2018.04.005

Jin, M., Choi, J. K., Choi, Y. A., Kim, Y. Y., Baek, M. C., Lee, B. H., et al. (2016). 1,2,4,5-tetramethoxybenzene Suppresses House Dust Mite-Induced Allergic Inflammation in BALB/c Mice. *Int. Arch. Allergy Immunol.* 170 (1), 35–45. doi:10.1159/000446510

Jo, B. G., Park, N. J., Jegal, J., Choi, S., Lee, S. W., Jin, H., et al. (2018). A New Flavonoid from *Stellera Chamaejasme* L., Stechamone, Alleviated 2,4-Dinitrochlorobenzene-Induced Atopic Dermatitis-like Skin Lesions in a Murine Model. *Int. Immunopharmacol.* 59, 113–119. doi:10.1016/j.intimp.2018.04.008

Jo, B. G., Park, N. J., Jegal, J., Choi, S., Lee, S. W., Yi, L. W., et al. (2019). *Stellera Chamaejasme* and its Main Compound Luteolin 7-O-Glucoside Alleviates Skin Lesions in Oxazolone- and 2,4-Dinitrochlorobenzene-Stimulated Murine Models of Atopic Dermatitis. *Planta Med.* 85 (7), 583–590. doi:10.1055/a-0746-8698

Ju Ho, P., Jun Sung, J., Ki Cheon, K., and Jin Tae, H. (2018). Anti-inflammatory Effect of *Centella asiatica* Phytosome in a Mouse Model of Phthalic Anhydride-Induced Atopic Dermatitis. *Phytomedicine* 43, 110–119. doi:10.1016/j.phymed.2018.04.013

Jung, J. W., Kim, S. J., Ahn, E. M., Oh, S. R., Lee, H. J., Jeong, J. A., et al. (2014). *Ribes Fasciculatum* Var. *Chinense* Attenuated Allergic Inflammation In Vivo and In Vitro. *Biomol. Ther. Seoul.* 22 (6), 547–552. doi:10.4062/biomolther.2014.015

Jung, M., Lee, T. H., Oh, H. J., Kim, H., Son, Y., Lee, E. H., et al. (2015). Inhibitory Effect of 5,6-Dihydroergosteol-Glucoside on Atopic Dermatitis-like Skin Lesions via Suppression of NF-Kb and STAT Activation. *J. Dermatol Sci.* 79 (3), 252–261. doi:10.1016/j.jdermsci.2015.06.005

Jung, Y., Kim, J. C., Park, N. J., Bong, S. K., Lee, S., Jegal, H., et al. (2018). Eupatilin, an Activator of PPARα, Inhibits the Development of Oxazolone-Induced Atopic Dermatitis Symptoms in Balb/c Mice. *Biochem. Biophys. Res. Commun.* 496 (2), 508–514. doi:10.1016/j.bbrc.2018.01.098

Kang, S. Y., Jung, H. W., Nam, J. H., Kim, W. K., Kang, J. S., Kim, Y. H., et al. (2017). Effects of the Fruit Extract of *Tribulus Terrestris* on Skin Inflammation in Mice with Oxazolone-Induced Atopic Dermatitis through Regulation of Calcium Channels, Orai-1 and TRPV3, and Mast Cell Activation. *Evid. Based Complement. Altern. Med.* 2017, 1–12. doi:10.1155/2017/8312946

Kang, Y. M., Lee, K. Y., and An, H. J. (2018). Inhibitory Effects of *Helianthus Tuberosus* Ethanol Extract on Dermatophagoides Farina Body-Induced Atopic Dermatitis Mouse Model and Human Keratinocytes. *Nutrients* 10 (11), 1657. doi:10.3390/nu10111657

Kawakami, T., Ando, T., Kimura, M., Wilson, B. S., and Kawakami, Y. (2009). Mast Cells in Atopic Dermatitis. *Curr. Opin. Immunol.* 21 (6), 666–678. doi:10.1016/j.coi.2009.09.006

Kee, J. Y., Jeon, Y. D., Kim, D. S., Han, Y. H., Park, J., Youn, D. H., et al. (2017). Korean Red Ginseng Improves Atopic Dermatitis-like Skin Lesions by Suppressing Expression of Proinflammatory Cytokines and Chemokines In Vivo and In Vitro. *J. Ginseng Res.* 41 (2), 134–143. doi:10.1016/j.jgr.2016.02.003

Kilkenny, C., Parsons, N., Kadyszewski, E., Festing, M. F., Cuthill, I. C., Fry, D., et al. (2009). Survey of the Quality of Experimental Design, Statistical Analysis and Reporting of Research Using Animals. *PloS one* 4 (11), e7824. doi:10.1371/journal.pone.0007824

Kim, D., Kobayashi, T., and Nagao, K. (2019). Research Techniques Made Simple: Mouse Models of Atopic Dermatitis. *J. Invest. Dermatol* 139 (5), 984–990. doi:10.1016/j.jid.2019.02.014

Kim H, H., Kim, J. R., Kang, H., Choi, J., Yang, H., Lee, P., et al. (2014). 7,8,4'-Trihydroxyisoflavone Attenuates DNCB-Induced Atopic Dermatitis-like Symptoms in NC/Nga Mice. *PLoS One* 9 (8), e104938. doi:10.1371/journal.pone.0104938

Kim, H. Y., Ahn, S. H., Yang, I. J., Park, S. Y., and Kim, K. (2020). Effect of Hataedock Treatment on Epidermal Structure Maintenance through Intervention in the Endocannabinoid System. *Evid. Based Complement. Altern. Med.* 2020, 3605153. doi:10.1155/2020/3605153

Kim, J., Lee, I. S., Park, S., and Choue, R. (2010). Effects of *Scutellariae* Radix and *Aloe Vera* Gel Extracts on Immunoglobulin E and Cytokine Levels in Atopic Dermatitis NC/Nga Mice. *J. Ethnopharmacol.* 132 (2), 529–532. doi:10.1016/j.jep.2010.08.049

Kim SR, S. R., Choi, H. S., Seo, H. S., Ku, J. M., Hong, S. H., Yoo, H. H., et al. (2014). Oral Administration of Herbal Mixture Extract Inhibits 2,4-Dinitrochlorobenzene-Induced Atopic Dermatitis in BALB/c Mice. *Mediat. Inflamm.* 2014, 319438. doi:10.1155/2014/319438

Kim, W. Y., Kim, H. G., Lee, H. W., Lee, J. S., Im, H. J., Kim, H. S., et al. (2015). A Herbal Formula, Atofreellage, Ameliorates Atopic Dermatitis-like Skin Lesions in an NC/Nga Mouse Model. *Molecules* 21 (1), 35. doi:10.3390/molecules21010035

Kong, L., Wu, J., Lin, Y., Wang, G., Wang, J., Liu, J., et al. (2015). BuShenYiQi Granule Inhibits Atopic Dermatitis via Improving Central and Skin Hypothalamic-Pituitary-Adrenal axis Function. *PLoS One* 10 (2), e0116427. doi:10.1371/journal.pone.0116427

Ku, J. M., Hong, S. H., Kim, H. I., Seo, H. S., Shin, Y. C., and Ko, S. G. (2017). Effects of *Angelicae Dahuricae Radix* on 2, 4-Dinitrochlorobenzene-Induced Atopic Dermatitis-like Skin Lesions in Mice Model. *BMC Complement. Altern. Med.* 17 (1), 98. doi:10.1186/s12906-017-1584-8

Ku, J. M., Hong, S. H., Kim, S. R., Choi, H-S., Kim, H. I., Kim, D. U., et al. (2018). The Prevention of 2,4-Dinitrochlorobenzene-Induced Inflammation in Atopic Dermatitis-like Skin Lesions in BALB/c Mice by Jawoongo. *BMC Complement. Altern. Med.* 18 (1), 1–5. doi:10.1186/s12906-018-2280-z

Kulka, M., and Befus, A. D. (2003). The Dynamic and Complex Role of Mast Cells in Allergic Disease. *Arch. Immunol. Ther. Exp.* 51 (2), 111–120.

Kwak, M. H., Kim, J. E., Go, J., Son, H. J., Lee, H. S., Hong, J. T., et al. (2017). Effects of Aqueous Extract from Red Liriope Platyphylla on Phthalic-Anhydride-Induced Atopic Dermatitis in Interleukin-4/Luciferase/Consensus Non-coding Sequence-1 Transgenic Mice Evaluated in Terms of Luciferase Signal and General Phenotype Biomarkers. *J. Traditional Chin. Med.* 37 (4), 475–485. doi:10.1016/S0254-6272(17)30154-1

Laughter, M. R., Maymone, M. B. C., Mashayekhi, S., Arents, B. W. M., Karimkhani, C., Langan, S. M., et al. (2021). The Global Burden of Atopic Dermatitis: Lessons from the Global Burden of Disease Study 1990-2017. *Br. J. Dermatol* 184 (2), 304–309. doi:10.1111/bjd.19580

Lebwohl, M. G., Del Rosso, J. Q., Abramovits, W., Berman, B., Cohen, D. E., Guttman, E., et al. (2013). Pathways to Managing Atopic Dermatitis: Consensus from the Experts. *J. Clin. Aesthet. Dermatol* 6 (7 Suppl. l), S2–S18.

Lee, B. H., Kim, H. K., Jang, M., Kim, H. J., Choi, S. H., Hwang, S. H., et al. (2017). Effects of Gintonin-Enriched Fraction in an Atopic Dermatitis Animal Model: Involvement of Autotaxin Regulation. *Biol. Pharm. Bull.* 40 (7), 1063–1070. doi:10.1248/bpb.b17-00124

Lee, H., Ha, H., Lee, J. K., Park, S. J., Jeong, S. I., and Shin, H. K. (2014). The Leaves of Broussonetia Kazinoki Siebold Inhibit Atopic Dermatitis-like Response on Mite Allergen-Treated NC/Nga Mice. *Biomol. Ther. Seoul.* 22 (5), 438–444. doi:10.4062/biomolther.2014.023

Lee Hj, H. J., Kim, M. H., Choi, Y. Y., Kim, E. H., Hong, J., Kim, K., et al. (2016). Improvement of Atopic Dermatitis with Topical Application of *Spirodela Polyrhiza*. *J. Ethnopharmacol.* 180, 12–17. doi:10.1016/j.jep.2016.01.010

Lee J, J., Choi, Y. Y., Kim, M. H., Han, J. M., Lee, J. E., Kim, E. H., et al. (2016). Topical Application of *Angelica Sinensis* Improves Pruritus and Skin Inflammation in Mice with Atopic Dermatitis-like Symptoms. *J. Med. Food* 19 (1), 98–105. doi:10.1089/jmf.2015.3489

Lee JH, J. H., Jo, E. H., Lee, B., Noh, H. M., Park, S., Lee, Y. M., et al. (2019). Soshiho-tang, a Traditional Herbal Medicine, Alleviates Atopic Dermatitis Symptoms via Regulation of Inflammatory Mediators. *Front. Pharmacol.* 10, 742. doi:10.3389/fphar.2019.00742

Lee, K. S., Jeong, E. S., Heo, S. H., Seo, J. H., Jeong, D. G., and Choi, Y. K. (2010). A Novel Model for Human Atopic Dermatitis: Application of Repeated DNCB Patch in BALB/c Mice, in Comparison with NC/Nga Mice. *Lab. Anim. Res.* 26 (1), 95–102. doi:10.5625/lar.2010.26.1.95

Lee, S., Park, N. J., Bong, S. K., Jegal, J., Park, S. A., Kim, S. N., et al. (2018). Ameliorative Effects of *Juniperus Rigida* Fruit on Oxazolone-And 2, 4-Dinitrochlorobenzene-Induced Atopic Dermatitis in Mice. *J. Ethnopharmacol.* 214, 160–167. doi:10.1016/j.jep.2017.12.022

Lee S, S., Jegal, H., Bong, S. K., Yoon, K. N., Park, N. J., Shin, M. S., et al. (2019). Anti-atopic Effect of Acorn Shell Extract on Atopic Dermatitis-like Lesions in Mice and its Active Phytochemicals. *Biomolecules* 10 (1), 57. doi:10.3390/biom10010057

Lee, S. Y., Park, N. J., Jegal, J., Jo, B. G., Choi, S., Lee, S. W., et al. (2020). Suppression of DNCB-Induced Atopic Skin Lesions in Mice by *Wikstroemia Indica* Extract. *Nutrients* 12 (1), 173. doi:10.3390/nu12010173

Li, M. (2014). Current Evidence of Epidermal Barrier Dysfunction and Thymic Stromal Lymphopoietin in the Atopic March. *Eur. Respir. Rev.* 23 (133), 292–298. doi:10.1183/09059180.00004314

Lim, H. S., Ha, H., Lee, H., Lee, J. K., Lee, M. Y., and Shin, H. K. (2014a). *Morus Alba* L. Suppresses the Development of Atopic Dermatitis Induced by the House Dust Mite in NC/Nga Mice. *BMC Complement. Altern. Med.* 14 (1), 139. doi:10.1186/1472-6882-14-139

Lim, H. S., Ha, H., Lee, M. Y., Jin, S. E., Jeong, S. J., Jeon, W. Y., et al. (2014b). *Saussurea Lappa* Alleviates Inflammatory Chemokine Production in HaCaT Cells and House Dust Mite-Induced Atopic-like Dermatitis in Nc/Nga Mice. *Food Chem. Toxicol.* 63, 212–220. doi:10.1016/j.fct.2013.10.050

Lim, H. S., Ha, H., Shin, H. K., and Jeong, S. J. (2015). The Genome-wide Expression Profile of *Saussurea Lappa* Extract on House Dust Mite-Induced Atopic Dermatitis in Nc/Nga Mice. *Mol. Cells* 38 (9), 765–772. doi:10.14348/molcells.2015.0062

Lim, J. M., Lee, B., Min, J. H., Kim, E. Y., Kim, J. H., Hong, S., et al. (2018). Effect of Peiminine on DNCB-Induced Atopic Dermatitis by Inhibiting Inflammatory Cytokine Expression In Vivo and In Vitro. *Int. Immunopharmacol.* 56, 135–142. doi:10.1016/j.intimp.2018.01.025

Liu, T., Zhang, L., Joo, D., and Sun, S. C. (2017). NF-κB Signaling in Inflammation. *Signal Transduct Target Ther* 2 (1), 17023. doi:10.1038/sigtrans.2017.23

Makino, T., Shiraki, Y., and Mizukami, H. (2014). Interaction of Gypsum and the Rhizome of *Anemarrhena Asphodeloides* Plays an Important Role in Anti-allergic Effects of Byakkokakeishito in Mice. *J. Nat. Med.* 68 (3), 505–512. doi:10.1007/s11418-014-0827-y

Malik, K., Heitmiller, K. D., and Czarnowicki, T. (2017). An Update on the Pathophysiology of Atopic Dermatitis. *Dermatol Clin.* 35 (3), 317–326. doi:10.1016/j.det.2017.02.006

Mechesso, A. F., Lee, S. J., Park, N. H., Kim, J. Y., Im, Z. E., Suh, J. W., et al. (2019). Preventive Effects of a Novel Herbal Mixture on Atopic Dermatitis-like Skin Lesions in BALB/C Mice. *BMC Complement Altern Med* 19 (1), 25. doi:10.1186/s12906-018-2426-z

Mekori, Y. A., Oh, C. K., and Metcalfe, D. D. (1995). The Role of C-Kit and its Ligand, Stem Cell Factor, in Mast Cell Apoptosis. *Int. Arch. Allergy Immunol.* 107 (1-3), 136–138. doi:10.1159/000236955

Meng, Y., Liu, Z., Zhai, C., Di, T., Zhang, L., Zhang, L., et al. (2019). Paeonol Inhibits the Development of 1-chloro-2, 4-Dinitrobenzene-Induced Atopic Dermatitis via Mast and T Cells in BALB/c Mice. *Mol. Med. Rep.* 19 (4), 3217–3229. doi:10.3892/mmr.2019.9985

Montes-Torres, A., Llamas-Velasco, M., Pérez-Plaza, A., Solano-López, G., and Sánchez-Pérez, J. (2015). Biological Treatments in Atopic Dermatitis. *J. Clin. Med.* 4 (4), 593–613. doi:10.3390/jcm4040593

Moon, P. D., Han, N. R., Lee, J. S., Hong, S., Yoo, M. S., Kim, H. J., et al. (2019). Use of Physcion to Improve Atopic Dermatitis-like Skin Lesions through Blocking of Thymic Stromal Lymphopoietin. *Molecules* 24 (8), 1484. doi:10.3390/molecules24081484

Mowobi, G. G., Abubakar, S., Osuji, C., Etim, V. N., Ogechi, N., and Egya, J. J. (2016). Ethnobotanical Survey of Medicinal Plants Used for the Treatment of Skin Disease in Keffi, Nigeria. *Am. J. Phytomedicine Clin. Ther.* 4 (2), 73–90.

Mukai, K., Urai, T., Asano, K., Nakajima, Y., and Nakatani, T. (2016). Evaluation of Effects of Topical Estradiol Benzoate Application on Cutaneous Wound Healing in Ovariectomized Female Mice. *PLoS One* 11 (9), e0163560. doi:10.1371/journal.pone.0163560

Ngo, H. T. T., Fang, M., Hwang, E., Kim, Y., Park, B., Seo, S. A., et al. (2020). Inhibitory Effects of *Urtica Thunbergiana* Ethanol Extract on Atopic Dermatitis-Induced NC/Nga Mice. *Antioxidants* 9 (3), 197. doi:10.3390/antiox9030197

Nygaard, U., Deleuran, M., and Vestergaard, C. (2017). Emerging Treatment Options in Atopic Dermatitis: Topical Therapies. *Dermatology* 233 (5), 333–343. doi:10.1159/000484407

Ok, S., Oh, S. R., Jung, T. S., Jeon, S. O., Jung, J. W., and Ryu, D. S. (2018). Effects of *Angelica gigas* Nakai as an Anti-inflammatory Agent in In Vitro and In Vivo Atopic Dermatitis Models. *Evid. Based Complement. Altern. Med.* 2018, 2450712. doi:10.1155/2018/2450712

Oladeji, O. S., Adelowo, F. E., Oluyori, A. P., and Bankole, D. T. (2020). Ethnobotanical Description and Biological Activities of *Senna alata*. *Evid. Based Complement. Altern. Med.* 2020, 2580259. doi:10.1155/2020/2580259

Osada-Oka, M., Hirai, S., Izumi, Y., Misumi, K., Samukawa, K., Tomita, S., et al. (2018). Red Ginseng Extracts Attenuate Skin Inflammation in Atopic Dermatitis through P70 Ribosomal Protein S6 Kinase Activation. *J. Pharmacol. Sci.* 136 (1), 9–15. doi:10.1016/j.jphs.2017.11.002

Park BK, B. K., Park, Y. C., Jung, I. C., Kim, S. H., Choi, J. E., Park, S., et al. (2014). Oral Administration of SSC201, a Medicinal Herbal Formula, Suppresses Atopic Dermatitis-like Skin Lesions. *J. Med. Food* 17 (4), 496–504. doi:10.1089/jmf.2013.2941

Park, B. K., Park, Y. C., Jung, I. C., Kim, S. H., Choi, J. J., Do, M., et al. (2015). Gamisasangja-tang Suppresses Pruritus and Atopic Skin Inflammation in the NC/Nga Murine Model of Atopic Dermatitis. *J. Ethnopharmacol.* 165, 54–60. doi:10.1016/j.jep.2015.02.040

Park J, J., Youn, D. H., Kang, J., Ahn, K. S., Kwak, H. J., and Um, J. Y. (2019). Taeumjowi-tang, a Traditional Korean Sasang Remedy, Improves Obesity-Atopic Dermatitis Comorbidity by Regulating Hypoxia-Inducible Factor 1 Alpha. *Front. Pharmacol.* 10, 1458. doi:10.3389/fphar.2019.01458

Park, J. G., Yi, Y. S., Han, S. Y., Hong, Y. H., Yoo, S., Kim, E., et al. (2018). Tabetri™(*Tabebuia Avellanedae* Ethanol Extract) Ameliorates Atopic Dermatitis Symptoms in Mice. *Mediat. Inflamm.* 2018, 9079527. doi:10.1155/2018/9079527

Park JH, J. H., Ahn, E. K., Ko, H. J., Lee, J. Y., Hwang, S. M., Ko, S., et al. (2019). Korean Red Ginseng Water Extract Alleviates Atopic Dermatitis-like Inflammatory Responses by Negative Regulation of Mitogen-Activated Protein Kinase Signaling Pathway In Vivo. *Biomed. Pharmacother.* 117 (109066), 109066. doi:10.1016/j.biopha.2019.109066

Park KH, K. H., Jeong, M. S., Park, K. J., Choi, Y. W., Seo, S. J., and Lee, M. W. (2014). Topical Application of *Rosa Multiflora* Root Extract Improves Atopic Dermatitis-like Skin Lesions Induced by Mite Antigen in NC/Nga Mice. *Biol. Pharm. Bull.* 37 (1), 178–183. doi:10.1248/bpb.b13-00619

Park, S. H., Jang, S., An, J. E., kil Choo, B., and Kim, H. K. (2020). *I. Inflexus* (Thunb.) Kudo Extract Improves Atopic Dermatitis and Depressive-like Behaviour in DfE-Induced Atopic Dermatitis-like Disease. *Phytomedicine* 67, 153137. doi:10.1016/j.phymed.2019.153137

Park SH, S. H., An, J. E., Jang, S., Kim, J. Y., Lee, J. W., and Kim, H. K. (2019). *Gardenia Jasminoides* Extract without Crocin Improved Atopic Dermatitis-like Skin Lesions via Suppression of Th2-Related Cytokines in DfE-Induced NC/Nga Mice. *J. Ethnopharmacol.* 241 (112015), 112015. doi:10.1016/j.jep.2019.112015

Qiu, C., Zhong, L., Huang, C., Long, J., Ye, X., Wu, J., et al. (2020). Cell-bound IgE and Plasma IgE as a Combined Clinical Diagnostic Indicator for Allergic Patients. *Sci. Rep.* 10 (1), 4700. doi:10.1038/s41598-020-61455-8

Renert-Yuval, Y., Thyssen, J. P., Bissonnette, R., Bieber, T., Kabashima, K., Hijnen, D., et al. (2021). Biomarkers in Atopic Dermatitis-A Review on Behalf of the International Eczema Council. *J. Allergy Clin. Immunol.* 147 (4), 1174–1190. doi:10.1016/j.jaci.2021.01.013

Ryu, K. J., Yoou, M. S., Seo, Y., Yoon, K. W., Kim, H. M., and Jeong, H. J. (2018). Therapeutic effects of *Artemisia scoparia* Waldst. et Kitaib in a murine model of atopic dermatitis. *Clin. Exp. Dermatol* 43 (7), 798–805. doi:10.1111/ced.13565

Sánchez, M., González-Burgos, E., Iglesias, I., and Gómez-Serranillos, M. P. (2020). Pharmacological Update Properties of *Aloe Vera* and its Major Active Constituents. *Molecules* 25 (6), 1324. doi:10.3390/molecules25061324

Shamseer, L., Moher, D., Clarke, M., Ghersi, D., Liberati, A., Petticrew, M., et al. (2015). Preferred Reporting Items for Systematic Review and Meta-Analysis Protocols (PRISMA-P) 2015: Elaboration and Explanation. *Bmj* 350, g7647. doi:10.1136/bmj.g7647

Shiohara, T., Hayakawa, J., and Mizukawa, Y. (2004). Animal Models for Atopic Dermatitis: Are They Relevant to Human Disease? *J. Dermatol Sci.* 36 (1), 1–9. doi:10.1016/j.jdermsci.2004.02.013

Siebenhaar, F., Redegeld, F. A., Bischoff, S. C., Gibbs, B. F., and Maurer, M. (2018). Mast Cells as Drivers of Disease and Therapeutic Targets. *Trends Immunol.* 39 (2), 151–162. doi:10.1016/j.it.2017.10.005

Silverberg, N. B., and Silverberg, J. I. (2015). Inside Out or outside in: Does Atopic Dermatitis Disrupt Barrier Function or Does Disruption of Barrier Function Trigger Atopic Dermatitis. *Cutis* 96 (6), 359–361.

Song-lin, Z., Tan, G. H., Feng-yin, H., Wang, H., Ying-ying, L., and Shuang-lin, C. (2014). Sanpao Herbs Inhibit Development of Atopic Dermatitis in Balb/c Mice. *Asian Pac. J. Allergy Immunol.* 32 (2), 140. doi:10.12932/ap0381.32.2.2013

Stone, K. D., Prussin, C., and Metcalfe, D. D. (2010). IgE, Mast Cells, Basophils, and Eosinophils. *J. Allergy Clin. Immunol.* 125 (2), S73–S80. doi:10.1016/j.jaci.2009.11.017

Sung, Y. Y., and Kim, H. K. (2018). Crocin Ameliorates Atopic Dermatitis Symptoms by Down Regulation of Th2 Response via Blocking of NF-Kb/stat6 Signaling Pathways in Mice. *Nutrients* 10 (11), 1625. doi:10.3390/nu10111625

Sung, Y. Y., Lee, A. Y., and Kim, H. K. (2016). *Forsythia Suspensa* Fruit Extracts and the Constituent Matairesinol Confer Anti-allergic Effects in an Allergic Dermatitis Mouse Model. *J. Ethnopharmacol.* 187, 49–56. doi:10.1016/j.jep.2016.04.015

Sung, Y. Y., Lee, A. Y., and Kim, H. K. (2014). The *Gardenia Jasminoides* Extract and its Constituent, Geniposide, Elicit Anti-allergic Effects on Atopic Dermatitis by Inhibiting Histamine In Vitro and In Vivo. *J. Ethnopharmacol.* 156, 33–40. doi:10.1016/j.jep.2014.07.060

Sur, B., Lee, B., Yoon, Y. S., Lim, P., Hong, R., Yeom, M., et al. (2017). Extract of *Polygala Tenuifolia* Alleviates Stress-Exacerbated Atopy-like Skin Dermatitis through the Modulation of Protein Kinase A and P38 Mitogen-Activated Protein Kinase Signaling Pathway. *Int. J. Mol. Sci.* 18 (1), 190. doi:10.3390/ijms18010190

Tak, P. P., and Firestein, G. S. (2001). NF-κB: a Key Role in Inflammatory Diseases. *J. Clin. Investigation* 107 (1), 7–11. doi:10.1172/JCI11830

Tanaka, A., Muto, S., Jung, K., Itai, A., and Matsuda, H. (2007). Topical Application with a New NF-Kb Inhibitor Improves Atopic Dermatitis in NC/NgaTnd Mice. *J. Investigative Dermatology* 127 (4), 855–863. doi:10.1038/sj.jid.5700603

Tao, Y., Wang, Y., Wang, X., Wang, C., Bao, K., Ji, L., et al. (2017). Calycosin Suppresses Epithelial Derived Initiative Key Factors and Maintains Epithelial Barrier in Allergic Inflammation via TLR4 Mediated NF-Kb Pathway. *Cell Physiol. Biochem.* 44 (3), 1106–1119. doi:10.1159/000485416

Thomsen, S. F. (2014). Atopic Dermatitis: Natural History, Diagnosis, and Treatment. *ISRN Allergy* 2014, 354250. doi:10.1155/2014/354250

Tsang, M. S., Jiao, D., Chan, B. C., Hon, K. L., Leung, P. C., Lau, C., et al. (2016). Anti-inflammatory Activities of Pentaherbs Formula, Berberine, Gallic Acid and Chlorogenic Acid in Atopic Dermatitis-like Skin Inflammation. *Molecules* 21 (4), 519. doi:10.3390/molecules21040519

Wald, C., and Wu, C. (2010). Biomedical Research. Of Mice and Women: the Bias in Animal Models. *Science* 327 (5973), 1571–1572. doi:10.1126/science.327.5973.1571

Wan, H. L., Chen, H. Z., and Shi, X. Q. (2016). Study on Effect of Traditional Chinese Medicine Jianpi Chushi Decoction and Ointment on Chronic Eczema. *Asian Pac J. Trop. Med.* 9 (9), 920–923. doi:10.1016/j.apjtm.2016.07.019

Wang, Q., Gao, S., Wu, G. Z., Yang, N., Zu, X. P., Li, W. C., et al. (2018). Total Sesquiterpene Lactones Isolated from *Inula Helenium* L. Attenuates 2, 4-Dinitrochlorobenzene-Induced Atopic Dermatitis-like Skin Lesions in Mice. *Phytomedicine* 46, 78–84. doi:10.1016/j.phymed.2018.04.036

Wang, X., Jiang, X., Yu, X., Liu, H., Tao, Y., Jiang, G., et al. (2017). Cimifugin Suppresses Allergic Inflammation by Reducing Epithelial Derived Initiative Key Factors via Regulating Tight Junctions. *J. Cell Mol. Med.* 21 (11), 2926–2936. doi:10.1111/jcmm.13204

Williams, C. M., and Galli, S. J. (2000). The Diverse Potential Effector and Immunoregulatory Roles of Mast Cells in Allergic Disease. *J. Allergy Clin. Immunol.* 105 (5), 847–859. doi:10.1067/mai.2000.106485

Wu, C. T., Huang, K. S., Yang, C. H., Chen, Y. C., Liao, J. W., Kuo, C. L., et al. (2014). Inhibitory Effects of Cultured *Dendrobium Tosaense* on Atopic Dermatitis Murine Model. *Int. J. Pharm.* 463 (2), 193–200. doi:10.1016/j.ijpharm.2013.08.015

Wu, S., Yu, D., Liu, W., Zhang, J., Liu, X., Wang, J., et al. (2020). Magnoflorine from *Coptis Chinese* Has the Potential to Treat DNCB-Induced Atopic Dermatitis by Inhibiting Apoptosis of Keratinocyte. *Bioorg. Med. Chem.* 28 (2), 115093. doi:10.1016/j.bmc.2019.115093

Xiao-Tong, W. A., Hai-Liang, L. I., Xi, Y. U., Can, W. A., Gu, L., Xiao-Yu, W. A., et al. (2019). Chinese Medicine *Yu-Ping-Feng-San* Attenuates Allergic Inflammation by Regulating Epithelial Derived Pro-allergic Cytokines. *Chin. J. Nat. Med.* 17 (7), 525–534. doi:10.1016/S1875-5364(19)30074-3

Yan, F., Zhang, J., Li, X., Mo, X., Liu, J., Ye, S., et al. (2019). Therapeutic Effects of Chinese Herbal Formula (PTQX) on NC/Nga Mice with Atopic Dermatitis-like Skin Lesions. *Evid. Based Complement. Altern. Med.* 2019, 8359252. doi:10.1155/2019/8359252

Yang G, G., An, D., Lee, M. H., Lee, K., Kim, B., Suman, C. K., et al. (2016). Effect of *Acer Tegmentosum* Bark on Atopic Dermatitis-like Skin Lesions in NC/Nga Mice. *J. Ethnopharmacol.* 177, 53–60. doi:10.1016/j.jep.2015.10.033

Yang Hj, H. J., Kim, M. J., Kang, S., Moon, N. R., Kim, D. S., Lee, N. R., et al. (2017). Topical Treatments of *Saussurea costus* Root and *Thuja Orientalis* L. Synergistically Alleviate Atopic Dermatitis-like Skin Lesions by Inhibiting Protease-Activated Receptor-2 and NF-Kb Signaling in HaCaT Cells and Nc/Nga Mice. *J. Ethnopharmacol.* 199, 97–105. doi:10.1016/j.jep.2017.01.055

Yang Ij, I. J., Lee, D. U., and Shin, H. M. (2016). Inhibitory Effect of Valencene on the Development of Atopic Dermatitis-like Skin Lesions in NC/Nga Mice. *Evid. Based Complement. Altern. Med.* 2016, 9370893. doi:10.1155/2016/9370893

Yang J, J., Xiong, Y. A., Xiao, S. J., and Xu, Y. S. (2017). Anti-inflammatory Effects of Saxifrage Cream in Hapten-Induced Chronic Dermatitis-Eczema in Mice. *Chin. Herb. Med.* 9 (2), 176–182. doi:10.1016/S1674-6384(17)60092-3

Yang JH, J. H., Yoo, J. M., Cho, W. K., and Ma, J. Y. (2016). Ethanol Extract of Sanguisorbae Radix Inhibits Mast Cell Degranulation and Suppresses 2, 4-Dinitrochlorobenzene-Induced Atopic Dermatitis-like Skin Lesions. *Mediat. Inflamm.* 2016, 2947390. doi:10.1155/2016/2947390

Yang, J. H., Lee, E., Lee, B., Cho, W. K., Ma, J. Y., and Park, K. I. (2018). Ethanolic Extracts of *Artemisia Apiacea* Hance Improved Atopic Dermatitis-like Skin Lesions In Vivo and Suppressed TNF-alpha/IFN-Gamma–Induced Proinflammatory Chemokine Production In Vitro. *Nutrients* 10 (7), 806. doi:10.3390/nu10070806

Zari, S. T., and Zari, T. A. (2015). A Review of Four Common Medicinal Plants Used to Treat Eczema. *J. Med. Plants Res.* 9 (24), 702–711. doi:10.5897/JMPR2015.5831

Zhanxue, S., Jingjun, W., Yuhong, K., Nan, L., Xiaoyuan, J., Ting, C., et al. (2018). Effect of Yupingfeng Granules on the Skin Barrier in Atopic Dermatitis Mice Models. *J. Traditional Chin. Med.* 38 (6), 872–878. doi:10.1016/S0254-6272(18)30986-5

Zheng, J., Wang, X., Tao, Y., Wang, Y., Yu, X., Liu, H., et al. (2019). *Yu-Ping-Feng-San* Ameliorates Recurrent Allergic Inflammation of Atopic Dermatitis by Repairing Tight Junction Defects of the Epithelial Barrier. *Phytomedicine* 54, 214–223. doi:10.1016/j.phymed.2018.09.190

15

Established and Emerging Treatments of Skin GvHD

Cornelia S. Link-Rachner[1,2]*, Katja Sockel*[1] *and Catharina Schuetz*[3*]

[1] *Medizinische Klinik und Poliklinik I, Medizinische Fakultät Carl Gustav Carus, Technische Universität Dresden, Dresden, Germany,* [2] *Center for Regenerative Therapies Dresden, Technische Universität Dresden, Dresden, Germany,* [3] *Klinik und Poliklinik für Kinder- und Jugendmedizin, Medizinische Fakultät Carl Gustav Carus, Technische Universität Dresden, Dresden, Germany*

Correspondence:
Catharina Schuetz
catharina.schuetz@ukdd.de

Graft-versus-host disease (GvHD) of the skin is a severe allo-immune reaction and complication following allogeneic stem cell transplantation. Over the past years, intensive pre-clinical research has led to an improved understanding of the pathophysiology of acute and to a lesser extend chronic GvHD. This has translated into the approval of several new agents for the treatment of both forms of GvHD. This review summarizes the most recent advances in underlying pathomechanisms, clinical trials and newly approved agents for GvHD, with a special focus on skin involvement.

Keywords: Graft-versus-host disease, cutaneous GvHD, acute skin GvHD, chronic skin GvHD, cell-based therapy, targeted therapy, GvHD treatment, GvHD therapies

INTRODUCTION

Graft-versus-host disease (GvHD) remains a frequent complication following allogeneic stem cell transplantation (HSCT). Despite better pretransplant conditioning, prophylaxes and graft manipulation, treatment refractory GvHD accounts for 5-30% (1). Skin is the first and most frequently affected organ by GvHD. While local treatment may be sufficient for mild manifestations, systemic immunomodulatory or immunosuppressive therapies are inevitable in moderate and severe forms.

CUTANEOUS GvHD: CLINICAL PRESENTATION

While up to 50% of patients after allogeneic HSCT are affected by any type of GvHD (2), cutaneous lesions are often the first sign of GvHD. A maculopapular rash starting on the décolleté and neck, palms and soles generally spreads to the trunk and extremities as erythroderma. At worst epidermal injury may present itself as bullae which resemble second degree burns or toxic epidermal necrolysis. Itching is one of the first symptoms even before cutaneous lesions occur. Chronic GvHD is more variable in its presentation and may resemble several autoimmune disorders. Cutaneous pathologies include interface dermatitis, lichenoid manifestations, sclerosing dermatitis or panniculitis and fasciitis (3). Sclerodermatous GvHD may evolve toward a scleroderma-like disease with severe functional impairment, some patients becoming wheel-chair bound due to contractures. In addition, chronic cutaneous GvHD is often associated with disturbed wound healing, loss of body hair or alopecia. Advances in the management of skin GvHD are propelled by studies dissecting some of the pathomechanisms underlying GvHD in preclinical models (4).

BASIC PATHOMECHANISMS OF CUTANEOUS GvHD

Pathomechanisms driving GvHD need to be discussed in light of host and donor characteristics. Host predisposing factors refer to the inflammatory milieu at the time of HSCT. A certain degree of skin toxicity, i.e. inflammation or damage, will inevitably follow treatment with chemotherapeutic agents. Upon infusion of donor stem cells, the presence of chronic viral infection and an altered host microbiome may further contribute to a favorable host environment facilitating GvHD.

In acute GvHD, besides T cell mediated inflammation, innate immune cells like neutrophils and monocytes also trigger inflammation through a number of mechanisms including ROS production, release of proinflammatory signals *via* pathogen-associated molecular patterns (PAMP) and danger-associated molecular patterns (DAMP, e.g. ATP, uric acid) released from injured cells (2). DAMPs activate the NLRP3 inflammasome and promote IL-1β-driven cell injury (5). Proinflammatory cytokines and chemokines directly damage epithelial cells, e.g. TNFα or activate donor T cells (6). These migrate to lymphoid tissues where they encounter host antigen-presenting cells (APCs) early after HSCT – as well as emerging donor APCs in the later post-transplant HSCT phase – which will detect antigen histo-incompatibilities (7). So-called "allo"reactive cytotoxic T cells then migrate to the skin causing tissue injury. Of note, various cell types mentioned above may also have regulatory functions preventing or limiting GvHD induced tissue damage.

While aGvHD is mostly T cell and cytokine driven, the pathophysiology of cGvHD is much more complex. Standardization of nomenclature in order to group different GvH-variants is key to deciphering the following main mechanisms: inflammatory vs. allo/autoimmune-mediated vs. mechanisms resulting in skin fibrosis (8). Moreover, thymic dysregulation leading to poor negative selection, tissue infiltration and injury by Th17 cytotoxic T cells, lack of regulatory T cells and also B cellular hyperactivity with auto/allo-antibody production as well reflect some of the complex mechanisms involved in cGvHD (7) as illustrated in **Figure 1A**.

CLASSIFICATION, STAGING, GRADING AND SCORING FOR GvHD

According to the current National Institutes of Health (NIH) classification system, acute GvHD may occur as classic aGvHD within the first 100 days post HSCT, or persistent/recurrent or late-onset aGvHD, reflecting clinical signs of acute GvHD beyond 100 days following HSCT. The latter is typically observed after reduction of immunosuppressive therapy. Chronic GvHD can be divided into the classic form, without signs of aGvHD and the overlap syndrome, combining features of chronic and acute GvHD (9).

In aGvHD the extent or severity of organ involvement falls into 4 stages, and categories are defined for skin, gut and liver (10, 11). For skin involvement, staging reflects the extent of affected body surface area with <25%, 25-50%, >50% and generalized erythroderma plus bullous formation and desquamation >5% from stage 1 to 4. Histopathological grades I-IV describe the epithelial damage ranging from vacuolation of epidermal basal cells to confluent areas of keratinocyte necrosis or even sloughing (12). As for cGvHD, the grading is more detailed with organ specific assessment (13). Notably, so-called "diagnostic" clinical features including poikilodermia, lichen planus, lichen sclerosis and sclerosis are sufficient to establish a clinical diagnosis of cGvHD, while a diagnostic biopsy is mandatory in case of "distinctive" clinical features of cGvHD such as papulosquamous lesions, oral ulcers, onycholysis, or possible alternative diagnoses. **Supplementary Table 1** provides information on how to score severity for cGvHD of the skin.

ESTABLISHED TREATMENTS OF CUTANEOUS GvHD

While highly desired, there is currently no available tool to predict the occurrence of GvHD safely. A standard GvHD prophylaxis for patients following transplantation consists of a combination of immunosuppressive agents (14). For many years the most common combinations used in Europe consisted of a calcineurin inhibitor such as cyclosporine A in combination with methotrexate. In some institutions cyclosporine A has been replaced by tacrolimus following the finding of 2 phase III trials in which the incidence of grade II-IV acute GvHD was lower with tacrolimus (15). More recently, antithymocyte globulin (ATG) or post-transplant cyclophosphamide have been used as GvHD prophylaxis (16).

Acute GvHD

The choice of treatment greatly depends on the grade and localization of GvHD. For locally restricted forms of grade I acute skin GvHD, the initial treatment approach will consist of a topical steroid (17). Low-potency topical steroid should be preferred in thinner skin areas (face). Upon grade 2 systemic treatment is required. Standard first-line treatment are systemic corticosteroids such as prednisolone, frequently used at a dosage of 1-2 mg/kg body weight per day (14). A lower dose (< 1 mg/kg) might be sufficient in less severe forms of acute skin GvHD (body surface involvement <50%) and associated with less side effects. Indeed, while being effective in many cases, high dose steroids have numerous adverse effects on metabolism and organs such as bone (18) and steroid-resistance remains an issue that correlates with increasing GvHD severity (19). The treatment of steroid refractory skin GvHD (14) is especially challenging as there are no standardized guidelines available for second-line treatment and trial results of available agents are often limited to single arm studies lacking direct comparability.

A well-established therapeutic option is extracorporeal photopheresis (ECP) (20). Particularly for the treatment of skin-predominant forms of acute GvHD, ECP has been proven to be effective while reducing the cumulative amount of systemic

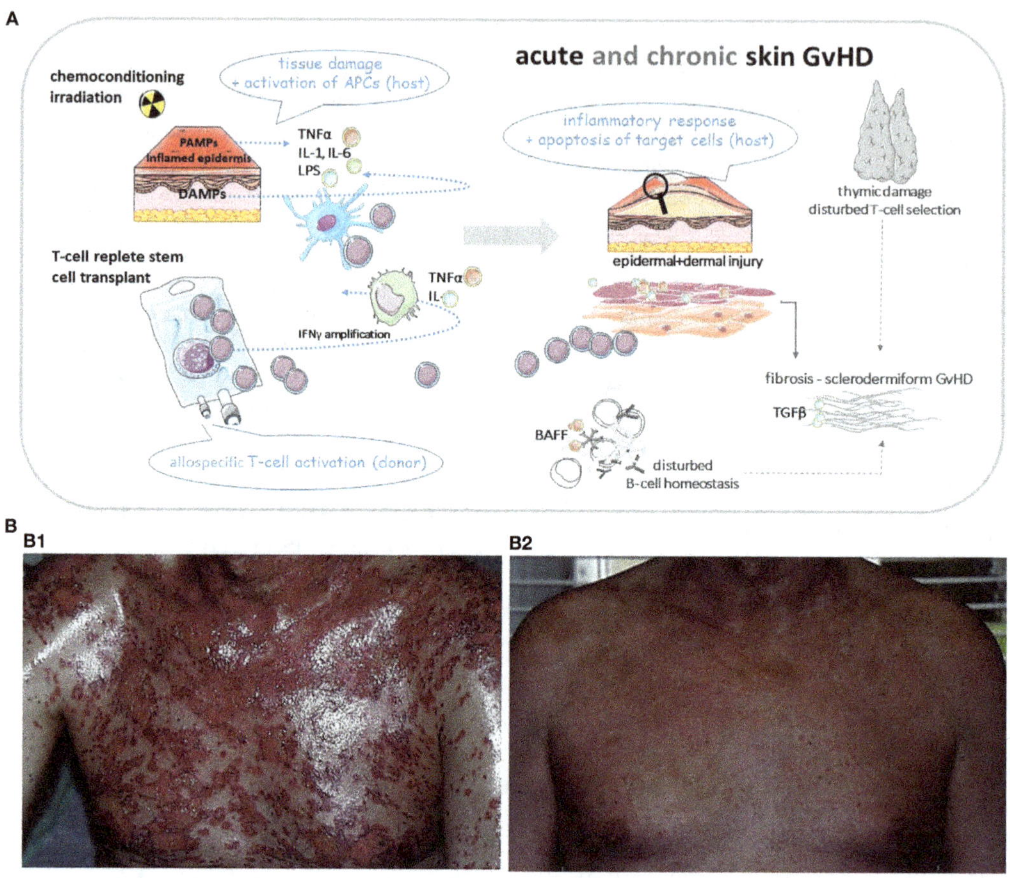

FIGURE 1 | **(A)** Cartoon of basic pathomechanisms in acute and chronic GvHD of the skin. In aGvHD proinflammatory cytokines (TNFα, IL-1 and IL-6) are released from injured tissue following pretransplant conditioning. Increased release of PAMPs (from pathogens within the microbiome) and DAMPs (from damaged cells) drive inflammation through induction of host APCs. These APCs amplify the inflammatory cascade by recruiting cells of the adaptive immune system, e.g. donor T cells and directing T cell migration to lymphoid tissues. Alloreactive T cells differentiate into Th1 and Th17 cells which secrete cytokines like TNFα and INFγ driving alloimmunity. Cytotoxic donor T cells infiltrate the skin or other target organs. In cGvHD cytokines activate the innate and adaptive immune systems or result in direct tissue damage. Thymic injury by alloreactive T cells results in disturbed self-tolerance characterized by decreased regulatory T cells and release of self-reactive T cells. Delayed and dysregulated B cell reconstitution and increased *B cell–activating factor (BAFF)* levels foster aberrant antibody production to host antigens. Finally aberrant repair of inflamed or damaged skin layers is promoted by activated macrophages, which induce fibroblasts and produce growth factors like TGFβ, resulting in skin fibrosis. APC, antigen presenting cell; BAFF, B cell activating factor; DAMP, damage associated molecular pattern; GvHD, graft-versus-host-disease (aGvHD for acute; cGvHD for chronic); IL, interleukin; INF, interferon; PAMP, pathogen associated molecular pattern; Th, T-helper cell; TNF, tumor necrosis factor. **(B1)** Patient with severe acute skin GvHD (III°). **(B2)** The same patient three weeks after treatment with mesenchymal stem cells. Pictures were provided by Prof. Martin Bornhäuser (MK1, UKD TU Dresden).

steroids required in clinical trials (12) and real world settings (21). Complete response rates of cutaneous GvHD of >80% have been reported, which also translated into an improved survival and reduction in mortality (12). Importantly, there is increasing data to suggest that an early initiation, preferably within 35 days of onset of aGvHD, achieved an even better response rate (22). In a systemic analysis of 9 studies and >300 patients an overall response rate of 69% was observed across all patients with the highest rate of 84% in cutaneous aGvHD (23). As a limitation this meta-analysis only contained 1 randomized controlled trial indicating the difficulty there is in comparing study results due to a lack of high quality randomized controlled trials. Systemic treatment of acute GvHD may vary depending on local protocols but recent advances in clinical trials and guidelines have aimed at standardizing treatment (17). For localized cutaneous aGvHD manifestations UVA-1 and UVB based phototherapy may be beneficial, resulting in complete response rates of 70% and partial response rates of 24,3% for UVA-1, (24); 57% and 21% for UVB therapy (25). However, treatment response may take weeks to set in.

Antithymocyte globulin (ATG) is also commonly used in patients with steroid-refractory aGvHD. While some older studies have presented data that may indicate a less than expected effect and a higher rate of infections, more recent studies have shown better outcomes [summarized and discussed in (26)]. Recently a study design with a gradual dose escalation scheme has been published with promising outcome, which may be one option in reducing the risk of infectious complications (27). There are no clear guidelines for the second-line therapy of acute skin GvHD in line with the complexity of the disease. Individualized solutions include switching to a different calcineurin inhibitor, (re)introducing mycophenolate mofetil or the mTor inhibitor sirolimus (28).

Chronic GvHD

The lack of an internationally accepted primary endpoint in clinical trials of cGvHD makes the comparability of previously published trials difficult and the chosen primary endpoints may not automatically translate into a clinical benefit. While this issue has been increasingly addressed in the past years and we are now starting to obtain data from RCTs and discussions on defining a gold standard for the endpoint of these trials (29). Furthermore, in 2014 the NIH re-defined criteria for clinical trials in cGvHD (13).

First-line therapy in the case of a mild cGvHD are topical steroids, mostly higher potency steroids (e.g., clobetasol propionate 0.05%). Cutaneous atrophy or local infections may occur during long-term use of topical steroids; topical calcineurin inhibitors (tacrolimus and pimecrolimus) may spare steroids in some of these patients (30).

Systemic steroids alone or in combination with calcineurin inhibitors are required for severe cGvHD (31). However, the adverse events associated with chronic steroid treatment become particularly apparent in this situation and alternative approaches to spare steroids are especially important. In cGvHD, the use of ECP is one of the best investigated treatment options (29). In a phase 2 trial, ECP resulted in a significantly higher proportion of the subjects achieving partial or complete response of skin manifestations ($p < 0.001$). A limiting factor was that this assessment was conducted in a non-blinded manner. However, the initial blinded assessment of the total skin score and reduction in steroid use also favored the ECP over the standard care (32).

In a more recent randomized control trial in cGvHD, ECP was added to the standard of care in a first line setting of patients newly diagnosed with moderate or severe cGvHD (33). At 28 weeks, ORR was 74.1% in the ECP arm, compared to 66.7% in the standard of care arm. In addition, quality of life was maintained in the ECP group but declined in the control group.

In an extensive review of 27 studies, where ECP was used in steroid-resistant or dependent cGvHD, the mean response rate for cutaneous cGvHD was 74% (34). A comparable response rate of 64% (ORR) and 27% (CRR) for cutaneous involvement has been previously published in a different meta-analyses (35).

Notably, a recent systematic review of adverse events in second- and third-line treatments for acute and chronic GvHD revealed a lower incidence of infectious adverse events in acute GvHD and lower number of grade 3-5 adverse events in cGvHD in patients on ECP compared to any pharmaceutical management highlighting the safety aspect of this form of treatment (36).

Another therapeutic approach is the use of Rituximab. The anti-CD20 monoclonal antibody is widely used especially in sclerosing cGvHD of the skin, fasciitis, musculoskeletal cGvHD. Clinical responses up to 70% have been described (37). In addition, the tyrosine kinase inhibitor imatinib has been applied for severe, sclerodermic cGVHD (38). Imatinib targets the PDGFR and TGF-β pathways which are involved in skin fibrosis. Besides pharmaceutic interventions, physiotherapy is one of the most useful adjunctive treatments in patients with fasciitis or contractures due to sclerodermiformic GvHD and should always be part of a comprehensive treatment approach (39).

EMERGING TREATMENTS FOR CUTANEOUS GvHD

In the past years a number of novel agents have been tested in advanced clinical trials in acute or chronic GvHD and some of these drugs are now available for clinical use. While none of these trials was specifically designed only to assess the effect on skin GvHD, a large percentage of subjects included in these trials were affected by skin GvHD (**Table 1**).

Acute GvHD

JAK Inhibitors

Ruxolitinib, an inhibitor of the Janus kinase (JAK) 1/2, was approved for the treatment of steroid-refractory acute GvHD in 2019. JAK signaling plays an important role in regulating the underlying immune cells relevant for GvHD such as dendritic cells, macrophages as well as B- and T cells. Most importantly, there is preclinical evidence to suggest that inhibition of the JAK pathway does not negatively impact the GvL effect [as summarized in (40)].

Approval followed a successful open-label, single arm, phase 2 trial (NCT02953678) (41). Of the 70 patients enrolled, 36 had signs of skin GvHD and the overall response rate (ORR) on day 28 was 61% with 25% of patients experiencing a CR. A

TABLE 1 | Emerging treatments for steroid refractory GvHD (sr = steroid refractory).

Drug	Target	sr-aGvHD	sr-cGvHD	Approved	Reference
Ruxolitinib	JAK inhibitor	✓	✓	sr-aGvHD sr-cGvHD	(40–42) and (43, 44)
Itacitinib	JAK inhibitor	✓			(45)
IL-2R antibodies	Interleukin-2 receptor	✓			(46–49)
TNFa antibodies	Tumor necrosis factor alpha	✓			(50–54)
MSCs	T cell proliferation and T cell response	✓			(55–59)
Ibrutinib	Bruton tyrosine kinase (B cells) and interleukin-2-inducible kinase (T cells)		✓	sr-cGvHD	(60)
Belumosudil	Rho-associated coiled-coil-containing kinase 2		✓	sr-cGvHD	(61)
Tregs	T cell subset with immunosuppressive and immunoregulatory functions		✓		(62, 63)

subsequent phase 3 trial with 309 patients assigned to ruxolitinib (10 mg twice daily) or investigator's choice of therapy (control arm) was conducted more recently. ORR at day 28 was higher in the ruxolitinib group than in the control group (62% vs. 39%; OR 2.64. 95%CI 1.65-4.22, p<0.001). Overall survival was 11.1 in the ruxolitinib group compared to 6.5 months in the control arm (HR 0.83; 95%CI 0.60-1.15). In this trial the majority (54%) of patients had skin involvement (42). Since ruxolitinib impairs viral specific T cell response, careful monitoring for viral reactivation (including HSV, VZV, CMV) is mandatory. Itacitinib, another JAK1 inhibitor has currently revealed promising results in a phase-1 study on aGvHD, with an overall response rate of about 70% in steroid-refractory aGVH patients (45).

IL-2R Antibodies

A number of IL-2R antibodies, namely daclizumab, basiliximab and inolimomab, have been tested in clinical trials for the treatment of aGvHD. These agents generally showed some level of clinical activity in treating aGvHD, especially in cases where skin or gut was involved, (46, 47). However, despite initially promising results, data from subsequent studies were clouded by high rates of infectious complications and in some cases poor long-term survival. In a phase III trial, inolimomab was compared to ATG in patients with steroid-refractory aGvHD (48). The primary endpoint was not met, but long-term follow-up of this study pointed towards a survival benefit of inolimomab (31%) versus ATG [20%, HR 0.572, p=0.03) (49)].

Anti-TNFa-Antibodies

The TNFa antibodies infliximab and etanercept have both been investigated for the treatment of aGvHD. Studies with infliximab have delivered mixed results with a modest effect but a generally high rate of infectious complications, (50, 51). There are more studies available for etanercept although the majority of these have yielded a higher response rate than seen in studies with infliximab, but no clear survival benefit has been described (52, 53).

Combining TNFa with IL-2R blocking may be attractive. A prospective trial assessing patients treated with basiliximab in combination with etanercept had an ORR at day 28 of 91% and a two-year OS rate of 55% (54).

Mesenchymal Stem Cells (MSC)

A cell-based therapeutic approach is the use of mesenchymal stromal cells (MSCs) in patients with steroid refractory GvHD (**Figure 1B**). MSCs have immunomodulatory properties as inhibitors of T cell proliferation and T cell response (55, 56). Several studies show promising results with an overall response on day 28 ranging from 42% to 100% and a complete response ranging from 8%-75% (57). In a prospective study of 69 patients, the ORR was 83% (58). Most recently, a phase III study in pediatric patients was published (59). ORR at day 28 was 70.4% and OS was 74.1% at day 100, with the OR at day 28 being highly predictive of improved survival. An example of a patient with GvHD III° prior and following treatment with MSCs is shown in **Figure 1B**.

Chronic GvHD

In addition to the well-established first-line treatment with prednisolone and CNIs, several new agents have recently been approved for the treatment of cGvHD.

Ibrutinib

In 2017 ibrutinib was approved as a second-line treatment for steroid-resistant cGvHD. Approval came following a successful phase I/II trial (NCT02195869). Forty-two patients with active cGvHD were enrolled who had previously failed 1 to 3 prior treatments. After a median follow-up of 13.9 months the best OR was 67% (60). Notably, analysis by organ domain showed similar responses in the skin (88%) as in the other organs. A phase III trial (NCT02959944) has been completed, but its results have not yet been published.

Ruxolitinib

In addition to its positive clinical activity in aGvHD, there are data from a retrospective survey, which indicates that ruxolitinib leads to a high response and 6-month survival rates in heavily pretreated patients afflicted with chronic GvHD (43). Based on these data and the successful trials in aGvHD the prospective, randomized REACH3 trial (NCT03112603) was conducted in 329 steroid-refractory cGVHD patients who received either ruxolitinib or control therapy (44). At 24 weeks OR was 49.7% in the ruxolitinib group (OR 2.99, p<0.001) and failure-free survival was significantly longer (>18.6 months vs. 5.7 months). In this trial approx. 70% of patients had skin involvement, with ~60% having a skin score of greater than or equal to 2. Skin response at week 24 was 41.2% in the ruxolitinib group compared to 15.2% in the control arm. Based on these data the FDA approved ruxolitinib for cGvHD in September 2021 with a recommended starting dose of 10mg given orally twice a day. Studies evaluating the JAK1 Inhibitor itacitinib in the cGVHd setting are currently underway (NCT04200365, NCT035845169). In addition to the systemic use of JAK inhibitors, recent publications point to the benefits of topical application of ruxolitinib by suppressing IFN-γ signaling and T cell infiltration into the skin (64) while sparing systemic side effects. Topical ruxolitinib is currently investigated in clinical trials for cGVHD (NCT03395340, NCT03954236).

Belumosudil

Belumosudil is a serine/threonine kinase inhibitor blocking the activity of Rho-associated coiled-coil kinase 2 (ROCK2). The efficacy of belumosudil was evaluated in a phase 2 randomized multicentre trial in cGvHD-patients who had receive 2-5 prior lines of therapy (NCT03640481). Primary endpoint of this study of the best ORR, which was 74% and 77% for belumosudil at 200 mg daily and at 200 mg twice daily, respectively (61). Of note, 38 patients previously treated with ruxolitinib showed a response rate of 68% when treated with belumosudil. In this study 83% of patients had skin involvement and ORR was reported at 37%, with 16% classified as complete responders. Belumosudil was approved by the FDA in 2021 for the treatment of cGvHD after failure of at least two prior lines of systemic treatment.

Regulatory T Cells

An innovative cellular approach in the treatment of GvHD is the adoptive transfer of regulatory T cells (Tregs). Tregs are a subset of CD4 T cells with an immunosuppressive and immunoregulatory function (65, 66). The first patients with cGvHD, including skin GvHD, treated with Tregs showed an improvement of GvHD symptoms and systemic immunosuppression could be reduced significantly (62). Adoptive transfer of Tregs was used in a series of five patients with refractory cGvHD (all with a skin GvHD III °). Two of five patients showed improvement of their GvHD symptoms and in four patients immunosuppressive treatment was reduced. Nevertheless, one patient was diagnosed with malignant melanoma and one with Bowen skin cancer several months after the Treg infusion (63).

SUMMARY AND OUTLOOK

Mild acute GvHD of the skin can usually be controlled with standardized treatment protocols. Severe acute skin GvHD requires more aggressive conventional treatments, but newer approaches including cellular therapies are now available. Chronic forms of skin GvHD are the transplant physician's enemies. Functional impairment and decreased quality of life need to be avoided strenuously. Marked improvement may be obtained with extracorporal photopheresis. Drugs targeting either B cells or the JAK-STAT pathway have opened new treatment perspectives. Regulatory T cells may reverse cGvHD of the skin, but data are still preliminary. It is encouraging that patients who have overcome cGVHD, experience a health status and quality of life similar to those HSCT patients without a history of cGvHD (67).

AUTHOR CONTRIBUTIONS

All authors have contributed equally in designing the review article, writing and revising. All authors contributed to the article and approved the submitted version.

SUPPLEMENTARY MATERIAL

Supplementary Table 1 | Skin scoring of chronic GvHD [adapted from (9)]

REFERENCES

1. Gooptu M, Koreth J. Translational and Clinical Advances in Acute Graft-Versus-Host Disease. *Haematologica* (2020) 105:2550–60. doi: 10.3324/haematol.2019.240309
2. Zeiser R, Blazar BR. Acute Graft-Versus-Host Disease - Biologic Process, Prevention, and Therapy. *N Engl J Med* (2017) 377:2167–79. doi: 10.1056/NEJMra1609337
3. Ziemer M, Haeusermann P, Janin A, Massi D, Ziepert M, Wolff D, et al. Histopathological Diagnosis of Graft-Versus-Host Disease of the Skin: An Interobserver Comparison. *J Eur Acad Dermatol Venereol* (2014) 28:915–24. doi: 10.1111/jdv.12215
4. Teshima T, Hill GR. The Pathophysiology and Treatment of Graft-Versus-Host Disease: Lessons Learnt From Animal Models. *Front Immunol* (2021) 12:715424. doi: 10.3389/fimmu.2021.715424
5. Chen S, Smith BA, Iype J, Prestipino A, Pfeifer D, Grundmann S, et al. Microrna-155-Deficient Dendritic Cells Cause Less Severe GVHD Through Reduced Migration and Defective Inflammasome Activation. *Blood* (2015) 126:103–12. doi: 10.1182/blood-2014-12-617258
6. Zeiser R. Advances in Understanding the Pathogenesis of Graft-Versus-Host Disease. *Br J Haematol* (2019) 187:563–72. doi: 10.1111/bjh.16190
7. Strong Rodrigues K, Oliveira-Ribeiro C, de Abreu Fiuza Gomes S, Knobler R. Cutaneous Graft-Versus-Host Disease: Diagnosis and Treatment. *Am J Clin Dermatol* (2018) 19:33–50. doi: 10.1007/s40257-017-0306-9
8. Cooke KR, Luznik L, Sarantopoulos S, Hakim FT, Jagasia M, Fowler DH, et al. The Biology of Chronic Graft-Versus-Host Disease: A Task Force Report From the National Institutes of Health Consensus Development Project on Criteria for Clinical Trials in Chronic Graft-Versus-Host Disease. *Biol Blood Marrow Transplant* (2017) 23:211–34. doi: 10.1016/j.bbmt.2016.09.023
9. Filipovich AH, Weisdorf D, Pavletic S, Socie G, Wingard JR, Lee SJ, et al. National Institutes of Health Consensus Development Project on Criteria for Clinical Trials in Chronic Graft-Versus-Host Disease: I. Diagnosis and Staging Working Group Report. *Biol Blood Marrow Transplant* (2005) 11:945–56. doi: 10.1016/j.bbmt.2005.09.004
10. Harris AC, Young R, Devine S, Hogan WJ, Ayuk F, Bunworasate U, et al. International, Multicenter Standardization of Acute Graft-Versus-Host Disease Clinical Data Collection: A Report From the Mount Sinai Acute GVHD International Consortium. *Biol Blood Marrow Transplant* (2016) 22:4–10. doi: 10.1016/j.bbmt.2015.09.001
11. Glucksberg H, Storb R, Fefer A, Buckner CD, Neiman PE, Clift RA, et al. Clinical Manifestations of Graft-Versus-Host Disease in Human Recipients of Marrow From HL-a-Matched Sibling Donors. *Transplantation* (1974) 18:295–304. doi: 10.1097/00007890-197410000-00001
12. Greinix HT, Knobler RM, Worel N, Schneider B, Schneeberger A, Hoecker P, et al. The Effect of Intensified Extracorporeal Photochemotherapy on Long-Term Survival in Patients With Severe Acute Graft-Versus-Host Disease. *Haematologica* (2006) 91:405–8.
13. Jagasia MH, Greinix HT, Arora M, Williams KM, Wolff D, Cowen EW, et al. National Institutes of Health Consensus Development Project on Criteria for Clinical Trials in Chronic Graft-Versus-Host Disease: I. The 2014 Diagnosis and Staging Working Group Report. *Biol Blood Marrow Transplant* (2015) 21:389–401.e1. doi: 10.1016/j.bbmt.2014.12.001
14. Ruutu T, Gratwohl A, de Witte T, Afanasyev B, Apperley J, Bacigalupo A, et al. Prophylaxis and Treatment of GVHD: EBMT-ELN Working Group Recommendations for a Standardized Practice. *Bone Marrow Transplant* (2014) 49:168–73. doi: 10.1038/bmt.2013.107
15. Nash RA, Antin JH, Karanes C, Fay JW, Avalos BR, Yeager AM, et al. Phase 3 Study Comparing Methotrexate and Tacrolimus With Methotrexate and Cyclosporine for Prophylaxis of Acute Graft-Versus-Host Disease After Marrow Transplantation From Unrelated Donors. *Blood* (2000) 96:2062–8.
16. Luznik L, O'Donnell PV, Symons HJ, Chen AR, Leffell MS, Zahurak M, et al. HLA-Haploidentical Bone Marrow Transplantation for Hematologic Malignancies Using Nonmyeloablative Conditioning and High-Dose, Posttransplantation Cyclophosphamide. *Biol Blood Marrow Transplant* (2008) 14:641–50. doi: 10.1016/j.bbmt.2008.03.005
17. Penack O, Marchetti M, Ruutu T, Aljurf M, Bacigalupo A, Bonifazi F, et al. Prophylaxis and Management of Graft Versus Host Disease After Stem-Cell Transplantation for Haematological Malignancies: Updated Consensus Recommendations of the European Society for Blood and Marrow Transplantation. *Lancet Haematol* (2020) 7:e157–67. doi: 10.1016/S2352-3026(19)30256-X
18. Rachner TD, Link-Rachner CS, Bornhäuser M, Hofbauer LC. Skeletal Health in Patients Following Allogeneic Hematopoietic Cell Transplantation. *Bone* (2020) 10:115684. doi: 10.1016/j.bone.2020.115684

19. Holler E, Greinix H, Zeiser R. Acute Graft-Versus-Host Disease. In: E Carreras, C Dufour, M Mohty, N Kröger, editors. *The EBMT Handbook: Hematopoietic Stem Cell Transplantation and Cellular Therapies*. Cham (CH: Springer Copyright 2019, EBMT and the Author(s (2019). p. 323–30.
20. Mankarious M, Matthews NC, Snowden JA, Alfred A. Extracorporeal Photopheresis (ECP) and the Potential of Novel Biomarkers in Optimizing Management of Acute and Chronic Graft vs. Host Disease (Gvhd). *Front Immunol* (2020) 11:81. doi: 10.3389/fimmu.2020.00081
21. Sestili S, Eder S, Belhocine R, Dulery R, Battipaglia G, Brissot E, et al. Extracorporeal Photopheresis as First-Line Strategy in the Treatment of Acute Graft-Versus-Host Disease After Hematopoietic Stem Cell Transplantation: A Single-Center Experience. *Cytotherapy* (2020) 22:445–9. doi: 10.1016/j.jcyt.2020.03.003
22. Perfetti P, Carlier P, Strada P, Gualandi F, Occhini D, Van Lint MT, et al. Extracorporeal Photopheresis for the Treatment of Steroid Refractory Acute GVHD. *Bone Marrow Transplant* (2008) 42:609–17. doi: 10.1038/bmt.2008.221
23. Abu-Dalle I, Reljic T, Nishihori T, Antar A, Bazarbachi A, Djulbegovic B, et al. Extracorporeal Photopheresis in Steroid-Refractory Acute or Chronic Graft-Versus-Host Disease: Results of a Systematic Review of Prospective Studies. *Biol Blood Marrow Transplant* (2014) 20:1677–86. doi: 10.1016/j.bbmt.2014.05.017
24. Schlaak M, Schwind S, Wetzig T, Maschke J, Treudler R, Basara N, et al. UVA (UVA-1) Therapy for the Treatment of Acute GVHD of the Skin. *Bone Marrow Transplant* (2010) 45:1741–8. doi: 10.1038/bmt.2010.230
25. Feldstein JV, Bolaños-Meade J, Anders VL, Abuav R. Narrowband Ultraviolet B Phototherapy for the Treatment of Steroid-Refractory and Steroid-Dependent Acute Graft-Versus-Host Disease of the Skin. *J Am Acad Dermatol* (2011) 65:733–8. doi: 10.1016/j.jaad.2010.08.006
26. Malard F, Huang XJ, Sim JPY. Treatment and Unmet Needs in Steroid-Refractory Acute Graft-Versus-Host Disease. *Leukemia* (2020) 34:1229–40. doi: 10.1038/s41375-020-0804-2
27. Nishimoto M, Nakamae H, Koh H, Nakamae M, Hirose A, Hayashi Y, et al. Response-Guided Therapy for Steroid-Refractory Acute GVHD Starting With Very-Low-Dose Antithymocyte Globulin. *Exp Hematol* (2015) 43:177–9. doi: 10.1016/j.exphem.2014.11.008
28. Wolff D, Ayuk F, Elmaagacli A, Bertz H, Lawitschka A, Schleuning M, et al. Current Practice in Diagnosis and Treatment of Acute Graft-Versus-Host Disease: Results From a Survey Among German-Austrian-Swiss Hematopoietic Stem Cell Transplant Centers. *Biol Blood Marrow Transplant* (2013) 19:767–76. doi: 10.1016/j.bbmt.2013.01.018
29. Martin PJ, Storer BE, Inamoto Y, Flowers MED, Carpenter PA, Pidala J, et al. An Endpoint Associated With Clinical Benefit After Initial Treatment of Chronic Graft-Versus-Host Disease. *Blood* (2017) 130:360–7. doi: 10.1182/blood-2017-03-775767
30. Dignan FL, Scarisbrick JJ, Cornish J, Clark A, Amrolia P, Jackson G, et al. Organ-Specific Management and Supportive Care in Chronic Graft-Versus-Host Disease. *Br J Haematol* (2012) 158:62–78. doi: 10.1111/j.1365-2141.2012.09131.x
31. Wolff D, Gerbitz A, Ayuk F, Kiani A, Hildebrandt GC, Vogelsang GB, et al. Consensus Conference on Clinical Practice in Chronic Graft-Versus-Host Disease (GVHD): First-Line and Topical Treatment of Chronic GVHD. *Biol Blood Marrow Transplant* (2010) 16:1611–28. doi: 10.1016/j.bbmt.2010.06.015
32. Flowers ME, Apperley JF, van Besien K, Elmaagacli A, Grigg A, Reddy V, et al. A Multicenter Prospective Phase 2 Randomized Study of Extracorporeal Photopheresis for Treatment of Chronic Graft-Versus-Host Disease. *Blood* (2008) 112:2667–74. doi: 10.1182/blood-2008-03-141481
33. Jagasia M, Scheid C, Socié G, Ayuk FA, Tischer J, Donato ML, et al. Randomized Controlled Study of ECP With Methoxsalen as First-Line Treatment of Patients With Moderate to Severe Cgvhd. *Blood Adv* (2019) 3:2218–29. doi: 10.1182/bloodadvances.2019000145
34. Alfred A, Taylor PC, Dignan F, El-Ghariani K, Griffin J, Gennery AR, et al. The Role of Extracorporeal Photopheresis in the Management of Cutaneous T-Cell Lymphoma, Graft-Versus-Host Disease and Organ Transplant Rejection: A Consensus Statement Update From the UK Photopheresis Society. *Br J Haematol* (2017) 177:287–310. doi: 10.1111/bjh.14537
35. Pierelli L, Perseghin P, Marchetti M, Messina C, Perotti C, Mazzoni A, et al. Extracorporeal Photopheresis for the Treatment of Acute and Chronic Graft-Versus-Host Disease in Adults and Children: Best Practice Recommendations From an Italian Society of Hemapheresis and Cell Manipulation (Sidem) and Italian Group for Bone Marrow Transplantation (GITMO) Consensus Process. *Transfusion* (2013) 53:2340–52. doi: 10.1111/trf.12059
36. Velickovic VM, McIlwaine E, Zhang R, Spelman T. Adverse Events in Second- and Third-Line Treatments for Acute and Chronic Graft-Versus-Host Disease: Systematic Review. *Ther Adv Hematol* (2020) 11:2040620720977039. doi: 10.1177/2040620720977039
37. Cutler C, Miklos D, Kim HT, Treister N, Woo SB, Bienfang D, et al. Rituximab for Steroid-Refractory Chronic Graft-Versus-Host Disease. *Blood* (2006) 108:756–62. doi: 10.1182/blood-2006-01-0233
38. Olivieri A, Locatelli F, Zecca M, Sanna A, Cimminiello M, Raimondi R, et al. Imatinib for Refractory Chronic Graft-Versus-Host Disease With Fibrotic Features. *Blood* (2009) 114:709–18. doi: 10.1182/blood-2009-02-204156
39. Molés-Poveda P, Comis LE, Joe GO, Mitchell SA, Pichard DC, Rosenstein RK, et al. Rehabilitation Interventions in the Multidisciplinary Management of Patients With Sclerotic Graft-Versus-Host Disease of the Skin and Fascia. *Arch Phys Med Rehabil* (2021) 102:776–88. doi: 10.1016/j.apmr.2020.10.141
40. Schroeder MA, Choi J, Staser K, DiPersio JF. The Role of Janus Kinase Signaling in Graft-Versus-Host Disease and Graft Versus Leukemia. *Biol Blood Marrow Transplant* (2018) 24:1125–34. doi: 10.1016/j.bbmt.2017.12.797
41. Jagasia M, Perales MA, Schroeder MA, Ali H, Shah NN, Chen YB, et al. Ruxolitinib for the Treatment of Steroid-Refractory Acute GVHD (REACH1): A Multicenter, Open-Label Phase 2 Trial. *Blood* (2020) 135:1739–49. doi: 10.1182/blood.2020004823
42. Zeiser R, von Bubnoff N, Butler J, Mohty M, Niederwieser D, Or R, et al. Ruxolitinib for Glucocorticoid-Refractory Acute Graft-Versus-Host Disease. *N Engl J Med* (2020) 382:1800–10. doi: 10.1056/NEJMoa1917635
43. Zeiser R, Burchert A, Lengerke C, Verbeek M, Maas-Bauer K, Metzelder SK, et al. Ruxolitinib in Corticosteroid-Refractory Graft-Versus-Host Disease After Allogeneic Stem Cell Transplantation: A Multicenter Survey. *Leukemia* (2015) 29:2062–8. doi: 10.1038/leu.2015.212
44. Zeiser R, Polverelli N, Ram R, Hashmi SK, Chakraverty R, Middeke JM, et al. Ruxolitinib for Glucocorticoid-Refractory Chronic Graft-Versus-Host Disease. *N Engl J Med* (2021) 385:228–38. doi: 10.1056/NEJMoa2033122
45. Schroeder MA, Khoury HJ, Jagasia M, Ali H, Schiller GJ, Staser K, et al. A Phase 1 Trial of Itacitinib, a Selective JAK1 Inhibitor, in Patients With Acute Graft-Versus-Host Disease. *Blood Adv* (2020) 4:1656–69. doi: 10.1182/bloodadvances.2019001043
46. Przepiorka D, Kernan NA, Ippoliti C, Papadopoulos EB, Giralt S, Khouri I, et al. Daclizumab, a Humanized Anti-Interleukin-2 Receptor Alpha Chain Antibody, for Treatment of Acute Graft-Versus-Host Disease. *Blood* (2000) 95:83–9. doi: 10.1182/blood.V95.1.83
47. Massenkeil G, Rackwitz S, Genvresse I, Rosen O, Dörken B, Arnold R. Basiliximab Is Well Tolerated and Effective in the Treatment of Steroid-Refractory Acute Graft-Versus-Host Disease After Allogeneic Stem Cell Transplantation. *Bone Marrow Transplant* (2002) 30:899–903. doi: 10.1038/sj.bmt.1703737
48. Socié G, Vigouroux S, Yakoub-Agha I, Bay JO, Fürst S, Bilger K, et al. A Phase 3 Randomized Trial Comparing Inolimomab vs Usual Care in Steroid-Resistant Acute GVHD. *Blood* (2017) 129:643–9. doi: 10.1182/blood-2016-09-738625
49. Socié G, Milpied N, Yakoub-Agha I, Bay JO, Fürst S, Bilger K, et al. Long-Term Follow-Up of a Phase 3 Clinical Trial of Inolimomab for the Treatment of Primary Steroid Refractory Agvhd. *Blood Adv* (2019) 3:184–6. doi: 10.1182/bloodadvances.2018028282
50. Yalniz FF, Hefazi M, McCullough K, Litzow MR, Hogan WJ, Wolf R, et al. Safety and Efficacy of Infliximab Therapy in the Setting of Steroid-Refractory Acute Graft-Versus-Host Disease. *Biol Blood Marrow Transplant* (2017) 23:1478–84. doi: 10.1016/j.bbmt.2017.05.001
51. Nygaard M, Andersen NS, Moser CE, Olesen G, Schjødt IM, Heilmann C, et al. Evaluation of Infliximab as Second-Line Treatment of Acute Graft Versus Host Disease -Validating Response on Day 7 and 28 as Predictors of Survival. *Bone Marrow Transplant* (2018) 53:844–51. doi: 10.1038/s41409-018-0099-3

52. De Jong CN, Saes L, Klerk CPW, van der Klift M, Cornelissen JJ, Broers AEC. Etanercept for Steroid-Refractory Acute Graft-Versus-Host Disease: A Single Center Experience. *PloS One* (2017) 12:e0187184. doi: 10.1371/journal.pone.0187184
53. Park JH, Lee HJ, Kim SR, Song GW, Lee SK, Park SY, et al. Etanercept for Steroid-Refractory Acute Graft Versus Host Disease Following Allogeneic Hematopoietic Stem Cell Transplantation. *Korean J Intern Med* (2014) 29:630–6. doi: 10.3904/kjim.2014.29.5.630
54. Tan Y, Xiao H, Wu D, Luo Y, Lan J, Liu Q, et al. Combining Therapeutic Antibodies Using Basiliximab and Etanercept for Severe Steroid-Refractory Acute Graft-Versus-Host Disease: A Multi-Center Prospective Study. *Oncoimmunology* (2017) 6:e1277307. doi: 10.1080/2162402X.2016.1277307
55. Aggarwal S, Pittenger MF. Human Mesenchymal Stem Cells Modulate Allogeneic Immune Cell Responses. *Blood* (2005) 105:1815–22. doi: 10.1182/blood-2004-04-1559
56. von Dalowski F, Kramer M, Wermke M, Wehner R, Röllig C, Alakel N, et al. Mesenchymal Stromal Cells for Treatment of Acute Steroid-Refractory Graft Versus Host Disease: Clinical Responses and Long-Term Outcome. *Stem Cells* (2016) 34:357–66. doi: 10.1002/stem.2224
57. Kelly K, Rasko JEJ. Mesenchymal Stromal Cells for the Treatment of Graft Versus Host Disease. *Front Immunol* (2021) 12. doi: 10.3389/fimmu.2021.761616
58. Bader P, Kuçi Z, Bakhtiar S, Basu O, Bug G, Dennis M, et al. Effective Treatment of Steroid and Therapy-Refractory Acute Graft-Versus-Host Disease With a Novel Mesenchymal Stromal Cell Product (MSC-FFM). *Bone Marrow Transplant* (2018) 53:852–62. doi: 10.1038/s41409-018-0102-z
59. Kurtzberg J, Abdel-Azim H, Carpenter P, Chaudhury S, Horn B, Mahadeo K, et al. A Phase 3, Single-Arm, Prospective Study of Remestemcel-L, *Ex Vivo* Culture-Expanded Adult Human Mesenchymal Stromal Cells for the Treatment of Pediatric Patients Who Failed to Respond to Steroid Treatment for Acute Graft-Versus-Host Disease. *Biol Blood Marrow Transplant* (2020) 26:845–54. doi: 10.1016/j.bbmt.2020.01.018
60. Miklos D, Cutler CS, Arora M, Waller EK, Jagasia M, Pusic I, et al. Ibrutinib for Chronic Graft-Versus-Host Disease After Failure of Prior Therapy. *Blood* (2017) 130:2243–50. doi: 10.1182/blood-2017-07-793786
61. Cutler C, Lee SJ, Arai S, Rotta M, Zoghi B, Lazaryan A, et al. Belumosudil for Chronic Graft-Versus-Host Disease After 2 or More Prior Lines of Therapy: The Rockstar Study. *Blood* (2021) 138:2278–89. doi: 10.1182/blood.2021012021
62. Trzonkowski P, Bieniaszewska M, Juścińska J, Dobyszuk A, Krzystyniak A, Marek N, et al. First-in-Man Clinical Results of the Treatment of Patients With Graft Versus Host Disease With Human *Ex Vivo* Expanded CD4+CD25 +CD127- T Regulatory Cells. *Clin Immunol* (2009) 133:22–6. doi: 10.1016/j.clim.2009.06.001
63. Theil A, Tuve S, Oelschlägel U, Maiwald A, Döhler D, Oßmann D, et al. Adoptive Transfer of Allogeneic Regulatory T Cells Into Patients With Chronic Graft-Versus-Host Disease. *Cytotherapy* (2015) 17:473–86. doi: 10.1016/j.jcyt.2014.11.005
64. Takahashi S, Hashimoto D, Hayase E, Ogasawara R, Ohigashi H, Ara T, et al. Ruxolitinib Protects Skin Stem Cells and Maintains Skin Homeostasis in Murine Graft-Versus-Host Disease. *Blood* (2018) 131:2074–85. doi: 10.1182/blood-2017-06-792614
65. Duggleby R, Danby RD, Madrigal JA, Saudemont A. Clinical Grade Regulatory Cd4+ T Cells (Tregs): Moving Toward Cellular-Based Immunomodulatory Therapies. *Front Immunol* (2018) 9. doi: 10.3389/fimmu.2018.00252
66. Guo WW, Su XH, Wang MY, Han MZ, Feng XM, Jiang EL. Regulatory T Cells in GVHD Therapy. *Front Immunol* (2021) 12:697854. doi: 10.3389/fimmu.2021.697854
67. Baker KS, Fraser CJ. Quality of Life and Recovery After Graft-Versus-Host Disease. *Best Pract Res Clin Haematol* (2008) 21:333–41. doi: 10.1016/j.beha.2008.03.002

16

Successful Treatment of Acute Generalized Exanthematous Pustulosis with Secukinumab

Liangliang Zhang [1†], Qiuyun Xu [1†], Tingting Lin [1†], Shifan Ruan [1], Mengting Lin [1], Chengbei Bao [1], Jing Zhang [1], Tao Liu [2], Ting Gong [1] and Chao Ji [1*]*

[1] *Department of Dermatology, The First Hospital of Fujian Medical University, Fuzhou, China,* [2] *Department of Medical Affairs, Beijing Novartis Pharma Company Limited, Shanghai, China*

Correspondence:
Ting Gong
tinggongyou@126.com
Chao Ji
jichaofy@fjmu.edu.cn

† These authors have contributed equally to this work

Acute generalized exanthematous pustulosis is a severe, usually drug-related reaction, characterized by an acute onset of mainly small non-follicular pustules on an erythematous base. Most cases of acute generalized exanthematous pustulosis (AGEP) clear quickly with a systemic corticosteroid, but severe or recalcitrant cases may need other systemic therapies. In this case, a man in his 40 s with a history of psoriasis consulted a physician about widespread erythema, pustules, target lesions, and fever after the administration of a quadruple antituberculosis drug. Routine laboratory testing revealed elevated white blood cell count and C-reactive protein. The histopathology showed subcorneal pustules, spongiosis as well as lymphocyte and eosinophils infiltration in the dermis. The patient was diagnosed with definitive AGEP according to the diagnostic score from the EuroSCAR study. Cutaneous lesions especially pustules and erythema multiforme-like lesions on the upper arms and palms are crucial for distinguishing AGEP from Generalized pustular psoriasis. The patient was treated with secukinumab as a result of his failure to respond to topical corticosteroids and constrain of systemic steroids. Remission with secukinumab therapy was safe without increased risks of infections. This case indicates that secukinumab is a potential therapy that can rapidly improve the clinical symptoms of AGEP.

Keywords: AGEP, secukinumab, biologic, interleukin-17A inhibition, drug eruption

INTRODUCTION

Acute generalized exanthematous pustulosis is a rare disease, therefore there are no high-quality evidence-based therapeutic recommendations. As it is, treatment is mainly potent topical or systemic steroids. However, a minority of cases fail to respond to them, highlighting the need for additional treatment options for these refractory cases (1). Secukinumab is an interleukin (IL)-17 inhibitor that is approved to treat psoriasis. However, the efficacy of secukinumab on acute generalized exanthematous pustulosis (AGEP) is unclear. In this review, we reported the successful use of secukinumab in a patient with AGEP.

REPORT OF A CASE

A 41-year-old man presented with a 1-day history of rapidly growing erythema and pustules on the face, trunk, and extremities. One day before, he took isoniazid, rifampicin, ethambutol, and

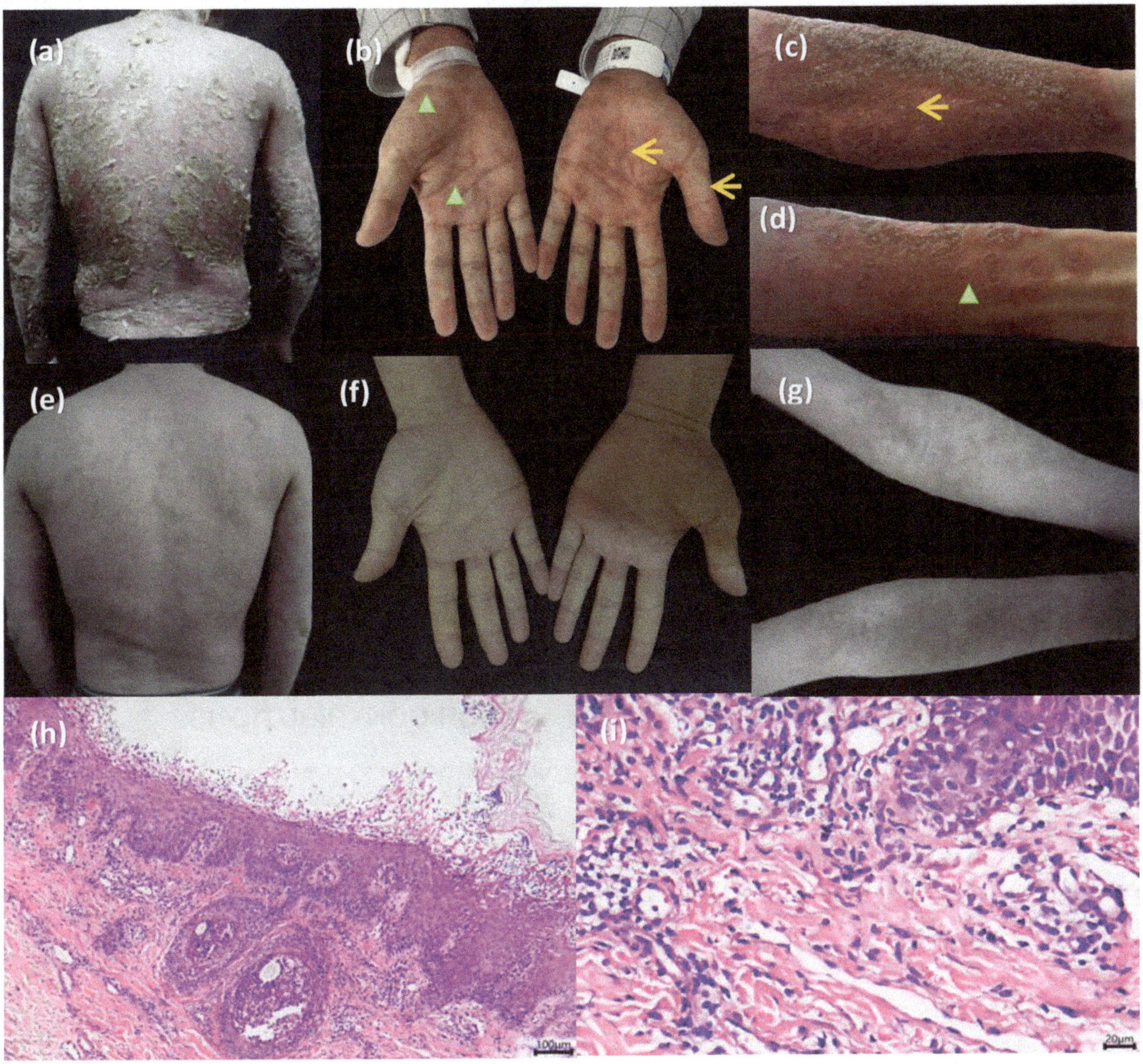

FIGURE 1 | (a) The patient presented with diffuse erythema and dried-up lakes of pus on the back. **(b–d)** Pinpoint pustules and erythema multiforme-like lesions were diffusely spread over the upper arms and palms (pinpoint pustules, yellow arrowhead; target lesions, green arrowhead). **(h,i)** Biopsy results demonstrated subcorneal pustules, spongiosis as well as lymphocyte and eosinophils infiltration in the dermis. **(e–g)** All pustules faded 3 days later and erythema substantially darkened.

pyrazinamide to treat pulmonary tuberculosis in lazaretto. At admission, the patient was febrile to a temperature of 40°C. He also had a 2-year history of plaque psoriasis with no history of smoking. Routine laboratory testing revealed white blood cell count of 13,890/μl (normal range, 1,214–5,110/μl) and serum levels of C-reactive protein (CRP) of 7.75 mg/dl (normal range, 0–0.2 mg/dl). Physical examination revealed widespread erythema and dried-up lakes of pus, taking up body surface area of 80%. Pustules and erythema multiforme-like lesions were diffusely spread over the upper arms and palms (**Figures 1a–d**). Biopsies of pustule and erythema multiforme-like lesions on the arms were performed. The result demonstrated subcorneal pustules, spongiosis as well as lymphocyte and eosinophils infiltration in the dermis (**Figures 1h,i**).

The patient was assessed using a diagnostic score according to the EuroSCAR study. The final score was nine, which was defined as the definitive AGEP. The patient was subsequently treated with expectant treatment and topic potent steroids for 4 days, followed by no improvement. However, given the patient's femoral head necrosis, systemic glucocorticoid was not recommended. Repeated computed tomography on the chest showed multiple calcifications and thus excluded the possibility of active tuberculosis. Other infections including hepatitis B and hepatitis C were also excluded. The patient received secukinumab 300 mg after being informed of impersonal medical risks (**Supplementary Figure**). After the first therapy of secukinumab, all pustules faded at day 3, and erythema substantially darkened with defervescence (**Figures 1e–g**). The Dermatology life quality index (DLQI) decreased rapidly from 25 to 1 at week 4. There were no clinical symptoms and radiological data related to the progression of latent tuberculosis infection.

DISCUSSION

In this case, the patient had a medication history of quadruple anti-tuberculosis drugs, specific exanthem of erythema multiforme-like lesion, abnormal laboratory results of white blood cell count and C-reactive protein, dermatologic evidence of spongiosis, and subcorneal pustule and eosinophils infiltration. He was then diagnosed with definitive AGEP according to the diagnostic score from the EuroSCAR study. Generalized pustular psoriasis, either the "Annular variant" or "Exanthematic variant," can also present a similar acute eruption following initiation of medications. The common disease-causing medications include TNF-α inhibitors, lithium, interferons, antimalarials, beta-blockers, rapid withdrawal of systemic corticosteroids. This case provides some clinical reasonings of differential diagnosis between AGEP and GPP. First, cutaneous lesions especially pustules and erythema multiforme-like lesions on the upper arms and palms are crucial for differential diagnosis in this case. Besides, dermatologic evidence of spongiosis, as well as eosinophils infiltration in pathology, favors a diagnosis of AGEP. Finally, the rapid resolution of pustular eruption with secukinumab is suggestive of the diagnosis being AGEP.

Owing to his failure to respond to topical corticosteroids and constrain of systemic steroids, the patient was treated with secukinumab for 1 month. Disease progression was then controlled promptly, with a resolution of pustules and erythema. The great improvement of dermatology-specific health-related quality of life was also observed. Prior to clinical admission to our department, the patient was misdiagnosed as active TB and was sequentially prescribed isoniazid, rifampicin, ethambutol, and pyrazinamide in lazaretto. At admission, active tuberculosis was excluded based on clinical symptoms and results of repeated chest computed tomography. We confirmed that the patient only had latent tuberculosis infection. Thus, this patient did not receive any treatment for his latent TB. The chest radiography was done 1 month later and then every 6 months over a 2-year follow-up. The results showed no change in the lung pathology (calcification). As reported in the literature, patients with latent TB who received no chemoprophylaxis could be safely treated with secukinumab (1, 2).

The underlying mechanism of action of secukinumab on AGEP is related to IL-17. AGEP has been classified as a T cell-related sterile neutrophilic inflammatory response with a predominant T-helper (Th) 1 cell and Th17 (3–5). Th17 cells release IL-17, which affects neutrophil recruitment (6, 7). Therefore, the IL-17 pathway is a potential therapeutic target shown to be implicated in AGEP. Further clinical trials are needed to corroborate the safety and efficacy of secukinumab in AGEP.

AUTHOR CONTRIBUTIONS

All authors listed have made a substantial, direct, and intellectual contribution to the work and approved it for publication.

ACKNOWLEDGMENTS

We thank all study participants involved in facilitating and running this study.

REFERENCES

1. Hadavand MA, Kaffenberger B, Cartron AM, Trinidad JCL. Clinical presentation and management of atypical and recalcitrant acute generalized exanthematous pustulosis. *J Am Acad Dermatol.* (2020) 11. doi: 10.1016/j.jaad.2020.09.024
2. Shu D, Zhang Z, Zhou EY, Ma X, Zhao Y. Is chemoprophylaxis necessary for all latent tuberculosis infection patients receiving IL-17 inhibitors? A cohort study. *Dermatol Ther.* (2020) 33:e14512. doi: 10.1111/dth.14512
3. Britschgi M, Pichler WJ. Acute generalized exanthematous pustulosis, a clue to neutrophil-mediated inflammatory processes orchestrated by T cells. *Curr Opin Allergy Clin Immunol.* (2002) 2:325–31. doi: 10.1097/00130832-200208000-00006
4. Britschgi M, Steiner UC, Schmid S, Depta JP, Senti G, Bircher A, et al. T-cell involvement in drug-induced acute generalized exanthematous pustulosis. *J Clin Investig.* (2001) 107:1433–41. doi: 10.1172/JCI12118
5. Schmid S, Kuechler PC, Britschgi M, Steiner UC, Yawalkar N, Limat A, et al. Acute generalized exanthematous pustulosis: role of cytotoxic T cells in pustules formation. *Am J Pathol.* (2002) 161:2079–86. doi: 10.1016/S0002-9440(10)64486-0
6. Schaerli P, Britschgi M, Keller M, Steiner UC, Steinmann LS, Moser B, et al. Characterization of human T cells that regulate neutrophilic skin inflammation. *J Immunol.* (2004) 173:2151–8. doi: 10.4049/jimmunol.173.3.2151
7. Kakeda M, Schlapbach C, Danelon G, Tang MM, Cecchinato V, Yawalkar N, et al. Innate immune cells express IL-17A/F in acute generalized exanthematous pustulosis and generalized pustular psoriasis. *Arch Dermatol Res.* (2014) 306:933–8. doi: 10.1007/s00403-014-1488-0

17

Combined Effect of Microneedling and Platelet-Rich Plasma for the Treatment of Acne Scars

*Cheng Kang and Dakai Lu**

Department of Otolaryngology-Head and Neck Surgery, HuaMei Hospital, University of Chinese Academy of Sciences, Ningbo, China

***Correspondence:**
Dakai Lu
nbludakai_920@21cn.com

Background: Microneedling is a promising method for the treatment of acne scars, while the effect of microneedling combined with platelet-rich plasma (PRP) remains unknown. We performed a meta-analysis of controlled studies to compare the efficacy and safety of microneedling treatment with and without additional PRP in patients with acne scars.

Methods: Randomized and non-randomized controlled studies were identified by search of Medline, Embase, and Cochrane's Library databases. Results were pooled with a random-effects model, incorporating the possible heterogeneity.

Results: Four randomized and 10 split-face non-randomized controlled studies with 472 patients were included. Compared to microneedling therapy without PRP, combined treatment with microneedling and PRP was associated with increased odds of clinical improvement of >50% in Goodman's qualitative scale [GQS: odds ratio (OR): 2.97, 95% confidence interval (CI): 1.96–4.51, $p < 0.001$; $I^2 = 0\%$], and a significantly improved mean GQS score (mean difference: −0.32, 95% CI: −0.44 to −0.20, $p < 0.001$; $I^2 = 0\%$). Combined treatment was associated with a higher patient satisfying rate (OR: 4.15, 95% CI: 2.13 to 8.09, $p < 0.001$; $I^2 = 53\%$), while the incidence of severe adverse events such as severe erythema (OR: 1.59, 95% CI:.73 to 3.46, $P = 0.24$; $I^2 = 0\%$) and severe edema (OR: 1.14, 95% CI: 0.47 to 2.76, $P = 0.77$; $I^2 = 0\%$) were not significantly different.

Conclusions: Combined treatment with microneedling with PRP is more effective than microneedling without PRP for patients with acne scars.

Keywords: acne scar, microneedling treatment, platelet-rich plasma, controlled studies, meta-analysis

INTRODUCTION

Acne vulgaris is a chronic inflammatory disease of skins, which mainly involves the hair follicles and sebaceous glands (1, 2). Acne is common, which could affect up to 80% of the adolescents (3, 4). The most common sequela of acne is acne scars, which could be formed in about 50% of people with acne, most commonly in highly visible areas such as faces and cheeks (5). Atrophic acne scars are the most common type of acne scars, which significantly affect the beauty of the patients and also impair the quality of life for some patients (6, 7). The pathogenesis of atrophic acne scars is complicated, which mainly involves the degradation of inflammatory mediators, collagen fibers, and subcutaneous fat, ultimately leading to the change of subcutaneous collagen deposition (8, 9). Multiple treatment strategies have been developed for the clinical management of acne scars (10, 11). Among them, microneedling is well-applied as an effective and minimally invasive technology for the treatment of atrophic acne scars *via* creation of skin microwounds to induce collagen production and dermal remodeling (12, 13). Besides, platelet-rich plasma (PRP), which contains various growth factors and bioactive cytokines, has also been applied as adjuvant therapy for acne scars (14, 15). Some small-scale clinical studies have observed the role of combined treatment with microneedling and PRP for patients with atrophic acne scars (16–29). However, the efficacy and safety of microneedling treatment combined with PRP in patients with atrophic acne scars have rarely been comprehensively evaluated. Accordingly, we performed a meta-analysis of controlled studies to systematically compare the efficacy and safety of microneedling treatment with and without additional PRP in patients with acne scars.

METHODS

The PRISMA (Preferred Reporting Items for Systematic Reviews and Meta-Analyses) statement (30) and the Cochrane Handbook guidelines (31) were followed during the designing and implementation of the study.

Search Strategy

Medline, Embase, and the Cochrane's Library (Cochrane Center Register of Controlled Trials) databases were searched for relevant studies with a combined strategy of: (1) "platelet-rich

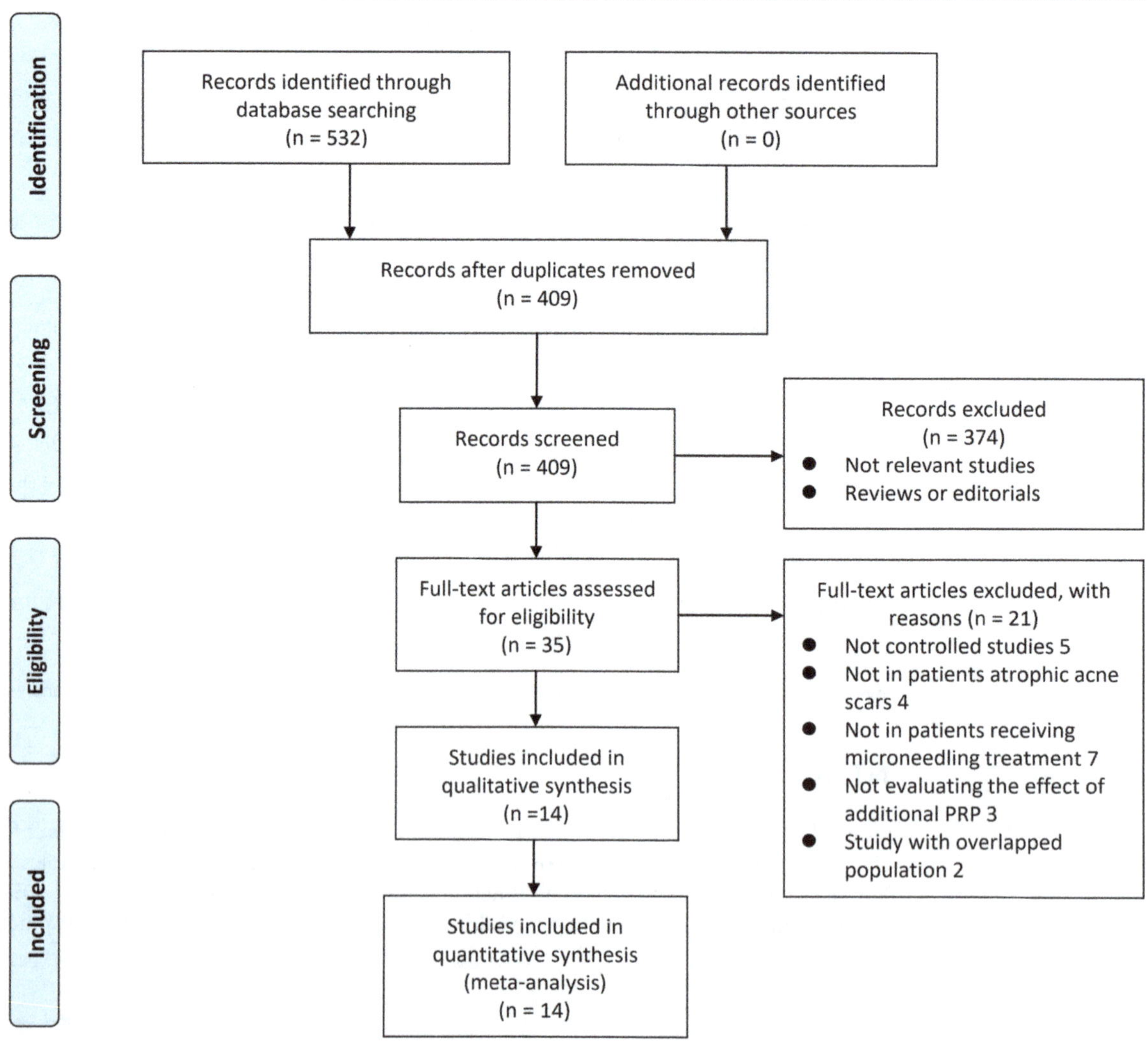

FIGURE 1 | A flow chart of literature search. From Moher et al. (35).

TABLE 1 | Characteristics of the included studies.

References	Country	Design	No. of patients	Scar characteristics	Age (years)	Male (%)	Details of MN	PRP preparation	Intervention	Control	Sessions	Follow-up duration (weeks)	Outcome assessment
Fabbrocini et al. (16)	Italy	NRCT, Split-face study	12	Acne scars	32.2	41.7	Using rolling barrel 1-mm wide, equipped with 96 needles in 4 rows	70–80 ml autologous whole blood centrifuged at 1,200 g for 15 min, then further centrifuged at 1,800 g for 10 min, to get a 4.5× PRP	MN + PRP	MN only	2	32	Rate of GQS improvement and changes of GQS
Chawla (17)	India	NRCT, Split-face study	27	Grade 2–4 acne scars	27.5	70	Using rolling drum of 192 needles	10 ml autologous whole blood centrifuged at 1500 rpm for 10 min, then further centrifuged at 3700 rpm for 10 min, to get a 4.5x PRP	MN + PRP	MN + Vitamin C	3	4	Rate of GQS improvement and patient satisfying
Asif et al. (18)	India	NRCT, Split-face study	50	Grade 2–4 acne scars	25.7	50	Using a standard roller device with 192 needles, each of 1.5 mm in size	17 ml autologous whole blood centrifuged at 294 g for 5 min, then further centrifuged at 691 g for 17 min, to get a 5.2× PRP	MN + PRP	MN + distilled water	3	12	Rate of GQS improvement and patient satisfying
Ibrahim et al. (19)	Egypt	RCT, OL	36	Acne scars	26.3	49	Using an automated microneedling device (dermapen 3) with nine microneedles of 0.25 mm to 2.5 mm length	20 ml autologous whole blood centrifuged at 1,419 g for 7 min, then further centrifuged at 2,522 g for 5 min, to get a 10× PRP	MN + PRP	MN only	6	12	Rate of GQS improvement and incidence of severe side effect

(Continued)

TABLE 1 | Continued

References	Country	Design	No. of patients	Scar characteristics	Age (years)	Male (%)	Details of MN	PRP preparation	Intervention	Control	Sessions	Follow-up duration (weeks)	Outcome assessment
Porwal et al. (22)	India	RCT, OL	55	Grade 2–4 acne scars	26	46.2	Using a dermaroller with 192 needles of 1.5 mm length	20 ml autologous whole blood centrifuged at 1,200 rpm for 15 min, then further centrifuged at 2,000 rpm for 10 min, to get a PRP	MN + PRP	MN only	3	4	Changes of GQS and incidence of severe side effect
El-Domyati et al. (20)	Egypt	NRCT, Split-face study	24	Acne scars	27.3	25	Using a dermaroller with 600 needles of 1.5 mm length	10 ml autologous whole blood centrifuged at 252 g for 10 min, then further centrifuged at 1,792 g for 5 min, to get a PRP	MN + PRP	MN only	2	12	Rate of GQS improvement
Ibrahim et al. (21)	Egypt	NRCT, Split-face study	35	Acne scars	24.7	NR	Using a dermaroller with 192 needles of 1.5 mm length	10 ml autologous whole blood centrifuged at 2,500 rpm for 10 min, then further centrifuged at 3,500 rpm for 10 min, to get a PRP	MN + PRP	MN only	4	12	Changes of GQS and rate of patient satisfying
Bhargava et al. (23)	India	RCT, SB	30	Grade 4 acne scars	27.7	36.7	Using a dermaroller with 192 needles of 1.5 mm length	10 ml autologous whole blood centrifuged at 1,500 rpm for 10 min, then further centrifuged at 3,700 rpm for 10 min, to get a 4.5× PRP	MN + PRP	MN only	3	12	Rate of GQS improvement and patient satisfying

(Continued)

TABLE 1 | Continued

References	Country	Design	No. of patients	Scar characteristics	Age (years)	Male (%)	Details of MN	PRP preparation	Intervention	Control	Sessions	Follow-up duration (weeks)	Outcome assessment
Elfar and Hasby (24)	Egypt	RCT, SB	40	Grade 2–4 acne scars	27.2	30	Using a dermaroller with 540 needles of 2.0 mm length	10 ml autologous whole blood centrifuged at 72 g for 15 min, then further centrifuged at 1,006 g for 5 min, to get a PRP	MN + PRP	MN only	4	12	Rate of GQS improvement
Sharma et al. (29)	India	NRCT, Split-face study	40	Grade 2–4 acne scars	25.3	32.5	Using a dermaroller with 192 needles of 1.5 mm length	10 ml autologous whole blood centrifuged at 1,500 rpm for 10 min, then further centrifuged at 3,700 rpm for 10 min, to get a 4.5× PRP	MN + PRP	MN + NS	4	24	Rate of GQS improvement, changes of GQS, and incidence of severe side effect
Amer et al. (25)	Egypt	NRCT, Split-face study	41	Grade 2–4 acne scars	28	31.7	Using a dermaroller	10 ml autologous whole blood centrifuged at 1,600 rpm for 10 min, then further centrifuged at 4,000 rpm for 15 min, to get a PRP	MN + PRP	MN + HA	4	4	Rate of GQS improvement and patient satisfying
Pawar and Singh (28)	India	NRCT, Split-face study	16	Acne scars	24.7	43.8	Using a dermaroller with 192 needles of 1.5 mm length	10 ml autologous whole blood centrifuged at 1,500 rpm for 10 min, then further centrifuged at 3,700 rpm for 10 min, to get a 4.5× PRP	MN + PRP	MN + insulin	4	12	Changes of GQS and incidence of severe side effect
Gupta et al. (26)	India	NRCT, Split-face study	36	Acne scars	23.7	47.2	Using a dermaroller with 192 needles of 2.0 mm length	8.5 ml autologous whole blood centrifuged at 1,400 rpm for 10 min, then further centrifuged at 3,500 rpm for 10 min, to get a PRP	MN + PRP	MN only	4	24	Changes of GQS

(Continued)

TABLE 1 | Continued

References	Country	Design	No. of patients	Scar characteristics	Age (years)	Male (%)	Details of MN	PRP preparation	Intervention	Control	Sessions	Follow-up duration (weeks)	Outcome assessment
Nandini et al. (27)	India	NRCT, Split-face study	30	Grade 2–4 acne scars	25	60	Using a dermaroller with 192 needles of 2.0 mm length	6 ml autologous whole blood centrifuged at 3,600 rpm for 15 min to get a PRP	MN + PRP	MN only	4	12	Rate of GQS improvement and patient satisfying

MN, microneedling; PRP, platelet-rich plasma; NRCT, nonrandomized controlled trials; RCT, randomized controlled trials; OL, open-label; SB, single-blind; HA, hyaluronic acid; GQS, Goodman's qualitative scale; NR, not reported; NS, normal saline.

plasma" OR "PRP" OR "platelet-rich plasma" OR "platelet concentrate" OR "platelet concentrates"; (2) "needle" OR "microneedle" OR "microneedling"; and (3) "scar" OR "scars." This expanded search strategy was used to avoid missing possible relevant studies. Only clinical studies in humans and published in English were considered. The references of related reviews and original articles were also searched as complementation. The final database search was conducted on June 10, 2021.

Study Selection

Studies that fulfilled the following criteria were included: (1) articles published as full-length articles in English; (2) designed as split-fact non-randomized controlled studies or parallel-group randomized controlled trials (RCTs); (3) included patients with atrophic acne scars allocated to an interventional group with microneedling and PRP and a control group with microneedling without PRP; and (4) reported at least one of the following outcomes, including the rate of significant clinical improvement defined as >50% improvement in Goodman's qualitative scale (GQS), changes of mean GQS from the baseline, the rate of patient satisfaction, and incidence of severe adverse events. The clinical improvement was assessed by the dermatologists based on GQS. Reviews, studies not including patients with atrophic acne scars, without interventions of microneedling or PRP, without a control group, or studies that did not report the outcomes of interest were excluded.

Data Extraction and Quality Assessment

Database search, data extraction, and quality evaluation were conducted by two independent authors. If disagreement occurred, it was resolved by consensus between the authors. We extracted data on study information (first author, publication year, and study country), study design (randomized or non-randomized), patient information (number of participants, the range of age, and sex), intervention and control (details of microneedling applied, PRP preparation, and sessions), follow-up duration, and outcomes reported. For RCTs, quality evaluation was achieved using the Cochrane's Risk of Bias Tool (31) according to the following aspects: (1) random sequence generation; (2) allocation concealment; (3) blinding of participants and personnel; (4) blinding of outcome assessors; (5) incomplete outcome data; (6) selective outcome reporting; and (7) other potential bias. For non-randomized studies, quality evaluation was performed with the Newcastle—Ottawa Scale (NOS) (32), which included three domains, such as defining of study groups, between-group comparability, and validation of the outcome. The NOS totally scored from 1 to 9 stars, with 9 stars indicating the highest study quality level.

Statistical Analysis

Incidence of significant clinical improvement, patient satisfaction, and adverse events were separately evaluated *via* odds ratios (ORs) and their 95% confidence intervals

(CIs) in this meta-analysis, while changes of mean GQS from the baseline were evaluated with mean difference (MD) and corresponding 95% CI. We used Cochrane's Q test to detect the heterogeneity (33). The I^2 statistic was also calculated, and an $I^2 > 50\%$ reflected significant heterogeneity. Pooled analyses were calculated using a random-effects model because this method incorporates the influence of potential heterogeneity and retrieves a more generalized result (31). Sensitivity analysis was performed to compare the treatments between microneedling and PRP with microneedling alone (31). Predefined subgroup analyses were used to evaluate the possible influences of study design on the outcomes. Publication bias was evaluated by visual inspection of funnel plots, and Egger's regression asymmetry test (34). $P < 0.05$ were considered statistically significant. The RevMan (Version 5.1; Cochrane, Oxford, UK) and Stata software (Version 12.0; Stata, College Station, TX) were applied for statistical analyses.

RESULTS

Search Results

The process of database search and study identification is shown in **Figure 1**. Briefly, 532 articles were obtained through the database search, and 409 were retrieved after exclusion of duplicated records. Among them, 374 articles were subsequently excluded based on titles and abstracts, primarily because these studies were irrelevant to the aim of the meta-analysis. Of the 35 articles that underwent full-text review, 21 were further excluded for the reasons presented in **Figure 1**. Finally, 14 studies, including four RCTs (19, 22–24) and 10 non-randomized controlled studies (16–18, 20, 21, 25–29) were included.

Study Characteristics

Table 1 shows the characteristics of the included studies. Overall, four RCTs (19, 22–24) and 10 face-split non-randomized controlled studies (16–18, 20, 21, 25–29) with 472 patients were included in the meta-analysis. The studies were published between 2011 and 2021. The studies were mostly performed in India (17, 18, 22, 23, 26–29) and Egypt (19–21, 24, 25), as well as one study in Italy (16). All of the studies included patients with acne scars. The mean ages varied between 23 and 33 years, and the proportions of men ranged between 25 and 70%. The details of PRP preparation are also summarized in **Table 1**, which typically included two steps of centrifugation of the autologous whole blood, except for one study (27), which applied a one-step centrifugation method. For the comparisons, interventions of combined microneedling and PRP were compared with controls of microneedling alone in nine studies (16, 19–24, 26, 27), with microneedling and distilled water or normal saline in two studies (18, 29), and with microneedling and vitamin C, hyaluronic acid, and insulin in the other three studies (17, 25, 28). For each treatment, two to six sessions were applied, with the follow-up durations varying from 4 to 32 weeks.

TABLE 2 | Quality evaluation *via* the Newcastle—Ottawa Scale for non-randomized controlled studies.

References	Representativeness of the exposed cohort	Selection of the non-exposed cohort	Ascertainment of exposure	Demonstration that outcome of interest was not present at start of study	Comparability-age and gender	Comparability-other factors	Assessment of outcome	Was follow-up long enough for outcomes to occur	Adequacy of follow-up of cohorts	Total
Fabbrocini et al. (16)	1	1	1	1	1	1	1	1	1	9
Chawla (17)	1	1	1	1	1	1	1	1	0	8
Asif et al. (18)	1	1	1	1	1	1	1	1	1	9
El-Domyati et al. (20)	1	1	1	1	1	1	1	1	0	8
Ibrahim et al. (21)	1	1	1	1	1	1	1	1	1	9
Sharma et al. (29)	1	1	1	1	1	1	1	1	1	9
Amer et al. (25)	1	1	1	1	1	1	1	1	1	9
Pawar and Singh (28)	1	1	1	1	1	1	1	1	0	8
Gupta et al. (26)	1	1	1	1	1	1	1	1	0	8
Nandini et al. (27)	1	1	1	1	1	1	1	1	1	9

TABLE 3 | Quality evaluation for the randomized controlled trials *via* the Cochrane's Risk of Bias Tool.

References	Random sequence generation	Allocation concealment	Blinding of participants	Blinding of outcome assessment	Incomplete outcome data addressed	Selective reporting	Other sources of bias	Total
Ibrahim et al. (19)	Unclear	Unclear	High	High	Low	Low	Low	3
Porwal et al. (22)	Unclear	Unclear	High	High	Low	Low	Low	3
Bhargava et al. (23)	Unclear	Unclear	High	Low	Low	Low	Low	4
Elfar and Hasby (24)	Low	Low	High	Low	Low	Low	Low	6

Data Quality

Table 2 shows the details of the study quality of the included non-randomized studies (16–18, 20, 21, 25–29). The NOS varied between 8 and 9 stars, indicating generally good study quality. **Table 3** shows the details of study quality of the included RCTs (19, 22–24). Two of the RCTs were open-label (19, 22), and the other two were single-blinded (23, 24). The method of random sequence generation and information of allocation concealment was reported in only one RCT (24). The overall quality score varied between 3 and 7, indicating moderate to good study quality.

Meta-Analysis Results

Pooled results of 10 studies (16–20, 23–25, 27, 29) showed that combined treatment with microneedling and PRP was associated with increased odds of significant clinical improvement as compared with microneedling therapy without PRP (OR: 2.97, 95% CI: 1.96 to 4.51, $p < 0.001$; **Figure 2A**) without significant heterogeneity (P for Cochrane's Q-test $= 0.45$, $I^2 = 0\%$). Sensitivity analysis showed consistent results limited to the comparisons between the combined treatment and microneedling alone (OR: 4.58, 95% CI: 2.49 to 8.42, $p < 0.001$; $I^2 = 0\%$). Subgroup analyses according to the study design showed both significant results in non-randomized studies and RCTs, while the effect was more remarkable in RCTs than in non-randomized studies (OR: 7.85 vs. 3.02, P for subgroup difference $= 0.02$; **Figure 2A**). In addition, combined treatment with microneedling and PRP was associated with a significantly improved mean GQS score (six studies MD: −0.32, 95% CI: −0.44 to −0.20, $p < 0.001$; $I^2 = 0\%$; **Figure 2B**) and a higher patient satisfying rate (six studies, OR: 4.15, 95% CI: 2.13 to 8.09, $p < 0.001$; $I^2 = 53\%$; **Figure 2C**) compared to treatment with microneedling without PRP. Subgroup analyses showed that difference in study design did not significantly affect the results (P for subgroup difference $= 0.22$ and 0.63, respectively). Meta-analyses of three and two studies showed that the incidence of severe adverse events such as severe erythema (OR: 1.59, 95% CI: 0.73 to 3.46, $P = 0.24$; $I^2 = 0\%$; **Figure 3A**) and severe edema (OR: 1.14, 95% CI: 0.47 to 2.76, $P = 0.77$; $I^2 = 0\%$; **Figure 3B**) were not significantly different between the two treatment groups.

Publication Bias

The funnel plots for the meta-analyses of outcomes of the significant clinical improvement rate, changes of GQS, and the patient satisfying rate are shown in **Figures 4A–C**, respectively. These plots were symmetrical, suggesting low risk of publication biases among the outcomes. Egger's regression tests also showed low risks of publication biases for these meta-analyses (P for Egger's regression test $= 0.534$, 0.328, and 0.297, respectively).

DISCUSSION

In this meta-analysis, by pooling the results of 14 non-randomized studies and RCTs, we found that a combined treatment with microneedling and PRP was associated with better improvement of atrophic acne scars than microneedling without PRP. The efficacy of a combined treatment was evidenced by the higher rate of significant improvement and better improved GQS evaluated by dermatologists and the higher satisfying rate from the patients. Besides, pooled results of limited datasets suggested no significant difference in the incidence of severe adverse events between groups, such as severe erythema and edema. Taken together, the results of our meta-analysis indicated that combined treatment with microneedling with PRP is more effective than microneedling without PRP for patients with acne scars, without further increasing the risk of adverse events. These findings support PRP as an adjuvant therapy for patients with acne scars receiving microneedling therapy.

To the best of our knowledge, few meta-analyses were performed to evaluate the efficacy and safety of additional PRP as an adjuvant therapy for patients with acne scars receiving microneedling therapy. A previous meta-analysis, including five comparative studies before 2019 with 226 patients with atrophic scars showed that a combined treatment with microneedling and PRP may confer better efficacy in patients with atrophic acne scars than treatment with microneedling alone. However, the results were based on limited studies, and other efficacy outcomes, such as changes of GQS, were unable to be determined (36). Our study has several strengths compared to the previous one (36). Firstly, an up-to-date and compressive literature search was performed. With the expanded literature search strategy, we identified 14 comparative studies, including 472 patients, which were much larger than the previous one. Moreover, the relatively larger number of studies enables us to evaluate the efficacy of a combined therapy with microneedling and PRP in a multidimensional manner, including the outcomes of the significant clinical improvement rate, between-group difference of GQS changes, and the patient satisfying rate. All of these outcomes consistently indicated a better efficacy of the combined therapy with PRP compared to microneedling without PRP for

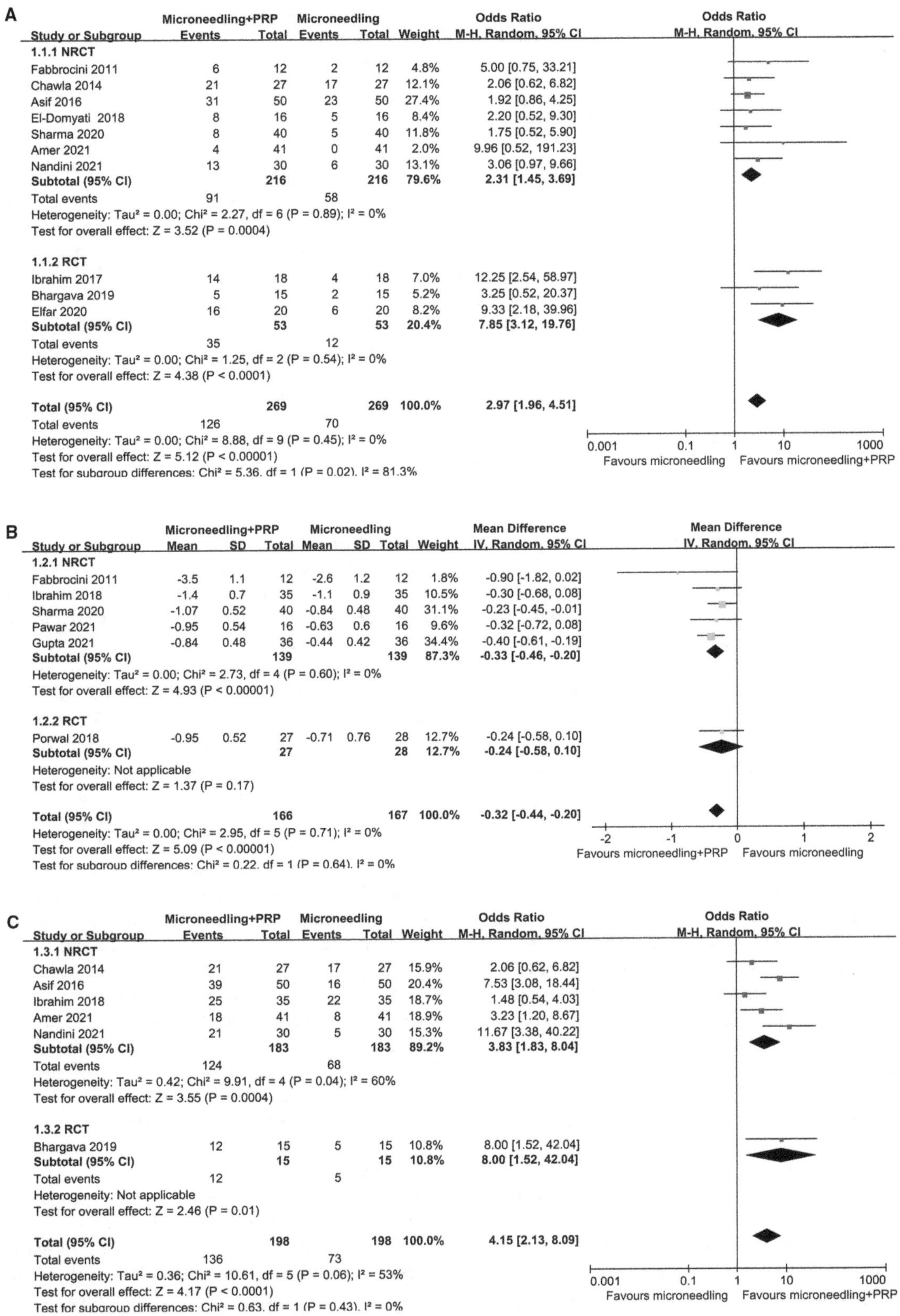

FIGURE 2 | Forest plots for the meta-analyses, comparing the effect of combined treatment with microneedling and PRP vs. microneedling without PRP for patients with acne scars; **(A)** the rate of significant clinical improvement; **(B)** difference of changes of GQS after treatment; and **(C)** the rate of patient satisfaction.

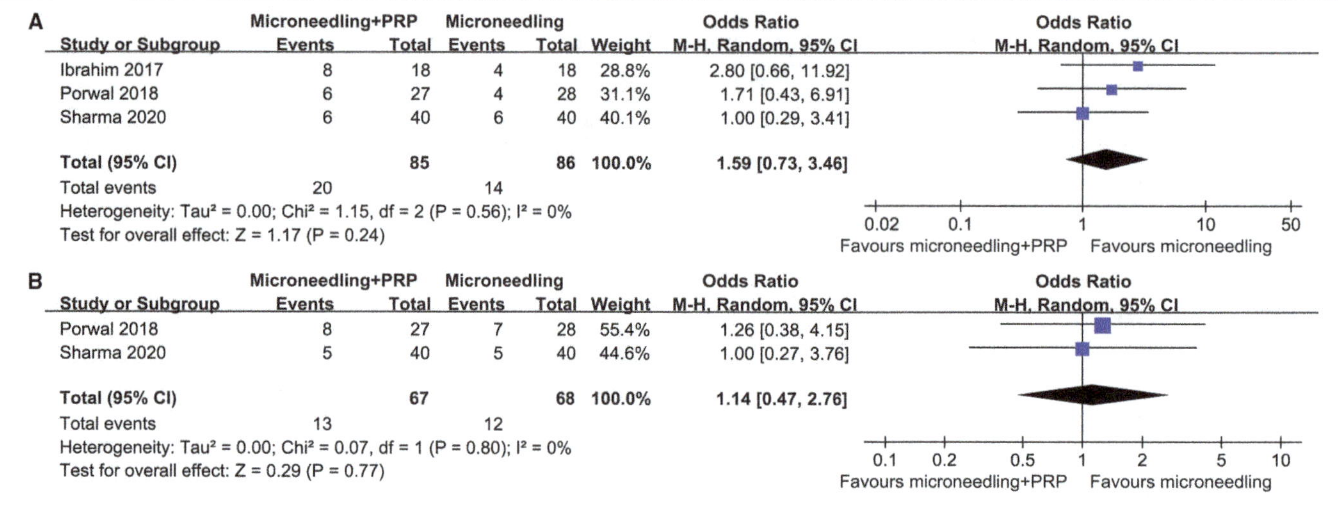

FIGURE 3 | Forest plots for the meta-analyses, comparing the safety of combined treatment with microneedling and PRP vs. microneedling without PRP for patients with acne scars; **(A)** incidence of severe erythema; and **(B)** incidence of severe edema.

acne scars. In addition, safety outcomes were also explored, which did not show that additional use of PRP was associated with an increased risk of severe adverse events. Finally, sensitivity analysis and subgroup analysis according to the design of the studies were performed, and the consistent results further assured the stability of the findings.

The possible synergistic effect of PRP on the basis of microneedling treatment for atrophic acne scars may be explained by multiple mechanisms (37). The primary mechanisms for the microneedling treatment are the formation of skin microwounds to induce collagen production and dermal remodeling (12, 13). Previous studies have confirmed that PRP contains multiple active cytokines and growth factors that are primarily released from the a-granules of platelets and actively involved in the process of dermal remodeling, such as the dermal-transforming growth factor, the platelet-derived growth factor, the vascular endothelial growth factor, and the fibroblast growth factor (38, 39). The skin microwounds resulting from the microneedling therapy may also enhance the absorption of the above active cytokines in PRP by the skin (12, 13). However, studies evaluating the mechanisms underlying the synergetic therapeutic efficacy of microneedling and PRP are limited. Interestingly, a recent study has shown that, compared to the use of microneedling alone, combined treatment with microneedling and PRP was associated with a marked excellent improvement of the skin lesions, a more significant deposition of collagen and elastic fibers, and an increased proliferative activity in the epidermis in people with striae distensa, which may also reflect the synergetic benefits of action microneedling and PRP on scar formation and collagen/dermal remodeling (40). Interestingly, the efficacy of combined treatment with microneedling and PRP has also been observed in people with androgenetic alopecia (41) and melisma (42). The exact molecular mechanisms underlying the benefits of a combined therapy with microneedling and PRP for atrophic acne scars should be further evaluated.

Some limitations of the current meta-analysis should be considered when the results are interpreted. Firstly, the numbers of available studies and the included patients for some outcomes were limited. For example, meta-analysis of adverse events only involved 2–3 studies; the results of which should be validated in large-scale RCTs. In addition, the limited number of available datasets may also reduce the reliability of funnel plots for the estimation of publication biases. In particular, it has been suggested that visual interpretation of funnel plots is too subjective to be useful (31), and it has been pointed out that the researchers had only a limited ability to identify correctly funnel plots for meta-analyses that were subject to bias due to missing results (43). Moreover, quality scores of the included RCTs were moderate, and 10/14 of the included studies were non-randomized face-split studies, although subgroup analysis according to study design was performed. Accordingly, high-quality large-scale RCTs with adequate statistical power are warranted to verify our findings. In addition, the optimal PRP formulation remains unknown, and the influence of PRP formulation on the outcomes was not performed because most of the included studies did not provide adequate details related with PRP preparation. Finally, most of the studies were performed in India and Egypt. Studies from the other regions of the world are warranted to validate the findings.

In conclusion, the results of our meta-analysis indicated that combined treatment with microneedling with PRP is more effective than microneedling without PRP for patients with acne scars, without further increasing the risk of adverse events. Although large-scale RCTs are warranted to confirm these results, the findings of the meta-analysis support using PRP as an adjuvant therapy for patients with acne scars receiving microneedling therapy.

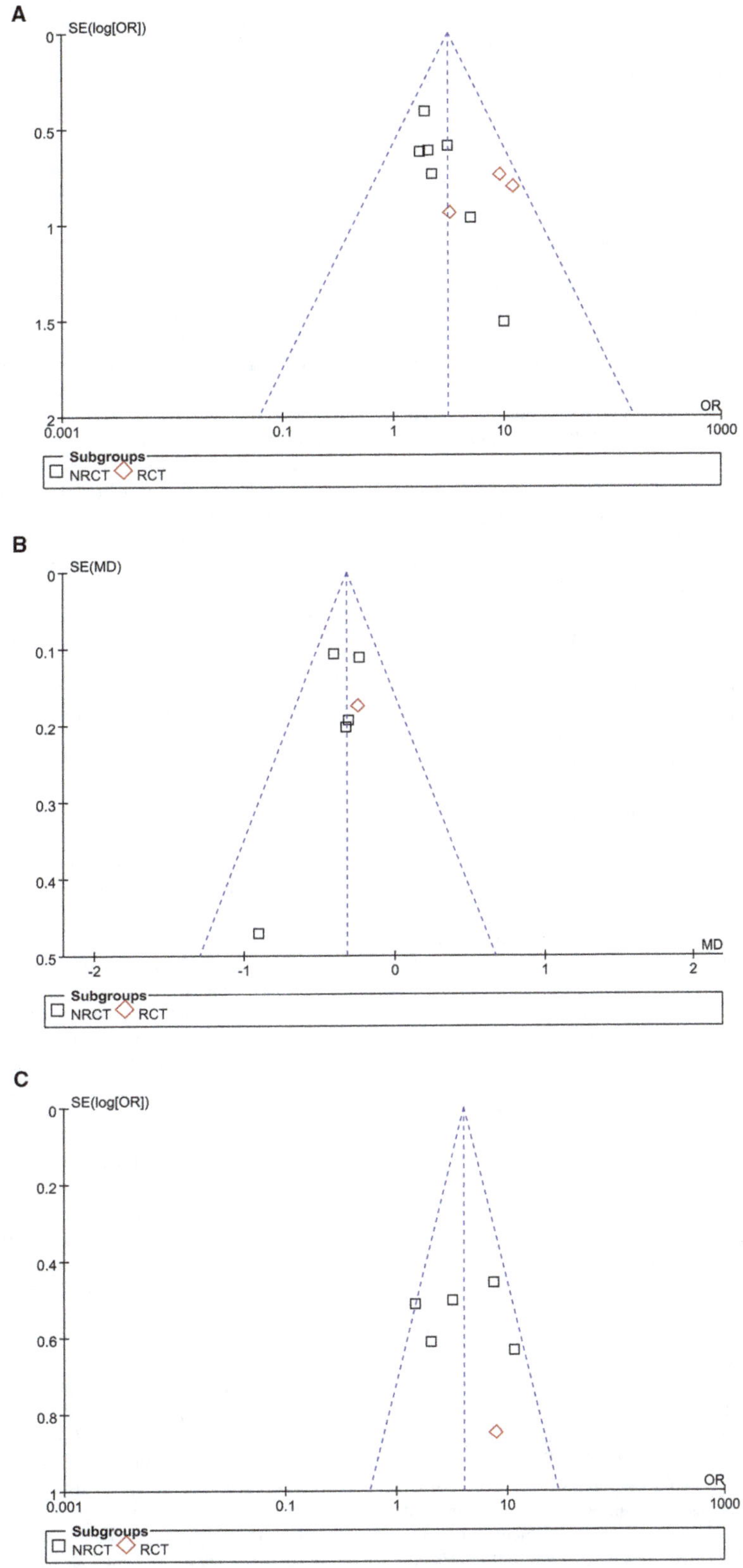

FIGURE 4 | Funnel plots for the publication bias within the meta-analyses, comparing the effect of combined treatment with microneedling and PRP vs. microneedling without PRP for patients with acne scars; **(A)** funnel plots for the rate of significant clinical improvement; **(B)** funnel plots for the difference of changes of GQS after treatment; and **(C)** funnel plots for the rate of patient satisfaction.

AUTHOR CONTRIBUTIONS

CK and DL designed the study, performed database search, data extraction, statistical analyses, and interpretation of the results. CK drafted the manuscript. DL critically revised the manuscript. All authors approved the submission of the manuscript.

REFERENCES

1. Zaenglein AL, Pathy AL, Schlosser BJ, Alikhan A, Baldwin HE, Berson DS, et al. Guidelines of care for the management of acne vulgaris. *J Am Acad Dermatol.* (2016) 74:945–73.e933. doi: 10.1016/j.jaad.2015.12.037
2. Berry K, Lim J, Zaenglein AL. Acne vulgaris: treatment made easy for the primary care physician. *Pediatr Ann.* (2020) 49:e109–15. doi: 10.3928/19382359-20200211-01
3. Tan JK, Bhate K. A global perspective on the epidemiology of acne. *Br J Dermatol.* (2015) 172(Suppl 1):3–12. doi: 10.1111/bjd.13462
4. Layton AM, Thiboutot D, Tan J. Reviewing the global burden of acne: how could we improve care to reduce the burden? *Br J Dermatol.* (2021) 184:219–25. doi: 10.1111/bjd.19477
5. Boen M, Jacob C. A review and update of treatment options using the acne scar classification system. *Dermatol Surg.* (2019) 45:411–22. doi: 10.1097/DSS.0000000000001765
6. Gieler U, Gieler T, Kupfer JP. Acne and quality of life - impact and management. *J Eur Acad Dermatol Venereol.* (2015) 29(Suppl 4):12–4. doi: 10.1111/jdv.13191
7. Dreno B, Amici JM, Demessant-Flavigny AL, Wright C, Taieb C, Desai SR, et al. The impact of acne, atopic dermatitis, skin toxicities and scars on quality of life and the importance of a holistic treatment approach. *Clin Cosmet Investig Dermatol.* (2021) 14:623–32. doi: 10.2147/CCID.S315846
8. Connolly D, Vu HL, Mariwalla K, Saedi N. Acne scarring-pathogenesis, evaluation, and treatment options. *J Clin Aesthet Dermatol.* (2017) 10:12–23.
9. Tan J, Thiboutot D, Gollnick H, Kang S, Layton A, Leyden JJ, et al. Development of an atrophic acne scar risk assessment tool. *J Eur Acad Dermatol Venereol.* (2017) 31:1547–54. doi: 10.1111/jdv.14325
10. Zaleski-Larsen LA, Fabi SG, Mcgraw T, Taylor M. Acne scar treatment: a multimodality approach tailored to scar type. *Dermatol Surg.* (2016) 42(Suppl 2):S139–49. doi: 10.1097/DSS.0000000000000746
11. Bhargava S, Cunha PR, Lee J, Kroumpouzos G. Acne scarring management: systematic review and evaluation of the evidence. *Am J Clin Dermatol.* (2018) 19:459–77. doi: 10.1007/s40257-018-0358-5
12. Juhasz MLW, Cohen JL. Microneedling for the treatment of scars: an update for clinicians. *Clin Cosmet Investig Dermatol.* (2020) 13:997–1003. doi: 10.2147/CCID.S267192
13. Schoenberg E, O'connor M, Wang JV, Yang S, Saedi N. Microneedling and PRP for acne scars: a new tool in our arsenal. *J Cosmet Dermatol.* (2020) 19:112–4. doi: 10.1111/jocd.12988
14. Zhang M, Park G, Zhou B, Luo D. Applications and efficacy of platelet-rich plasma in dermatology: a clinical review. *J Cosmet Dermatol.* (2018) 17:660–5. doi: 10.1111/jocd.12673
15. Hesseler MJ, Shyam N. Platelet-rich plasma and its utility in medical dermatology: a systematic review. *J Am Acad Dermatol.* (2019) 81:834–46. doi: 10.1016/j.jaad.2019.04.037
16. Fabbrocini G, De Vita V, Pastore F, Panariello L, Fardella N, Sepulveres R, et al. Combined use of skin needling and platelet-rich plasma in acne scarring treatment. *Cosmetic Dermatol.* (2011) 24:177–83.
17. Chawla S. Split face comparative study of microneedling with PRP versus microneedling with vitamin c in treating atrophic post acne scars. *J Cutan Aesthet Surg.* (2014) 7:209–12. doi: 10.4103/0974-2077.150742
18. Asif M, Kanodia S, Singh K. Combined autologous platelet-rich plasma with microneedling verses microneedling with distilled water in the treatment of atrophic acne scars: a concurrent split-face study. *J Cosmet Dermatol.* (2016) 15:434–43. doi: 10.1111/jocd.12207
19. Ibrahim ZA, El-Ashmawy AA, Shora OA. Therapeutic effect of microneedling and autologous platelet-rich plasma in the treatment of atrophic scars: a randomized study. *J Cosmet Dermatol.* (2017) 16:388–99. doi: 10.1111/jocd.12356
20. El-Domyati M, Abdel-Wahab H, Hossam A. Microneedling combined with platelet-rich plasma or trichloroacetic acid peeling for management of acne scarring: a split-face clinical and histologic comparison. *J Cosmet Dermatol.* (2018) 17:73–83. doi: 10.1111/jocd.12459
21. Ibrahim MK, Ibrahim SM, Salem AM. Skin microneedling plus platelet-rich plasma versus skin microneedling alone in the treatment of atrophic post acne scars: a split face comparative study. *J Dermatolog Treat.* (2018) 29:281–6. doi: 10.1080/09546634.2017.1365111
22. Porwal S, Chahar YS, Singh PK. A Comparative study of combined dermaroller and platelet-rich plasma versus dermaroller alone in acne scars and assessment of quality of life before and after treatment. *Indian J Dermatol.* (2018) 63:403–8. doi: 10.4103/ijd.IJD_118_17
23. Bhargava S, Kroumpouzos G, Varma K, Kumar U. Combination therapy using subcision, needling, and platelet-rich plasma in the management of grade 4 atrophic acne scars: a pilot study. *J Cosmet Dermatol.* (2019) 18:1092–7. doi: 10.1111/jocd.12935
24. Elfar NN, Hasby EA. Efficacy and safety of plasma gel as a new modality in treatment of atrophic acne scars. *Int J Dermatol.* (2020) 59:620–6. doi: 10.1111/ijd.14815
25. Amer A, Elhariry S, Al-Balat W. Combined autologous platelet-rich plasma with microneedling versus microneedling with non-cross-linked hyaluronic acid in the treatment of atrophic acne scars: Split-face study. *Dermatol Ther.* (2021) 34:e14457. doi: 10.1111/dth.14457
26. Gupta M, Barman KD, Sarkar R. A comparative study of microneedling alone versus along with platelet-rich plasma in acne scars. *J Cutan Aesthet Surg.* (2021) 14:64–71.
27. Nandini AS, Sankey SM, Sowmya CS, Sharath Kumar BC. Split-face comparative study of efficacy of platelet-rich plasma combined with microneedling versus microneedling alone in treatment of post-acne scars. *J Cutan Aesthet Surg.* (2021) 14:26–31. doi: 10.4103/JCAS.JCAS_160_18
28. Pawar M, Singh M. Microneedling with autologous platelet-rich plasma versus microneedling with topical insulin in the treatment of postacne atrophic scars: a simultaneous split-face comparative study. *J Am Acad Dermatol.* (2021) 84:810–1. doi: 10.1016/j.jaad.2020.05.152
29. Sharma S, Kaur T, Bassi R. A split face comparative study to evaluate the efficacy of skin microneedling and platelet rich plasma (PRP) combination versus skin microneedling alone for treatment of post acne scars. *J Pakistan Assoc Dermatol.* (2021) 30:449–55.
30. Moher D, Liberati A, Tetzlaff J, Altman DG. Preferred reporting items for systematic reviews and meta-analyses: the PRISMA statement. *BMJ.* (2009) 339:b2535. doi: 10.1136/bmj.b2535
31. Higgins, J., and Green, S. (2011). *Cochrane Handbook for Systematic Reviews of Interventions Version 5.1.0.* The Cochrane Collaboration. Available online at: www.cochranehandbook.org (accessed August 20, 2021).
32. Wells GA, Shea B, O'connell D, Peterson J, Welch V, Losos M, et al. *The Newcastle-Ottawa Scale (NOS) for Assessing the Quality of Nonrandomised Studies in Meta-Analyses.* (2010). Available online at: http://www.ohri.ca/programs/clinical_epidemiology/oxford.asp (accessed August 20, 2021).
33. Higgins JP, Thompson SG. Quantifying heterogeneity in a meta-analysis. *Stat Med.* (2002) 21:1539–58. doi: 10.1002/sim.1186
34. Egger M, Davey Smith G, Schneider M, Minder C. Bias in meta-analysis detected by a simple, graphical test. *BMJ.* (1997) 315:629–34. doi: 10.1136/bmj.315.7109.629
35. Moher D, Liberati A, Tetzlaff J, Altman DG. Preferred reporting items for systematic reviews and meta-analyses: the PRISMA statement. *PLoS Med.* (2009) 6:e1000097. doi: 10.1371/journal.pmed1000097
36. Chang HC, Sung CW, Lin MH. Combination therapy with microneedling and platelet-rich plasma for acne scarring: a systematic review and meta-analysis.

Dermatol Surg. (2020) 46:1118–22. doi: 10.1097/DSS.0000000000002033
37. Hashim PW, Levy Z, Cohen JL, Goldenberg G. Microneedling therapy with and without platelet-rich plasma. *Cutis.* (2017) 99:239–42.
38. Mussano F, Genova T, Munaron L, Petrillo S, Erovigni F, Carossa S. Cytokine, chemokine, and growth factor profile of platelet-rich plasma. *Platelets.* (2016) 27:467–71. doi: 10.3109/09537104.2016.1143922
39. Samadi P, Sheykhhasan M, Khoshinani HM. The use of platelet-rich plasma in aesthetic and regenerative medicine: a comprehensive review. *Aesthetic Plast Surg.* (2019) 43:803–14. doi: 10.1007/s00266-018-1293-9
40. Abdel-Motaleb AA, Zedan H, Mostafa MM, Abu-Dief EE, Gebril SM, Abdelwahed Hussein MR. Combined microneedling with topical application of platelet-rich plasma versus microneedling alone in the treatment of stria distensae: clinicopathological analysis. *J Dermatolog Treat.* (2020) 31:1–12. doi: 10.1080/09546634.2020.1782323
41. Strazzulla LC, Avila L, Lo Sicco K, Shapiro J. An Overview of the Biology of Platelet-Rich Plasma and Microneedling as Potential Treatments for Alopecia Areata. *J Investig Dermatol Symp Proc.* (2018) 19:S21–4. doi: 10.1016/j.jisp.2017.10.002
42. Zhao L, Hu M, Xiao Q, Zhou R, Li Y, Xiong L, et al. Efficacy and safety of platelet-rich plasma in melasma: a systematic review and meta-analysis. *Dermatol Ther.* (2021) 11:1587–97. doi: 10.1007/s13555-021-00575-z
43. Terrin N, Schmid CH, Lau J. In an empirical evaluation of the funnel plot, researchers could not visually identify publication bias. *J Clin Epidemiol.* (2005) 58:894–901. doi: 10.1016/j.jclinepi.2005.01.006

18

Clearance of Chronic Actinic Dermatitis with Dupilumab Therapy in Chinese Patients

Kamran Ali [1†], Liming Wu [2†], HaiYue Lou [2†], Jianbo Zhong [2], YunMi Qiu [2], JiaYang Da [3], JingPeng Shan [2] and KaiNing Lu [3]*

[1] Department of Dermatology, International Education College of Zhejiang Chinese Medical University, Hangzhou, China, [2] Department of Dermatology, Affiliated Hangzhou First People's Hospital, Zhejiang University School of Medicine, Hangzhou, China, [3] Department of Oncological Surgery, Affiliated Hangzhou First People's Hospital, Zhejiang University School of Medicine, Hangzhou, China

***Correspondence:**
Liming Wu
18957118053@163.com

† These authors have contributed equally to this work and share first authorship

Chronic actinic dermatitis (CAD) is a rare chronic immunological photo-dermatosis resulting in pruritic eczematous eruption on sun-exposed skin to ultraviolet (UV) light. The disease mechanism may include a delay-type hypersensitivity reaction to an endogenous photo-induced antigen, postulated to be UVR-altered DNA, but the exact pathophysiology is unknown. Minimum erythema dosing and patch testing are diagnostic tools of CAD. There are limited safe and effective treatment options for CAD. Herein, a case series of three patients with severe recalcitrant CAD is presented after being treated with dupilumab off-label. The patients in this study had persistent severe disease and taken the first-line management plan, which consists of topical calcineurin inhibitors (TCI), topical corticosteroids (TCS), and strict photoprotection. However, the above treatment options were not able to control the symptoms. The patients were treated with dupilumab 600 mg first dose, 300 mg biweekly subcutaneously (SC), and hydroxychloroquine. Dupilumab showed excellent clinical benefits, including safe and well-tolerated in chronic actinic dermatitis. Further studies are required to be carried out before being applied in clinical practice.

Keywords: chronic actinic dermatitis, dupilumab, photo-dermatoses, hydroxychloroquine, photodermatitis

INTRODUCTION

Chronic actinic dermatitis (CAD) was previously known as photosensitive dermatitis, eczema, actinic reticuloid (AR), and immunological-mediated photo-dermatosis. CAD is defined as chronic pruritus eczematous lesions and often lichenified plaques

predominantly upon sun-exposed skin areas in patients above 50 years old, who often have outdoor activities (1). Chronic actinic dermatitis is seen in all skin types, more prevalent in patients of lower skin phenotypes. However, in Fitzpatrick, skin Types V and VI are most likely seen in younger patients (2). There are limited treatment options available for CAD, and it has inadequate therapeutic effects and severe side effects. Dupilumab is an IgG human monoclonal antibody (mAB) that binds to the IL-4 receptor (IL-4R-alpha), inhibits the lL-4 and IL-13 cytokines signaling pathway, and reduces the level of Th2 biomarkers. Dupilumab has promisingly improved skin barrier function and the health-related quality of life HRQoL in the clinical trial for atopic dermatitis (AD). Dupilumab has been approved by the food and drug administration (FDA) for moderate-to-severe AD, and CAD shared the similar Th2-mediated inflammatory pathogenesis as atopic dermatitis (AD) (3, 4). This study presents a case series of patients with CAD treated with **Dupilumab,** Hydroxychloroquine, and topical calcineurin inhibitors (0.3% tacrolimus ointment) to overcome the disease severity. Following treatment showed a significant outcome, and no side effects were observed during the follow-up period.

METHODS

Patients and Assessments

The patients were clinically diagnosed as chronic actinic dermatitis, and we took the complete medical and family history. Photo testing indicated UVA-MED negative for one patient, and the other two patients showed positive at 24 h, and UVB-MED was positive at 24 h. A complete blood count and the erythrocyte sedimentation rate were normal. Anti-SSA, antinuclear antibodies (ANA), and anti-SSB antibodies were negative. The patients were recalcitrant to topical and systemic therapy and were injected 600 mg initial dose of dupilumab, followed by 300 mg biweekly with the combination of hydroxychloroquine 100 mg BID per oral (PO). Patients continued strict photoprotective measures and topical medications. No additional systematic immunosuppressant therapy was added to the treatment. The dupilumab outcome was observed and recorded based on clinical presentation. Treatment outcomes were recorded as well as any side effects of dupilumab. Follow-up was done biweekly to observe the change in lesion and disease progress. In addition, we extracted the data on the history of CAD treatment and systemic comorbidities from patients' previous medical records. Data of patients with CAD treated with dupilumab and hydroxychloroquine were retrospectively analyzed from February 2021 to October 2021.

RESULTS

Case Presentation

Three male patients with CAD were diagnosed clinically and treated in our dermatology department since February, 2021 to October, 2021. The patients had a history of mild chronic eczematous, scaly, and excoriated papules. They presented with pruritic edematous red plaques on the sun-exposed areas, including scalp, forehead, ears, face, and dorsa of hands, but no lesions were observed on the shaded areas of the body (**Table 1; Figures 1a, 2a**). They have experienced increased symptoms in summer on sun-exposed skin, but less in winter. Upon examination, the clinical presentations were consistent with chronic actinic dermatitis. The patients were diagnosed based on clinical presentation and MED results. One patient had a history of atopic dermatitis (AD). The patients have been treated with topical mometasone furoate and oral antihistamines and diligent photoprotection without significant improvement. Systematic treatment was initiated due to topical therapy's worsening symptoms and failure to photoprotective clothing and sunscreen. Methotrexate, hydroxychloroquine, and azathioprine did not show satisfactory results (**Table 1**). After discussion with the patients, dupilumab was initiated off-label at a 600-mg loading dose and 300 mg subcutaneously (SC) biweekly with the concomitant of hydroxychloroquine 100 mg two times a day for 8–20 weeks. All other systemic treatments were discontinued. However, strict photoprotection and topical ointment were continued. The efficacy and adverse events were analyzed.

All three patients showed reduced lichenified edematous plaques and decreased pruritus after 1 month of treatment with dupilumab and hydroxychloroquine. Patients 1 and three experienced reduced edematous plaques, scaling, erythema, and pruritus associated with the affected area in 4 weeks. The lesions were nearly cleared after 16- week of treatment. No adverse events were observed. Patient two had exacerbations of the erythematous lesion after the initial dose, but edematous flares were cleared with continued treatment with dupilumab for 12 weeks (**Figures 1b, 2b**); he did not receive any other systemic therapy. Post-treatment photo-testing was not performed or patients' denial to do repeating photo-testing. However, patients resumed their daily activities without photoprotection and did not complain about disease severity and photosensitivity during the treatment. The patients provided informed photo consent before collecting the images. Details are described in **Table 1.**

DISCUSSION

The pathogenesis of chronic actinic dermatitis (CAD) remains unknown. Due to a loss of photo-immunosuppression ability, allowing the photo-induced antigen to activate the hypersensitive reaction, it is more likely to be delayed-type hypercreativity reaction, the more rigorously photo-allergic reaction in allergic contact dermatitis (ACD). These allergens develop when photo-induction (UV-radiation) causes molecular changes in patients with CAD, and some research has suggested that these allergens are driven by or related to UVR-altered DNA (5, 6).

Management of chronic actinic dermatitis and photo-dermatoses is involved in strict sun protection, photoprotective clothing, UVA, and UVB protective sunscreen (physical or sunscreen) but also includes topical and systemic corticosteroids and PUVA therapy. Narrowband ultraviolet B (NB UVB) phototherapy has shown remarkable therapeutic effects and a safety profile in Chinese patients (7). Azathioprine, cyclosporine, mycophenolate mofetil, and hydroxyurea are the steroid-sparing agents that have efficacy in CAD. Long-term use of these drugs has significant health-related risks and side effects; so new safe and effective treatment options are necessary (1, 2). The above case series demonstrated the comprehensive therapeutic option for chronic actinic dermatitis with dupilumab and hydroxychloroquine. None of our patients reported any adverse effects.

Furthermore, in the literature review, we identify three reports with a total of 10 patients (8–10). All the patients showed a moderate-to-complete reduction in disease severity. Two patients developed conjunctivitis and were successfully treated with ophthalmic corticosteroids (20% of the cases) (8). Only one patient had to suspend the treatment with dupilumab because of the DFR (dupilumab facial redness). About 10% of the total reported cases (10). Dupilumab is an IgG4 human mAB that binds to the IL-4 receptor (IL-Rα), inhibiting the transmission of

TABLE 1 | Patients with chronic actinic dermatitis (CAD) treated with dupilumab ($n = 3$).

	Patient 1	Patient 2	Patient 3
Age	58	77	69
Sex	Male	Male	Male
Duration of CAD (Years)	>10	4	1
Clinical presentation	Well-demarcated Erythematous excoriated lichenified pruritic plaques on sun-exposed areas (face, fore arm, dorsa of hands and scalp), increased symptoms in summer during outdoor activities. Spared shaded areas.	Pruritic edematous excoriated lichenified plaques on sun-exposed areas (face, upper chest, dorsa of hands and scalp), increased symptoms in summer specially during outdoor activities. Shaded areas are spared.	Well-demarcated phot-induced eczematous on sun-exposed areas (face, upper chest, fore arm, dorsa of hands and scalp), increased symptoms in summer during outdoor activities. No lesion were found on the shaded areas of the body.
Serum IgE levels	150 IU/mL (normal 20–200 IU/mL)	88 IU/mL (normal 20–200 IU/mL)	Not done
Severity measurement tools (IGA, EASI, Pruritic-NRS)	IGA: $4^{v0}/1^{A}$ EASI: $10.3^{v0}/1^{A}$ BSA:$21^{v0}/6^{A}$ Pruritic-NRS: $7^{v0}/2^{A}$	IGA: $4^{v0}/1^{A}$ EASI: $13^{v0}/1.7^{A}$ BSA:$20^{v0}/8^{A}$ Pruritic-NRS: $8^{v0}/1^{A}$	IGA: $4^{v0}/2^{A}$ EASI: $11^{v0}/2^{A}$ BSA:$26^{v0}/10^{A}$ Pruritic-NRS: $8^{v0}/3^{A}$
Previous treatment	Corticosteroid (T, PO), TCI, methotrexate, antihistamine, hydroxychloroquine (2)	Corticosteroid (T, PO), TCI, methotrexate, Azathioprine, hydroxychloroquine, mycophenolate mofetil (2)	Corticosteroids (T), TCI, antihistamines and hydroxychloroquine (2)
Photo-testing (MED)	UVA: positive at 7 mJ/cm2 at 24 h (normal range: ≥10 mJ/cm2) UVB: positive at 25 mJ/cm2 at 24 h (normal range: ≥40 mJ/cm2)	UVA: negative at 24 h UVB: positive at 15 mJ/cm2 at 24 h (normal range: ≥40 mJ/cm2)	UVA: positive at 3 mJ/cm2 at 24 h (normal range: ≥10 mJ/cm2) UVB: positive at 18 mJ/cm2 at 24 h (normal range: ≥40 mJ/cm2)
Treatment with Dupilumab	Dupilumab 600 mg, 300 mg biweekly+ hydroxychloroquine	Dupilumab 600 mg, 300 mg biweekly+ hydroxychloroquine	Dupilumab 600 mg, 300 mg biweekly+ hydroxychloroquine
Treatment duration	16 weeks (continued)	20 weeks (continued)	8 weeks (continued)
Follow up	Clearance of lesions	Nearly clearance of lesions.	Significant reduced pruritus and rash
Overall effects	↑↑↑	↑↑↑	↑↑
Complications	none	none	none
Comments	History of AD Yes	no	no

PO, per oral; T, topical; TCIs, topical calcineurin inhibitors; MED, minimal erythema dose; V0, visit zero; A, after treatment; overall effects: →, none; ↑, mild; ↑↑, moderate; ↑↑↑, complete.

the interleukin (IL-4) and interleukin (IL-13) cytokines signaling. Dupilumab is the first systemic biological agent to treat moderate to severe AD.

In previous studies, it was found that 85 percent of patients with atopic dermatitis (AD) treated with dupilumab had a significant reduction in the Eczema Area and Severity Index score (EASI) when compared to patients who received a placebo (35%) (2, 11). It is challenging to speculate the precise mechanism of action through which dupilumab improved the disease severity in patients with CAD. However, durable and long-lasting responses reveal that dupilumab targets vital inflammatory pathways of atopic dermatitis (AD) and other Th2 cell-mediated inflammatory skin diseases, such as CAD, As Ko et al. have recently suggested that T cells may play a role in the dysbalance of Th1/Th2 in CAD, in atopic dermatitis, there is an over-activation of the Th2 in the acute stage. However, the chronic phase is manifested by Thl immune response and sustained Th2 -cells activation (12, 13). According to the study, UVB-induced CD3+, CD4+, and $CD8^{-}$ regulatory T cells suppress the immune system through the release of the immune-regulatory cytokines IL-4 and IL-10 (14). Stephen E. Ullrich et al. demonstrated that UV irritation suppresses the antigen-presenting capacity to T helper-1 T (Th1) cells, whereas antigen presentation to T helper-2 type T (Th2) cells is enhanced (4). Despite the fact that the immunological pathways of atopic dermatitis and chronic actinic dermatitis are not the same, however, there is overlapping. Russell SC, et al. first reported seven young British patients with AD, who were photosensitive (15). Subsequently, Creamer D, et al. and Ogboli MI, et al. also reported CAD in young sufferers with a history of atopic dermatitis (16, 17). Nevertheless, an extensive long-term study would be necessary to determine the direct efficacy of this drug on CAD and reveal the similar inflammatory nature of CAD and AD. In the pieces of literature mentioned above, 3 out of 10 patients (30%) had a history of AD.

Hydroxychloroquine belongs to the 4-aminoquinoline derivatives type antimalarial drug, which has antiproliferative, anti-inflammatory, photoprotective, and immunomodulatory effects. It inhibits UV-induced reactions, effectively alleviates the rash, and plays an excellent role in sun protection (18). Our patients were treated with hydroxychloroquine alone or with other immunosuppression, but the results were unsatisfactory. It is suggested that dupilumab inhibits the IL-4 and IL-13 transmission and may interact with the CAD pathogenic cascade, potentially implicating Th2 in the pathophysiology

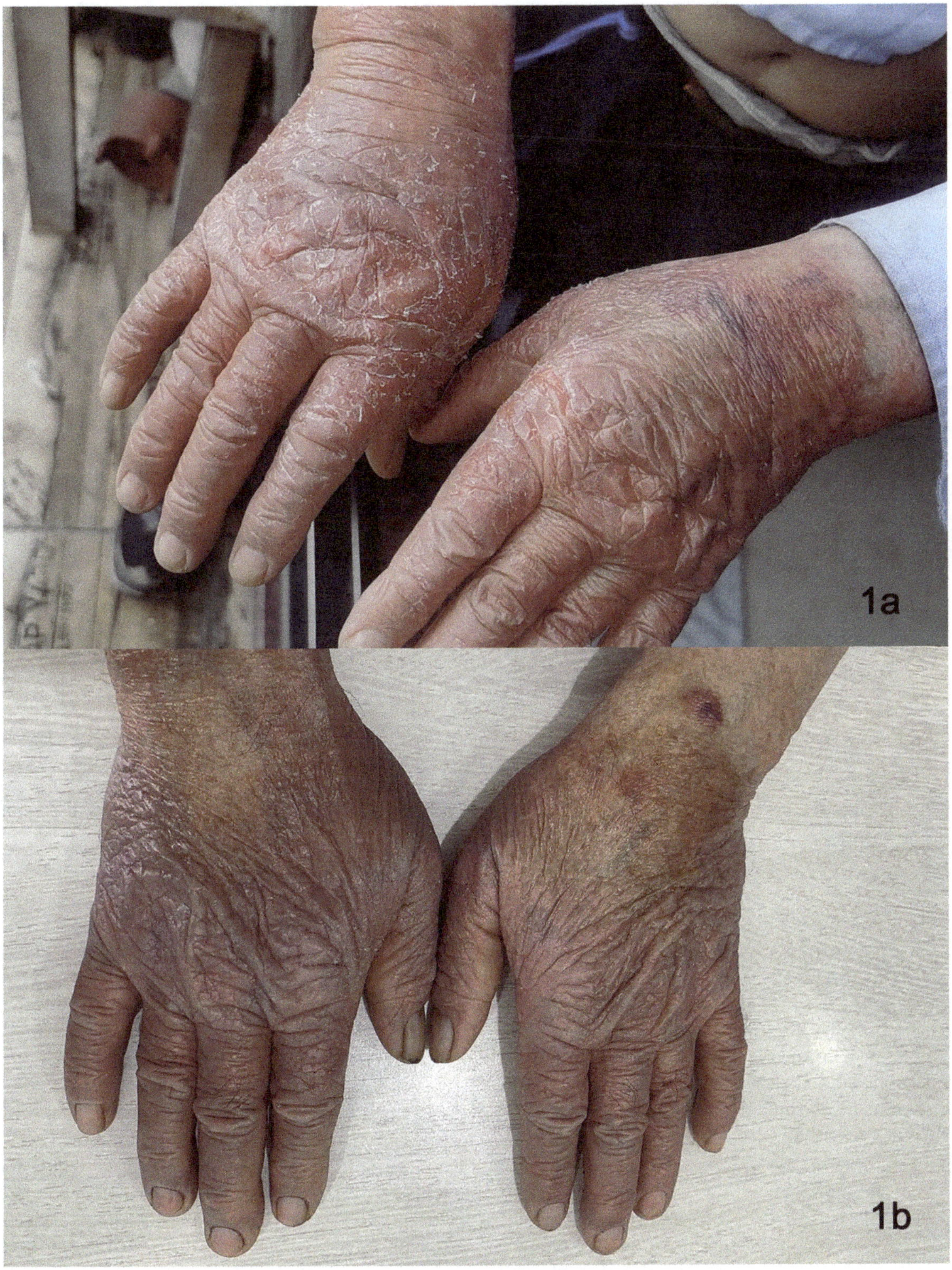

FIGURE 1 | Lesions on dorsa of hands of Patient 2 before dupilumab therapy **(a)**, remarkably improved lesions on dorsal hands after treatment **(b)**.

of CAD. However, hydroxychloroquine has photoprotective effects, and it can inhibit UV-induced reactions, which have an important role in CAD pathogeneses. We speculated that the concomitant dupilumab and hydroxychloroquine increase the primary outcome of disease control in patients with CAD.

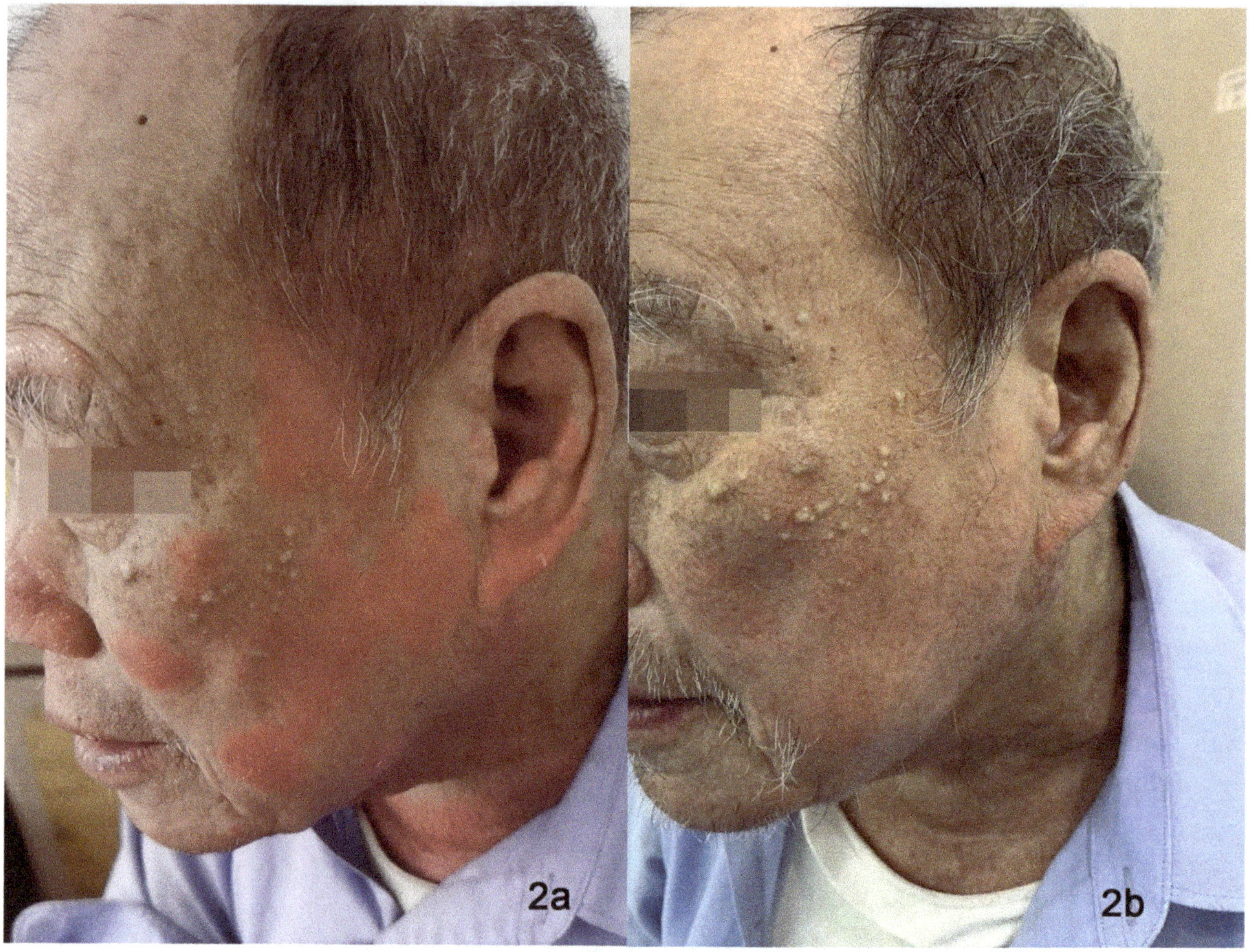

FIGURE 2 | Eczematous, scaly, and excoriated plaques on the face of Patient 2 before treatment **(a)**. Nearly clearance of lesions after dupilumab treatment **(b)**.

In conclusion, the treatment of chronic actinic dermatitis is complicated, and there are no standard and safe therapeutic options. Our case study is small; meanwhile, we presented this case series to provide the clinician with another potential therapeutic option to treat CAD. Hence, dupilumab and hydroxychloroquine showed excellent outcomes in our study, and combination therapy could be considered in managing compliant CAD. Further studies are needed to carry out to use in clinical practice.

CONCLUSION

Chronic actinic dermatitis treatment is complicated, and currently available therapeutic options have limited efficacy and safety concerns. Dupilumab has shown significant improvement in patients with CAD in our study. Further clinical trials are needed to confirm the long-term safety and efficacy of dupilumab in CAD before adding it to a standard treatment option.

AUTHOR CONTRIBUTIONS

KA: wrote the original paper. LW: edit and correct the paper. HL: collect case data. JZ and JS: literature search. YQ: language editing. JD: images editing. KL: provided article ideas and article review. All authors contributed to the article and approved the submitted version.

REFERENCES

1. Paek SY, Lim HW. Chronic actinic dermatitis. *Dermatol Clin.* (2014)0.32:355–61, viii-ix. doi: 10.1016/j.det.2014.03.007

2. Lim HW, Morison WL, Kamide R, Buchness MR, Harris R, Soter NA, et al. Chronic actinic dermatitis an analysis of 51 patients evaluated in the United States and Japan. *Arch Dermatol.* (1994) 130:1284–9. doi: 10.1001/archderm.130.10.1284

3. Eshtiaghi P, Gooderham MJ. Dupilumab: an evidence-based review of its potential in the treatment of atopic dermatitis. *Core Evid.* (2018) 13:13–20. doi: 10.2147/CE.S133661
4. Ullrich SE. Does exposure to UV radiation induce a shift to a Th-2-like immune reaction? *Photochem Photobiol.* (1996) 64:254–8. doi: 10.1111/j.1751-1097.1996.tb02454.x
5. Beach RA, Pratt MD. Chronic actinic dermatitis: clinical cases, diagnostic workup, therapeutic management. *J Cutan Med Surg.* (2009) 13:121–8. doi: 10.2310/7750.2008.08018
6. Hawk JL. Chronic actinic dermatitis. *Photodermatol Photoimmunol Photomed.* (2004) 20:312–4. doi: 10.1111/j.1600-0781.2004.00129.x
7. Ma L, Zhang Q, Hu Y, Luo X. Evaluation of narrow band ultraviolet B phototherapy in the treatment of chronic actinic dermatitis in Chinese patients. *Dermatol Ther.* (2017) 30. doi: 10.1111/dth.12528
8. Patel N, Konda S, Lim HW. Dupilumab for the treatment of chronic actinic dermatitis. *Photodermatol Photoimmunol Photomed.* (2020) 36:398–400. doi: 10.1111/phpp.12566
9. Verma L, Pratt M. A case report of therapeutically challenging chronic actinic dermatitis. *SAGE Open Med Case Rep.* (2019) 7. doi: 10.1177/2050313X19845235
10. Smith MP, Ly K, Thibodeaux Q, Beck K, Berger T, Khodosh R, et al. Dupilumab for the treatment of severe photodermatitis. *JAAD Case Rep.* (2019) 5:614–6. doi: 10.1016/j.jdcr.2019.05.006
11. Beck LA, Thaçi D, Hamilton JD, Graham NM, Bieber T, Rocklin R, et al. Dupilumab treatment in adults with moderate-to-severe atopic dermatitis. *N Engl J Med.* (2014) 371:130–9. doi: 10.1056/NEJMoa1314768
12. Ko DY, Choi SH, Ha SM, Kim TH, Song KH, Kim KH, et al. The clinical severity score of chronic actinic dermatitis correlates with in vivo photoallergic reactions and the immunologic parameters related to a shift towards Th2 immunity from the Th2/Th1 balanced status in patients with chronic actinic dermatitis. *Photodermatol Photoimmunol Photomed.* (2016) 32:199–206. doi: 10.1111/phpp.12244
13. Kim J, Kim BE, Leung DYM. Pathophysiology of atopic dermatitis: clinical implications. *Allergy Asthma Proc.* (2019) 40:84–92. doi: 10.2500/aap.2019.40.4202
14. Rivas JM, Ullrich SE. The role of IL-4, IL-10, and TNF-alpha in the immune suppression induced by ultraviolet radiation. *J Leukoc Biol.* (1994) 56:769–75. doi: 10.1002/jlb.56.6.769
15. Russell SC, Dawe RS, Collins P, Man I, Ferguson J. The photosensitivity dermatitis and actinic reticuloid syndrome (chronic actinic dermatitis) occurring in seven young atopic dermatitis patients. *Br J Dermatol.* (1998) 138:496–501. doi: 10.1046/j.1365-2133.1998.02132.x
16. Creamer D, McGregor JM, Hawk JL. Chronic actinic dermatitis occurring in young patients with atopic dermatitis. *Br J Dermatol.* (1998) 139:1112–3. doi: 10.1046/j.1365-2133.1998.2576c.x
17. Ogboli MI, Rhodes LE. Chronic actinic dermatitis in young atopic dermatitis sufferers. *Br J Dermatol.* (2000) 142:845. doi: 10.1046/j.1365-2133.2000.03457.x
18. Sardana K, Sinha S, Sachdeva S. Hydroxychloroquine in dermatology and beyond: recent update. *Indian Dermatol Online J.* (2020) 11:453–64. doi: 10.4103/idoj.IDOJ_280_20

Permissions

All chapters in this book were first published Frontiers; hereby published with permission under the Creative Commons Attribution License or equivalent. Every chapter published in this book has been scrutinized by our experts. Their significance has been extensively debated. The topics covered herein carry significant findings which will fuel the growth of the discipline. They may even be implemented as practical applications or may be referred to as a beginning point for another development.

The contributors of this book come from diverse backgrounds, making this book a truly international effort. This book will bring forth new frontiers with its revolutionizing research information and detailed analysis of the nascent developments around the world.

We would like to thank all the contributing authors for lending their expertise to make the book truly unique. They have played a crucial role in the development of this book. Without their invaluable contributions this book wouldn't have been possible. They have made vital efforts to compile up to date information on the varied aspects of this subject to make this book a valuable addition to the collection of many professionals and students.

This book was conceptualized with the vision of imparting up-to-date information and advanced data in this field. To ensure the same, a matchless editorial board was set up. Every individual on the board went through rigorous rounds of assessment to prove their worth. After which they invested a large part of their time researching and compiling the most relevant data for our readers.

The editorial board has been involved in producing this book since its inception. They have spent rigorous hours researching and exploring the diverse topics which have resulted in the successful publishing of this book. They have passed on their knowledge of decades through this book. To expedite this challenging task, the publisher supported the team at every step. A small team of assistant editors was also appointed to further simplify the editing procedure and attain best results for the readers.

Apart from the editorial board, the designing team has also invested a significant amount of their time in understanding the subject and creating the most relevant covers. They scrutinized every image to scout for the most suitable representation of the subject and create an appropriate cover for the book.

The publishing team has been an ardent support to the editorial, designing and production team. Their endless efforts to recruit the best for this project, has resulted in the accomplishment of this book. They are a veteran in the field of academics and their pool of knowledge is as vast as their experience in printing. Their expertise and guidance has proved useful at every step. Their uncompromising quality standards have made this book an exceptional effort. Their encouragement from time to time has been an inspiration for everyone.

The publisher and the editorial board hope that this book will prove to be a valuable piece of knowledge for researchers, students, practitioners and scholars across the globe.

List of Contributors

Xiaoqi Jin
School of Pharmacy, Hubei University of Chinese Medicine, Wuhan, China

Hongfeng Xu, Chuanqi Huang, Haoran Ma, Xin Xiong, Lu Cheng and Fuqian Wang
Department of Pharmacy, Wuhan Hospital of Traditional Chinese and Western Medicine, Wuhan, China

Geng Zhang
School of Pharmacy, Hubei University of Chinese Medicine, Wuhan, China
Department of Pharmacy, Wuhan Hospital of Traditional Chinese and Western Medicine, Wuhan, China

Yan Feng
Department of Pathology, Wuhan Hospital of Traditional Chinese and Western Medicine, Wuhan, China

Ju Hyun Lee
Department of Korean Medicine Ophthalmology and Otolaryngology and Dermatology, Wonkwang University Korean Medicine Hospital, Iksan, South Korea

Eun Heui Jo
Department of Acupuncture and Moxibustion, Wonkwang University Korean Medicine Hospital and Research Center of Traditional Korean Medicine, Wonkwang University, Deokjingu, South Korea

Jee Youn Jung and Mi-Ju Son
Clinical Medicine Division, Korea Institute of Oriental Medicine, Daejeon, South Korea

Young-Eun Kim
Future Medicine Division, Korea Institute of Oriental Medicine, Daejeon, South Korea

Su Jin Kang
Department of Korean Medicine Obstetrics and Gynecology, Wonkwang University Korean Medicine Hospital, Iksan, South Korea

Geum Jin Yang and Yu Hwa Shim
Korean Medicine Dermatology Clinical Research Center of Wonkwang University, Iksan, South Korea

Min Cheol Park
Department of Korean Medicine Ophthalmology and Otolaryngology and Dermatology, Wonk wang University Korean Medicine Hospital and Research Center of Traditional Korean Medicine, Wonkwang University, Iksan, South Korea
Research Center of Traditional Korean Medicine, Wonkwang University, Iksan, South Korea
Department of Korean Medical Ophthalmology & Otolaryngology & Dermatology, College of Korean Medicine, Wonkwang University, Iksan, South Korea

Jiang-Min Liu, Quan-Xin Jin, Fang-Fang Li, Lin-Bo Jin, Ran Yu, Fan-Ping Meng and Gui-Hua Jin
Department of Immunology and Pathogenic Biology, Yanbian University Medical College, Yanji, China

Manabu Fujimoto
Department of Dermatology, Graduate School of Medicine, Osaka University; Laboratory of Cutaneous Immunology, Osaka University Immunology Frontier Research Center, Osaka, Japan

Guang-Hai Yan
Jilin Key Laboratory for Immune and Targeting Research on Common Allergic Diseases, Yanbian University Medical College, Yanji, China

Lian-Hua Zhu
Department of Dermatology, Yanbian University Hospital, Yanji, China

Qing-Gao Zhang
Chronic Disease Research Center, Dalian University, Dalian, China

Weiwen Chen
Beijing Hospital of Traditional Chinese Medicine, Capital Medical University, Beijing, China

Jingxia Zhao, Yan Wang, Jing Fu, Tingting Di, Cong Qi, Zhaoxia Chen and Ping Li
Beijing Hospital of Traditional Chinese Medicine, Capital Medical University, Beijing, China
Beijing Key Laboratory of Clinic and Basic Research with Traditional Chinese Medicine on Psoriasis, Beijing Institute of Traditional Chinese Medicine, Beijing, China

Yu Liu
Beijing Hospital of Traditional Chinese Medicine, Capital Medical University, Beijing, China
Beijing Key Laboratory of Clinic and Basic Research with Traditional Chinese Medicine on Psoriasis, Beijing Institute of Traditional Chinese Medicine, Beijing, China
Beijing University of Chinese Medicine, Beijing, China

Tingting Chen, Zhaoming Zhu, Qunqun Du, Zhuxian Wang, Wenfeng Wu, Yaqi Xue, Yuan Wang, Yufan Wu, Quanfu Zeng, Cuiping Jiang, Chunyan Shen, Li Liu and Qiang Liu
School of Traditional Chinese Medicine, Southern Medical University, Guangzhou, China

Hongxia Zhu
Integrated Hospital of Traditional Chinese Medicine, Southern Medical University, Guangzhou, China

Kang Nien How
Dermatology Unit, Faculty of Medicine and Health Sciences, Universiti Putra Malaysia, Serdang, Malaysia

Wei Hsum Yap, Calvin Lai Hock Lim and Zee Wei Lai
Faculty of Medical and Health Sciences, School of Biosciences, Taylor's University, Subang Jaya, Malaysia

Bey Hing Goh
College of Pharmaceutical Sciences, Zhejiang University, Hangzhou, China
Biofunctional Molecule Exploratory Research Group (BMEX), School of Pharmacy, Monash University Malaysia, Bandar Sunway, Malaysia

Wei-Jen Cheng
Graduate Institute of Clinical Medical Sciences, College of Medicine, Chang Gung University, Taoyuan, Taiwan
School of Traditional Chinese Medicine, College of Medicine, Chang Gung University, Taoyuan, Taiwan
Center for Traditional Chinese Medicine, Chang Gung Memorial Hospital, Taoyuan, Taiwan

Chung-Yuan Hsu
Center for Traditional Chinese Medicine, Chang Gung Memorial Hospital, Taoyuan, Taiwan

Chih-Chao Chiang
Graduate Institute of Clinical Medical Sciences, College of Medicine, Chang Gung University, Taoyuan, Taiwan
Puxin Fengze Chinese Medicine Clinic, Taoyuan, Taiwan

Cheng-Yu Lin, Yann-Lii Leu, Jia-Yu Sie and Wen-Ling Chen
Graduate Institute of Natural Products, College of Medicine, Chang Gung University, Taoyuan, Taiwan

Yu-Li Chen
Research Center for Chinese Herbal Medicine, Research Center for Food and Cosmetic Safety, Graduate Institute of Health Industry Technology, College of Human Ecology, Chang Gung University of Science and Technology, Taoyuan, Taiwan

Jong-Jen Kuo
School of Traditional Chinese Medicine, College of Medicine, Chang Gung University, Taoyuan, Taiwan
Center for Traditional Chinese Medicine, Chang Gung Memorial Hospital, Taoyuan, Taiwan
Graduate Institute of Traditional Chinese Medicine, School of Traditional Chinese Medicine, College of Medicine, Chang Gung University, Taoyuan, Taiwan

Tsong-Long Hwang
Graduate Institute of Natural Products, College of Medicine, Chang Gung University, Taoyuan, Taiwan
Research Center for Chinese Herbal Medicine, Research Center for Food and Cosmetic Safety, Graduate Institute of Health Industry Technology, College of Human Ecology, Chang Gung University of Science and Technology, Taoyuan, Taiwan
Department of Anesthesiology, Chang Gung Memorial Hospital, Taoyuan, Taiwan
Department of Chemical Engineering, Ming Chi University of Technology, New Taipei City, Taiwan

Lipeng Tang, Ying Zhu, Bing Feng and Zuqing Su
State Key Laboratory of Dampness Syndrome of Chinese Medicine, The Second Clinical College of Guangzhou University of Chinese Medicine, Guangzhou, China
Guangdong-Hong Kong-Macau Joint Lab on Chinese Medicine and Immune Disease Research, The Second Clinical College of Guangzhou University of Chinese Medicine, Guangzhou, China
Department of Pharmacology of Traditional Chinese Medicine, The Second Clinical College of Guangzhou University of Chinese Medicine, Guangzhou, China

Bowen Zhang, Laijun Yang and Hongxia Li
Department of Pharmacology of Traditional Chinese Medicine, The Second Clinical College of Guangzhou University of Chinese Medicine, Guangzhou, China

Tong Li
State Key Laboratory of Dampness Syndrome of Chinese Medicine, The Second Clinical College of Guangzhou University of Chinese Medicine, Guangzhou, China
Guangdong-Hong Kong-Macau Joint Lab on Chinese Medicine and Immune Disease Research, The Second Clinical College of Guangzhou University of Chinese Medicine, Guangzhou, China
Department of Pharmacology of Traditional Chinese Medicine, The Second Clinical College of Guangzhou University of Chinese Medicine, Guangzhou, China
Department of Pharmacy, The Second Clinical College of Guangzhou University of Chinese Medicine, Guangzhou, China

Ben Li
Department of Pharmacy, The Second Clinical College of Guangzhou University of Chinese Medicine, Guangzhou, China

Zihao Zhang and Xiaoyi Sun
School of Life Sciences and Biopharmaceutics, Guangdong Pharmaceutical University, Guangzhou, China

Huazhen Liu, Yuchao Chen and Zhenhua Dai
Section of Immunology, Guangdong Provincial Academy of Chinese Medical Sciences, Guangzhou, China

Xirun Zheng, Mingxian Li, Chutian Li, Jie Zhao and Han Liu
Department of Pathology, The Second Clinical College of Guangzhou University of Chinese Medicine, Guangzhou, China

Guangjuan Zheng
State Key Laboratory of Dampness Syndrome of Chinese Medicine, The Second Clinical College of Guangzhou University of Chinese Medicine, Guangzhou, China
Guangdong-Hong Kong-Macau Joint Lab on Chinese Medicine and Immune Disease Research, The Second Clinical College of Guangzhou University of Chinese Medicine, Guangzhou, China
Department of Pharmacology of Traditional Chinese Medicine, The Second Clinical College of Guangzhou University of Chinese Medicine, Guangzhou, China
Department of Pathology, The Second Clinical College of Guangzhou University of Chinese Medicine, Guangzhou, China

Xinmin Qiu
Genetic Testing Lab, The Second Clinical College of Guangzhou University of Chinese Medicine, Guangzhou, China

Shuyan Ye
Department of Dermatology, The Second Clinical College of Guangzhou University of Chinese Medicine, Guangzhou, China

Chuanjian Lu
State Key Laboratory of Dampness Syndrome of Chinese Medicine, The Second Clinical College of Guangzhou University of Chinese Medicine, Guangzhou, China
Guangdong-Hong Kong-Macau Joint Lab on Chinese Medicine and Immune Disease Research, The Second Clinical College of Guangzhou University of Chinese Medicine, Guangzhou, China
Department of Dermatology, The Second Clinical College of Guangzhou University of Chinese Medicine, Guangzhou, China
Guangdong Provincial Key Laboratory of Clinical Research on Traditional Chinese Medicine Syndrome, The Second Clinical College of Guangzhou University of Chinese Medicine, Guangzhou, China

Ji-Hyun Lee, Ji-Ye Lim and Dae-Ki Kim
Department of Immunology and Institute of Medical Sciences, Medical School, Chonbuk National University, Jeonju, South Korea

Eun Hee Jo
Research Center of Traditional Korean Medicine, Wonkwang University, Iksan, South Korea
Department of Acupuncture and Moxibustion, College of Korean Medicine, Wonkwang University, Iksan, South Korea

Hyeon Min Noh
Korean Traditional Medicine Institute, Wonkwang University, Iksan, South Korea

Sunggu Park
Department of Korean Medical Ophthalmology & Otolaryngology & Dermatology, College of Korean Medicine, Wonkwang University, Iksan, South Korea

Jaemoo Chun, You Mee Ahn, Sarah Shin and Jeeyoun Jung
KM Science Research Division, Korea Institute of Oriental Medicine, Daejeon, South Korea

So Min Lee
KM Convergence Research Division, Korea Institute of Oriental Medicine, Daejeon, South Korea

Min-Gyung Baek
Interdisciplinary Program in Precision Public Health, Korea University, Seoul, South Korea
Department of Public Health Sciences, Korea University, Seoul, South Korea

Hana Yi
School of Biosystems and Biomedical Sciences, Korea University, Seoul, South Korea

Pei Du, Wenqian Zhang, Shuang Lu and Ming Zhao
Department of Dermatology, Second Xiangya Hospital, Central South University, Changsha, China
Hunan Key Laboratory of Medical Epigenomics, Second Xiangya Hospital, Central South University, Changsha, China
Research Unit of Key Technologies of Diagnosis and Treatment for Immune-related Skin Diseases, Chinese Academy of Medical Sciences, Changsha, China
Clinical Medical Research Center of Major Skin Diseases and Skin Health of Hunan Province, Changsha, China

Haobo Cui and Wei He
Department of Pharmacy, The Third Xiangya Hospital, Central South University, Changsha, China

Sujie Jia
Hunan Key Laboratory of Medical Epigenomics, Second Xiangya Hospital, Central South University, Changsha, China
Department of Pharmacy, The Third Xiangya Hospital, Central South University, Changsha, China

Dali Gan, Li Wu and Meixian Xiang
School of Pharmaceutical Sciences, South-Central University for Nationalities, Wuhan, China

Qiyuan Su
Department of Statistics, University of Illinois at Urbana-Champaign, Urbana, IL, United States

Hanwen Su
Department of Clinical Laboratory, Renmin Hospital of Wuhan University, Wuhan, China

Jun Chen
Department of Pharmacy, Wuhan No.1 Hospital (Wuhan Hospital of Traditional Chinese and Western Medicine), Wuhan, China

Bing Han
Department of Pathology, Penn State College of Medicine, Milton S. Hershey Medical Center, Hershey, PA, United States

Yaobin Pang, Shi Wu, Yingjie He, Qing Nian, Jing Lei, Yejing Yao and Jing Guo
Dermatological Department, Hospital of Chengdu University of Traditional Chinese Medicine, Chengdu, China

Jinhao Zeng
Geriatric Department, Hospital of Chengdu University of Traditional Chinese Medicine, Chengdu, China
TCM Regulating Metabolic Diseases Key Laboratory of Sichuan Province, Hospital of Chengdu University of Traditional Chinese Medicine, Chengdu, China

Vivi Nur Khalieda Mohd Kasim, Kong Yen Liew, Daud Ahmad Israf and Chau Ling Tham
Department of Biomedical Science, Faculty of Medicine and Health Sciences, Universiti Putra Malaysia, Serdang, Malaysia

Siti Mahirah Noble and Ji Wei Tan
School of Science, Monash University Malaysia, Subang Jaya, Malaysia

Katja Sockel
Medizinische Klinik und Poliklinik I, Medizinische Fakultät Carl Gustav Carus, Technische Universität Dresden, Dresden, Germany

Cornelia S. Link-Rachner
Medizinische Klinik und Poliklinik I, Medizinische Fakultät Carl Gustav Carus, Technische Universität Dresden, Dresden, Germany
Center for Regenerative Therapies Dresden, Technische Universität Dresden, Dresden, Germany

Catharina Schuetz
Klinik und Poliklinik für Kinder- und Jugendmedizin, Medizinische Fakultät Carl Gustav Carus, Technische Universität Dresden, Dresden, Germany

Liangliang Zhang, Qiuyun Xu, Tingting Lin, Shifan Ruan, Mengting Lin, Chengbei Bao, Jing Zhang, Ting Gong and Chao Ji
Department of Dermatology, The First Hospital of Fujian Medical University, Fuzhou, China

Tao Liu
Department of Medical Affairs, Beijing Novartis Pharma Company Limited, Shanghai, China

Cheng Kang and Dakai Lu
Department of Otolaryngology-Head and Neck Surgery, HuaMei Hospital, University of Chinese Academy of Sciences, Ningbo, China

Kamran Ali
Department of Dermatology, International Education College of Zhejiang Chinese Medical University, Hangzhou, China

Liming Wu, HaiYue Lou, Jianbo Zhong, YunMi Qiu and JingPeng Shan
Department of Dermatology, Affiliated Hangzhou First People's Hospital, Zhejiang University School of Medicine, Hangzhou China

JiaYang Da and KaiNing Lu
Department of Oncological Surgery, Affiliated Hangzhou First People's Hospital, Zhejiang University School of Medicine, Hangzhou, China

Index

www.ingramcontent.com/pod-product-compliance
Lightning Source LLC
LaVergne TN
LVHW082217200926
848484LV00008B/2270